Basics of Anesthesia

THIRD EDITION

Robert K. Stoelting, M.D.
Professor and Chair
Department of Anesthesia
Indiana University School of Medicine
Indianapolis, Indiana

Ronald D. Miller, M.D.
Professor and Chair
Department of Anesthesia
Professor
Department of Pharmacology
University of California, San Francisco
School of Medicine
San Francisco, California

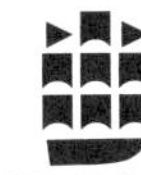

Churchill Livingstone
New York, Edinburgh, London, Melbourne, Tokyo

Library of Congress Cataloging-in-Publication Data

Stoelting, Robert K.
Basics of anesthesia / Robert K. Stoelting, Ronald D. Miller —
3rd ed.
p. cm.
Includes bibliographical references and index.
ISBN 0-443-08962-0
1. Anesthesia I. Miller, Ronald D., date. II. Title.
[DNLM: 1. Anesthesia. WO 200 S872b 1994]
RD81.S86 1994
617.9′6—dc20
DNLM/DLC
for Library of Congress 94-2905
CIP

Distributed in the United Kingdom by Churchill Livingstone, Robert Stevenson House, 1–3 Baxter's Place, Leith Walk, Edinburgh EH1 3AF, and by associated companies, branches, and representatives throughout the world.

Accurate indications , adverse reactions, and dosage schedules for drugs are provided in this book, but it is posisble that they may change. The reader is urged to review the package information data of the manufacturer of the medications mentioned.

The Publishers have made every effort to trace the copyright holders for borrowed material. If they have inadvertently overlooked any, they will be pleased to make the necessary arrangements at the first opportunity.

Acquisitions Editor: *Toni M. Tracy*
Copy Editor: *Bridgett L. Dickinson*
Production Supervisor: *Christina Hippeli*
Desktop Coordinator: *Jo-Ann Demas*
Cover Design: *Jeanette Jacobs*

Printed in the United States of America

First published in 1994 7 6 5 4 3 2

Preface to the Third Edition

Basics of Anesthesia was first published in 1984 with the stated goal of providing a concise source of information for the entire spectrum of students of anesthesia—medical students, physicians in training, and the established practitioner. This third edition of *Basics of Anesthesia* continues to pursue this goal. An in-depth and highly referenced textbook has never been our intention. Rather, we continue to believe that it is possible and desirable to develop an introductory textbook that succinctly presents pertinent information relevant to our specialty.

Unlike the previous two editions, this edition of *Basics of Anesthesia* reflects the emergence of acute postoperative pain management, organ transplantation, and anesthesia for procedures performed outside the operating room as important components of the anesthesiologist's professional practice. The importance of these topics is emphasized by their presentation as new chapters in this third edition. The anesthetic management of the trauma patient is a new part of the chapter on Critical Care Medicine. Figures and tables have undergone extensive revision in an attempt to improve the ability of the reader to both understand and visualize information in the written text.

We wish to acknowledge the excellent secretarial support provided by Deanna M. Walker and the editorial review provided by Stephen F. Dierdorf, M.D., both of Indiana University. As in the past, the authors recognize and appreciate the support of the staff of Churchill Livingstone in the preparation of this third edition. In particular, we are grateful for the continued support of Toni M. Tracy, President of Churchill Livingstone.

Robert K. Stoelting, M.D.
Ronald D. Miller, M.D.

Preface to the First Edition

Basics of Anesthesia is intended to provide the student and beginning trainee with introductory information pertinent to the wide spectrum (operating room, intensive care, pain management, cardiopulmonary resuscitation) of the practice of anesthesiology. Likewise, the advanced trainee and practitioner should find the concise but thorough description of anesthetic practice a useful review as well as a reference source for fundamental questions.

An in-depth and highly referenced presentation is not the goal of *Basics of Anesthesia.* Nevertheless, we believe it is possible, in a concise manner, to achieve an accurate and pertinent presentation of essential information for the practice of anesthesiology. References are limited in number but should direct the reader to classic articles or more detailed discussions of the specific topic.

The editors wish to acknowledge the superb editorial and technical assistance of Deanna M. Walker of Indiana University and Susan M.S. Ishida of the University of California, San Francisco. The staff of Churchill Livingstone provided the necessary encouragement and flexibility to ensure timely progression of the textbook to its final form. In particular, Donna Balopole guided this project through the important publication steps.

Robert K. Stoelting, M.D.
Ronald D. Miller, M.D.
1984

Contents

Section IV Special Anesthetic Considerations

Section V Recovery Period

Section VI Consultant Anesthetic Practice

Section VII Appendices

Section I
Introduction

1

History and Scope of Anesthesia

Since its beginning in 1842, anesthesiology has evolved into a recognized medical specialty providing continuing improvement in patient care based on the introductions of new drugs and techniques made possible in large part by research in the basic and clinical sciences (Table 1-1). The scope of anesthesiology extends beyond the operating room to include respiratory therapy, treatment of acute postoperative pain, management of chronic pain problems, and care of critically ill patients in intensive care units. As with other medical specialties, anesthesiology is represented by professional societies, scientific journals, a Residency Review Committee that establishes compliance of anesthesia residency training programs with published standards, and a medical specialty board that establishes criteria for becoming a certified specialist in anesthesiology (Table 1-1).

DISCOVERY OF ANESTHESIA

The discovery of anesthesia represents a totally American contribution to medicine.[1] Dr. Crawford W. Long, a medical practitioner in rural Georgia, was the first physician known to administer the vapor of ether by inhalation to produce surgical anesthesia, in 1842. This finding was not publicized. Thus, 4 years later a dentist, Dr. William T. Morton, from Hartford, Connecticut, administered the vapor of ether to Mr. Gilbert Abbott for the removal of a tumor from below the mandible by the well-known surgeon Dr. John C. Warren. The successful anesthesia took place at Massachusetts General Hospital on Friday, October 16, 1846, in front of an audience that included surgeons, medical students, and a newspaper reporter. Indeed, an account of the "ether demonstration" appeared the next day in the Boston Daily Journal. Within a few weeks the discovery of surgical anesthesia was known worldwide.

In England, Dr. James Y. Simpson, a highly respected obstetrician, administered ether to a parturient in 1847 to relieve the pain of labor. The use of chloroform in England for obstetric analgesia gained public acceptance when another English physician, Dr. John Snow, administered this drug to Queen Victoria during the birth of Prince Leopold in 1853. Dr. Snow qualifies as the first anesthesiologist because he was the first to devote his medical practice to the administration of anesthesia.

Another American dentist, Dr. Horace Wells, was the first to recognize the potential of nitrous oxide as an anesthetic. Although nitrous oxide was isolated in 1772 and its anesthetic properties described in 1799, it was not until 1844, when Dr. Wells allowed nitrous oxide to be administered to him by Gardner C. Colton (an itinerant showman) while a fellow dentist painlessly extracted one of Dr. Wells' teeth, that the anesthetic potential of this gas was realized. Unfortunately, the use of nitrous oxide for medical purposes temporarily fell into disrepute when Dr. Wells, who did not appreciate the lack of potency of nitrous oxide, failed in an attempt to produce anesthesia for surgery during a demonstration before a group of his colleagues at Massachusetts General Hospital. It was not until 1868, when a Chicago surgeon, Dr. Edmond W. Andrews, popularized the use

Table 1-1. History of Anesthesia

Year	Event
1842	Diethyl ether used by Long to produce surgical anesthesia
1844	Nitrous oxide used by Wells to produce dental analgesia
1846	Diethyl ether used publicly by Morton to produce surgical anesthesia
1847	Chloroform popularized for surgical anesthesia in England
1853	Chloroform administered by Snow to Queen Victoria for the birth of Prince Leopold; this removed the stigma attached to pain relief for childbirth
1854	Hollow metallic needle invented by Wood
1868	Administration of nitrous oxide with oxygen introduced by Andrews
1871	Cylinders of compressed nitrous oxide introduced by Brothers
1884	Cocaine used by Koller to produce topical anesthesia
1885	Nerve block and infiltration anesthesia by injection of cocaine introduced by Halsted Epidural anesthesia introduced by Corning
1893	London Society of Anaesthetists founded
1898	Spinal anesthesia introduced by Bier
1904	Buchanan appointed first professor of anesthesia in the United States at the New York Medical College
1905	Procaine synthesized by Einhorn Long Island Society of Anesthetists founded by Erdmann
1911	Long Island Society of Anesthetists becomes the New York Society of Anesthetists
1914	*American Journal of Anesthesia and Analgesia* first published as a quarterly supplement to the *American Journal of Surgery*
1917	Oxygen mask developed by Poulton
1919	National Anesthesia Research Society founded by McMechan
1920	Guedel published data on signs of anesthesia Tracheal tubes for delivery of inhaled anesthetics introduced by Magill
1922	The journal *Current Researches in Anesthesia and Analgesia* first published
1923	Mary A. Ross, M.D. becomes the first postgraduate trainee (Iowa) in anesthesiology in the United States *British Journal of Anaesthesia* first published
1924	National Anesthesia Research Society becomes the International Anesthesia Research Society
1926	*American Journal of Anesthesia and Analgesia* ceases publication
1927	Waters appointed as the first university professor of anesthesia in the United States at the University of Wisconsin Anesthetists Travel Club founded
1930	Circle anesthetic breathing and carbon dioxide absorption system described by Sword
1932	Association of Anaesthetists of Great Britain and Ireland founded
1933	Cyclopropane used by Waters to produce surgical anesthesia
1934	Thiopental used by Lundy for induction of anesthesia
1935	Rovenstine organized a department of anesthesia at Bellevue Hospital in New York
1936	New York Society of Anesthetists becomes the American Society of Anesthetists
1938	The American Board of Anesthesiology founded
1940	The journal *Anesthesiology* first published
1942	*d*-Tubocurarine used by Griffith and Johnson to produce skeletal muscle relaxation during general anesthesia
1943	Lidocaine synthesized by Lofgren
1945	American Society of Anesthetists becomes the American Society of Anesthesiologists
1946	The journal *Anaesthesia* first published
1949	Succinylcholine used clinically by Phillips and Fusco
1952	The journal *der Anaesthetist* first published
1953	Association of University Anesthetists founded Residency Review Committee in Anesthesiology established
1954	*Canadian Anaesthetists' Society Journal* first published Anesthetists' Travel Club becomes the Academy of Anesthesiology
1956	Halothane used clinically by Johnson
1957	The journal *Survey of Anesthesiology* first published The journal *Acta Anesthesiologica Scandinavica* first published *Current Researches in Anesthesia and Analgesia* becomes *Anesthesia and Analgesia, Current Researches*
1958	"Audio Digest Anesthesiology" first recorded
1959	Methoxyflurane used clinically by Artusio and Van Poznak
1968	Society of Academic Anesthesia Chairman founded
1972	Enflurane used clinically

(Continues)

Table 1-1. History of Anesthesia *(Continued)*

1973	The journal *Critical Care Medicine* first published
1975	In-training examination in anesthesiology initiated
	American Society of Regional Anesthesia refounded
1976	The journal *Regional Anesthesia* first published
1979	*Anesthesia and Analgesia, Current Researches* becomes *Anesthesia and Analgesia*
1981	Isoflurane used clinically
1985	Anesthesia Patient Safety Foundation established
1986	Foundation for Anesthesia Education and Research established
1989	Propofol used clinically
1992	Desflurane used clinically

(Information derived in part from a chart prepared by William H. G. Dornette, M.D., for the Ohio Chemical and Surgical Equipment Company, Madison, WI, 1962.)

of nitrous oxide with oxygen, that the full value of this gas as an anesthetic began to be appreciated. Between 1844 and 1868, nitrous oxide continued to be used by itinerant showmen who staged public displays of the exhilarating effects of this gas on the sensorium. Likewise, ether was often used for nonmedical purposes described as "ether frolics." Indeed, it is likely that Dr. Long saw ether used in this way during his medical student days in Philadelphia before 1842.

ANESTHESIA AFTER ETHER

The discovery of the anesthetic properties of ether, chloroform, and nitrous oxide satisfied the immediate needs to provide analgesia during surgery. Indeed, no significant new inhaled anesthetics were introduced during the next 80 years (Fig. 1-1).[2] The search for new inhaled anesthetics began in the 1920s, when the expanding scientific basis of anesthesia and surgery demanded drugs with greater flexibility and fewer side effects than currently provided by ether and chloroform. As such, cyclopropane, because of its low blood solubility and support of the circulation, became the most important new inhaled anesthetic in the 1930s.

Until the 1950s, all the available inhaled anesthetics possessed at least one of two defects: explosive in oxygen (ether, ethylene, vinethene, cyclopropane) or toxic (chloroform, vinethene, trichloroethylene). The evolution of fluorine technology, stimulated originally by the need to separate uranium isotopes for the development of the atomic bomb, led to a new generation of fluorinated inhaled anesthetics in the 1950s. For example, combining fluorine with carbon decreased the flammability while the stability of this bond tended to decrease metabolism and thus organ toxicity. The first of the new fluorinated inhaled anesthetics, introduced in 1954, was fluroxene. Fluroxene had several desirable characteristics, including low blood solubility and a minimal tendency to depress cardiovascular function or sensitize the heart to exogenous epinephrine. Fluroxene, however, frequently caused nausea and vomiting and at higher anesthetic concentrations was flammable. Later work also suggested this inhaled anesthetic could, on rare occasions, be hepatotoxic and might also be carcinogenic.[3] Fluroxene was voluntarily withdrawn from the market in 1975, mainly because of its flammability.

Modern Inhaled Anesthetics

Presently, one gas (nitrous oxide) and the vapors of four volatile liquids (halothane, enflurane, isoflurane, desflurane) represent the commonly used inhaled anesthetics. These drugs differ in their physical and chemical characteristics (see Chapter 2) and their pharmacology (see Chapter 4).

Halothane

Halothane was introduced in 1956 after pharmacologists had predicted that its halogenated chemical structure would provide nonflammability, low blood solubility, molecular stability (trifluorocarbon molecule), and anesthetic potency (chlorine and bromine) (Fig. 1-2).[4] This drug was found to produce a rapid and pleasant induction of anesthesia, bronchodilation, skeletal muscle relaxation, a prompt return to consciousness, and minimal postoperative nausea and vomiting. These attributes and the subsequent clinical popularity of halothane temporarily halted the search for new inhaled anesthetics. With continued use of halothane, however, its limitations (depression of ventilation and circulation, enhancement of cardiac dysrhythmogenic

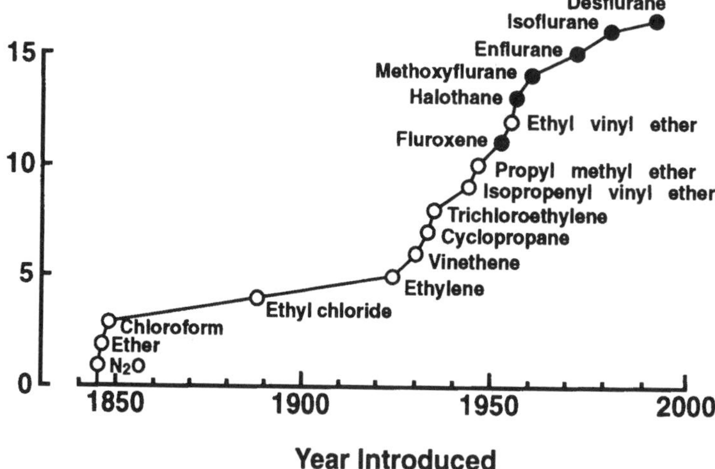

Figure 1-1. Anesthetics used in clinical practice. The history of anesthesia began with the introduction of nitrous oxide, ether, and chloroform. After 1950, all introduced drugs, with the exception of ethyl vinyl ether, have contained fluorine (solid circles). (Modified from Eger,[2] with permission.)

effects of epinephrine, rare potential to produce hepatotoxicity) led to renewed interest in the search for other inhaled anesthetics.[5]

Methoxyflurane

The search for new inhaled anesthetics focused on methyl ethyl ether derivatives, since ether derivatives do not increase the incidence of cardiac dsyrhythmias. Methoxyflurane, introduced in 1959, was the first of the methyl ethyl ethers to be used clinically (Fig. 1-2).6 This drug did not increase myocardial irritability and seemed to be less depressant to the circulation than halothane. Methoxyflurane, however, was extensively metabolized, particularly to inorganic fluoride, introducing the potential for fluoride nephrotoxicity. In addition, its high blood (blood:gas partition coefficient 13) and tissue solubility resulted in slow induction of anesthesia and in the potential for delayed awakening, especially after prolonged administration. These undesirable characteristics have led to the infrequent use of methoxyflurane despite its continued clinical availability.

Enflurane

Enflurane, introduced in 1972, was the next methyl ethyl ether derivative to become available for use as an inhaled anesthetic (Fig. 1-2).[7] This drug provided stable cardiac rhythm and produced excellent skeletal muscle relaxation. Metabolism to inorganic fluoride is substantially lower following administration of enflurane than following administration of methoxyflurane and fluoride-induced nephrotoxicity seems unlikely. Seizure activity on the electroencephalogram and evidence of peripheral skeletal muscle movement may accompany administration of high doses (more than 2 MAC [minimum alveolar

Characteristics of an Ideal Inhaled Anesthetic

Absence of flammability
Easily vaporized at ambient temperature
Potent
Low blood solubility to ensure rapid induction and recovery from anesthesia
Minimal metabolism
Compatible with epinephrine
Skeletal muscle relaxation
Suppression of excessive sympathetic nervous system activity
Not irritating to airways
Bronchodilation
Absence of excessive myocardial depression
Absence of cerebral vasodilation
Absence of hepatic and renal toxicity

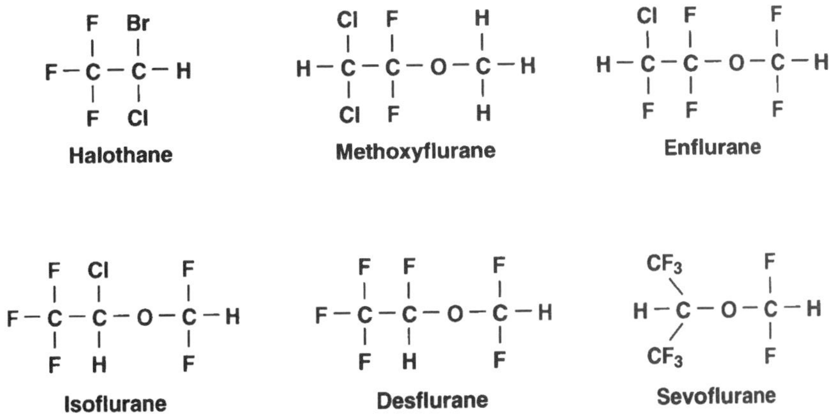

Halothane Methoxyflurane Enflurane

Isoflurane Desflurane Sevoflurane

Figure 1-2. Chemical structures of volatile anesthetics. Halothane is an alkane derivative, whereas the other volatile anesthetics are derivatives of methyl ethyl ether. Isoflurane is the chemical isomer of enflurane.

concentration]) of enflurane, especially if the $PaCO_2$ is less than 30 mmHg. There is no evidence this drug-induced seizure activity poses an increased risk to patients.

Isoflurane

Isoflurane was introduced for patient use in 1981 and rapidly became the most commonly administered volatile anesthetic (Fig. 1-2).[8] In contrast to enflurane, isoflurane undergoes less metabolism, does not evoke evidence of seizure activity on the electroencephalogram, and is somewhat less soluble in blood. Like enflurane, its pungency limits its usefulness for inhalation induction of anesthesia. Despite modest airway irritability effects, isoflurane appears to produce bronchodilation similar to halothane.

Desflurane

Desflurane was introduced for patient use in 1992.[9] This fluorinated methyl ethyl ether differs from isoflurane only by substitution of fluorine for the chlorine found on the alpha-ethyl component of isoflurane (Fig. 1-2). Its solubility characteristics resemble those of nitrous oxide, resulting in a rapid onset of anesthesia followed by prompt recovery. The high vapor pressure of desflurane (669 mmHg at 20°C) necessitates the utilization of a specially constructed heated and pressurized vaporizer for delivery of this anesthetic. Pungency causes airway irritability, thus limiting the usefulness of desflurane for inhalation induction of anesthesia. Metabolism of desflurane to trifluoroacetic acid and inorganic fluoride is about 10-fold lower than that of isoflurane. To put this in perspective, it is estimated that less than 0.02% of the amount of desflurane absorbed is ultimately metabolized. The likelihood of liver damage due to prior sensitization from exposure to other volatile anesthetics (halothane, enflurane, isoflurane) also metabolized to trifluoroacetic acid (covalent reaction of trifluoroacetic acid with a liver protein to form a neoantigen and evoke formation of antibodies) seems remote considering the minimal production of trifluoroacetic acid from the metabolism of desflurane (see Chapter 20). Its advantages include prompt recovery, which is considered particularly desirable in patients undergoing surgical procedures as outpatients.

Sevoflurane

Sevoflurane is a fluorinated methyl ethyl ether that was initially evaluated in the 1970s but was discarded principally because of its metabolism to inorganic fluoride (similar to enflurane) and instability in soda lime (questionable clinical significance) (Fig. 1-2).[9,10] Renewed interest in this anesthetic is based on its low blood solubility (0.62), its potency (MAC 1.71), and the lack of airway irritation. The vapor pressure of sevoflurane (160 mmHg at 20°C) permits its administration using a conventional vaporizer, which contrasts with the requirement for a heated and pressurized vaporizer necessary for the delivery of desflurane.

Regional Anesthesia

The introduction of regional anesthesia awaited the development of a hollow metal needle in 1854 and the discovery of local anesthetics. In 1884, Dr. Carl

Koller discovered the local anesthetic effects of cocaine when applied topically to the eye. In 1885, Dr. William S. Halsted, a surgeon, introduced the concept of nerve block anesthesia and infiltration anesthesia by the injection of cocaine. Also in 1885, Dr. Leonard Corning, a neurologist, was the first to produce lumbar epidural anesthesia by the injection of cocaine. In 1898, Dr. August Bier demonstrated the feasibility of spinal anesthesia by the injection of cocaine into the subarachnoid space of a patient undergoing a foot amputation. Procaine, synthesized in 1905 by Einhorn, replaced cocaine for producing regional anesthesia. Today the most frequently used local anesthetics are tetracaine (topical anesthesia, spinal anesthesia), lidocaine (topical anesthesia, infiltration anesthesia, peripheral nerve block, epidural anesthesia, spinal anesthesia, treatment of ventricular cardiac dysrhythmias), and bupivacaine (peripheral nerve block, epidural anesthesia, spinal anesthesia) (see Chapter 6).

Injected Drugs

Induction of anesthesia with the intravenous injection of thiopental was introduced by Dr. John S. Lundy in 1934. The popularity of thiopental for rapid intravenous induction of anesthesia was not seriously challenged by the subsequent availability of new drugs (methohexital, ketamine, diazepam, midazolam, etomidate) until 1989, when the introduction of propofol provided a drug with an onset time similar to that of thiopental but with a more rapid and complete dissipation of drug effects. The introduction of *d*-tubocurarine into clinical anesthesia in 1942 revolutionized the methods by which skeletal muscle relaxation during surgery was produced.[11] Opioids, used for many years in combination with nitrous oxide to produce general anesthesia, can also be used as the sole anesthetic (high-dose fentanyl) for critically ill patients who cannot tolerate even minimal cardiac depression produced by inhaled drugs.

ANESTHESIA AS A MEDICAL SPECIALTY

Anesthesia as a medical specialty evolved differently in England and the United States. Chloroform, the standard anesthetic in England, was a potent ventilatory and cardiac depressant requiring great skills in its administration. As a result, only physicians were considered competent to administer chloroform. By contrast, ether remained the dominant anesthetic in the United States. Unlike chloroform, ether stimulated ventilation and maintained the circulation. For these reasons, ether was thought to have a built-in protection for the patient, and its administration was often relegated to an inexperienced physician or nurse. Indeed, it was more than 60 years after the demonstration of ether anesthesia by Dr. Morton before American physicians began to devote full-time medical practice to the administration of anesthetics. For example, the first department of anesthesia was created in 1904 at the New York Medical College, with Dr. Thomas D. Buchanan as professor and chair. Dr. Arthur E. Guedel, a 1908 graduate of Indiana University School of Medicine, described the stages and planes of anesthesia in a monograph published in 1920. In 1923, Dr. Mary A. Ross became the first formal postgraduate trainee in anesthesiology in the United States, receiving a certificate from the University of Iowa for her year of training after graduation from medical school. Dr. John S. Lundy organized a department of anesthesia at the Mayo Clinic in 1924, and Dr. Ralph M. Waters arrived at the University of Wisconsin for the same purpose in 1927. Graduates of training programs directed by Drs. Lundy and Waters continued to expand the scope of anesthesiology. Among those graduates was Dr. Emory A. Rovenstine, who in 1935 left Wisconsin to develop a department of anesthesia at Bellevue, the teaching hospital of New York University. During the next 25 years, over 30 graduates of Dr. Rovenstine's program became directors of departments of anesthesia.

American Society of Anesthesiologists (ASA)

The first anesthesia organization in the United States was the Long Island Society of Anesthetists organized in 1905 by Dr. A. Frederick Erdmann and eight physician colleagues from the New York City area. The stated goal of this society was to "promote the art and science of anesthesia," and annual dues were $1.00. Only the London Society of Anaesthetists, founded in 1893, preceded this first society in the United States. The Long Island Society of Anesthetists grew in membership, becoming the New York Society of Anesthetists in 1911. The society became the American Society of Anesthetists in 1935, with 487 members and annual dues of $5.00. In 1945, the name was changed to the American Society of Anesthesiologists. This name change was intended to reflect more accurately the membership of the society, which consists of physicians with postgraduate training in anesthesia, (anesthesiologists) in contrast to nonphysicians (anesthetists) who also administer anesthesia (see the section *Certified Registered Nurse Anesthetist*). This semantic distinction is observed most consistently in the United States, whereas in other areas of the world where only physicians administer anesthesia, the terms tend to be used interchangeably. Today, the American Society of Anesthesiologists has over 30,000 members, making anesthesia the sixth largest among the American medical specialties.

Anesthesiology, the official journal of the American Society of Anesthesiolgists, was first published in July 1940, with Dr. Henry S. Ruth as the editor. This initial issue was sent to 568 members of the society and 300 additional nonmember subscribers. Today this highly respected peer-review journal has a monthly worldwide circulation that exceeds 38,000.

International Anesthesia Research Society (IARS)

At the same time that the New York Society of Anesthetists was evolving into the American Society of Anesthesiologists, another important organization was developing under the direction of Dr. Francis H. McMechan, a physician practicing in Cincinnati, Ohio. In 1919, Dr. McMechan established the National Anesthesia Research Society. This society held annual meetings, and in August 1922 the first medical journal devoted entirely to the specialty of anesthesiology, *Current Researches in Anesthesia and Analgesia*, appeared, with Dr. McMechan as editor. Previously, the only other source of scientific information for anesthesiology was the *American Journal of Anesthesia and Analgesia*, published since 1914 as a quarterly supplement to the *American Journal of Surgery*. In 1925, the National Anesthesia Research Society was renamed the International Anesthesia Research Society, which today continues to sponsor an annual scientific meeting and publish the journal *Anesthesia and Analgesia*.

American Society of Regional Anesthesia (ASRA)

The American Society of Regional Anesthesia was founded in 1923 to provide a forum for physicians interested in regional anesthesia. This society was absorbed into the American Society of Anesthetists in 1941, only to again become an independent organization in 1975. The official journal of this society, *Regional Anesthesia*, was first published in October 1976.

The American Board of Anesthesiology (ABA)

The American Board of Anesthesiology was incorporated as an affiliate of The American Board of Surgery in 1938. After the first voluntary examinations, 87 physicians were certified as Diplomates of The American Board of Anesthesiology. The American Board of Anesthesiology was recognized as an independent board by The American Board of Medical Specialties in 1941. To date, over 20,000 anesthesiologists have been certified as Diplomates of The American Board of Anesthesiology.

Certified Registered Nurse Anesthetist (CRNA)

In the past, nearly 50% of the anesthetics given in the United States each year were administered by certified registered nurse anesthetists, most often with the supervision of a physician. To become a nurse anesthetist, the candidate must earn a Registered Nurse degree, spend 1 year as a critical care nurse, and then complete 2 years of anesthesia training in an approved nurse anesthesia training program. At present, the American Association of Nurse Anesthetists (AANA) remains responsible for the curriculum of most nurse anesthesia training programs, as well as for the establishment of criteria for certification as a nurse anesthetist. The activities of nurse anesthetists are usually confined to the operating room, working with the supervision (medical direction) of an anesthesiologist. This physician-nurse team approach (anesthesia care team) is consistent with the concept that the administration of anesthesia is the practice of medicine.

Postgraduate (Residency) Training in Anesthesiology

Postgraduate training in anesthesiology consists of 4 years of supervised experience in an approved program after the degree of Doctor of Medicine or Osteopathy has been obtained. The first year of postgraduate training in anesthesiology consists of nonanesthesia experience (Clinical Base Year) in patient care-related specialties. The second, third, and fourth postgraduate years (Clinical Anesthesia 1–3) are spent in learning all aspects of clinical anesthesia, including subspecialty experiences in obstetric anesthesia, pediatric anesthesia, cardiac anesthesia, neuroanesthesia, pain management, and critical care medicine. Six months during the Clinical Anesthesia 3 year may be elected by the resident for pursuit of research interests. Alternatively, residents who plan a career as an academic investigator may combine research (18 months) and clinical anesthesia training (18 months) following completion of the Clinical Anesthesia 1 year.

The content of the educational experience during the clinical anesthesia years reflects the wide-ranging scope of anesthesiology as a medical specialty. At present, anesthesiology is defined in the booklet of information of The American Board of Anesthesiology as a practice of medicine dealing with but not limited to

1. The assessment of, consultation for, and preparation of patients for anesthesia.
2. The provision of insensibility to pain during surgical, obstetric, therapeutic, and diagnostic procedures, and the management of patients so affected.
3. The monitoring and restoration of homeostasis during the perioperative period, as well as homeostasis in the critically ill, injured, or otherwise seriously ill patient.
4. The diagnosis and treatment of painful syndromes.
5. The clinical management and teaching of cardiac and pulmonary resuscitation.
6. The evaluation of respiratory function and application of respiratory therapy in all its forms.
7. The supervision, teaching, and evaluation of performance of both medical and paramedical personnel involved in anesthesia, respiratory, and critical care.
8. The conduct of research at the clinical and basic science levels to explain and improve the care of patients.
9. The administrative involvement in hospitals, medical schools, and outpatient facilities necessary to implement these responsibilities.

This definition emphasizes the continued major role of the anesthesiologist in the operating room. Indeed, the anesthesiologist should function as the clinical pharmacologist and internist or pediatrician in the operating room. Furthermore, the definition emphasizes that the scope of anesthesiology extends beyond the operating room to include acute and chronic pain management (see Chapters 32 and 34), critical care medicine (see Chapter 33), cardiopulmonary resuscitation (see Chapter 35), and research. Indeed, much remains to be learned, and even the mechanism of general anesthesia remains unknown.

Approximately 160 postgraduate training programs in anesthesiology are approved by the Accreditation Council for Graduate Medical Education of the American Medical Association. These training programs offer more than 5700 postgraduate positions in anesthesiology. Approved postgraduate training programs are visited periodically by a representative of the Residency Review Committee to ensure continued compliance with the published standards of quality medical education. The Residency Review Committee consists of members appointed by the American Medical Association, American Society of Anesthesiologists, and The American Board of Anesthesiology.

After completion of the required postgraduate training in anesthesiology, the physician can voluntarily enter the examination system of The American Board of Anesthesiology. Successful completion of a written and then an oral examination results in the issuance of a primary certificate confirming that the physician is a Diplomate ("Board certified") of The American Board of Anesthesiology. A certificate of special qualifications in Anesthesiology Critical Care Medicine and a certificate of added qualifications in Anesthesiology Pain Management are available to Diplomates of The American Board of Anesthesiology who spend an additional year of training after completion of the 4-year continuum and pass a written examination. The primary certificate and critical care medicine certificate are valid for the entire professional life of the Diplomate. The certificate for pain management is valid for 10 years following its issuance (time-limited) and can be renewed by meeting specific credentialing requirements and passing a written examination. A Diplomate is also eligible to voluntarily participate in a process known as Continued Demonstration of Qualifications (CDQ), which includes a credentialing process and a written examination designed to demonstrate current practice and knowledge.

HAZARDS OF WORKING IN THE OPERATING ROOM

Anesthesiologists spend long hours in an environment (operating room) associated with exposure to vapors from chemicals (volatile anesthetics, methylmethacrylate), ionizing radiation, and infectious agents (hepatitis viruses, human immunodeficiency virus). There is psychological stress resulting from constant vigilance required for care of patients during anesthesia and from the interactions with members of the operating team (surgeons, nurses). Removal of waste anesthetic gases (scavenging) has decreased exposure to trace concentrations of these gases, although evidence that this practice has improved the health of anesthesia personnel is lacking. Universal precautions are recommended in caring for every patient in an attempt to prevent transmission of blood-borne infections.[12] The risk of an anesthesiologist becoming infected with human immunodeficiency virus through an accidental needle stick during a 30-year career has been estimated to be 0.05% to 4.50% based on geographic location.[13] Substance abuse, mental illness (depression), and suicide seem to occur with increased frequency among anesthesiologists, perhaps reflecting the impact of occupational stress.

PROFESSIONAL LIABILITY

The anesthesiologist is responsible for the management of and recovery from anesthesia. Physicians administering anesthetics are not expected to guarantee a favorable outcome to the patient but are required to exercise ordinary or reasonable care or skill compared with other anesthesiologists. That the anticipated result does not follow or that complications occur does not imply negligence (practice below the standard of care). Furthermore, an anesthesiologist is not responsible for an error in judgment unless it is so gross as to be inconsistent with the skill expected of every physician. As a specialist, however, an anesthesiologist is responsible for making medical judgments that are consistent with national, not local, standards. Anesthesiologists carry professional liability (malpractice) insurance that provides financial protection should a court judgment against them occur. The best protection for the anesthesiologist against medicolegal action lies in the thorough and up-to-date practice of anesthesia coupled with interest in the patient by virtue of preoperative and postoperative visits plus detailed records of the course of anesthesia.

A nurse anesthetist can be held legally responsible for the technical aspects of the administration of anesthesia. It is likely, however, that legal responsibilities for the actions of the nurse anesthetist will be shared by the physician responsible for supervising the administration of anesthesia. If an anesthesiologist employs the nurse anesthetist or advises the hospital as to the qualifications or conditions of employment, the anesthesiologist may be held

Universal Precautions

1. All needles, blades, and sharp instruments should be handled with a view to preventing accidental injuries, and all should be considered potentially infected. Disposable sharp items should be placed in puncture-resistant containers located as close as practical to the area in which they are used. Needles should not be recapped, bent, broken, or removed from disposable syringes before being placed in appropriate disposable containers.
2. Gloves should be worn when touching mucous membranes or open skin of all patients. When the possibility exists of exposure to blood, body fluids, or items soiled with these, gloves should be used. With some procedures, such as endoscopy, when aerosolization or

(Continues)

Universal Precautions

(Continued)

splashes of blood or secretions are likely to occur, masks, eye coverings, and gowns are indicated. Gloves and body coverings should be removed and disposed of properly after patient contact.

3. Frequent handwashing, especially between patient contact and after removal of gloves, should be encouraged. If hands are accidentally contaminated with blood or other body fluids, they should be washed as soon as possible.
4. Ventilation devices for resuscitation should be available at appropriate locations to prevent the need for emergency mouth-to-mouth resuscitation.
5. Health-care workers who have exudative lesions or weeping dermatitis should not participate in direct patient care activity until the condition resolves.

(From Centers for Disease Control,[12] with permission.)

responsible for the nurse anesthetist's actions even though not directly concerned in supervision at the time of an alleged act of negligence.

Medical students and resident physicians are not immune to court action and should be protected by professional liability insurance in the same manner as the anesthesiologist or nurse anesthetist. Insurance coverage for the medical student or resident physician is most often provided by the institution that provides the course for credit for the medical student or employs the resident physician.

Most patients and/or families are understanding and are satisfied by frank discussion of problems related to the administration of anesthesia. In the event of an accident or complication related to the administration of anesthesia, the anesthesiologist should immediately document the facts on the patient's medical record. Patient treatment should be noted and consultation with other physicians sought when appropriate. The anesthesiologist should provide the hospital and the company that writes the physician's professional liability insurance with a complete account of the incident. Should a lawsuit be threatened or legal inquiry be made concerning a patient, the anesthesiologist should immediately notify the insurance company and, when appropriate, seek legal assistance.

Malpractice is a theory arising from tort law. A tort is a civil (not criminal) wrong for which a patient can seek compensation through legal action for an alleged act of negligence by the anesthesiologist. The patient who claims injury obtains legal counsel and files a malpractice suit. Discovery depositions are taken by attorneys for both sides to elicit plaintiffs', defendants', and witnesses' opinions as to the facts of the event; a court hearing is arranged, usually with a jury present; and witnesses, including experts, for the defendant (physician) and plaintiff (patient) give testimony. The judge explains the points of law to the jury, and the jury then makes a decision and recommendation of compensation for damages. This chain of events may be interrupted at any point. For example, the plaintiff may drop the suit, or the defendant may be advised by counsel to make a settlement. A settlement can be arranged with the aid of the judge at any time during the trial before the jury verdict. Indeed, about 80% of malpractice suits are settled out of court and, of those that go to court trial, physicians win more than they lose.

Risk of Anesthesia

An estimated 20 to 25 million anesthetics are administered annually in the United States. The risk of mortality due solely to the administration of anesthesia is extremely rare (about 1 in 10,000 administrations or 0.01%).[14] For the relatively healthy patient having a simple elective operation, the risk is even lower, perhaps in the range of 1 in 50,000 to 100,000 anesthetic administrations. Regardless of the risk of anesthesia, it is estimated that 50% to 75% of anesthetic-related deaths are preventable. When adverse events do occur, it is often difficult to establish the exact mechanism. In many instances, it is impossible to separate an adverse event due to an inappropriate action of the anesthesiologist ("lapse of vigilance," below the standard of care) from an unavoidable mishap (maloccurrence, coincidental event) that occurred despite optimal care.[15] Although anesthetic medical liability claims make up only about 3% to 4% of the total in medicine, the indemnity paid exceeds 10%, emphasizing the perceived severity of the associated injuries.

Common mechanisms of avoidable adverse events include (1) inadequate ventilation of the lungs, (2) unrecognized esophageal intubation, (3) unrecognized extubation of the trachea, (4) unrecognized ventilator disconnections, (5) relative or absolute drug overdoses, and (6) injuries related to positioning during surgery.[16–18] It is hoped that improved monitoring of anesthetized patients will serve to further enhance the vigilance of the anesthesiologist and decrease the role of human error in anesthetic morbidity and mortality. At the same time, it is important to recognize that not all adverse events during anesthesia are a result of human error and therefore preventable. For example, postoperative ulnar nerve palsy may occur despite appropriate padding and positioning during surgery.[17,18]

Risk Management (Quality Improvement)

Risk management is a program within each hospital that is intended to prevent patient injury and ensure the practice of high-quality medicine. With respect to anesthesia, the key factors in the prevention of patient injury are vigilance, up-to-date knowledge, and adequate monitoring. Clearly, it is important to follow the standards endorsed by the American Society of Anesthesiologists (see Appendix 1). In this regard, American anesthesiology has been the unquestioned leader within organized medicine in the development and implementation of formal, published standards of practice.[19] These standards have significantly influenced how anesthesia is practiced in the United States.

On a departmental level, review based on established patterns of care criteria and anesthesia-related morbidity and mortality data should be an ongoing process. A regular schedule for equipment maintenance and procedures to follow when equipment malfunction occurs or is suspected should be established. The National Practitioner Data Bank is a nationwide information system that gathers information (medical malpractice payments, license actions by medical boards, clinical privileges actions taken by hospitals) and is intended to provide licensing boards and hospitals with a better means of detecting adverse information about physicians.

REFERENCES

1. Greene NM. Anesthesia and the development of surgery (1846–1896). Anesth Analg 1979;58:5–12.
2. Eger EI II. Isoflurane (Forane). A Compendium and Reference. Madison, WI, Anaquest, a division of BOC, Inc. 1985;1–4.
3. Baden JM, Kelley M, Wharton RS, Hitt BA, Simmon VF, Mazze RI. Mutagenicity of halogenated ether anesthetics. Anesthesiology 1977;46:346–50.
4. Raventos J. Action of Fluothane—New volatile anesthetic. Br J Pharmacol 1956;11:394–410.
5. Summary of the national halothane study. JAMA 1966;197:775–88.
6. Artusio JF, Van Poznak A, Hunt RE, Tiers FM, Alexander M. A clinical evaluation of methoxyflurane in man. Anesthesiology 1960;21:512–7.
7. Dobkin AB, Heinrich RG, Israel JS, Levy AA, Neville JF, Ounkasem K. Clinical and laboratory evaluation of a new inhalation agent. Compound 347 (CHF_2OCF_2CHFCl). Anesthesiology 1968;29:275–87.
8. Vitcha JF. A history of Forane. Anesthesiology 1971; 35:4–7.
9. Jones RM. Desflurane and sevoflurane: Inhalation anesthetics for this decade? Br J Anaesth 1990; 65:527–36.
10. Frink EJ, Malan TP, Morgan SE, Brown EA, Malcomson M, Brown BR. Quantification of the degradation products of sevoflurane in two CO_2 absorbants during low-flow anesthesia in surgical patients. Anesthesiology 1992;77:1064–9.
11. Griffith HR, Johnson GG. Use of curare in general anesthesia. Anesthesiology 1942;3:418–20.
12. Centers for Disease Control: Update: Universal precautions for prevention of transmission of human immunodeficiency virus, hepatitis B virus, and other bloodborne pathogens in health-care settings. MMWR 1988;37:377–88.
13. Buergler JM, Kim R, Thisted RA, Cohn SJ, Lichtor JL, Roizen MF. Risk of human immunodeficiency virus in surgeons, anesthesiologists, and medical students. Anesth Analg 1992;75:118–24.
14. Deaths during general anesthesia. J Health Care Technol 1985;1:155–75.
15. Keats AS. Anesthesia mortality—A new mechanism. Anesthesiology 1988;68:2–4.
16. Cheney FW, Posner KL, Caplan RA. Adverse respiratory events infrequently leading to malpractice suits. A closed claims analysis. Anesthesiology 1991;75:932–9.
17. Kroll DA, Caplan RA, Posner K, et al. Nerve injury associated with anesthesia. Anesthesiology 1990;73:202–7.
18. Stoelting RK. Postoperative ulnar nerve palsy—Is it a preventable complication? Anesth Analg 1993;76:7–9.
19. Eichhorn JH. Pulse oximetry as a standard of practice in anesthesia. Anesthesiology 1993;78:423–6.

Section II

Pharmacology

2
Basic Pharmacologic Principles

Basic principles of pharmacology are derived from an understanding of pharmacokinetics and pharmacodynamics.[1] Pharmacokinetics describes the absorption, distribution, metabolism, and excretion of inhaled or injected drugs (what the body does to the drug). Pharmacodynamics describes the responsiveness of receptors to drugs and the mechanism by which these effects occur (what the drug does to the body). Receptors are the components of the cell that interact with drugs to initiate a chain of events leading to pharmacologic effects. Selectivity of drug action is also determined by receptors that recognize specific drugs. Termination of a drug's effect is by metabolism, excretion, and/or its redistribution to inactive tissue sites.

TERMINOLOGY AND DEFINITIONS

Drugs (dobutamine) that activate receptors are called agonists. Antagonists are drugs (propranolol) that bind to receptors without activating them while at the same time preventing agonists from stimulating them. Competitive antagonism is present when increasing concentrations of an antagonist (nondepolarizing muscle relaxants) progressively inhibit responses to unchanging concentrations of an agonist (acetylcholine). High concentrations of an agonist, however, can overcome competitive antagonism. Noncompetitive antagonism is present when even high concentrations of an agonist cannot completely overcome antagonism.

An additive effect means that a second drug acting with the first drug will produce an effect equal to algebraic summation. For example, the anesthetic effects of two inhaled anesthetics are additive as reflected by minimum alveolar concentration (MAC) equivalents[2] (see the section *Minimum Alveolar Concentration*). A synergistic effect means that two drugs interact to produce an effect greater than that expected from algebraic summation. For example, aminoglycoside antibiotics do not produce clinically significant neuromuscular blockade by themselves but greatly enhance that produced by nondepolarizing muscle relaxants.

Hyperreactive and hyporeactive individuals are those in whom the usual dose of drug produces increased or decreased effects, respectively. Hyporeactivity acquired from chronic exposure to a drug is often termed tolerance. Cross-tolerance commonly develops between drugs of different classes that produce similar pharmacologic effects (inhaled anesthetics and chronic alcohol ingestion). Tolerance that develops acutely with only a few doses of a drug such as ephedrine is termed tachyphylaxis. Idiosyncrasy is present when an unusual effect of a drug occurs in uniquely susceptible patients regardless of the dose, most probably reflecting hypersensitivity (allergy) or genetic differences.

Dose-Response Curves

Dose-response curves depict the relationship between the dose of drug administered (or the resulting plasma concentration) and the resulting pharmacologic effect (Fig. 2-1). Logarithmic transformation of dosage is frequently used, because it permits display of a large range of doses. Dose-

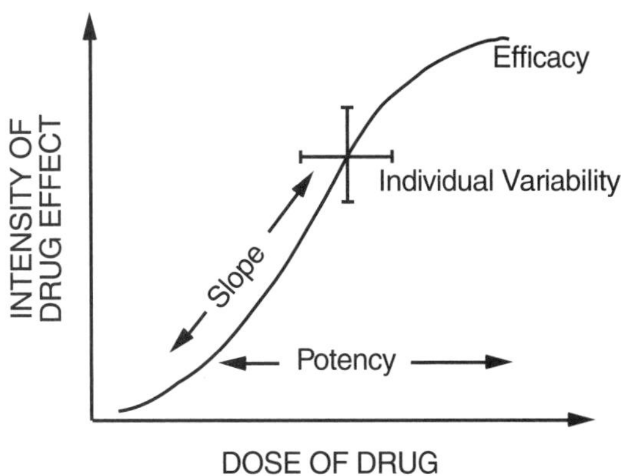

Figure 2-1. Dose-response curves are characterized by differences in potency, slope, efficacy, and individual responses.

response curves are characterized by differences in potency, slope, efficacy, and individual responses.

Potency

The potency of a drug is depicted by its location along the dose axis of the dose-response curve. Doses required to produce a specified effect are designated as the effective dose (ED) necessary to produce that effect in a given percentage of patients (ED_{50}, ED_{90}). Increased affinity of a drug for its receptors moves the dose-response curve to the left. For clinical purposes, the potency of a drug makes little difference as long as the necessary dose of the drug can be administered conveniently.

Slope

The slope of the dose-response curve is influenced by the number of receptors that must be occupied before a drug effect occurs. If a drug must occupy a majority of receptors before an effect occurs, the slope of the dose-response curve will be steep (characteristic of muscle relaxants and inhaled anesthetics). This means that small increases in dose evoke large increases in drug effect. For example, a 1 MAC concentration of a volatile anesthetic prevents skeletal muscle movement in response to a surgical skin incision in 50% (ED_{50}) of patients, whereas a further modest increase to about 1.3 MAC prevents movement in at least 95% (ED_{95}) of patients. Furthermore, when the dose-response curve is steep, the difference between a therapeutic and a toxic concentration may be small. This is true for volatile anesthetics that are characterized by small differences between the doses that produce desirable degrees of central nervous system depression and undesirable degrees of cardiopulmonary depression.

Efficacy

The maximal effect of a drug reflects its efficacy as depicted by the plateau in dose-response curves. Undesirable side effects of a drug may limit dosage to below the concentration associated with its maximal effect. Efficacy and potency of a drug are not necessarily related.

Individual Responses

Individual responses to a drug may vary as reflections of differences in pharmacokinetics (renal function, liver function, cardiac function, patient age) and/or pharmacodynamics (enzyme activity, genetic differences).

PHARMACOKINETICS OF INHALED ANESTHETICS

Pharmacokinetics of inhaled anesthetics describes their uptake (absorption) from alveoli into the systemic circulation, distribution in the body, and eventual elimination via the lungs or metabolism principally in the liver.[3] By controlling the inspired partial pressure (PI) (same as concentration when referring to the gas phase) of an inhaled anesthetic, a gradient is created such that the anesthetic is delivered from the anesthetic machine to its site of action, the brain. The primary objective of inhalation anesthesia is to achieve a constant and optimal partial pressure of the anesthetic in the brain (Pbr).

The brain and all other tissues equilibrate with the partial pressure of the inhaled anesthetic delivered to them by the arterial blood (Pa). Likewise, the blood equilibrates with the alveolar partial pressure (PA) of the anesthetic:

$$PA \leftrightarrows Pa \leftrightarrows Pbr$$

Therefore, maintaining a constant and optimal PA becomes an indirect but useful method for controlling the Pbr. The PA of an inhaled anesthetic mirrors its Pbr and is the reason the PA is used as an index of anesthetic depth, a reflection of the rate of induction and recovery from anesthesia, and a measure of equal potency (see the section *Minimum Alveolar Concentration*).

Summary of Factors Determining Partial Pressure Gradients Necessary for Establishment of Anesthesia

- Transfer of inhaled anesthetic from anesthetic machine to alveoli
  - Inspired partial pressure
  - Alveolar ventilation
  - Characteristics of anesthetic breathing system
- Transfer of inhaled anesthetic from alveoli to arterial blood
  - Blood:gas partition coefficient
  - Cardic output
  - Alveolar-to-venous partial pressure difference
- Transfer of inhaled anesthetic from arterial blood to brain
  - Brain:blood partition coefficient
  - Cerebral blood flow
  - Arterial-to-venous partial pressure difference

Understanding the factors that determine the PA and thus the Pbr allows the anesthesiologist to skillfully control and adjust the dose of inhaled anesthetic delivered to the brain.

Factors that Determine the Alveolar Partial Pressure

The PA and ultimately the Pbr of an inhaled anesthetic is determined by input (delivery) into the alveoli minus uptake (loss) of the drug from the alveoli into the arterial blood. Input of the inhaled anesthetic is dependent on the (1) PI, (2) alveolar ventilation (VA), and (3) characteristics of the anesthetic breathing system. Uptake of the inhaled anesthetic is dependent on the (1) solubility, (2) cardiac output (CO), and (3) alveolar-to-venous partial pressure difference (A-vD). These six factors act simultaneously to determine the PA. Metabolism and percutaneous loss of inhaled anesthetics do not significantly influence PA during induction and maintenance of anesthesia.

Inspired Anesthetic Partial Pressure

A high PI is necessary during initial administration of an inhaled anesthetic. This initial high PI (input) offsets the impact of uptake into the blood and thus accelerates induction of anesthesia as reflected by the rate of increase in the PA. This effect of the PI is known as the concentration effect. Clinically, the range of concentrations necessary to produce a concentration effect is possible only with nitrous oxide (Fig. 2-2).[4]

With time, as uptake into the blood decreases, the PI should be decreased to match the decreased anesthetic uptake. Indeed, decreasing the PI to match decreasing uptake with time is crucial if one is to achieve the goal of maintaining a constant and optimal Pbr. For example, if the PI were maintained constant with time (input constant), the PA (and Pbr) would progressively increase as uptake of the anesthetic into the blood diminished.

Second Gas Effect. The second gas effect is a distinct phenomenon that occurs independently of the concentration effect.[5] The ability of the large vol-

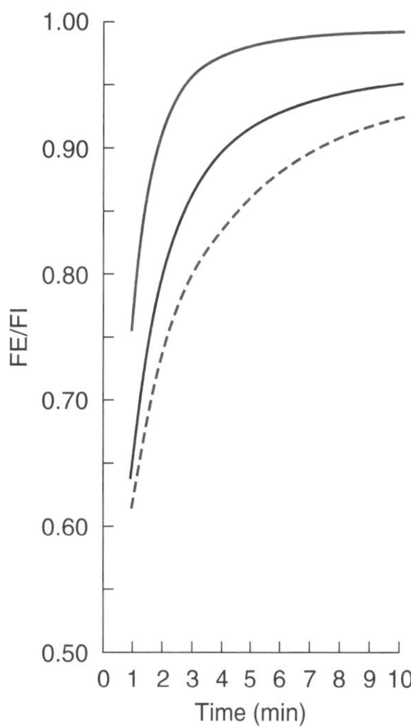

Figure 2-2. The impact of the inspired concentration (%) (FI) on the rate of increase of the alveolar (end-tidal) concentration (FE) is known as the concentration effect. Solid red line, 85%; black line, 50%; dashed red line, 10%. (From Eger,[4] with permission.)

ume uptake of one gas (first gas) to accelerate the rate of increase of the PA of a concurrently administered companion gas (second gas) is known as the second gas effect. For example, the initial large volume uptake of nitrous oxide accelerates the uptake of companion gases such as volatile anesthetics and oxygen. Indeed, the transient increase (about 10%) in PaO_2 that accompanies the early phase of nitrous oxide administration reflects the second gas effect. This increase in PaO_2 has been designated as alveolar hyperoxygenation. Increased tracheal inflow of all inhaled gases (first and second gases) and concentration of the second gases in a smaller lung volume (concentrating effect) owing to the high volume uptake of the first gas are the explanations for the second gas effect.[6] Although the second gas effect may produce detectable alterations in the PA, it probably should not be considered clinically significant.

Alveolar Ventilation

Increased VA, like PI, promotes input of inhaled anesthetics to offset uptake into the blood. The net effect is a more rapid rate of increase in the PA and induction of anesthesia. Predictably, hypoventilation has the opposite effect, acting to slow the induction of anesthesia.

Controlled ventilation of the lungs that results in hyperventilation and decreased venous return accelerates the rate of increase of the PA by virtue of increased input (increased VA) and decreased uptake (decreased CO) (see the section *Cardiac Output*). As a result, the risk of anesthetic overdose may be increased during controlled ventilation of the lungs. For this reason, it may be appropriate to decrease the PI of volatile anesthetics when ventilation of the lungs is changed from spontaneous to controlled so as to maintain the PA similar to that present during spontaneous ventilation.

Another effect of hyperventilation is decreased cerebral blood flow owing to any associated decrease in the $PaCO_2$. Conceivably, the impact of increased input on the rate of increase of the PA would be offset by decreased delivery of anesthetic to the brain. Theoretically, coronary blood flow may remain unchanged, such that increased input produces myocardial depression, and decreased cerebral blood flow prevents a concomitant onset of central nervous system depression.

Anesthetic Breathing System

Characteristics of the anesthetic breathing system that influence the rate of increase of the PA include the (1) volume of the system, (2) solubility of inhaled anesthetics in the rubber or plastic components of the system, and (3) gas inflow from the anesthetic machine. The volume of the anesthetic breathing system acts as a buffer to slow attainment of the PA. High gas inflow from the anesthetic machine negates this buffer effect. Solubility of inhaled anesthetics in the components of the anesthetic breathing system initially slows the rate at which the PA increases. At the conclusion of an anesthetic, reversal of the partial pressure gradient in the anesthetic breathing system results in elution of the anesthetics that slows the rate at which the PA decreases. Subsequent reuse of the same anesthetic breathing system on another patient results in exposure of that patient to trace concentrations of that anesthetic, even if another drug or technique has been selected.

Solubility

The solubility of inhaled anesthetics in blood and tissues is denoted by partition coefficients (Table 2-1). A partition coefficient is a distribution ratio describing how the inhaled anesthetic distributes itself between two phases at equilibrium (when the partial pressures are identical). For example, a blood:gas partition coefficient of 10 means that the concentration of the inhaled anesthetic is 10 in the blood and 1 in the alveolar gas when the partial pressures of that anesthetic in these two phases are identical. It is important to recognize that partition coefficients are temperature-dependent. For example, the solubility of a gas in a liquid is increased when the temperature of the liquid decreases. Unless otherwise stated, partition coefficients are for 37°C.

Blood:Gas Partition Coefficients. High blood solubility means that a large amount of inhaled anesthetic must be dissolved (undergo uptake) in the blood before equilibrium with the gas phase is reached. The blood can be considered a pharmacologically inactive reservoir, the size of which is determined by the solubility of the anesthetic in the blood. When the blood:gas partition coefficient is high, a large amount of anesthetic must be dissolved in the blood before the Pa equilibrates with the PA (Fig. 2-3).[7] Clinically, the impact of high blood solubility on the rate of increase of the PA can be offset

Table 2-1. Comparative Characteristics of Inhaled Anesthetics

	Isoflurane	Enflurane	Halothane	Desflurane	Sevoflurane	Nitrous Oxide
Blood:gas partition coefficient	1.4	1.9	2.4	0.42	0.68	0.46
Brain:blood partition coefficient	1.6	1.5	1.9	1.3	1.7	1.1
Muscle:blood partition coefficient	2.9	1.7	3.4	2.0	3.1	1.2
Fat:blood partition coeficient	45	36	51	27	48	2.3
MAC (volumes %, 30–55 years old)	1.15	1.68	0.75	7.25	2.05	105–110
Vapor pressure (mmHg, 20°C)	240	172	244	669	160	
Molecular weight	184.5	184.5	197.4	168	200	44
Stable in soda lime	Yes	Yes	No	Yes	No	Yes

to some extent by increasing the PI. When blood solubility is low, minimal amounts of the anesthetic have to be dissolved in the blood before equilibrium is reached such that the rate of increase of the PA and thus that of the Pa and Pbr are rapid (Fig. 2-3).[7]

Tissue:Blood Partition Coefficients. Tissue:blood partition coefficients determine the time necessary for equilibration of the tissue with the Pa (Table 2-1). This time can be predicted by calculating a time constant (amount of inhaled anesthetic that can be dissolved in the tissue divided by tissue blood flow) for each tissue. Brain:blood partition coefficients for volatile anesthetics such as isoflurane result in time constants of about 3 to 4 minutes. Complete equilibration of any tissue, including the brain, with the Pa requires at least three time constants. This is the rationale for maintaining the PA of these volatile anesthetics constant for 10 to 15 minutes before assuming that the Pbr is similar. Three time constants for those inhaled anesthetics with brain:blood partition coefficients between 0.42 to 0.68 are about 6 minutes.

Nitrous Oxide Transfer to Closed Gas Spaces. The blood:gas partition coefficient of nitrous oxide (0.46) is 34 times greater than that of nitrogen (0.014). This differential solubility means that nitrous oxide can leave the blood to enter an air-filled cavity 34 times more rapidly than nitrogen can leave the cavity to enter the blood.[8] As a result of this preferential transfer of nitrous oxide, the volume or pressure of the air-filled cavity increases. The entrance of nitrous oxide into an air-filled cavity surrounded by a compliant wall (intestinal gas, pneumothorax, pulmonary blebs, air embolism) causes the gas space to expand. Conversely, entrance of nitrous oxide into an air-filled cavity surrounded by a noncompliant wall (middle ear, cerebral ventricles, supratentorial subdural space) causes an increase in pressure.

The magnitude of volume or pressure increase is influenced by the PA of nitrous oxide, blood flow to the air-filled cavity, and duration of nitrous oxide administration. In an animal model, the inhalation of 75% nitrous oxide doubles the volume of a pneumothorax in 10 minutes (Fig. 2-4).[8] Therefore, the presence of a closed pneumothorax is a contraindication to the administration of nitrous oxide. Indeed, decreasing pulmonary compliance during administration of nitrous oxide to patients with histories of chest trauma (rib fractures) may reflect nitrous oxide-induced expansion of a previously unrecognized pneumothorax.

In contrast to the rapid expansion of a pneumothorax, the increase in bowel gas volume produced by nitrous oxide is slow. The question of whether to administer nitrous oxide to patients undergoing intra-abdominal surgery is of little importance if the operation is short. Limiting the inhaled concentration of nitrous oxide to 50%, however, may be a prudent recommendation when bowel gas volume is increased (bowel obstruction) preoperatively. Following this guideline, bowel gas volume, at most, would double even with prolonged operations.[8]

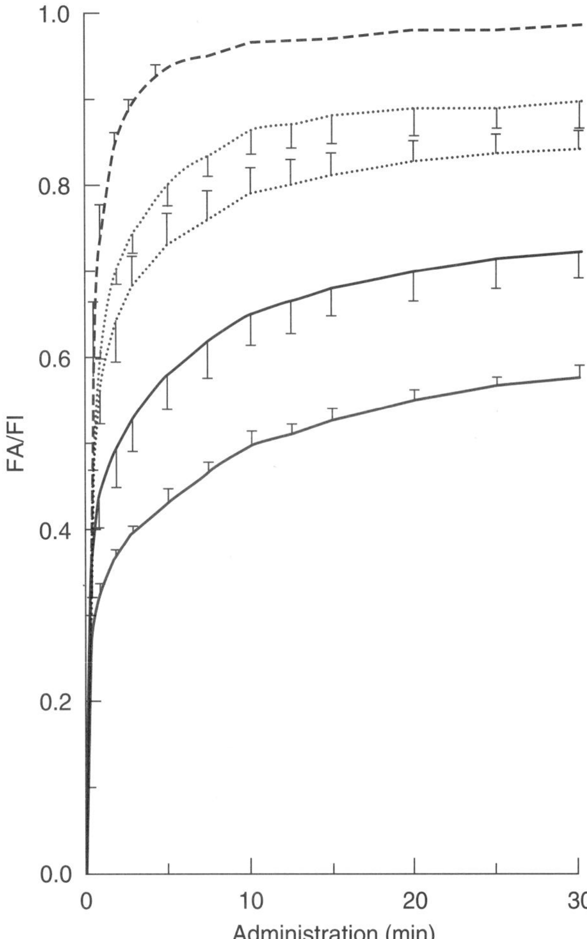

Figure 2-3. The blood:gas partition coefficient is the principal determinant of the rate at which the alveolar concentration (FA) increases toward a constant inspired concentration (FI). The rate of induction of anesthesia is paralleled by the rate of increase in the FA. Despite similar blood solubility (Table 2-1), the rate of increase of FA is more rapid for nitrous oxide (dashed black line) than for desflurane (dotted red line) or sevoflurane (dotted black line), reflecting the impact of the concentration effect on nitrous oxide (Fig. 2-2). Greater tissue solubility of desflurane and sevoflurane may also contribute to a slower rate of increase in the FA of these drugs compared with nitrous oxide. On the basis of its blood solubility, the curve for enflurane would be between the curves for halothane (solid red line) and isoflurane (solid black line). (From Yasuda et al.,[7] with permission.)

Cardiac Output

The CO influences uptake into the blood and therefore, PA, by carrying away more or less anesthetic from the alveoli. A high CO (fear) results in more rapid uptake, such that the rate of increase in the PA, and thus the induction of anesthesia, is slowed. A low CO (shock) speeds the rate of increase of the PA since there is less uptake into the blood to oppose input. Indeed, a common clinical impression is that induction of anesthesia in patients in shock is rapid.

Shunt. A right-to-left intracardiac or intrapulmonary shunt slows the rate of induction of anesthsia. This slowing reflects the dilutional effect of shunted blood containing no anesthetic on the partial pressure of anesthetic in blood coming from ventilated alveoli. A similar mechanism is responsible for the decrease in PaO_2 in the presence of a right-to-left shunt.

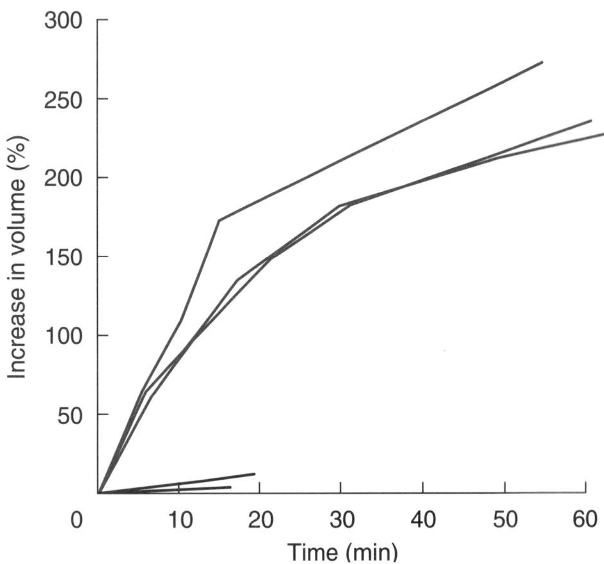

Figure 2-4. Inhalation of 75% nitrous oxide in oxygen (red lines) but not oxygen alone (black lines) rapidly increases the volume of a pneumothorax. (From Eger and Saidman,[8] with permission.)

A left-to-right tissue shunt (arteriovenous fistula, volatile anesthetic-induced increases in cutaneous blood flow) results in delivery to the lungs of venous blood containing a higher partial pressure of anesthetic than that present in venous blood that has passed through the tissues. As a result, a left-to-right tissue shunt offsets the dilutional effect of a right-to-left shunt on the Pa. Indeed, the effect of a left-to-right shunt on the rate of increase in the Pa is detectable only if there is the concomitant presence of a right-to-left shunt. Likewise, the dilutional effect of a right-to-left shunt will be greatest in the absence of a left-to-right shunt. All factors considered, it seems unlikely that the impact of a right-to-left shunt would be apparent clinically.

Wasted Ventilation. Ventilation of unperfused alveoli will not influence the rate of induction of anesthesia since a dilutional effect on the Pa is not produced. The principal effect of wasted ventilation is the production of a difference between the PA and Pa of the inhaled anesthetic. A similar mechanism is responsible for the difference often observed between the end-tidal PCO_2 and $PaCO_2$.

Alveolar-to-Venous Partial Pressure Differences

The A-vD reflects tissue uptake of inhaled anesthetics. Highly perfused tissues (brain, heart, kidneys, liver) account for less than 10% of body mass but receive about 75% of the CO (Table 2-2). As a result, these highly perfused tissues equilibrate rapidly with the Pa. Indeed, after three time constants (6 to 15 minutes for inhaled anesthetics), about 75% of the returning venous blood is at the same partial pressure as the PA (narrow A-vD). For this reason, uptake of volatile anesthetics from the alveoli is greatly decreased after 6 to 15 minutes, as reflected by a narrowing of the PI-to-PA difference. After this time, the inhaled concentrations of volatile anesthetic should be decreased so as to maintain a constant PA in the presence of decreased uptake.

Skeletal muscle and fat represent about 70% of the body mass but receive less than 25% of the CO (Table 2-2). Therefore, these tissues continue to act as inactive reservoirs for anesthetic uptake for several hours. Indeed, equilibration of fat with inhaled anesthetics in the arterial blood is probably never achieved.

Table 2-2. Body Tissue Compartments

	Body Mass (% of a 70-kg Adult)	Blood Flow (% of Cardiac Output)
Vessel-rich group	10	75
Muscle group	50	19
Fat group	20	5
Vessel-poor group	20	1

Recovery from Anesthesia

Recovery from anesthesia can be defined as the rate at which the PA decreases with time (Fig. 2-5).[7] In many respects, recovery is the inverse of induction of anesthesia. For example, VA, solubility, and CO determine the rate at which the PA decreases. Conversely, recovery from anesthesia is also influenced by factors unique to this phase of the anesthetic.

Differences from Induction

Recovery from anesthesia differs from induction of anesthesia with respect to (1) the absence of a concentration effect on recovery (the PI cannot be less than zero), (2) variable tissue concentrations of anesthetics at the start of recovery, and (3) the potential importance of metabolism on the rate of decrease in the PA.

Tissue Concentrations. Tissue concentrations of inhaled anesthetics serve as a reservoir to maintain the PA when the partial pressure gradient is reversed by decreasing the PI to or near zero at the conclusion of anesthesia. The impact of tissue storage will depend on the duration of anesthesia and solubility of the anesthetics in various tissue components. The variable concentrations of anesthetics in different tissues at the conclusion of anesthesia contrasts with induction of anesthesia, when all tissues initially have the same zero concentration of anesthetic.

Metabolism. An important difference between induction of anesthesia and recovery from anesthesia is the potential impact of metabolism on the rate of decrease in the PA at the conclusion of anesthesia. In this regard, metabolism is a principal determinant of the rate of decrease in the PA of highly

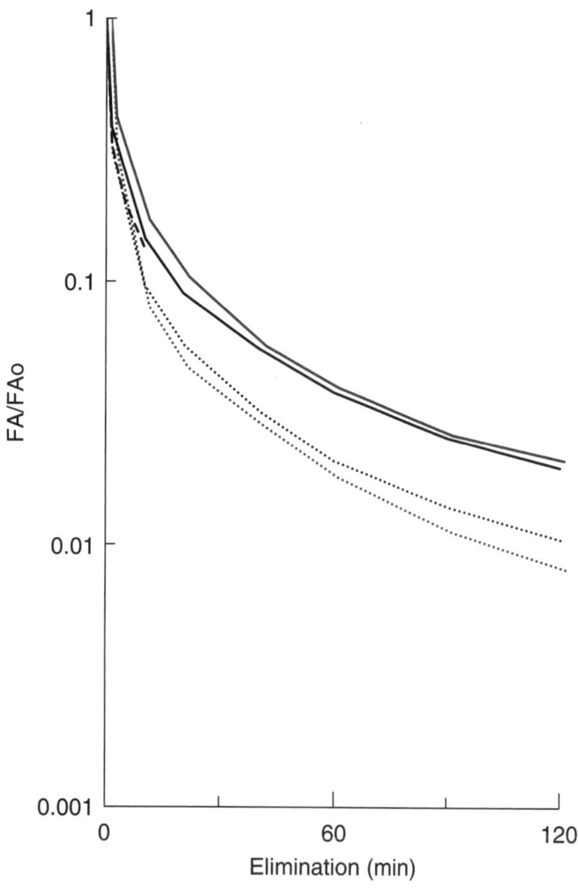

Figure 2-5. Elimination of inhaled anesthetics is reflected by the decrease in the alveolar concentration (FA) compared with the concentration present at the conclusion of anesthesia (FAo). Awakening from anesthesia is paralleled by these curves. Solid red line, halothane; solid black line, isoflurane; dashed black line, nitrous oxide; dotted red line, desflurane; dotted black line, sevoflurane. (From Yasuda et al.,[7] with permission.)

lipid soluble methoxyflurane. Metabolism and VA are equally important in the rate of decrease in the PA of halothane, whereas the rate of decrease in the PA of less lipid soluble enflurane, isoflurane, and desflurane is due principally to VA.[9]

Diffusion Hypoxia. Diffusion hypoxia may occur at the conclusion of nitrous oxide administration if patients are allowed to inhale room air. The initial high volume outpouring of nitrous oxide from the blood into the alveoli when inhalation of this gas is discontinued can so dilute the PAO_2 that the PaO_2 decreases.[3] The occurrence of diffusion hypoxia is prevented by filling the patient's lungs with oxygen at the conclusion of nitrous oxide administration.

PHARMACODYNAMICS OF INHALED ANESTHETICS

Minimum Alveolar Concentration

MAC is the minimum alveolar concentration (partial pressure) of an inhaled anesthetic at 1 atmosphere that prevents skeletal muscle movement in response to a noxious stimulus (surgical skin incision) in 50% of patients.[10] As such, MAC represents one point on the dose-response curve of effects produced by inhaled anesthetics. That MAC reflects the partial pressure at the anesthetic site of action (Pbr) has made it the most useful index of anesthetic equal potency.

Use of equally potent doses (comparable MACs) of inhaled anesthetics is mandatory for comparing effects of these drugs on vital organ function. For example, despite equivalent depression of the central nervous system, 1 MAC enflurane (1.68%) decreases CO more than an equally potent concentration of isoflurane (1.15%) (see Chapter 4). That the dose-response curves for different inhaled anesthetics are not parallel with respect to vital organ depression is an important observation. Specifically, the alveolar anesthetic concentration producing a given effect (blood pressure decrease, depression of ventilation, potentiation of nondepolarizing muscle relaxants) divided by MAC can be calculated (therapeutic index) for all the inhaled anesthetics. Each anesthetic possesses unique qualities with respect to these anesthetic side effects, yet similar MACs all produce equivalent depression of the central nervous system. Such information is helpful for the safe and rational selection of specific inhaled anesthetics for individual patients, as well as the dose of drug that is administered.

MAC values for combinations of inhaled anesthetics are additive. For example, 0.5 MAC nitrous oxide plus 0.5 MAC isoflurane has the same effect at the brain as either drug alone at 1 MAC. That the nitrous oxide MAC is higher than 100%, however, means that this anesthetic cannot be used alone at 1 atmosphere and still provide a minimum of 21% oxygen. Therefore, 50% to 75% inhaled nitrous oxide is commonly administered, with the remaining anesthesia being provided by volatile anesthetics and/or opioids. A guideline is that MAC for volatile anesthetics is decreased about 1% for every 1% alveolar nitrous oxide concentration. An important reason for administering nitrous oxide with volatile anesthetics is the observation that depression of ventilation and circulation is smaller when nitrous oxide is substituted for an equivalent MAC dose of the volatile drug (see Chapter 4).

Clinically, more than 1 MAC is necessary because, by definition, 50% of patients would move with surgical stimulation at 1 MAC. Administration of approximately 1.3 MAC prevents skeletal muscle movement in nearly all patients during surgery.

In addition to its value as an index of equal potency, the MAC concept allows a quantitative analysis of the impact of various pharmacologic and physiologic factors on anesthetic requirements.[2] Likewise, factors that do not influence MAC can be determined.[2] MAC is also useful as a tool to understanding better the mechanism by which anesthetics produce anesthesia.

Impact of Physiologic and Pharmacologic Factors on Minimum Alveolar Concentration

No change in MAC
- Duration of anesthesia
- Gender
- Anesthetic metabolism
- Thyroid gland dysfunction
- Hyperkalemia or hypokalemia
- $PaCO_2$ 15–95 mmHg
- PaO_2 >38 mmHg
- Blood pressure >40 mmHg

Increase in MAC
- Hyperthermia
- Drugs that increase CNS cateholamines (monoamine oxidase inhibitors, tricyclic antidepressants, cocaine, acute amphetamine ingestion)
- Infants
- Hypernatremia
- Chronic ethanol abuse (?)

Decrease in MAC
- Hypothermia
- Preoperative medication
- Intravenous anesthetics
- Neonates
- Elderly
- Pregnancy
- Alpha-2 agonists
- Acute ethanol ingestion
- Lithium
- Cardiopulmonary bypass
- Neuraxial opioids (?)
- PaO_2 <38 mmHg

Mechanism of Anesthesia

The mechanism by which inhaled anesthetics produce reversible and sometimes selective depression of the central nervous system (especially the reticular activating system) is not known.[11] Inhaled anesthetics have multiple effects, including alterations in membrane properties, neurotransmitter activity, receptor responsiveness, and chemical- and voltage-gated ion channels and enzymes. Genes that alter sensitivity to volatile anesthetics have been identified, emphasizing the importance of the molecular composition of the site of action of anesthetics. With all these possible effects, it is difficult to define precisely the mechanisms of general anesthesia. Although a single theory to explain the mechanism of anesthesia seems unlikely, several unitary theories have been proposed to explain the production of anesthesia by inhaled drugs.

Meyer-Overton Theory (Critical-Volume Hypothesis)

This theory recognizes the close correlation between the lipid solubility of inhaled anesthetics (oil:gas partition coefficient) and their potencies (MAC). Such a correlation suggests that anesthesia occurs when a sufficient number of anesthetic molecules dissolve (critical volume) in crucial hydrophobic sites, such as lipid cell membranes. Conceptually, expansion of hydrophobic membranes by dissolved anesthetic molecules could exert pressure on ion channels necessary for sodium flux and the subsequent development of action potentials for synaptic transmission. Indeed, membrane expansion by a critical volume of 0.4% results in anesthesia. Furthermore, high pressures (40 to 100 atmospheres) partially antagonize the action of inhaled anesthetics (pressure reversal), presumably by returning (compressing) lipid membranes to their "awake" contour. Universal acceptance of this theory, however, is prevented by the observation that some lipid soluble compounds are not anesthetics and, in fact, may be convulsants.

Protein (Receptor) Hypothesis

This theory proposes hydrophobic regions of specific proteins (receptors) in the central nervous system as the site of action of inhaled anesthetics. Evidence to support this theory includes the steep nature of anesthetic dose-response curves (1 MAC prevents movement in 50% of subjects, whereas 1.3 MAC is effective in about 95%), suggesting a crucial receptor occupancy. Receptor specificity is also suggested by conversion of an anesthetic to a nonanesthetic by increasing the molecular weight despite corresponding increases in lipid solubility.

In animals, the dextro isomer of medetomidine, an alpha-2 agonist, produces dose-dependent and stereospecific decreases in halothane MAC (Fig. 2-6).[12] The stereospecificity of this MAC-decreasing property suggests an effect on a homogenous receptor population such as alpha-2 receptors in the central nervous system (see the section *Stereospecificity*). It is possible that alpha-2 stimulation supplements the anesthetized state by producing an increase in potassium conductance (hyperpolarizes) with subsequent depression of neuronal excitability.

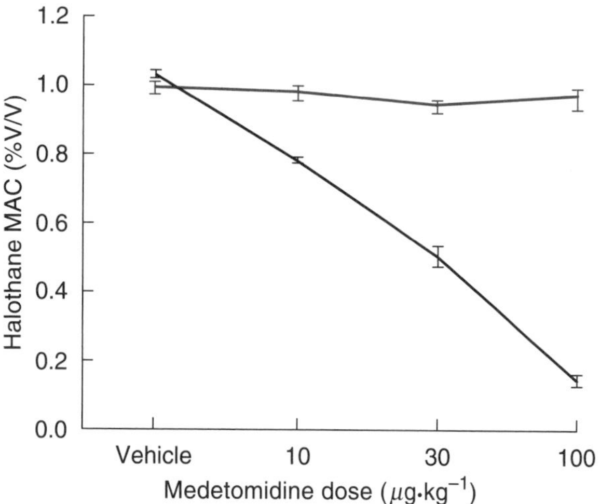

Figure 2-6. Effect of stereoisomers (red line, levomedetomidine; black line, dexmedetomidine) of the alpha-2 adrenergic agonist medetomidine on halothane MAC in animals. (From Segal et al.,[12] with permission.)

Alteration in Neurotransmitter Availability

Inhaled anesthetics may interfere with the metabolic breakdown of the inhibitory neurotransmitter gamma-aminobutyric acid (GABA). This inhibition leads to increased brain concentrations of GABA and the speculation that anesthesia may reflect enhanced synaptic inhibition by GABA.

PHARMACOKINETICS OF INTRAVENOUS DRUGS

Pharmacokinetics of intravenous drugs are influenced by the volume of distribution for that drug (Vd) and the clearance of that drug from the body. The rate at which the plasma concentration of a drug decreases with time (elimination half-time) is determined by the Vd and clearance of the drug. It must be recognized that pharmacokinetic characteristics of drugs measured in healthy and ambulatory adults may be different in patients with chronic diseases (especially renal and/or hepatic dysfunction) and at various extremes of age, hydration, nutrition, and skeletal muscle mass.

Knowledge of the pharmacokinetics and pharmacodynamics of intravenous drugs clearly defines the dose-response relationships of a drug and its comparisons with other drugs.[13] Furthermore, the influence of altered physiologic states (aging) on drug effect can be determined. Likewise, new approaches to drug administration (computer-driven infusion pumps, patient controlled analgesia) can be established.

Volume of Distribution

Vd is a calculated number (dose of drug administered intravenously divided by the plasma concentration) that reflects the apparent volumes of the compartments that constitute the compartmental model for that drug (Fig. 2-7).[1] Binding to plasma proteins, a high degree of ionization, and low lipid solubility limit passage of drugs to tissues (peripheral compartments), thus maintaining a high plasma concentration (central compartment) and a small calculated Vd. Examples of drugs with a small Vd similar to that of extracellular fluid are muscle relax ants. Nonionized lipid soluble drugs readily pass into tissues (peripheral compartments) from the circulation (central compartment) such that plasma concentrations are low and the calculated Vd is large. Examples of such drugs are thiopental and diazepam. It is important to recognize that Vd does not refer to absolute anatomic volumes.

Clearance

Clearance is the volume of plasma (central compartment) cleared of drug ($ml \cdot min^{-1}$) by renal excretion and/or metabolism in the liver or other organs. Clearance is one of the most important pharmacokinetic variables to be considered when defining a constant rate of intravenous drug infusion. When the rate of drug infusion exceeds clearance, the plasma concentration increases progressively and cumulative drug effects occur.

Renal Elimination

The kidneys are the most important organs for clearance of unchanged drugs or their metabolites. Water soluble compounds that are not bound to proteins are excreted more efficiently than protein-bound, lipid soluble drugs. This emphasizes the important role of metabolism in converting lipid soluble drugs to water soluble metabolites. Creatinine clearance or serum creatinine concentrations are useful clinical indicators of the ability of the kidneys to eliminate drugs. The magnitude of increase of these indices provides an estimate of the downward adjustment in drug dosage required to prevent accumulation of a drug in the plasma.

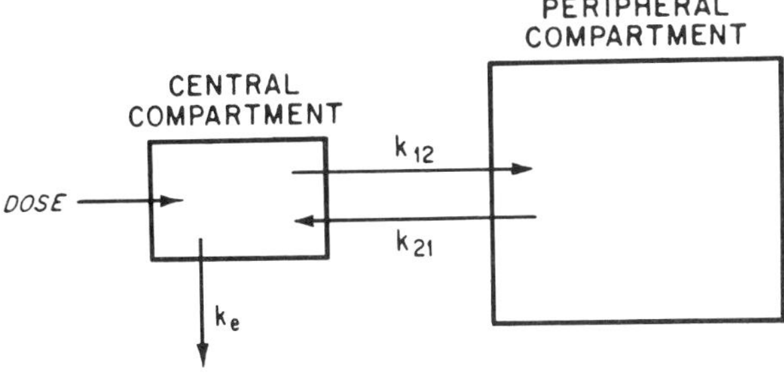

Figure 2-7. A two compartment pharmacokinetic model. The transfer of drugs between compartments (k12, k21) and elimination (clearance) from the central compartment (ke) is depicted by rate constants. (From Stanski and Watkins,[1] with permission.)

Metabolism

Metabolism (principally in the liver but to some extent also in the kidneys, lungs, and gastrointestinal tract) converts pharmacologically active lipid soluble drugs to water soluble and often inactive metabolites. Increased water solubility decreases the Vd of a drug and enhances its renal excretion. A lipid soluble drug is poorly excreted because of the ease of reabsorption from the lumens of renal tubules into pericapillary fluid.

Microsomal enzymes that participate in the metabolism of many drugs are located principally in hepatic smooth endoplasmic reticulum. The term microsomal enzymes is derived from the fact that centrifugation of homogenized hepatocytes concentrates fragments of the disrupted smooth endoplasmic reticulum in what is designated as the microsomal fraction. The microsomal fraction contains the cytochrome P-450 system, which is likely to be a large number of protein enzymes responsible for metabolism of many foreign compounds. Enzyme induction is stimulation of microsomal enzyme activity by drugs (classically phenobarbital) leading to accelerated metabolism of other drugs. The principal determinant of microsomal enzyme activity, however, is likely to be genetic, emphasizing the predictable large individual variation in rate of metabolism of drugs among patients.

Plasma Concentration Curves

A graphic plot of the logarithm of the plasma concentration of drug versus time following rapid intravenous (bolus) injection depicts two distinct phases that characterize the distribution half-time and elimination half-time of that drug (Fig. 2-8).[1] The first phase is designated the distribution (alpha) phase corresponding to the initial distribution of drug from the circulation to tissues (peripheral compartments). The second phase is designated the elimination (beta) phase. This phase is characterized by a gradual decrease in the plasma concentration of drug and reflects its elimination from the central vascular compartment by renal and hepatic mechanisms.

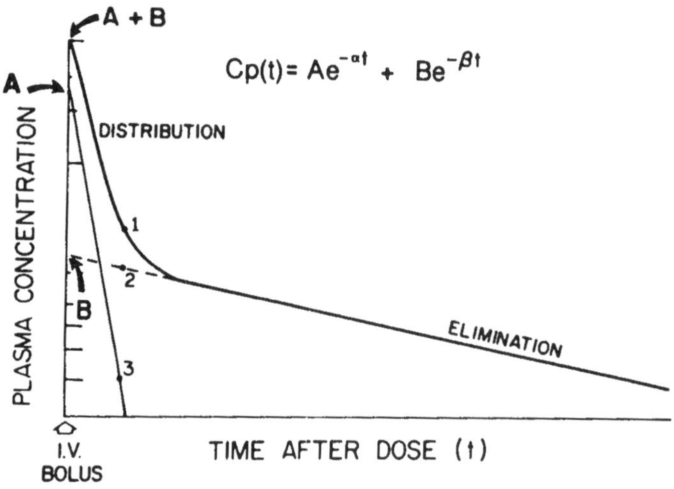

Figure 2-8. Schematic depiction of the decrease in the plasma concentration of drug with time following rapid intravenous injection into the central compartment (Fig. 2-7). The initial rapid decrease in plasma concentration reflects distribution to tissues, whereas the subsequent slow decrease in plasma concentration reflects drug elimination (clearance) by the liver and kidneys. The time necessary for the plasma concentration to decrease 50% during the distribution or elimination phase is the corresponding distribution or elimination half-time for that drug. (From Stanski and Watkins,[1] with permission.)

Elimination Half-Time

Elimination half-time is the time necessary for the plasma concentration of drug to decline 50% during the elimination phase (Fig. 2-8).[1] Five elimination half-times are required for almost complete elimination of a drug. Repeated doses of drug equivalent to the initial dose at intervals more frequent than five elimination half-times will result in cumulative drug effects. Drug accumulation continues until the rate of drug elimination equals the rate of drug administered. As with drug elimination, the time necessary for a drug to achieve a steady state plasma concentration (Cpss) with intermittent doses is about five elimination half-times. A common practice is to administer a large initial dose (loading dose) of drug intravenously to achieve a therapeutic concentration rapidly and then to give continuous or intermittent intravenous injections of decreased doses of drug to match the rate of elimination and thus maintain an optimal and unchanging plasma concentration. In most circumstances, this is most reliably achieved by continuous intravenous infusion techniques. The maintenance dose must be adjusted downward in the presence of renal or hepatic dysfunction so as to prevent drug accumulation due to a prolonged elimination half-time.

Ionization

The pharmacokinetics of a drug are highly dependent on the characteristics of the nonionized and ionized fraction of that drug (Table 2-3). The nonionized drug fraction tends to be pharmacologically active and lipid soluble, whereas the ionized fraction is inactive and water soluble. Lipid or water solubility also determines absorption and elimination characteristics of drugs.

The degree of ionization of a drug is a function of its pK and the pH of the surrounding fluid. When pK and pH are identical, 50% of the drug exists in the

Table 2-3. Characteristics of Nonionized and Ionized Drug Molecules

	Nonionized	Ionized
Pharmacologic effect	Active	Inactive
Solubility	Lipids	Water
Cross lipid barriers (renal tubules, gastrointestinal tract, placenta, blood-brain barrier)	Yes	No
Renal excretion	No	Yes
Hepatic metabolism	Yes	No

ionized form. Small changes in pH can result in large changes in the degree of ionization, especially if the pH and pK values are similar. Acidic drugs, such as barbiturates, tend to be highly ionized at an alkaline pH, whereas basic drugs, such as opioids and local anesthetics, are highly ionized at an acid pH.

Route of Administration

Intravenous administration of drugs ensures achievement of predictable plasma concentrations. Absorption of drugs after oral or intramuscular injection is often unpredictable and dependent on local blood flow. Drugs absorbed from the gastrointestinal tract (principally the small intestine) enter the portal venous blood and thus pass through the liver before entering the systemic circulation for delivery to tissue receptors (Fig. 2-9). This is known as the first-pass hepatic effect, and, for drugs that undergo extensive hepatic metabolism (propranolol, lidocaine), this is the reason for large differences between effective oral and intravenous (drug delivered to receptors before passing through the liver) doses. In addition to hepatic uptake, the lungs may have an important function in pharmacokinetics, as reflected by uptake of basic lipophilic amines (lidocaine, propranolol, fentanyl).[14] This first-pass pulmonary effect may influence the peak arterial concentration of these drugs and subsequently the lungs could serve as a reservoir to release drug back into the systemic circulation.

Redistribution

Following systemic absorption of drugs, the highly perfused tissues (brain, heart, kidneys, liver) receive a proportionally larger amount of the total dose (Table 2-2). For example, approximately 75% of the cardiac output is delivered to about 10% of the total body mass. This is consistent with the rapid onset of central nervous system effects of lipid soluble drugs (barbiturates, opioids) after their intravenous administration. As the plasma concentrations of drugs decrease below those in highly perfused tissues, the drugs leave these tissues to be delivered to less well-perfused sites, such as skeletal muscles and fat. This transfer of drug to inactive tissue sites, such as skeletal muscles, is known as redistribution. Redistribution of thiopental from the brain to inactive tissue sites is principally responsible for awakening after a single dose of this drug. Repeated doses of thiopental can saturate inactive tissue sites, leading to delayed awakening until metabolism can decrease plasma concentrations. Similarly, the normal short duration of action of fentanyl that is due to redistribution becomes a prolonged effect when single large doses, repeated doses, or continuous infusions saturate inactive tissue sites.

PHARMACODYNAMICS OF INTRAVENOUS DRUGS

The pharmacologic effects evoked by drugs administered intravenously reflect their interaction with specific receptors.

Receptors

Receptors are characterized as protein macromolecules that are present in cell membranes. Transmembrane signaling systems describe the mechanism by which receptors translate information imparted to them by neurotransmitters, hormones, or agonist drugs. For example, a receptor may be a protein channel (chloride channel) whose conductance is regulated by receptor activation

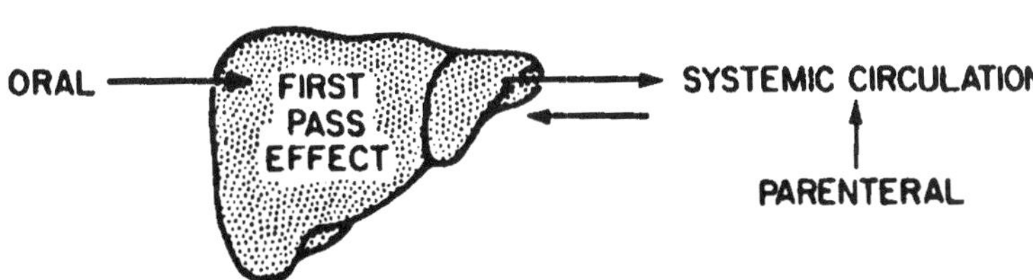

Figure 2-9. Drugs administered orally are absorbed from the gastrointestinal tract into the portal venous blood and pass through the liver (first-pass hepatic effect) before entering the systemic circulation for distribution to receptors. Conversely, intravenously administered drugs gain rapid access to the systemic circulation for delivery to receptors without an initial impact of metabolism in the liver.

(Fig. 2-10A).[15] A second type of transmembrane signaling system involves the coupling of three separate components that include a receptor protein, a guanine nucleotide binding protein (G protein), and an effector mechanism. Membrane-bound G proteins, as the most prevalent proteins in the central nervous system, may serve as target sites for anesthetic action. In some receptor-effector systems, the signal transduction pathway does not utilize intracellular messengers (muscarinic receptors controlling heart rate at the sinus node) (Fig. 2-10B).[15] Alternatively, the activity of an enzyme may be changed to generate a second messenger (specific intracellular signal molecule) (Fig. 2-10C).[15] For example, receptors may regulate the activity of adenylate cyclase in a positive manner (beta-adrenergic receptors) through a stimulatory G protein or a negative manner (alpha-2 receptors) through an inhibitory G protein, thus controlling the intracellular level of cyclic adenosine monophosphate (second messenger) (Fig. 2-10C).[15] Another membrane associated enzyme similar to adenylate cyclase is phospholipase C (alpha-1 receptors), which catalyzes reactions leading to second messengers that stimulate calcium release from intracellular stores (Fig. 2-10D).[15] Collectively, these receptor-induced responses most often result in a change in transmembrane voltage and hence neuronal excitability.

Receptors are identified and subsequently classified (alpha, beta, dopamine, histamine, mu) principally on the basis of effects of specific agonists and antagonists. Such classifications serve to summarize the pharmacologic effects of agonist drugs and the likely effects of antagonist drugs (see Table 3-1). Multiple subtypes of receptors (alpha-1, alpha-2, beta-1, beta-2, dopamine-1, dopamine-2, histamine-1, histamine-2, mu-1, mu-2) may exist.

Stereospecificity

Stereospecificity is often important in the interaction of a biologically active molecule (neurotransmitter, hormone, drug) with its receptor. Synthesis of drugs usually results in racemic mixtures containing 50% or more of either the dextro (*d*) or levo (*l*) isomer. It is important to recognize that stereoisomers are different chemicals often with distinct biologic properties (Fig. 2-6).[12,16] The inactive isomer can be considered an impurity that does not contribute to the pharmacologic effect of the drug but can contribute to the drug's side effects. For exam-

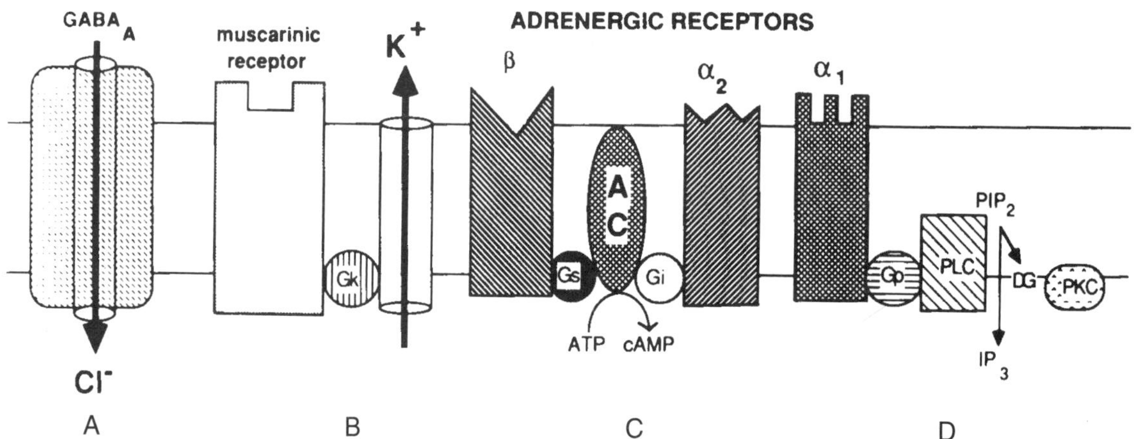

Figure 2-10. Schematic depiction of transmembrane signaling systems by which receptors translate information imparted to them by neurotransmitters, hormones, or agonist drugs. *(A)* Stimulation of the gamma-aminobutyric acid (GABA) receptor results in the flow of chloride ions into the cell through the associated ion channel. *(B)* Stimulation of the muscarinic receptor activates a coupling protein (Gk), leading to the flow of potassium ions (K^+) through a discrete ion channel. *(C)* Adenylate cyclase (AC) activity is enhanced via a stimulating G protein (Gs) following stimulation of a beta-adrenergic receptor. The activity of this enzyme can be attenuated via an inhibitory G protein (Gi) that is coupled to an alpha-2 receptor. *(D)* On stimulation of the alpha-1 receptor, the coupling protein (Gp) activates phospholipase C (PLC) to hydrolyze phosphatidylinositol biphosphate (PIP_2) into inositol triphosphate (IP_3) and diacylglycerol (DG), which then activates protein kinase C (PKC). ATP, adenosine triphosphate; cAMP, cyclic adenosine monophosphate. (From Maze,[15] with permission.)

ple, *d*-ketamine is predominantly hypnotic and analgesic, whereas *l*-ketamine is the likely source of this drug's unwanted side effects. *d*-Propranolol acts as a beta antagonist but both isomers contribute to its local anesthetic effects. Too often, data on drugs are presented as if only the active isomer were involved when, in fact, mixtures of stereoisomers (racemates) were studied.[16]

Number of Receptors

The number of receptors in lipid cell membranes is dynamic, either increasing (up-regulation) or decreasing (down-regulation) in response to specific stimuli. For example, prolonged administration of beta agonists, as in the treatment of asthma, is associated with tachyphylaxis and a concomitant decrease in the number of beta receptors. Conversely, chronic interference with activity of receptors as produced by beta antagonists may result in increased numbers of beta receptors such that an exaggerated response occurs if the blockade is abruptly reversed by discontinuation of drug therapy, as might occur in the preoperative period. Changes in responsiveness of receptors in the absence of an increase or decrease in the number of receptors may occur with aging. Indeed, more isoproterenol is necessary to increase heart rate in the elderly compared with younger patients despite an unchanged number of receptors with aging (see Chapter 27). Variable pharmacologic responses evoked by drugs in individual patients become more predictable when dynamic changes in concentrations of receptors or alterations in responsiveness of receptors are considered.

Relationship Between Receptor Concentration and Drug Effect

During steady state conditions, plasma concentrations of drugs are probably proportional, if not equal, to receptor concentrations of drugs. Certainly, pharmacokinetic factors that influence plasma concentrations of drugs (tissue uptake, renal excretion, hepatic metabolism) will also influence the concentration of drugs at receptors. Pharmacodynamics is usually expressed by relating the plasma concentration of a drug to the pharmacologic response elicited. For example, the demonstration that the Cpss of a nondepolarizing muscle relaxant that produces 50% depression of twitch response (ED_{50}) is similar in young adults and elderly patients suggests that the pharmacodynamics of the neuromuscular junction does not change with aging (see Chapter 7).

REFERENCES

1. Stanski DR, Watkins WD. Drug Disposition in Anesthesia. Orlando, FL, Grune & Stratton 1982.
2. Quasha AL, Eger EI II, Tinker JH. Determination and application of MAC. Anesthesiology 1980;53:315–34.
3. Eger EI II. Uptake of inhaled anesthetics: The alveolar to inspired anesthetic difference. In: Eger EI II, ed. Anesthetic Uptake and Action. Baltimore, Williams & Wilkins 1974;77–96.
4. Eger EI. Effect of inspired anesthetic concentration on the rate of rise of alveolar concentration. Anesthesiology 1963;24:153–7.
5. Epstein RM, Rackow H, Salanitre E, Wolfe GL. Influence of the concentration effect on the uptake of anesthetic mixtures: The second gas effect. Anesthesiology 1964;25:364–71.
6. Stoelting RK, Eger EI II. An additional explanation for the second gas effect. Anesthesiology 1969;30:273–7.
7. Yasuda N, Lockhart SH, Eger EI, et al. Comparison of kinetics of sevoflurane and isoflurane in humans. Anesth Analg 1991;72:316–24.
8. Eger EI II, Saidman LJ. Hazards of nitrous oxide anesthesia in bowel obstruction and pneumothorax. Anesthesiology 1965;26:61–6.
9. Carpenter RL, Eger EI II, Johnson BH, Unadkat JD, Sheiner LB. The extent of metabolism of inhaled anesthetics in humans. Anesthesiology 1986;65:201–5.
10. Merkel G, Eger EI II. A comparative study of halothane and halopropane anesthesia. Including method for determining equipotency. Anesthesiology 1963;24:346–57.
11. Pocok G, Richards CD. Cellular mechanisms in general anaesthesia. Br J Anaesth 1991;66:116–28.
12. Segal IS, Vickery RG, Walton JK, Doze VA, Maze M. Dexmedetomidine diminishes halothane anesthetic requirements in rats through a postsynaptic alpha-2 adrenergic receptor. Anesthesiology 1988;69:818–23.
13. Stanski DR. The contribution of pharmacokinetics and pharmacodynamics to clinical anaesthesia care. Can J Anaesth 1988;35:542–5.
14. Roerig DL, Kotrly KJ, Vucins EJ, Ahlf SB, Dawson CA, Kampine JP. First pass uptake of fentanyl, meperidine, and morphine in the human lung. Anesthesiology 1987;67:466–72.
15. Maze M. Transmembrane signalling and the holy grail of anesthesia. Anesthesiology 1990;72:959–61.
16. Ariens EJ. Stereochemistry, a basis for sophisticated nonsense in pharmacokinetics and clinical pharmacology. Eur J Clin Pharmacol 1984;26:663–8.

3
Autonomic Nervous System

Anesthesiology has been described as the practice of autonomic nervous system medicine.[1] The pharmacologic effects of catecholamines, sympathomimetics, antihypertensives, beta-adrenergic agonists, beta-adrenergic antagonists, anticholinergics, and anticholinesterases involve the actions of these drugs on the central and peripheral autonomic nervous system. An appreciation of the anatomy and physiology of the autonomic nervous system is important for understanding the effects of these drugs and predicting potential adverse drug interactions in the perioperative period. Preoperatively, the most practical bedside test to evaluate autonomic nervous system function is to record the blood pressure and heart rate response when the patient changes from the supine to the upright posture. Autonomic nervous system dysfunction is suggested by orthostatic hypotension (systolic blood pressure decrease more than 30 mmHg) and the absence of an increase in heart rate on assuming the upright posture.[2]

ANATOMY AND PHYSIOLOGY OF THE AUTONOMIC NERVOUS SYSTEM

The central autonomic nervous system includes the hypothalamus (stress responses, blood pressure control, temperature regulation) and vital centers for hemodynamic and ventilatory control in the medulla and pons. The peripheral autonomic nervous system is divided into the sympathetic and parasympathetic nervous system (Fig. 3-1).[1] Preganglionic fibers of the sympathetic nervous system arise from cells in the thoracolumbar portions of the spinal cord, whereas craniosacral cells are the origin of preganglionic fibers of the parasympathetic nervous system. A number of cell bodies form the autonomic ganglion, which acts as the site of synapse between preganglionic and postganglionic fibers. Preganglionic fibers are myelinated (rapid conduction), whereas postganglionic fibers are nonmyelinated. The postganglionic fibers of the sympathetic nervous system are distributed throughout the body, whereas distribution of parasympathetic nervous system postganglionic fibers is more limited. The parasympathetic nervous system has its terminal ganglia near the organs innervated and thus is more discrete in its discharge of impulses, in contrast to the more generalized (mass reflex) response that may accompany sympathetic nervous system stimulation (Fig. 3-1).[1]

Sympathetic Nervous System

Adrenergic receptors are characterized as alpha, beta, and dopamine (Fig. 3-1; see Fig. 2-10).[1] Postganglionic fibers of the sympathetic nervous system that release norepinephrine as the neurotransmitter stimulate alpha- and beta-adrenergic receptors, whereas dopamine is the neurotransmitter released by postganglionic fibers supplying dopamine receptors. Alpha-2 receptors are usually presynaptic (except in the central nervous system and on platelets) and function in a negative feedback loop such that their activation inhibits subsequent release of neurotransmitter (Fig. 3-2).[3] Stimulation of alpha- and beta-adrenergic receptors

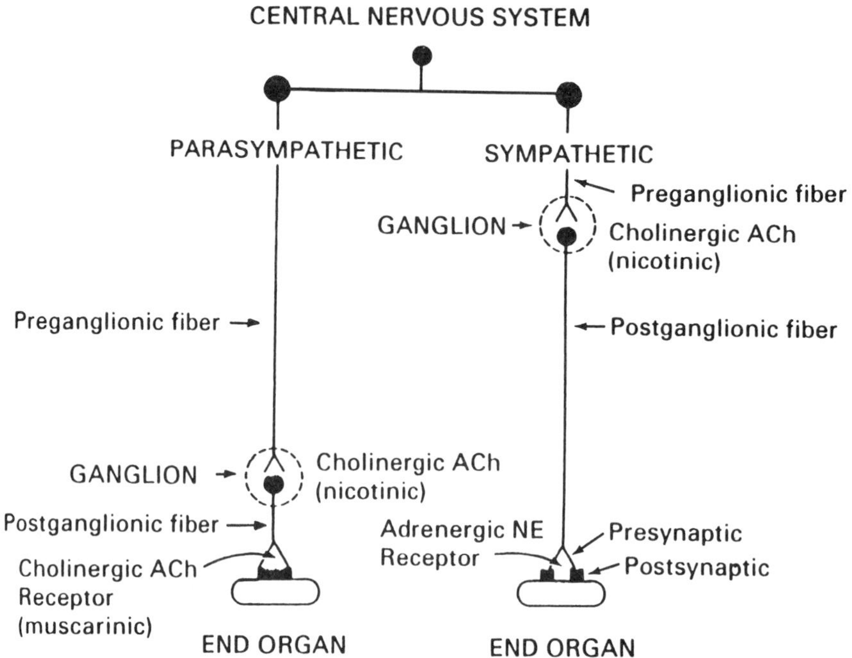

Figure 3-1. Schematic diagram of the peripheral autonomic nervous system. Preganglionic fibers and postganglionic fibers of the parasympathetic nervous system and preganglionic fibers of the sympathetic nervous system release acetylcholine (ACh) as the neurotransmitter. Postganglionic fibers of the sympathetic nervous system release norepinephrine (NE) as the neurotransmitter (exceptions are fibers to sweat glands, which release ACh). (From Lawson and Wallfisch,[1] with permission.)

by endogenous catecholamines or synthetic adrenergic agonists produces predictable pharmacologic responses (Table 3-1). An important factor in the pharmacologic responses elicited by drugs that act on these receptors is the density and sensitivity of alpha and beta receptors to neurotransmitters. Furthermore, there is an inverse relationship between circulating concentrations of neurotransmitters and the density of receptors. For example, increased plasma concentrations of norepinephrine

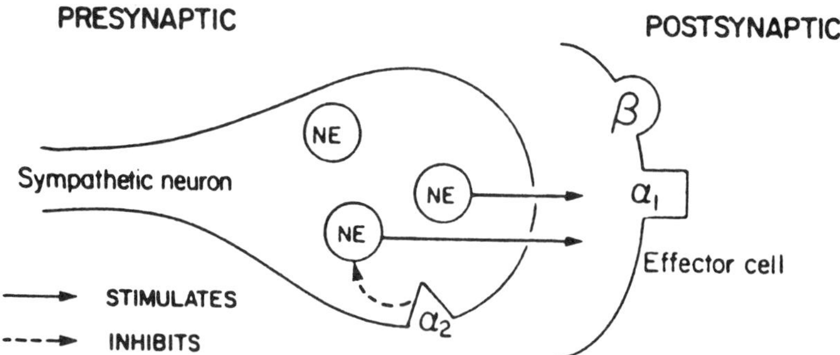

Figure 3-2. Schematic depiction of the postganglionic sympathetic nerve ending. Release of the neurotransmitter norepinephrine (NE) from the nerve ending results in stimulation of postsynaptic receptors that are classified as alpha-1, beta-1, and beta-2. Stimulation of presynaptic alpha-2 receptors results in inhibition of NE release from the nerve ending. (Modified from Ram and Kaplan,[3] with permission.)

result in decreases in the density or sensitivity (down-regulation) of beta receptors in cell membranes (see Chapter 2). The effects of alpha- and beta-adrenergic antagonists are predictable from a knowledge of responses evoked by stimulation of affected receptors (Table 3-1).

Termination of action of norepinephrine on responsive receptors is principally by uptake (reuptake) of this neurotransmitter from the receptors back into the postganglionic nerve ending. Following uptake, a small amount of norepinephrine is deaminated in the cytoplasm by the enzyme monoamine oxidase. Most of the norepinephrine, however, escapes breakdown and can be stored for subsequent release.

Parasympathetic Nervous System

Postganglionic fibers of the parasympathetic nervous system that release acetylcholine as the neurotransmitter are cholinergic, and postsynaptic receptors that respond to acetylcholine are classified as nicotinic and muscarinic (Fig. 3-1; see Fig. 2-10).[1] Stimulation of nicotinic or muscarinic receptors by acetylcholine or synthetic cholinergic agonists produces predictable pharmacologic responses (Table 3-1). The effects of cholinergic antagonists are predictable from a knowledge of responses evoked by stimulation of these receptors. The action of acetylcholine at responsive receptors is terminated by hydrolysis of this neurotransmitter by the enzyme acetylcholinesterase (true cholinesterase).

Table 3-1. Characteristics of the Autonomic Nervous System

			Synthetic Drugs	
Receptor	Effector Organ	Response to Stimulation	Agonist	Antagonist
Beta-1	Heart	Increased heart rate Increased contractility Increased conduction velocity	Dobutamine Dopamine Isoproterenol[a]	Metoprolol Esmolol Propranolol[a] Timolol[a] Labetalol[a,b]
	Fat cells	Lipolysis		
Beta-2	Blood vessels (especially skeletal and coronary arteries)	Dilation	Albuterol Ritodrine	Propranolol[a] Timolol[a] Labetalol[a,b]
	Bronchioles	Dilation		
	Uterus	Relaxation		
	Kidney	Renin secretion		
	Liver	Glycogenolysis Gluconeogenesis		
	Pancreas	Insulin secretion		
Alpha-1	Blood vessels	Constriction	Phenylephrine	Prazosin Phentolamine[b] Labetalol
	Pancreas	Inhibition of insulin secretion		
	Intestine and bladder	Relaxation Constriction of sphincters		
Alpha-2	Postganglionic (presynaptic sympathetic nerve ending)	Inhibition of norepinephrine release	Clonidine Dexmedetomidine	Yohimbine Phentolamine[b]
	Central nervous system (postsynaptic)	Increase in potassium conductance (?)		
	Platelets	Aggregation		
Dopamine-1	Blood vessels	Dilation	Dopamine	Droperidol
Dopamine-2	Postganglionic (presynaptic) sympathetic nerve ending	Inhibition of norepinephrine release	Dopamine	Domperidone

(Continues)

Table 3-1. Characteristics of the Autonomic Nervous System *(Continued)*

Receptor	Effector Organ	Response to Stimulation	Synthetic Drugs	
			Agonist	Antagonist
Muscarinic	Heart	Decreased heart rate Decreased contractility Decreased conduction velocity	Methacholine Carbachol	Atropine Scopolamine Glycopyrrolate
	Bronchioles	Constriction		
	Salivary glands	Stimulation of secretions		
	Intestine	Contraction Relaxation of sphincters Stimulation of secretions		
	Bladder	Contraction Relaxation of sphincter		
Nicotinic	Neuromuscular junction	Skeletal muscle contraction	Succinylcholine	Nondepolarizing muscle relaxants
	Autonomic ganglia	Sympathetic nervous system stimulation		

[a]Produces mixed beta-1 and beta-2 effects.
[b]Produces mixed alpha-1 and alpha-2 effects.

CATECHOLAMINES

Catecholamines are compounds with hydroxyl groups on the 3 and 4 positions of the benzene ring of phenylethylamine (Fig. 3-3). Endogenous catecholamines are dopamine, norepinephrine, and epinephrine. Catecholamines that do not occur endogenously are isoproterenol and dobutamine.

Pharmacologic effects produced by catecholamines reflect the ability of these substances to stimulate adrenergic receptors. Clinically, catecholamines are administered as continuous intravenous infusions to produce desirable pharmacologic effects manifesting predominantly on the cardiovascular system (Table 3-2).

Dopamine

Dopamine, depending on the dose, directly stimulates dopamine, beta-, and alpha-adrenergic recep-

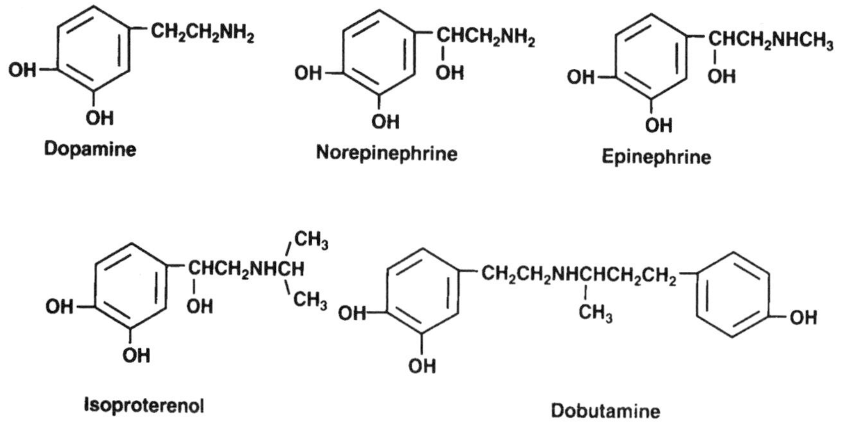

Figure 3-3. Chemical structures of endogenous (dopamine, norepinephrine, epinephrine) and exogenous (isoproterenol, dobutamine) catecholamines.

Table 3-2. Pharmacologic Effects and Therapeutic Doses of Catecholamines

Catecholamines	MAP	HR	CO	SVR	RBF	Preparation (mg in 250 ml)	Intravenous Dose (μg·kg^{-1}·min^{-1})
Dopamine	+	+	+++	+	+++	200 (800 μg·ml^{-1})	2–20
Norepinephrine	+++	–	–	+++	– – –	4 (16 μg·ml^{-1})	0.01–0.1
Epinephrine	+	++	++	++	– –	1 (4 μg·ml^{-1})	0.03–0.15
Isoproterenol	–	+++	+++	– –	–	1 (4 μg·ml^{-1})	0.03–0.15
Dobutamine	+	+	+++	±	++	250 (1000 μg·ml^{-1})	2–20

Abbreviations: MAP, mean arterial pressure; HR, heart rate; CO, cardiac output; SVR, systemic vascular resistance; RBF, renal blood flow; +, mild increase; ++ moderate increase; +++, marked increase; –, mild decrease; – –, moderate decrease; – – – , marked decrease.

tors. This catecholamine is unique among this class of drugs in its ability to stimulate dopamine receptors and redistribute blood flow to the kidneys. These renal effects predominate when the dose of dopamine is less than 3 μg·kg^{-1}·min^{-1} IV. This dose can also inhibit secretion of aldosterone, which, along with dopamine receptor stimulation, results in increased urine output. Beta-adrenergic stimulation characterized by increased myocardial contractility without marked changes in heart rate and blood pressure occurs when the dose of dopamine is 3 to 10 μg·kg^{-1}·min^{-1} IV. Dopamine also exerts part of its inotropic effect by evoking the release of endogenous stores of norepinephrine, which predisposes to cardiac dysrhythmias. Furthermore, this indirect stimulation may be an unreliable mechanism when cardiac catecholamine stores are depleted, as with chronic congestive heart failure. Beta- and alpha-adrenergic agonist effects occur when the dose of dopamine is between 10 and 20 μg·kg^{-1}·min^{-1} IV, whereas alpha-adrenergic effects of dopamine predominate with doses higher than 20 μg·kg^{-1}·min^{-1} IV. Intravenous infusion of dopamine interferes with the ventilatory response to hypoxemia, reflecting the role of dopamine as an inhibitory neurotransmitter at the carotid bodies. High doses of dopamine can inhibit the release of insulin, leading to hyperglycemia.

Dopamine is most often used in clinical situations characterized by decreased cardiac output, decreased blood pressure, increased left ventricular end-diastolic pressure, and oliguria. Rapid metabolism of dopamine mandates its use as a continuous intravenous infusion. Extravasation of dopamine, like norepinehrine, produces intense local vasoconstriction, which may be treated by local infiltration of phentolamine. The drug is prepared in a solution of 5% dextrose in water. More alkaline intravenous solutions may inactivate dopamine.

Norepinephrine

Norepinephrine, as the endogenous neurotransmitter for alpha- and beta-adrenergic receptors, is responsible for maintaining blood pressure by appropriate adjustments in systemic vascular resistance. Vasoconstriction induced by norepinephrine produces increases in systemic vascular resistance reflected by increases in systolic, diastolic, and mean arterial pressure. The beta-1 agonist effects of norepinephrine on the heart are overshadowed by the alpha-1 agonist effects of this catecholamine on the peripheral vasculature. Cardiac output may be decreased despite the increased blood pressure, reflecting the effect of increased ventricular afterload and baroreceptor-mediated reflex bradycardia. The beta-2 agonist effects of norepinephrine are minimal. Clinically, a continuous intravenous infusion of norepinephrine may be used to treat refractory hypotension as may occur in the early period following ligation of the vascular supply to a pheochromocytoma.

Epinephrine

Epinephrine stimulates alpha-1, beta-1, and beta-2 receptors. Low doses of epinephrine stimulate alpha-1 receptors in the skin, mucosa, and hepatorenal vasculature, producing vasoconstriction, whereas beta-2-induced vasodilation predominates in skeletal muscles. The net effect is decreased systemic vascular resistance and a preferential distribution of cardiac output to skeletal muscles. Renal blood flow is greatly decreased during infusion of epinephrine, even with an unchanged blood pressure.

Stimulation of beta-1 receptors increases heart rate and myocardial contractility, resulting in an increased cardiac output. Since the blood pressure is not greatly elevated, compensatory baroreceptor reflexes are not elicited and the cardiac output is increased. Beta-1 stimulation also increases the automaticity of the heart, which manifests as cardiac irritability, most often in the form of ventricular premature contractions.

Of all the catecholamines, epinephrine has the most significant effects on metabolism. For example, beta-adrenergic stimulation from epinephrine increases adipose tissue lipolysis and liver glycogenolysis, whereas alpha-1 stimulation inhibits release of insulin from the pancreas (Table 3-1). Epinephrine release in response to surgical stimulation is a likely explanation for the hyperglycemia that is often observed in the perioperative period.

Epinephrine may be used as a continuous intravenous infusion to treat decreased myocardial contractility. Subcutaneous epinephrine is also used in combination with local anesthetics to decrease systemic absorption and to provide local hemostasis. Epinephrine should be administered promptly intravenously in the treatment of life-threatening allergic reactions and refractory bradycardia as may accompany autonomic nervous system neuropathy (see Chapter 22). Along with oxygen, epinephrine administered intravenously is the most important initial pharmacologic treatment of cardiac arrest (see Chapter 35).

Isoproterenol

Isoproterenol is a synthetic catecholamine with potent stimulant effects on beta-1 and beta-2 receptors and no detectable effects on alpha-1 receptors. Myocardial contractility, heart rate, systolic blood pressure, and cardiac automaticity are increased, whereas systemic vascular resistance and diastolic blood pressure are decreased. The net effect is an increase in cardiac output and occasionally a decrease in mean arterial pressure. Bronchodilation is accompanied by significant cardiovascular effects because isoproterenol does not discriminate between beta-1 and beta-2 receptors (Table 3-1).

Excessive tachycardia and simultaneous diastolic hypotension may decrease coronary blood flow at the time myocardial oxygen requirements are increased by tachycardia. These events, combined with a high incidence of cardiac dysrhythmias and diversion of blood flow to skeletal muscles, detract from the value of isoproterenol, particularly in patients with ischemic heart disease. Clinical uses of isoproterenol include its continuous intravenous infusion to increase heart rate as following heart transplantation or in the presence of complete heart block (chemical pacemaker). Isoproterenol may be selected in patients with valvular heart disease in an attempt to decrease pulmonary vascular resistance.

Dobutamine

Dobutamine is a synthetic catecholamine with structural characteristics of dopamine and isoproterenol. Removal of the side-chain hydroxyl groups from the isoproterenol portion decreases cardiac dysrhythmogenicity but retains the inotropic properties. Dobutamine acts selectively on beta-1 receptors without exerting significant effects on beta-2 or alpha receptors. Unlike dopamine, this catecholamine does not act indirectly by evoking endogenous norepinephrine release, nor does it stimulate dopamine receptors to increase renal blood flow. The most prominent effect during the infusion of dobutamine (2 to 20 $\mu g \cdot kg^{-1} \cdot min^{-1}$ IV) is a dose-dependent increase in cardiac output, often with a decrease in systemic vascular resistance. This ability to increase myocardial contractility with minimal chronotropic or alpha stimulation is unique to dobutamine. Dobutamine may be ineffective for patients who need increased systemic vascular resistance to increase blood pressure. Since dobutamine lacks dopamine stimulating effects, it is reasonable to consider infusing this catecholamine with dopamine to patients who are hypotensive and oliguric. Dobutamine, like dopamine, can be inactivated when prepared in alkaline intravenous solutions, emphasizing the importance of preparing this drug in a 5% dextrose in water solution.

SYMPATHOMIMETICS

Sympathomimetics are synthetic drugs that are used as vasopressors to reverse downward trends in blood pressure that accompany vasodilation produced by spinal or epidural anesthesia. Likewise, hypotension produced by inhaled anesthetics may be treated with a sympathomimetic to ensure maintenance of an adequate perfusion pressure during the time needed to eliminate the excess inhaled drug.

Prolonged administration of sympathomimetics to support blood pressure in the presence of hypovolemia is not recommended. Despite the availability of several sympathomimetics, an understanding of the pharmacology of ephedrine and phenylephrine is probably sufficient for the management of most clinical situations (Table 3-3). Structurally, sympathomimetics resemble catecholamines except that hydroxyl groups are not present on both the 3 and 4 positions of the benzene ring (Fig. 3-4).

Classification

Sympathomimetics are classified according to their selectivity for stimulating alpha- and/or beta-adrenergic receptors (Table 3-3). Knowing the selectivity for either receptor permits selection of a drug to increase blood pressure principally by increased myocardial contractility (ephedrine) or peripheral vasoconstriction (phenylephrine). Alternatively, sympathomimetics may be classified as direct-acting (mimic effects of norepinephrine) or indirect-acting (evoke the release of endogenous norepinephrine) (Table 3-3).

Adverse Effects

Cardiac dysrhythmias that occur in association with administration of a sympathomimetic may reflect drug-induced beta-adrenergic stimulation. Conversely, a disadvantage of using a sympathomimetic that lacks beta-adrenergic effects is unopposed alpha-adrenergic receptor-induced peripheral vasoconstriction. Vasoconstriction results in increased diastolic blood pressure and associated baroreceptor reflex-mediated bradycardia and possible decreases in cardiac output. Antihypertensives that decrease sympathetic nervous system activity may decrease the pressor response elicited by an indirect-acting sympathomimetic, whereas the response to a direct-acting drug may be enhanced as receptors are sensitized (denervation hypersensitivity) by a lack of tonic impulses.

Treatment of patients with tricyclic antidepressants or monoamine oxidase inhibitors that increase the availability of endogenous norepinephrine introduces the potential for adverse drug interactions with sympathomimetics. For example, administration of an indirect-acting drug such as ephedrine could elicit an exaggerated blood pressure response. The risk of such an adverse response seems to be greatest during the first 14 to 21 days of treatment with tricyclic antidepressants or monoamine oxidase inhibitors.[4] If a sympathomimetic is required during this period, a decreased dose of a direct-acting drug such as phenylephrine may be useful. Should hypertension require treatment, a peripheral vasodilator is effective. After the period of acute treatment with antidepressants, there seems to be down-regulation of receptors and a decreased likelihood of exaggerated blood pressure responses following administration of a sympathomimetic. It is now accepted that tricyclic antidepressants or monoamine oxidase inhibitors may be continued throughout the perioperative period without introduction of an unacceptable risk of adverse drug interactions.[5]

Ephedrine

Ephedrine is an indirect-acting sympathomimetic that exerts its blood pressure effects principally by stimulating the release of norepinephrine. Ephedrine also has some direct-acting effects. Clinically, the cardiovascular effects of ephedrine

Table 3-3. Classification and Therapeutic Doses of Sympathomimetics

Sympathomimetic	Alpha-1	Alpha-2	Beta-1	Beta-2	Action	Intravenous Dose for an Adult (mg)
Ephedrine	++	?	++	+	I (some D)	10–25
Phenylephrine	+++	?	±	0	D	0.05–0.2
Metaraminol	+++	?	++	0	I (some D)	1.5–5
Mephentermine	+	?	++	+	I	10–25
Methoxamine	+++	?	0	0	D	5–10

Abbreviations: D, direct; I, indirect; 0, no change; +, mild stimulation; ++, moderate stimulation; +++, marked stimulation.

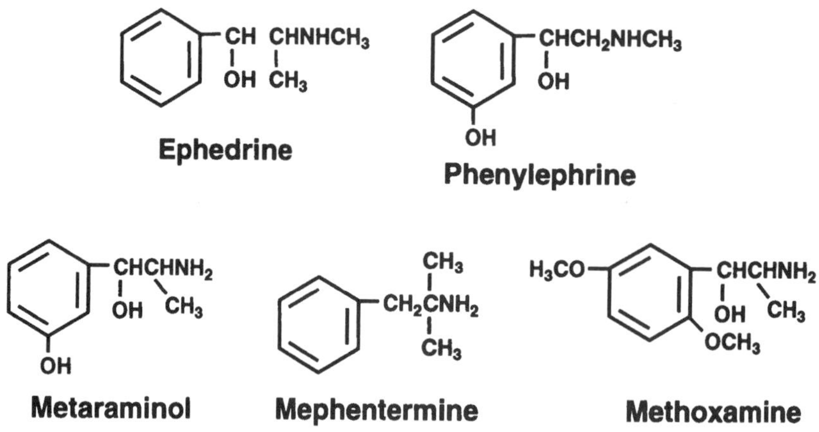

Figure 3-4. Chemical structures of sympathomimetics.

resemble those of epinephrine, but its blood pressure elevating response is less intense and lasts about 10 times longer. Intravenous administration of ephedrine results in increases in systolic and diastolic blood pressure, heart rate, and cardiac output. Beta-adrenergic stimulation may evoke cardiac dysrhythmias, especially in the presence of drugs that sensitize the heart to the effects of catecholamines. Systemic vascular resistance may be altered minimally because vasoconstriction (alpha-adrenergic stimulation) in some vascular beds is offset by vasodilation (beta-2 stimulation) in other areas. The principal mechanism for cardiovascular effects produced by ephedrine is increased myocardial contractility owing to stimulation of beta-1 receptors. In the presence of drug-induced beta-adrenergic blockade, the cardiovascular effects of ephedrine may resemble responses more typical of alpha-adrenergic receptor stimulation. Placental blood flow is preserved by ephedrine, making this drug useful for treating anesthetic-induced hypotension in parturients (see Fig. 25-3).

A second dose of ephedrine produces a less intense blood pressure response than the first dose (tachyphylaxis). Presumably, tachyphylaxis represents a persistent blockade of adrenergic receptors. For example, ephedrine-induced activation of adrenergic receptors persists even after blood pressure has returned to near predrug levels by virtue of compensatory cardiovascular changes. When ephedrine is administered at this time, the receptors still occupied by ephedrine limit available sites and the blood pressure response is less pronounced. Alternatively, tachyphylaxis may be due to depletion of norepinephrine stores.

Phenylephrine

Phenylephrine is a direct-acting sympathomimetic that increases systemic vascular resistance and blood pressure by stimulation of alpha-adrenergic receptors. It is devoid of significant beta-adrenergic receptor stimulation. Clinically, phenylephrine mimics the effects of norepinephrine but is less potent and longer lasting. The dose of phenylephrine necessary to stimulate alpha-1 receptors is lower than that needed to stimulate alpha-2 receptors. As a result, venoconstriction is greater than arterial constriction following administration of phenylephrine. Reflex bradycardia and an associated transient decrease in cardiac output is a possible response when blood pressure is increased by phenylephrine (Fig. 3-5).[6]

ANTIHYPERTENSIVES

Antihypertensives are useful in the treatment of essential hypertension to decrease blood pressure toward normal levels by selectively impairing sympathetic nervous system function at the heart and/or peripheral vasculature. Attenuation of sympathetic nervous system activity is reflected by orthostatic hypotension. During anesthesia, exaggerated decreases in blood pressure (as associated with hemorrhage, positive airway pressure, or sudden changes in body position) may reflect an impaired degree of

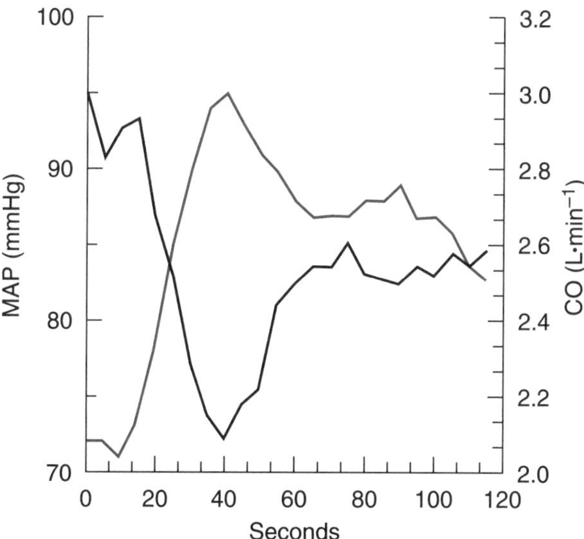

Figure 3-5. Hemodynamic responses to the rapid intravenous injection of phenylephrine. MAP, mean arterial pressure (red line); CO, cardiac output (black line). (Modified from Schwinn and Reves,[6] with permission.)

compensatory peripheral vascular vasoconstriction as a result of inhibitory effects of antihypertensives on sympathetic nervous system activity. The response to sympathomimetics may be modified by prior treatment with antihypertensives (see the section *Sympathomimetics*). Selective impairment of sympathetic nervous system activity by antihypertensives results in a predominance of parasympathetic nervous system tone, manifesting as bradycardia. Antihypertensives that decrease central nervous system sympathetic activity are associated with sedation and decreased anesthetic requirements (MAC).[7] Despite interference of antihypertensives with normal sympathetic nervous system activity, these drugs should be continued during the perioperative period so as to maintain optimal control of the blood pressure.

Clonidine

Clonidine is a centrally acting antihypertensive that stimulates alpha-2 receptors in the depressor area of the vasomotor center, leading to a decreased outflow of sympathetic nervous system impulses to the periphery. The net effect of this decreased sympathetic nervous system activity is a decrease in cardiac output, systemic vascular resistance, and blood pressure. Decreases in MAC of injected and inhaled drugs are produced by small doses of clonidine administered preoperatively, presumably reflecting the sedative and/or analgesic effects of this drug.[7] Sympathetic nervous system responses evoked by direct laryngoscopy and surgical stimulation are attenuated by prior treatment with clonidine. Bradycardia and dry mouth may accompany treatment with clonidine. The duration of action of a single dose of clonidine is 6 to 24 hours.

The most important adverse effect of chronic treatment with clonidine is the possibility of rebound hypertension when the drug is abruptly discontinued. Indeed, discontinuation of treatment

Antihypertensives Used in the Ambulatory Treatment of Essential Hypertension

- Central sympatholytics
  - Clonidine
  - Guanabenz
  - Alpha-methyldopa
- Peripheral sympatholytics
  - Guanethidine
  - Guanadrel
- Peripheral vasodilators
  - Minoxidil
  - Prazosin
  - Hydralazine
- Angiotensin converting enzyme inhibitors
  - Captopril
  - Enalapril
- Calcium entry blockers
  - Verapamil
  - Nifedipine
  - Diltiazem
  - Nicardipine
- Beta-adrenergic antagonists
  - Propranolol
  - Metoprolol
  - Nadolol
  - Atenolol
  - Timolol
- Alpha- and beta-adrenergic antagonists
  - Labetalol

with clonidine has been associated with the development of adverse increases in blood pressure before the induction of anesthesia, as well as in the early postoperative period.[8] The speculated mechanism for this rebound hypertension is an abrupt increase in systemic vascular resistance owing to the release of catecholamines. Rebound hypertension can usually be controlled or prevented by maintaining clonidine therapy (transdermal clonidine an alternative to oral administration) or substitution of alternative antihypertensive drugs. Antihypertensives that act independently of central and peripheral nervous system mechanisms (peripheral vasodilators, angiotensin-converting enzyme inhibitors) do not seem to be associated with rebound hypertension following sudden discontinuation of chronic therapy.[8]

Clonidine has been shown to be effective in suppressing the signs and symptoms of withdrawal from opioids. It is speculated that clonidine replaces opioid-mediated inhibition with alpha-2-mediated inhibition of central sympathetic nervous system activity. Clonidine lowers plasma catecholamine concentrations in normal patients but not in those with pheochromocytoma. Injection of clonidine into the epidural or subarachnoid space produces analgesia and, unlike opioids, does not produce depression of ventilation, pruritus, or nausea and vomiting. Bradycardia and sedation, however, may accompany this route of administration of clonidine.

Minoxidil

Minoxidil decreases blood pressure by direct relaxation of arteriolar smooth muscle. As with any peripheral vasodilator, minoxidil is associated with reflex tachycardia, sodium retention, and water retention. For these reasons, minoxidil is often administered in combination with a beta-adrenergic antagonist and diuretic. Pulmonary hypertension associated with minoxidil is more likely due to fluid retention than to a unique effect of this drug on pulmonary vasculature. Pericardial effusion and cardiac tamponade occur in a small number of patients treated with minoxidil, especially if renal dysfunction is present.[8] Minoxidil stimulates hair growth and a topical preparation may be used to treat baldness.

Prazosin

Prazosin lowers blood pressure by decreasing systemic vascular resistance due to selective postsynaptic alpha-1 receptor blockade. Absence of drug-induced presynaptic alpha-2 blockade leaves the normal inhibition of norepinephrine release intact. In addition to treating essential hypertension, prazosin may be of value for decreasing afterload in patients with congestive heart failure. It is also useful in the preoperative preparation of patients with pheochromocytoma. Fluid retention and orthostatic hypotension are prominent side effects of prazosin therapy.

Captopril

Captopril is an orally effective antihypertensive that acts by competitive inhibition of angiotensin I converting enzyme (ACE inhibitor). Patient compliance is high with captopril therapy, reflecting minimal side effects such as fatigue, lethargy, and mental depression compared with drugs acting on the central nervous system. Captopril may increase serum potassium levels, especially if it is administered with a potassium-sparing diuretic or if the patient's renal function is impaired. Appearance of cough and, in patients with chronic obstructive pulmonary disease, an exacerbation of dyspnea and wheezing may accompany the administration of captopril.

Verapamil

Verapamil, along with other calcium entry blockers, may be effective in the treatment of essential hypertension. Peripheral vasodilation produced by these drugs may be beneficial in patients with congestive heart failure related to chronic essential hypertension. Treatment with calcium entry blockers can be continued until the time of surgery without risk of significant drug interactions, especially with respect to conduction of cardiac impulses. Calcium entry blockers may potentiate the effects of muscle relaxants.

Labetalol

Labetalol lowers blood pressure by acting as a selective alpha-1 antagonist and nonselective beta-adrenergic receptor antagonist. Bronchospasm is less likely to occur than with other nonselective beta-antagonists, but orthostatic hypotension may be prominent.

BETA-ADRENERGIC AGONISTS

Catecholamines are examples of beta-1 agonists used to increase heart rate and myocardial contractility (Table 3-1) (see the section *Catecholamines*). Beta-2 agonists produce relaxation of bronchial, uterine, and vascular smooth muscle, reflecting selective stimulation of beta-2 receptors (Table 3-1). Beta-2 agonists are used to treat bronchial asthma and to stop premature labor.

Drugs selective for beta-2 receptors are less likely than beta-1 agonists to produce adverse cardiac effects such as tachycardia or cardiac dysrhythmias. Nevertheless, reflex tachycardia, presumably due to beta-2-mediated vasodilation and subsequent hypotension, has been observed after administration of these drugs.[9] Another serious hazard of continuous intravenous infusion of a beta-2 agonist, as used to stop premature labor, is hypokalemia.[10] Hypokalemia most likely reflects sustained beta-2 stimulation of the sodium pump with transfer of potassium intracellularly. Tachyphylaxis to the effects of beta-2 agonists is attributed to the decreased number or decreased sensitivity of beta receptors (down-regulation) that occurs with chronic stimulation of these receptors.

Albuterol is the selective beta-2 agonist that is becoming the preferred drug for the treatment of bronchospasm in anesthetized patients. Actuation of the metered-dose inhaler during a mechanically produced inspiration increases the amount of albuterol that passes beyond the distal end of the tracheal tube. Typically, the drug is delivered by two to three deep inhalations (each metered-aerosol actuation delivering about 90 μg) 1 to 5 minutes apart. The dose may be repeated every 4 to 6 hours, and the daily dose should not exceed 16 to 20 metered-aerosol actuations.

BETA-ADRENERGIC ANTAGONISTS

Beta antagonists may produce selective beta-1 blockade (decreased heart rate and myocardial contractility) or mixed responses that also reflect drug effects at beta-2 receptors (bronchial and vascular smooth muscle constriction) (Table 3-1). Beta antagonists may also possess membrane stabilizing activity and intrinsic sympathomimetic activity.

Beta antagonists probably decrease blood pressure by decreasing cardiac output. Heart rate slowing produced by beta antagonists lasts longer than negative inotropic effects, suggesting a possible subdivision of beta-1 receptors. Beta blockade attenuates baroreceptor-mediated increases in heart rate associated with vasodilator therapy. An important advantage of beta antagonists as used to treat essential hypertension is the absence of orthostatic hypotension. Fatigue and lethargy, however, are commonly associated with beta antagonist therapy. These drugs, however, do not alter anesthetic requirements (MAC).

In addition to treatment of essential hypertension, beta antagonists are effective in decreasing myocardial oxygen requirements by virtue of decreases in heart rate and myocardial contractility. These beta-1 antagonist effects more than offset any adverse effect of an increase in coronary vascular resistance caused by concomitant beta-2 receptor blockade. Evidence of decreased myocardial oxygen requirements in patients treated with beta antagonists is relief of angina pectoris. Indeed, beta antagonists may be effective in decreasing postmyocardial infarction mortality, as well as the incidence of myocardial reinfarction.

Adverse Effects

Hazards of beta blockade include excessive myocardial depression and bronchoconstriction. Additive myocardial depression with volatile anesthetics can occur, but this is not a clinically significant problem. When bronchoconstriction is a possible response, as in patients with bronchial asthma or chronic obstructive pulmonary disease, it may be useful to select beta antagonists with selective beta-1 blocking effects. Likewise, cardioselective drugs would be logical selections in patients with peripheral vascular disease so as to minimize the occurrence of vasoconstriction that accompanies beta-2 blockade (Table 3-1). Beta antagonists with intrinsic sympathomimetic activity may be logical selections for treatment of patients with depressed left ventricular function or bradycardia. Indeed, beta-adrenergic blockade may produce atrioventricular heart block.

Atropine is the initial drug recommended for treatment of signs of excessive drug-induced beta blockade manifesting as bradycardia or atrioventricular heart block. If signs of excessive beta blockade persist, a specific pharmacologic treatment is administration of a beta agonist such as isoproterenol or dobutamine. However, large doses of these drugs

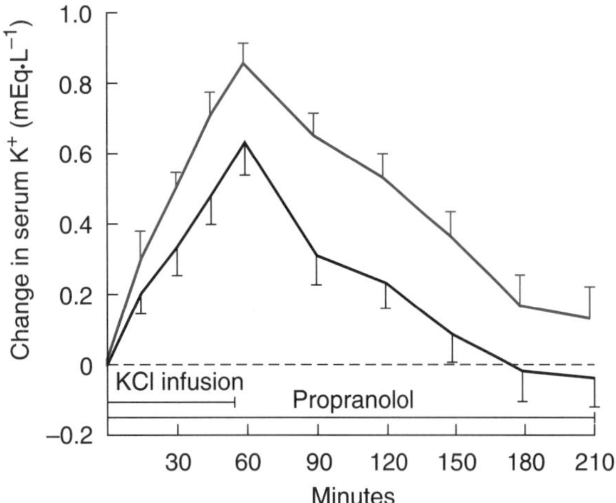

Figure 3-6. Increases in serum potassium (K^+) concentrations in response to infusion of potassium chloride (KCl) are greater in the presence of propranolol (red line) than in its absence (black line). Mean ± SE. (From Rosa et al.,[11] with permission.)

may be required to antagonize excessive beta blockade. Alternatively, calcium chloride administered intravenously antagonizes excessive beta blockade independently of any known effect mediated via beta-adrenergic receptors. As such, conventional doses of calcium chloride (5 to 10 mg·kg–1 IV) are likely to be effective.

It must be recognized that abrupt discontinuation of treatment with beta antagonists can be associated with excessive sympathetic nervous system activity manifesting as hypertension and myocardial ischemia. Presumably, this enhanced activity reflects an increase in the number or sensitivity of beta-adrenergic receptors (up-regulation) that occurs during chronic therapy. Therefore, treatment with these drugs should be maintained throughout the perioperative period. Continuous intravenous infusion of esmolol would also be effective in maintaining beta-adrenergic blockade in patients who cannot receive oral medications during the perioperative period.

Beta antagonists may accentuate increases in plasma concentrations of potassium associated with infusion of potassium chloride, presumably by interfering with the mechanism necessary for movement of this ion across cell membranes (Fig. 3-6).[11] Warning signs and symptoms of hypoglycemia are blunted by beta-adrenergic blockade, suggesting caution in the use of these drugs in patients with insulin-dependent diabetes mellitus. Cardioselective drugs would be logical selections when diabetes mellitus is present, since suppression of insulin secretion is produced by beta-2 blockade (Table 3-1).

ANTICHOLINERGICS

Anticholinergics (atropine, scopolamine, glycopyrrolate) prevent the muscarinic effects of acetylcholine by competing for the same receptors as are normally occupied by the neurotransmitter. Atropine and scopolamine are tertiary amines and can cross lipid barriers such as the blood-brain barrier and placenta. By contrast, glycopyrrolate acts principally on peripheral cholinergic receptors because its quaternary ammonium structure prevents it from crossing lipid barriers in significant amounts. The magnitude of anticholinergic effects may differ between drugs despite similar doses (see Table 9-6). The sensitivity of peripheral cholinergic receptors differs such that low doses of an anticholinergic may be sufficient to inhibit salivation but large doses are necessary for gastrointestinal effects.

ANTICHOLINESTERASES

Anticholinesterases are represented by quaternary ammonium (neostigmine, pyridostigmine, and edrophonium) and tertiary amine (physostigmine) drugs. These drugs inhibit the enzyme acetylcholinesterase (true cholinesterase), which is normally responsible for the rapid hydrolysis of acetylcholine after its release from cholinergic nerve endings. Therefore, in the presence of an anticholinesterase, acetylcholine accumulates at nicotinic and muscarinic receptor sites. Quaternary ammonium drugs cannot easily cross the blood-brain barrier such that accumulation of acetylcholine is predominantly at peripheral sites such as the nicotinic neuromuscular junction. Indeed, this is the principal mechanism for drug-assisted antagonism of nondepolarizing muscle relaxants (see Chapter 7). Conversely, physostigmine, with its tertiary amine structure, can cross the blood-brain barrier, making this an effective drug for treatment of the central anticholinergic syndrome that manifests as emergence delirium in the postanesthesia care unit (see Chapter 31).

REFERENCES

1. Lawson NW, Wallfisch HK. Cardiovascular pharmacology: A new look at the pressors. In: Stoelting RK, Barash PG, Gallagher TJ, eds. Advances in Anesthesia. Chicago, Year Book Medical Publishers 1986; 3:195–270.
2. Ebert TJ. Preoperative evaluation of the autonomic nervous system. In: Stoelting RK, Barash PG, Gallagher TJ, eds. Advances in Anesthesia. St. Louis, Mosby-Year Book 1993;10:49–68.
3. Ram CVS, Kaplan NM. Alpha- and beta-receptor blocking drugs in the treatment of hypertension. In: Harvey WP, et al., eds. Current Problems in Cardiology. Chicago, Year Book Medical Publishers 1979.
4. Braverman B, McCarthy RJ, Ivankovich AD. Vasopressor challenges during chronic MAOI or TCA treatment in anesthetized drugs. Life Sci 1987;40:2587–95.
5. Wells DG, Bjorksten AR. Monoamine oxidase inhibitors revisited. Can J Anaesth 1989;36:64–74.
6. Schwinn DA, Reves JG. Time course and hemodynamic effects of alpha-1 adrenergic bolus administration in anesthetized patients with myocardial disease. Anesth Analg 1989;68:571–8.
7. Engelman E, Lipszyc M, Gilbert E, et al. Effects of clonidine on anesthetic drug requirements and hemodynamic response during aortic surgery. Anesthesiology 1989;71:178–87.
8. Husserl FE, Messerli FH. Adverse effects of antihypertensive drugs. Drugs 1981;22:188–210.
9. Wheeler AS, Patel KF, Spain J. Pulmonary edema during beta-2 tocolytic therapy. Anesth Analg 1981;60:695–6.
10. Moravec MA, Hurlbert BJ. Hypokalemia associated with terbutaline administration in obstetrical patients. Anesth Analg 1980;59:917–20.
11. Rosa RM, Silva P, Young JB, et al. Adrenergic modulation of extrarenal potassium disposal. N Engl J Med 1980;302:431–4.

4

Effects of Inhaled Anesthetics on Ventilation and Circulation

Currently used inhaled anesthetics are represented by one gas (nitrous oxide) and four volatile liquids (halothane, enflurane, isoflurane, desflurane). These anesthetics have important and often differing pharmacologic effects on ventilation and circulation. Data from healthy volunteers breathing equally potent concentrations of these drugs have provided the foundation for establishing comparative differences of inhaled anesthetics on ventilation and circulation in the absence of extraneous influences.[1–4] It must always be appreciated, however, that surgical patients with other variables (co-existing diseases, drug therapy that influences the function of the autonomic nervous system, preoperative medication, surgical stimulation, altered intravascular fluid volume, extremes of age) can respond differently from healthy volunteers.

VENTILATION

Inhaled anesthetics produce dose-dependent and drug-specific depressant effects on ventilation. Anesthetic-induced depression of ventilation most likely reflects direct depressant effects of these drugs on the medullary ventilatory center and perhaps peripheral effects on intercostal muscle function. The incidence of postoperative pulmonary complications is not influenced by the inhaled anesthetics administered to maintain anesthesia.

Pattern of Breathing

Inhaled anesthetics, except for isoflurane, produce dose-dependent increases in the rate of breathing (Fig. 4-1).[4,5] Isoflurane increases the rate of breathing similarly to other inhaled anesthetics up to about 1 MAC, and above this dose the breathing frequency does not increase further. Nitrous oxide increases the rate of breathing more than other inhaled anesthetics at concentrations higher than 1 MAC. The effect of inhaled anesthetics on breathing frequency most likely reflects central nervous system stimulation and not, with the possible exception of nitrous oxide, stimulation of pulmonary stretch receptors.

Tidal volume is decreased in association with anesthetic-induced increases in the rate of breathing. The increase in rate of breathing is insufficient to offset the decrease in tidal volume, leading to a decrease in minute ventilation and an increase in $PaCO_2$ (Fig. 4-2)[1,4] (see the section *Arterial Partial Pressure of Carbon Dioxide*). Overall, the pattern of breathing during general anesthesia is characterized as rapid, shallow, regular, and rhythmic, in contrast to the awake pattern of intermittent deep breaths separated by varying intervals.

Arterial Partial Pressure of Carbon Dioxide

The resting $PaCO_2$ is the most frequently used index of the dose-dependent depression of ventilation produced by inhaled anesthetics. In healthy volunteers breathing equally potent concentrations of volatile anesthetics, the $PaCO_2$ is increased more by enflurane and desflurane and less by isoflurane and halothane (Fig. 4-2).[1,4] The presence of chronic obstructive pulmonary disease may accentuate the

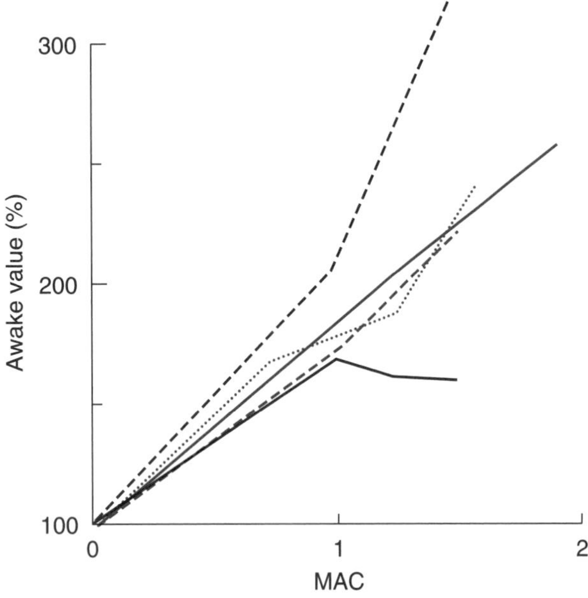

Figure 4-1. Inhaled anesthetics produce similar increases in the rate of breathing (percentage of awake value) up to doses of about 1 MAC. Increasing the dose above 1 MAC does not further increase the rate of breathing during inhalation of isoflurane. Solid red line, halothane; solid black line, isoflurane; dashed red line, enflurane; dashed black line, nitrous oxide; dotted red line, desflurane. (Data from Lockhart et al.[4] and Eger.[5])

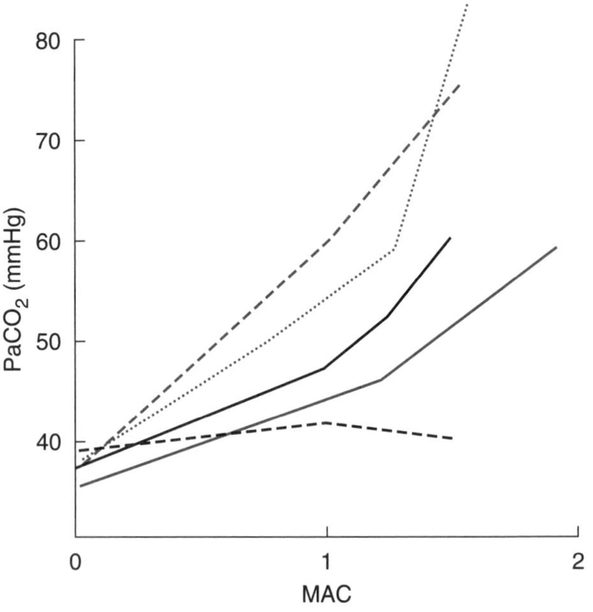

Figure 4-2. Increasing MAC levels of volatile anesthetics (halothane, [solid red line], isoflurane [solid black line], enflurane [dashed red line], desflurane [dotted red line]) produce dose-dependent increases in the $PaCO_2$ when administered to healthy volunteers. Nitrous oxide (dashed black line) was given in a hyperbaric chamber and did not increase the $PaCO_2$. (Data from Eger[1] and Lockhart et al.[4])

magnitude of increase in $PaCO_2$ produced by volatile anesthetics. Nitrous oxide administered to volunteers in a hyperbaric chamber does not alter $PaCO_2$ from awake levels. Indeed, substitution of nitrous oxide for an equivalent portion of the volatile anesthetic results in less increase of the $PaCO_2$ than that produced by the volatile anesthetic alone. Likewise, adding nitrous oxide without changing the inhaled concentration of volatile anesthetic does not further increase the $PaCO_2$, despite the greater depth of anesthesia in the presence of both inhaled drugs. The beneficial effect of nitrous oxide on limiting the increase in $PaCO_2$ is seen with all volatile anesthetics, but the greatest impact is present when nitrous oxide is used to replace an equivalent amount of enflurane or desflurane.

In addition to nitrous oxide, surgical stimulation and duration of administration may influence the magnitude of increase in $PaCO_2$ associated with the inhalation of volatile anesthetics. For example, surgical stimulation increases the tidal volume and breathing rate such that minute ventilation increases about 40%.[1] However, the $PaCO_2$ decreases only about 5 mmHg (10%) in response to surgical stimulation.[1] This discrepancy is presumed to reflect increased production of carbon dioxide by activation of the sympathetic nervous system in response to surgical stimulation. This increased production of carbon dioxide prevents the increase in ventilation from decreasing the $PaCO_2$ by the same magnitude. In addition, the magnitude of $PaCO_2$ increase produced by the same dose of volatile anesthetic is less after prolonged (more than 5 hours) than after brief (less than 1.5 hours) administration (Table 4-1).[4,6] The reason for this apparent lessening of depression of ventilation with time is not known.

Assisted ventilation of the lungs is not greatly effective in decreasing the $PaCO_2$ since the apneic threshold (the maximum $PaCO_2$ that does not initiate spontaneous ventilation) is only about 5 mmHg below the resting $PaCO_2$, regardless of the level of the resting $PaCO_2$. For example, patients inhaling a

Table 4-1. Recovery from Drug-Induced Ventilatory Depression with Time

Enflurane Concentration (MAC)	$PaCO_2$	
	1 Hour of Administration	5 Hours of Administration
1	61 mmHg	46 mmHg
2	Apnea	67 mmHg

(Data from Calverley et al.[6])

volatile anesthetic at a dose sufficient to increase the $PaCO_2$ to 50 mmHg would likely become apneic when assisted ventilation of the lungs decreased the $PaCO_2$ to about 45 mmHg. For this reason, assisted ventilation of the lungs is not a highly effective method to decrease the $PaCO_2$ during general anesthesia. Controlled ventilation of the lungs is the most predictable method for preventing increases in the $PaCO_2$ during inhalation of volatile anesthetics.

Ventilatory Response to Carbon Dioxide

Plotting the volume of ventilation at increasing levels of $PaCO_2$ (carbon dioxide response curve) is a sensitive method for quantitating the effects of drugs on ventilation. In awake humans, inhalation of carbon dioxide increases minute ventilation 1 to 3 $L \cdot min^{-1}$ for every 1-mmHg increase in $PaCO_2$. Inhaled anesthetics, including nitrous oxide, produce dose-dependent depression of the slope of the carbon dioxide response curve (Fig. 4-3).[1,4] In addition, the position of the carbon dioxide response curve is shifted to the right compared with the awake curve. A decreased slope reflects decreased sensitivity to the ventilatory stimulant effects of carbon dioxide, whereas rightward displacement depicts an attenuated responsiveness to carbon dioxide.

The depression of the ventilatory response to carbon dioxide implies that the drive to overcome resistance to breathing (upper airway obstruction, kinked endotracheal tube, airway secretions) could be decreased in the presence of these drugs. However, the slope and position of the carbon dioxide response curve during inhalation of volatile anesthetics returns toward normal (like the $PaCO_2$) after prolonged (more than 5 hours) administration of these drugs.

Ventilatory Response to Arterial Hypoxemia

Decreases in the PaO_2 to below 60 mmHg normally produce increases in minute ventilation. This response in humans is mediated by peripheral chemoreceptors known as the carotid bodies. Subanesthetic concentrations (0.1 MAC) of inhaled anesthetics greatly attenuate, and anesthetic concentrations (1 MAC) abolish, the ventilatory response to arterial hypoxemia (Table 4-2).[7] Conversely, subanesthetic concentrations of inhaled anesthetics do

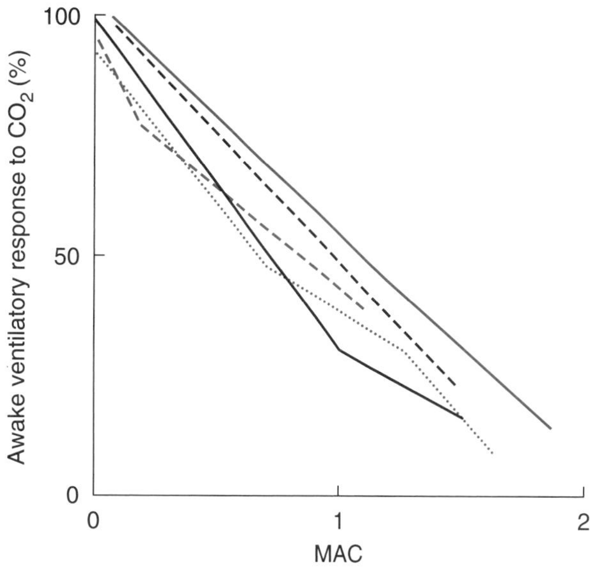

Figure 4-3. All inhaled anesthetics produce similar dose-dependent depression of the ventilatory response to carbon dioxide. Solid red line, halothane; solid black line, isoflurane; dashed red line, enflurane; dashed black line, nitrous oxide; dotted red line, desflurane. (Data from Eger[1] and Lockhart et al.[4])

not depress the ventilatory response to carbon dioxide to the same degree (Table 4-2).[7] Inhaled anesthetics also attenuate the usual synergistic effect of arterial hypoxemia and hypercapnia on stimulation of ventilation. The depression of hypoxic responsiveness by subanesthetic concentrations of inhaled drugs suggests that patients could manifest a diminished ventilatory response to arterial hypoxemia in the postanesthesia care unit (see Chapter 31).

Bronchodilation

Halothane and isoflurane administered at 1 MAC produce similar attenuation of antigen-induced bronchospasm in dogs (Fig. 4-4).[8] Despite these observations, there is no evidence that bronchodilating effects of volatile anesthetics are an effective method for treating status asthmaticus that is unresponsive to conventional bronchodilators. The relaxant effect of volatile anesthetics on bronchial smooth muscle most likely reflects anesthetic-induced decreases in afferent (vagal) nerve traffic from the central nervous system. For example, the effects of halothane and a beta-2 agonist, albuterol, are additive, emphasizing that the anesthetic acts principally by decreasing vagal tone.

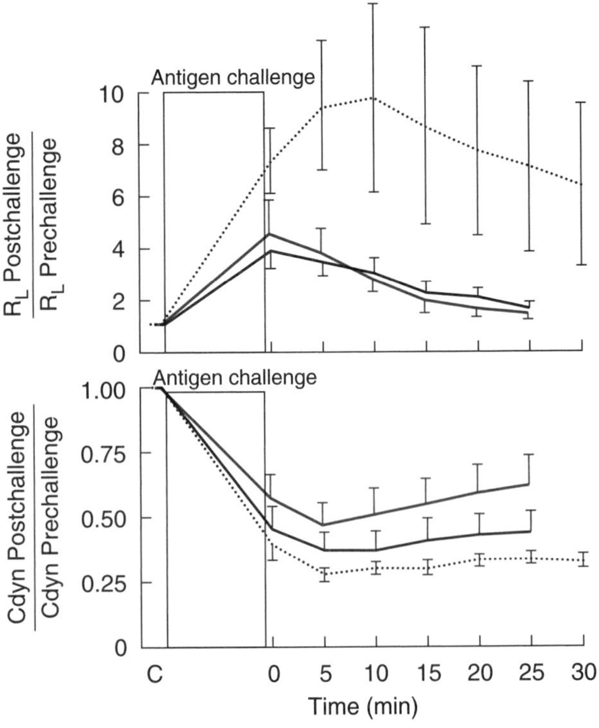

Figure 4-4. Halothane (solid red lines) and isoflurane (solid black lines) were equally effective in attenuating the antigen-induced increases in airway resistance (R_L) as compared with thiopental (dotted black lines). Conversely, halothane was somewhat more effective than isoflurane in minimizing concomitant decreases in pulmonary compliance (Cdyn). (From Hirshman et al.,[8] with permission.)

Airway Irritability

Isoflurane and desflurane are modest airway irritants, as reflected by occasional coughing, breath-holding, and production of secretions when administered for inhalation induction of anesthesia.[2] Although the low blood solubility of desflurane is a useful characteristic for rapid establishment of an anesthetizing concentration, its airway irritant effects may limit the rate at which it can be delivered. The addition of nitrous oxide and/or an opioid does not seem to greatly improve the acceptability of desflurane for inhalation induction. As a result of its airway irritant effects, desflurane is unlikely to replace halothane as the drug of choice for inhalation induction of anesthesia.

Table 4-2. Ventilatory Responses to Arterial Hypoxemia or Hypercapnia During Administration of Halothane to Humans

	Awake Response (%)	
Halothane Concentration (MAC)	Arterial Hypoxemia	Hypercapnia
0.1	31	100
1.1	0	36
2.0	0	17

(Data from Knill and Gelb.[7])

Hypoxic Pulmonary Vasoconstriction

Hypoxic pulmonary vasoconstriction is the reflex constriction of pulmonary arterioles in areas of atelectasis in attempts to decrease or prevent perfusion of unventilated alveoli. This reflex vasoconstriction is protective and its inhibition by inhaled anesthetics could adversely affect the PaO_2. Inhaled anesthetics directly inhibit regional hypoxic pulmonary vasoconstriction when studied in isolated lung models. Nevertheless, halothane and isoflurane do not further impair arterial oxygenation in anesthetized patients during one-lung ventilation, presumably reflecting the effects of compensatory mechanisms that would not be present in study preparations (see Fig. 19-5). In view of available data, it would seem premature to select one inhaled anesthetic over another on the basis of their presumed effects on hypoxic pulmonary vasoconstriction.

Respiratory Muscle Function

Optimal respiratory muscle function occurs when descent of the diaphragm is coupled with expansion of the rib cage produced by contraction of the intercostal muscles. Halothane produces preferential suppression of intercostal muscle function with relative sparing of the diaphragm.[9] Depression of intercostal muscle function interferes with rib cage expansion in response to chemical stimuli such as arterial hypoxemia or hypercapnia. Furthermore, depression of intercostal muscle function means that stabilization of the rib cage is decreased during spontaneous ventilation such that descent of the diaphragm tends to cause the chest to collapse inward, contributing to decreases in lung volumes, particularly the functional residual capacity. It is concluded that, in addition to depression of the medullary ventilatory center, halothane produces depression of ventilation by interfering with normal intercostal muscle function.[9] The effects of other inhaled anesthetics on intercostal muscle function have not been reported.

CIRCULATION

Inhaled anesthetics administered to healthy volunteers produce dose-dependent and drug-specific effects on the circulation (Fig. 4-5).[2,3] These data obtained during controlled ventilation of the lungs to maintain normocarbia permit isolation of circulatory changes due solely to the inhaled anesthetic. Surgical patients characterized by other variables that influence circulatory responses can respond differently from healthy volunteers (see the section *Other Variables that Influence Circulatory Variables*). As a generalization, the cardiovascular effects of isoflurane and desflurane may be considered to be similar.

Arterial Blood Pressure

Dose-dependent decreases of arterial blood pressure are produced by volatile anesthetics whereas nitrous oxide alone usually does not alter the blood pressure (Fig. 4-5).[2,3] Mixed venous oxyhemoglobin saturation is unchanged during administration of desflurane, indicating that adequate tissue perfusion is maintained despite decreases in perfusion pressure. Decreases in myocardial contractility and cardiac output are primarily responsible for decreases in blood pressure produced by inhalation of halothane and enflurane. Conversely, isoflurane- and desflurane-induced decreases in blood pressure are due principally to peripheral vasodilation and an associated decrease in systemic vascular resistance. Surgical stimulation and/or substitution of nitrous oxide for an equivalent portion of the volatile anesthetic results in less blood pressure decrease at the same anesthetic dose (Fig. 4-6).[1,2]

Heart Rate

Heart rate is unchanged by halothane and only minimally increased by nitrous oxide (Fig. 4-5).[2,3] Desflurane administered at less than 1 MAC does not change the heart rate, whereas deeper levels are associated with an increased heart rate (Fig. 4-5).[2,3] Heart rate is less likely to increase when desflurane is administered with nitrous oxide. Isoflurane-induced heart rate increases are more likely to occur in young adults than elderly patients and may be accentuated by the presence of other drugs (atropine, meperidine, pancuronium) that independently increase heart rate. Furthermore, inclusion of morphine in the preoperative medication or intravenous administration of fentanyl during induction of anesthesia prevents increases in heart rate associated with inhalation of volatile anesthetics, including isoflurane (see Fig. 9-2).[10] Enflurane is the only anesthetic that produces dose-dependent increases in heart rate in volunteers. In surgical patients, however, enflurane-induced heart rate changes have not been prominent.

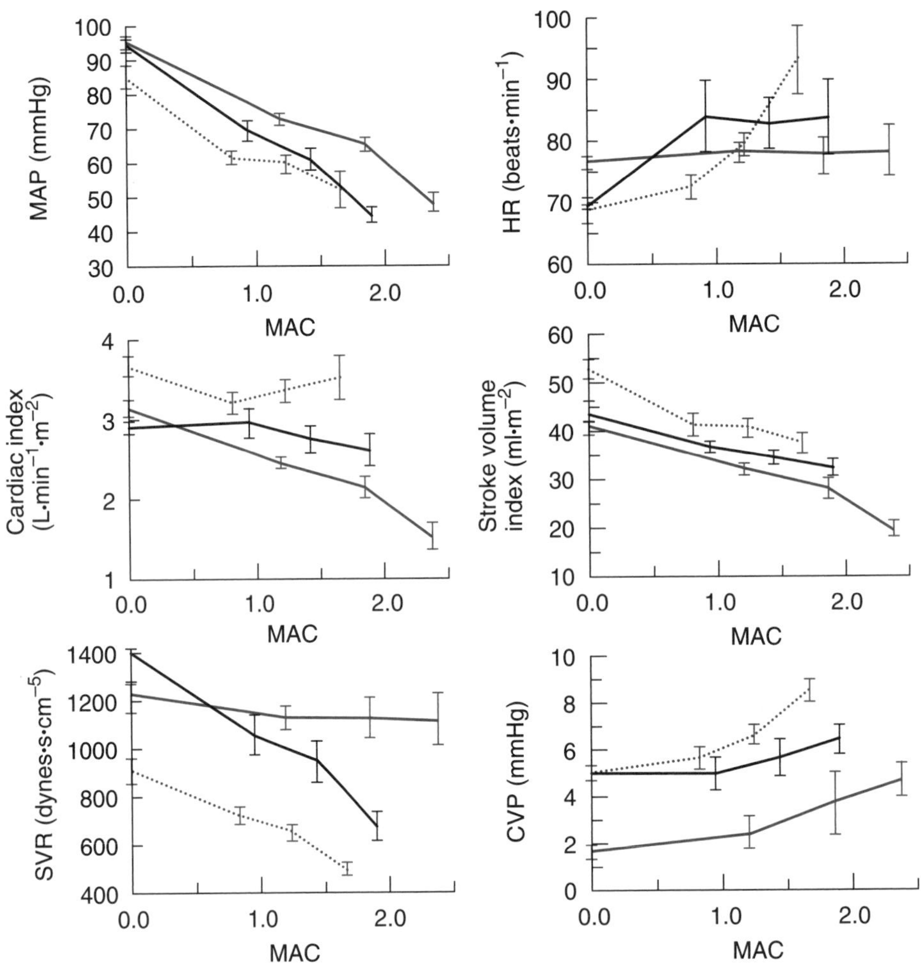

Figure 4-5. Comparison of the cardiovascular effects of volatile anesthetics (halothane [solid red line], isoflurane [solid black line], desflurane [dotted red line]) during mechanical ventilation of the lungs in otherwise healthy volunteers. MAP, mean arterial pressure; HR, heart rate; SVR, systemic vascular resistance; CVP, central venous pressure. (Adapted from Weiskopf et al.,[3] with permission.)

Anesthetic-induced decreases in blood pressure would tend to increase heart rate via stimulation of the carotid sinus baroreceptors. The presence of this reflex response is suggested by the increased heart rate that accompanies isoflurane-, desflurane-, and enflurane-induced decreases in blood pressure. By contrast, halothane inhibits the baroreceptor reflex response, and heart rate usually remains unchanged despite halothane-induced decreases in blood pressure.

Cardiac Output

Halothane and enflurane, but not desflurane and isoflurane, produce dose-dependent decreases in cardiac output (Fig. 4-5).[2,3] The depression of cardiac output produced by halothane and enflurane parallels the decreases in blood pressure produced by these drugs. In contrast to volatile anesthetics, nitrous oxide is associated with mild increases in cardiac output, presumably reflecting weak sympathomimetic effects of this drug.[1]

Stroke Volume

Volatile anesthetics produce dose-dependent decreases in calculated stroke volume (cardiac output divided by heart rate) (Fig. 4-5).[2,3] Stroke volume is not changed by nitrous oxide. Decreases in stroke volume are consistent with decreased myocardial contractility manifesting as a decreased cardiac output. It is also possible that cardiac output would not be as well maintained during inhalation of isoflurane and desflurane should increases in heart rate or decreases in systemic vascular resistance not accompany administration of these drugs (see the sections *Heart Rate* and *Systemic Vascular Resistance*). Increased heart rate during inhalation of isoflurane and desflurane offsets the decreased stroke volume, and cardiac output is unchanged. Increased heart rate associated with inhalation of enflurane is insufficient to offset the decrease in stroke volume, and cardiac output decreases.

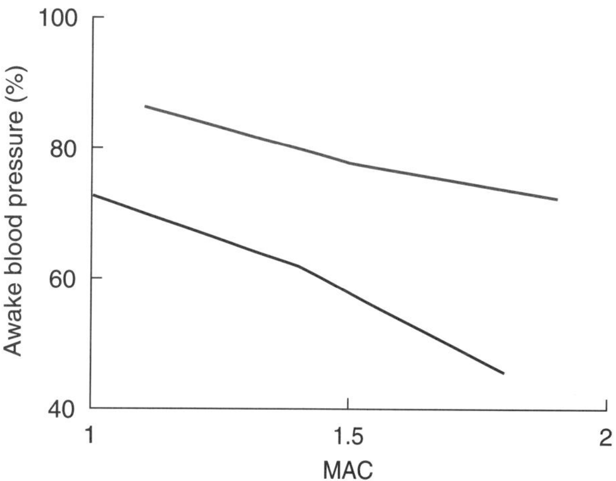

Figure 4-6. Blood pressure is decreased less when nitrous oxide is substituted for a portion of the isoflurane dose (red line) but with the total MAC kept the same as during administration of isoflurane alone (black line). (From Eger,[1] with permission.)

Myocardial Contractility

Inhaled anesthetics studied in vitro (isolated papillary muscle preparations) produce dose-dependent direct myocardial depression. Depression produced by nitrous oxide, however, is less than that produced by comparable concentrations of volatile anesthetics. Depression of myocardial contractility is greater in papillary muscles taken from animals in congestive heart failure than in cardiac muscle taken from normal animals. Therefore, patients with impaired myocardial contractility due to congestive heart failure might be particularly vulnerable to the direct myocardial depressant effects of inhaled anesthetics. Nevertheless, cardiac depression is not consistently seen in vivo, presumably because compensatory homeostatic mechanisms, particularly autonomic nervous system activity, can obscure these direct depressant effects.

Systemic Vascular Resistance

Isoflurane, desflurane, and, to a lesser extent, enflurane decrease calculated systemic vascular resistance (mean arterial pressure minus right arterial pressure divided by cardiac output), but no significant change is produced by halothane or nitrous oxide (Fig. 4-5).[2,3] Decreases in calculated systemic vascular resistance associated with inhalation of isoflurane and desflurane are predictable considering the decrease in blood pressure and unchanged cardiac output associated with administration of these drugs (Fig. 4-5).[2,3] Conversely, decreases in blood pressure associated with halothane administration parallel the decrease in cardiac output, and the calculated systemic vascular resistance is unchanged. This does not mean that halothane lacks vasodilating effects on specific organ systems. Indeed, the prominence of superficial cutaneous veins during inhalation of halothane and other volatile drugs reflects drug-induced venodilation. Anesthetic-induced increases in skin blood flow at the onset of anesthesia most likely reflect central inhibitory actions of these drugs on temperature-regulating mechanisms. All volatile anesthetics produce cerebral vasodilation and increase cerebral blood flow (halothane the most and isoflurane the least) regardless of their overall effects on calculated systemic vascular resistance. Isoflurane is unique in its ability to produce two- to threefold increases in skeletal muscle blood flow that contribute to decreases in systemic vascular resistance associated with administration of this drug. Skeletal muscle blood flow is not altered by nitrous oxide and is diminished by halothane, reflecting decreased perfusion pressure rather than vasoconstriction.

The decrease in systemic vascular resistance produced by isoflurane and desflurane is smaller when nitrous oxide is substituted for an equivalent amount of the volatile anesthetic. The lesser decrease in systemic vascular resistance is consistent with the attenuation of decreases in blood pressure produced by these drugs when administered with nitrous oxide (Fig. 4-6).[1,2]

Absence of changes in calculated systemic vascular resistance during the inhalation of halothane emphasizes that the depth of halothane anesthesia parallels cardiac depression as reflected by decreases in blood pressure. Conversely, decreases in blood pressure during administration of the other volatile anesthetics can occur at light levels of anesthesia, reflecting decreases in systemic vascular resistance rather than myocardial depression.

Coronary Vascular Resistance

Isoflurane, but not halothane or enflurane, selectively dilates coronary arterioles in animal models.[11] Theoretically, isoflurane-induced coronary arteriole vasodilation could result in diversion of blood flow from ischemic areas of myocardium (arterioles already maximally dilated) to areas with normally responsive vessels (coronary artery steal syndrome). Despite the ability of desflurane to produce mild coronary artery vasodilation similar to that caused by isoflurane, there is no evidence that desflurane evokes the coronary steal syndrome.[2] It is an inescapable clinical conclusion that most patients with ischemic heart disease do not develop myocardial ischemia during administration of volatile anesthetics, including isoflurane. This emphasizes that more important than the selection of a specific inhaled anesthetic is the avoidance of the drug-induced events that adversely alter myocardial oxygen delivery (hypotension) or myocardial oxygen requirements (tachycardia) (see Chapter 18). Autoregulation of coronary blood flow seems to be maintained during administration of inhaled anesthetics.

Right Atrial Pressure

Right atrial pressure is increased in a dose-dependent manner by inhaled anesthetics (Fig. 4-5).[2,3] Myocardial depression produced by volatile anesthetics would result in increases of right atrial pressures. Any peripheral vasodilating effect of a volatile drug could attenuate an increase in right atrial pressure produced by myocardial depression. Increased right atrial pressure during inhalation of nitrous oxide most likely reflects increased pulmonary vascular resistance due to sympathomimetic effects of this drug.[1]

Mechanism of Circulatory Effects

No single or predominant mechanism explains circulatory effects produced by inhaled anesthetics. Isoflurane is possibly unique among volatile anesthetics in possessing mild beta agonist properties. This property may oppose direct depressant effects of isoflurane on the heart and is consistent with maintenance of cardiac output, increased heart rate, elevated skeletal muscle blood flow, dilation of coronary arterioles, and decreased systemic vascular resistance associated with administration of this drug. Furthermore, isoflurane interferes with calcium influx and is less likely than enflurane or halothane to depress baroreceptor reflex responses. Another possible explanation for the lesser impact of isoflurane on myocardial contractility may be a greater anesthetic potency of isoflurane relative to halothane and enflurane (more favorable therapeutic index). The implication is that isoflurane may more readily depress the brain and thus, at a given MAC value, appear to spare the heart. Indeed, in animals, the ratio of fatal anesthetic concentration to MAC for isoflurane is 3.0 compared with 2.5 for desflurane and 2.0 for halothane.[2]

Proposed Mechanisms of Circulatory Effects Produced by Inhaled Anesthetics

- Direct myocardial depression
- Inhibition of sympathetic central nervous system activity
- Depression of transmission of impulses through autonomic ganglia
- Impaired baroreceptor reflex activity
- Decreased formation of cyclic adenosine monophosphate
- Increased formation of cyclic guanosine monophosphate
- Inhibition of calcium re-uptake by myocardial sarcoplasmic reticulum
- Decreased influx of calcium through slow channels

Nitrous oxide alone or when added to unchanged concentrations of volatile anesthetics produces signs of mild sympathomimetic stimulation characterized by increases in circulating plasma concentrations of catecholamines, mydriasis, and increased systemic and pulmonary vascular resistance.[12] Animal studies suggest that increases in systemic vascular resistance result from activation of the sympathetic nervous system due to the actions of nitrous oxide on suprapontine areas of the brain. Sympathomimetic effects of nitrous oxide are most evident when this drug is added to halothane. Conceivably, sympathetic nervous system stimulation produced by nitrous oxide alone or in combination with volatile drugs is responsible for the minimal to absent cardiac depression associated with inhalation of this drug. Plasma catecholamine concentrations usually do not increase during administration of volatile anesthetics, providing evidence that these drugs do not activate the sympathetic nervous system.

Cardiac Rhythm

Halothane decreases the amount of circulating epinephrine required to elicit ventricular premature contractions (Fig. 4-7).[13] By contrast, enflurane, isoflurane, and desflurane, as a reflection of their ether chemical structure (halothane is an alkane derivative), do not sensitize the heart to the effects of epinephrine. Children tolerate larger doses of subcutaneous epinephrine injected with or without lidocaine during halothane anesthesia. In animals, enhancement of the cardiac dysrhythmogenic potential of epinephrine is independent of the dose of halothane between alveolar concentrations of 0.5% and 2%. If true in patients, it is likely that therapeutic interventions other than decreasing the inhaled concentration of halothane will be required to promptly treat cardiac dysrhythmias caused by epinephrine.

Junctional rhythm leading to decreases in blood pressure is common during inhalation of halothane. The appearance of this cardiac rhythm disturbance most likely reflects suppression of sinus node activity by halothane.

Pulmonary Vasculature

The effect of volatile anesthetics on the pulmonary vasculature in the absence of any underlying pulmonary vascular abnormality is small.[12] Conversely, nitrous oxide can increase pulmonary vascular resistance particularly when administered to patients with co-existing pulmonary hypertension.[14]

Spontaneous Ventilation

Spontaneous ventilation during inhalation of volatile anesthetics leads to the accumulation of carbon dioxide. Accumulation of carbon dioxide may stimulate the sympathetic nervous system and produce peripheral vasodilation, thus altering circulatory effects produced by volatile anesthetics during spontaneous ventilation as compared with measurements obtained during controlled ventilation of the lungs and normocarbia. For example, heart rate and cardiac output are greater (sympathetic nervous system stimulation) and the systemic vascular resistance decreased more (peripheral vasodilation) during spontaneous inhalation of volatile anesthetics.[1] Despite these changes, the blood pressure is not altered from that observed during controlled ventilation of the lungs. In addition to affecting the cir-

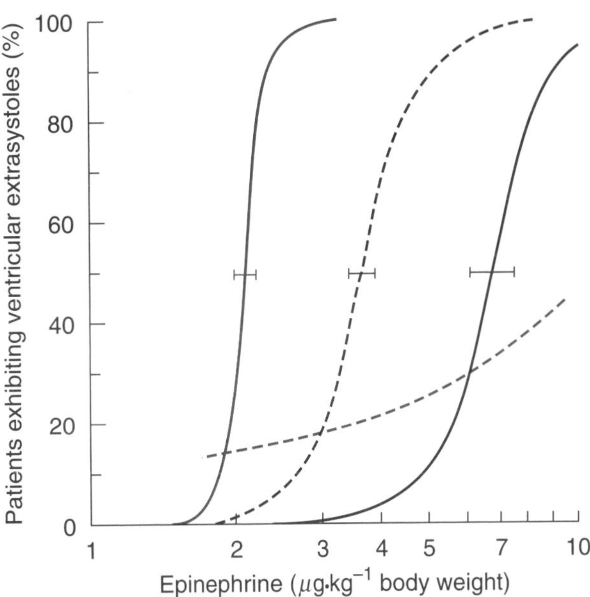

Figure 4-7. The dose (ED_{50}) of submucosal epinephrine necessary to produce ventricular premature contractions (ventricular extrasystoles) during 1.25 MAC anesthesia in adults was 2.1 $\mu g \cdot kg^{-1}$ for halothane (with saline, solid red line; with lidocaine, dashed black line) and 6.7 $\mu g \cdot kg^{-1}$ for isoflurane (solid black line). The flat nature of the enflurane (dashed red line) dose-response curve prevents calculation of an ED_{50} dose for this drug. (From Johnston et al.,[13] with permission.)

culation by allowing the accumulation of carbon dioxide, spontaneous ventilation of the lungs favors venous return to the heart.

Duration of Administration

Inhalation of volatile anesthetics for longer than 5 hours is associated with an increased heart rate, cardiac output, and right atrial pressure, and with decreased systemic vascular resistance compared with similar measurements after 1 to 1.5 hours of administration. Despite the increased cardiac output, blood pressure is unchanged with time, reflecting decreases in systemic vascular resistance. This recovery from the depressant effects of volatile anesthetics with time is most apparent during inhalation of halothane, intermediate with enflurane, and minimal with isoflurane and desflurane. Prior administration of propranolol attenuates or prevents these time-related changes, suggesting increased sympathetic nervous system activity as the mechanism.

Other Variables that Influence Circulatory Variables

Co-Existing Diseases

Co-existing diseases, particularly of the heart, may influence the significance of circulatory effects produced by inhaled anesthetics. For example, drug-induced decreases in myocardial contractility are additive with co-existing decreases in contractility associated with congestive heart failure. In patients with ischemic heart disease, inhalation of nitrous oxide produces evidence of myocardial depression that does not occur in patients without heart disease. Patients with stenotic lesions of the aortic or mitral valves may have poor tolerance of changes in blood pressure and systemic vascular resistance produced by inhaled anesthetics (see Chapter 18). Anemia does not predictably alter anesthetic-induced circulatory effects.

Prior Drug Therapy

Prior drug therapy that alters sympathetic nervous system activity (antihypertensives, beta-adrenergic antagonists) may exaggerate the magnitude of circulatory effects produced by inhaled anesthetics. For example, the magnitude of cardiac depression produced by enflurane, but not by isoflurane, seems to be accentuated by concomitant drug therapy with beta-adrenergic antagonists such as propranolol. Circulatory changes during inhalation of halothane in the presence of beta-adrenergic blockade are intermediate between those induced by isoflurane and enflurane. In an animal model, the effects of desflurane on blood pressure and myocardial contractility resembled those produced by isoflurane in the presence of drug-induced autonomic nervous system blockade.[2] Calcium entry blockers decrease myocardial contractility and thus render the heart more vulnerable to direct depressant effects of inhaled anesthetics. In animals, depressant effects of verapamil on cardiac output are greater during administration of enflurane than of isoflurane. Despite these differences, clinical experience has not suggested that a specific volatile anesthetic is indicated for administration to patients being treated with drugs that act on the heart or depress the sympathetic nervous system. Since additive depression may occur with these drugs, however, it may be necessary to decrease the dose of volatile anesthetics, especially when enflurane is being administered. Discontinuation of previously established efficacious drug therapy is not recommended as this practice may provoke an abrupt return of drug-suppressed symptoms such as hypertension or myocardial ischemia.

Surgical Stimulation

Surgical stimulation modifies the circulatory effects produced by inhaled anesthetics. Indeed, sympathetic nervous system stimulation produced by the surgical incision often results in increased blood pressure and heart rate. Volatile anesthetics oppose this response in a dose-dependent manner. For example, 1.47 MAC halothane or 1.63 MAC enflurane prevents blood pressure and heart rate responses evoked by surgical skin incision in 50% of patients.[15]

REFERENCES

1. Eger EI II. Isoflurane (Forane). A Compendium and Reference. Madison, WI, Anaquest, a division of BOC, Inc. 1986:1–160.
2. Warltier DC, Pagel PS. Cardiovascular and respiratory actions of desflurane: Is desflurane different from isoflurane? Anesth Analg 1992;75:S17–31.
3. Weiskopf RB, Cahalan MK, Eger EI, et al. Cardiovascular actions of desflurane in normocarbic volunteers. Anesth Analg 1991;73:143–56.

4. Lockhart SH, Rampil IJ, Yasuda N, Eger EI, Weiskopf RB. Depression of ventilation by desflurane in humans. Anesthesiology 1991;74:484–8.
5. Eger EI II. Respiratory effects of nitrous oxide. In: Nitrous Oxide. New York, Elsevier 1985:109–23.
6. Calverley RK, Smith NT, Jones CW, Prys-Roberts C, Eger EI II. Ventilatory and cardiovascular effects of enflurane anesthesia during spontaneous ventilation in man. Anesth Analg 1978;57:610–8.
7. Knill RL, Gelb AW. Ventilatory responses to hypoxia and hypercapnia during halothane sedation and anesthesia in man. Anesthesiology 1978;49:244–51.
8. Hirshman CA, Edelstein G, Peetz S, Wayne R, Downes H. Mechanism of action of inhalational anesthesia on airways. Anesthesiology 1982;56:107–11.
9. Tusiewicz K, Bryan AC, Froese AB. Contributions of changing rib cage-diaphragm interactions to the ventilatory depression of halothane anesthesia. Anesthesiology 1977;47:327–37.
10. Cahalan MK, Lurz FW, Eger EI II, Schwartz LA, Beaupre PN, Smith JS. Narcotics decrease heart rate during inhalation anesthesia. Anesth Analg 1987;66:166–70.
11. Sill JC, Bove AA, Nugent M, Blaise GA, Dewey JD, Grabau C. Effects of isoflurane on coronary arterioles in the intact dog. Anesthesiology 1987;66:273–9.
12. Hilgenberg JC, McCammon RL, Stoelting RK. Pulmonary and systemic vascular responses to nitrous oxide in patients with mitral stenosis and pulmonary hypertension. Anesth Analg 1980;59:323–6.
13. Johnston RR, Eger EI II, Wilson C. A comparative interaction of epinephrine with enflurane, isoflurane and halothane in man. Anesth Analg 1976;55:709–12.
14. Schulte-Sasse U, Hess W, Tarnow J. Pulmonary vascular responses to nitrous oxide in patients with normal and high pulmonary vascular resistance. Anesthesiology 1982;57:9–13.
15. Roizen MF, Horrigan RW, Frazer BM. Anesthetic doses blocking adrenergic (stress) and cardiovascular responses to incision-MAC BAR. Anesthesiology 1981;54:390–8.

5
Intravenous Anesthetics

Drugs classified as intravenous anesthetics are most often used to produce induction of anesthesia. Combined with inhaled anesthetics, these drugs may also be used for maintenance of anesthesia, by either intermittent bolus or constant intravenous infusion. Examples of intravenous anesthetics are barbiturates, benzodiazepines, opioids, and miscellaneous drugs such as ketamine, etomidate, and propofol.

BARBITURATES

Historically, barbiturates have been classified as long-acting, intermediate-acting, short-acting, and ultrashort-acting. This classification is no longer recommended as it incorrectly implies that the action of these drugs ends predictably after specified time intervals. This is not true as drug effects persist for several hours even after administration of thiopental, thiamylal, or methohexital (ultrashort-acting barbiturates) for induction of anesthesia. Thiopental is the most commonly used barbiturate and the drug with which all other drugs used for induction of anesthesia are compared.

General Pharmacology

Structure Activity Relationships

Barbiturates result from structural alterations at the number 2 and number 5 carbon atoms of barbituric acid (Fig. 5-1). Oxybarbiturates retain an oxygen atom on the number 2 carbon, whereas replacement of this atom with a sulfur atom results in more lipid soluble thiobarbiturates. Increased lipid solubility contributes to a more rapid onset and shorter duration of action. For example, thiopental and thiamylal have a more rapid onset and shorter duration of action than their less lipid soluble oxybarbiturate analogs, pentobarbital and secobarbital. Addition of a methyl group to the nitrogen atom of the barbituric acid ring results in a short duration of action as produced by methohexital.

Mechanism of Action

Barbiturates seem to be uniquely capable of depressing the reticular activating system, which is assumed to be important in the maintenance of wakefulness. This response may reflect the ability of barbiturates to decrease the rate of dissociation of the inhibitory neurotransmitter gamma-aminobutyric acid (GABA) from its receptors. GABA causes an increase in chloride conductance through ion channels, resulting in hyperpolarization and, consequently, inhibition of postsynaptic neurons. Barbiturates also selectively decrease transmission of impulses through sympathetic nervous system ganglia, which may contribute to the decreases in blood pressure that can accompany intravenous injection of barbiturates or that occur in association with a barbiturate overdose. Despite evidence that stereospecificity is important in the pharmacologic effects of barbiturates, there is no specific pharmacologic antagonist for barbiturate effects on the central nervous system.

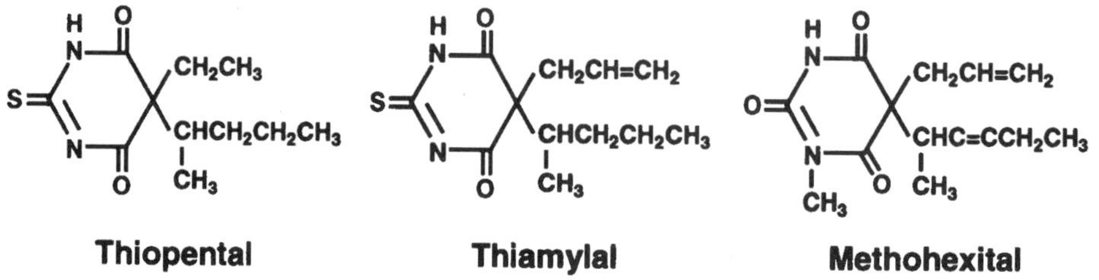

Thiopental | Thiamylal | Methohexital

Figure 5-1. Chemical structures of barbiturates administered intravenously most often for induction of anesthesia.

Cardiovascular System

Administration of barbiturates to produce induction of anesthesia typically produces modest decreases in blood pressure (10 to 20 mmHg) that are transient due to compensatory baroreceptor-mediated increases in heart rate (Fig. 5-2).[1] This blood pressure decrease is principally due to peripheral vasodilation, reflecting barbiturate-induced depression of the medullary vasomotor center and decreased sympathetic nervous system outflow from the central nervous system. Resulting dilation of peripheral capacitance vessels leads to pooling of blood, decreased venous return, and the potential for decreases in cardiac output and blood pressure. Indeed, hypovolemic patients, who are less able to compensate for peripheral vasodilating effects, are likely to experience exaggerated decreases in blood pressure when barbiturates are rapidly injected intravenously for the induction of anesthesia. Negative inotropic effects of barbiturates, which are readily demonstrated by using isolated heart preparations, are obscured in vivo by baroreceptor-mediated reflex responses.

Ventilation

Barbiturates depress medullary ventilatory centers as reflected by decreased responsiveness to ventilatory stimulant effects of carbon dioxide. Induction of anesthesia with barbiturates is likely to produce transient apnea requiring temporary controlled ventilation of the lungs. Apnea is particularly likely to occur when other depressant drugs such as opioids have been included in the preoperative medication. Resumption of spontaneous breathing after induction doses of barbiturates is characterized by a slow breathing rate and a decreased tidal volume. Laryngeal reflexes and cough reflexes are not greatly depressed by induction doses of barbiturates. Indeed, stimulation of the upper airway or trachea (secretions, laryngoscopy, intubation of the trachea) in the presence of inadequate depression of airway reflexes by barbiturates may result in laryngospasm

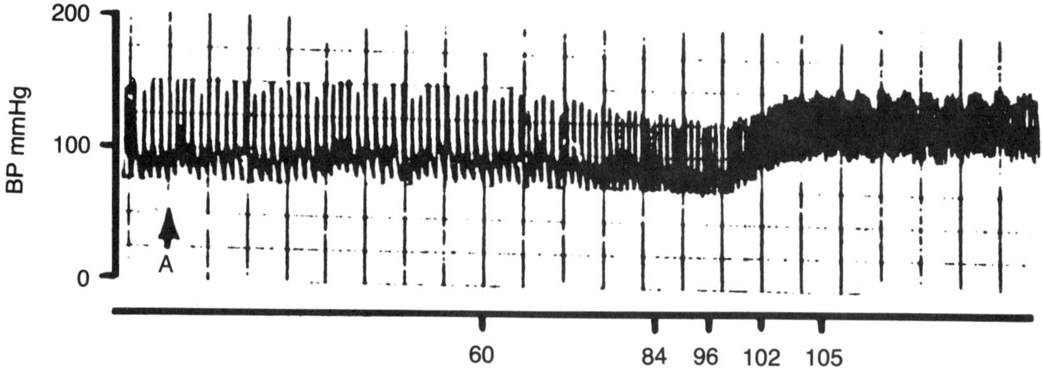

Figure 5-2. In normovolemic patients, the intravenous administration of thiopental (A) is followed by a modest decrease in blood pressure (BP), which is subsequently offset by a compensatory increase in heart rate (HR). (From Filner and Karliner,[1] with permission.)

or bronchospasm. This response should not be interpreted as unique to barbiturates but, rather, as an example of an adverse response to stimulation in the presence of inadequate drug-induced suppression of airway reflexes.

Central Nervous System

Barbiturates are potent cerebral vasoconstrictors, producing predictable decreases in cerebral blood flow, cerebral blood volume, and intracranial pressure (ICP). Cerebral metabolic oxygen requirements ($CMRO_2$) are decreased maximally when the electroencephalogram (EEG) is rendered isoelectric. The ability of barbiturates to decrease ICP and $CMRO_2$ makes these drugs useful in the management of anesthesia in patients with space-occupying intracranial lesions (see Chapter 23). An exception to the generalization that barbiturates decrease electrical activity on the EEG is methohexital, which activates epileptic foci, making their identification easier during surgery designed to ablate these sites. Barbiturates may provide protection of the brain from adverse effects produced by regional cerebral ischemia but not global cerebral ischemia, which is likely to accompany cardiac arrest (see Chapter 35).

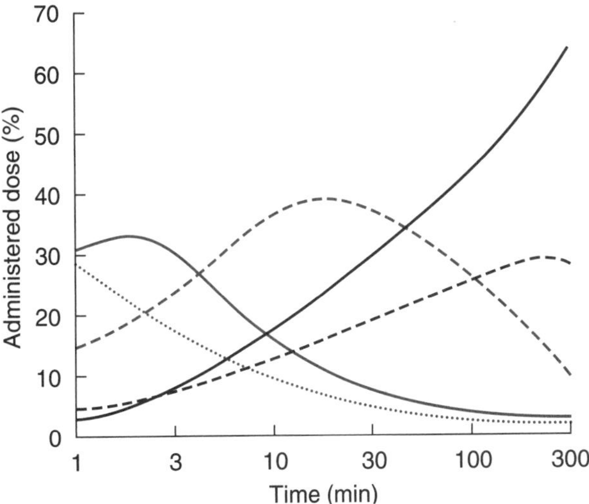

Figure 5-3. Following a rapid intravenous injection of thiopental, the percentage of the administered dose remaining in the blood (dotted red line) rapidly decreases as the drug moves from the blood to highly perfused vessel rich group (VRG) tissues (solid red line), especially the brain. Subsequently, thiopental is redistributed to skeletal muscles (dashed red line) and, to a lesser extent, to fat (dashed black line). Ultimately, most of the administered dose of thiopental undergoes metabolism (solid black line). (From Saidman,[2] with permission.)

Pharmacokinetics

Maximal brain uptake of barbiturates occurs within 30 seconds after their intravenous administration, accounting for the rapid induction of anesthesia (one or two circulation times) produced by these drugs (Fig. 5-3).[2] Prompt awakening following intravenous administration of thiopental, thiamylal, and methohexital reflects redistribution of these drugs from the brain to inactive tissues, especially skeletal muscles and fat. Ultimately, however, elimination of barbiturates from the body depends almost entirely on metabolism because less than 1% of the administered doses of these drugs are cleared unchanged by the kidneys. Large or repeated doses of lipid soluble barbiturates may saturate inactive tissue sites, resulting in prolonged effects of these usually short-acting drugs. The elimination half-time of methohexital is more rapid than that of thiopental, reflecting the greater hepatic metabolism of methohexital (Table 5-1).[3] These characteristics of methohexital should result in more rapid awakening than after administration of thiopental, especially if repeated doses of barbiturates are injected. For this reason, methohexital rather than thiopental is sometimes recommended for outpatient procedures when rapid awakening is especially important and a barbiturate is selected for induction of anesthesia.

Clinical Uses

Barbiturates are used most often for the intravenous induction of anesthesia (unconsciousness in less than 30 seconds) and occasionally to aid in the maintenance of anesthesia in combination with other inhaled drugs. When administered for induction of anesthesia, thiopental or thiamylal (3 to 5 $mg \cdot kg^{-1}$ IV) or methohexital (1 to 1.5 $mg \cdot kg^{-1}$ IV) is followed by succinylcholine or nondepolarizing muscle relaxants to produce skeletal muscle paralysis and facilitate subsequent intubation of the trachea. This approach is referred to as rapid sequence induction of anesthesia. An important advantage of rapid sequence induction of anesthesia is early tracheal intubation to provide protection against inhalation (pulmonary aspiration) of gastric fluid. Although rapid sequence induction of anesthesia is

Table 5-1. Pharmacokinetics of Barbiturates

	Thiopental	Methohexital
Equivalent dose ($mg \cdot kg^{-1}$)	3–5[a]	1–1.5
Elimination half-time (h)	11.6	3.9[b]
Clearance ($ml \cdot kg^{-1} \cdot min^{-1}$)	3.4	10.9[b]
Volume of distribution ($L \cdot kg^{-1}$)	2.2	2.5

[a]Same for thiamylal.
[b]Significantly different from thiopental.
(Data from Hudson et al.[3])

pleasant for the patient, it has associated hazards. For example, if the trachea cannot be promptly intubated, the paralyzed patient will be totally dependent on the anesthesiologist for adequate ventilation of the lungs. The need for prolonged manual ventilation of the lungs may increase the likelihood of inflating the patient's stomach with gas and associated hazards of regurgitation and aspiration. After anesthesia has been induced, it is maintained most often with combinations of inhaled (nitrous oxide and a volatile anesthetic) or injected (opioids, propofol) drugs, or both.

An alternative approach to rapid sequence induction of anesthesia is administration of small doses of barbiturates (thiopental 0.5 to 1 $mg \cdot kg^{-1}$ IV) followed by application of the anesthesia mask to the patient's face and delivery of inhaled anesthetics to complete the induction of anesthesia. The low dose of barbiturate improves patient acceptance of the anesthesia mask and the pungent volatile anesthetics, especially enflurane, isoflurane, and desflurane. This slow induction of anesthesia is not a likely selection for patients with a history of recent food ingestion who are considered to be at risk of aspiration of gastric contents. Rectal administration of barbiturates, especially methohexital (20 to 30 $mg \cdot kg^{-1}$), has been used to facilitate induction of anesthesia in uncooperative or young patients.

Barbiturates may be administered intravenously in high doses to decrease ICP, which remains elevated despite deliberate hyperventilation of the lungs and drug-induced diuresis. An isoelectric EEG confirms the presence of maximal barbiturate-induced depression of $CMRO_2$. A risk of high-dose barbiturate therapy as used to decrease ICP is hypotension, which can jeopardize the maintenance of an adequate cerebral perfusion pressure. Administration of thiopental is acceptable when the ability to monitor somatosensory evoked potentials is desirable.

Venous thrombosis following intravenous administration of barbiturates for induction of anesthesia presumably reflects deposition of barbiturate crystals (the pH of blood is too low to keep alkaline barbiturates in solution—thiopental pH 10.5) in veins. Accidental intra-arterial injection of barbiturates results in excruciating pain and intense vasoconstriction, often leading to gangrene despite aggressive therapy, including sympathetic nervous system blockade (stellate ganglion block) of the involved extremity. It is likely that barbiturate crystal formation results in occlusion of more distal small diameter arteries and arterioles. Barbiturate crystal formation in veins is less hazardous because of the ever increasing diameter of veins. Accidental subcutaneous injection (extravasation) of barbiturates results in local tissue irritation, emphasizing the importance of using dilute concentrations (thiopental and thiamylal 2.5%, methohexital 1.0%) of barbiturates. If extravasation occurs, some recommend local injection of 0.5% lidocaine (5 to 10 ml) in an attempt to dilute the barbiturate concentration. Life-threatening allergic reaction is a rare (estimated 1 in 30,000 patients) risk of induction of anesthesia by barbiturates.

BENZODIAZEPINES

Benzodiazepines commonly used in the perioperative period include diazepam, midazolam, and lorazepam (Fig. 5-4). In addition to their sedative and calming effects, their favorable pharmacologic characteristics include (1) impairment of the acquisition of new information (anterograde amnesia) with no predictable alteration of stored information (retrograde amnesia), (2) minimal depression of ventilation or the cardiovascular system, (3) specific site of action as anticonvulsants, (4) relative safety if taken in overdose, and (5) rarity of abuse or development of significant physical dependence. Another advantage is the ability to promptly antagonize the central nervous system effects of benzodiazepines with a selective benzodiazepine antagonist, flumazenil.

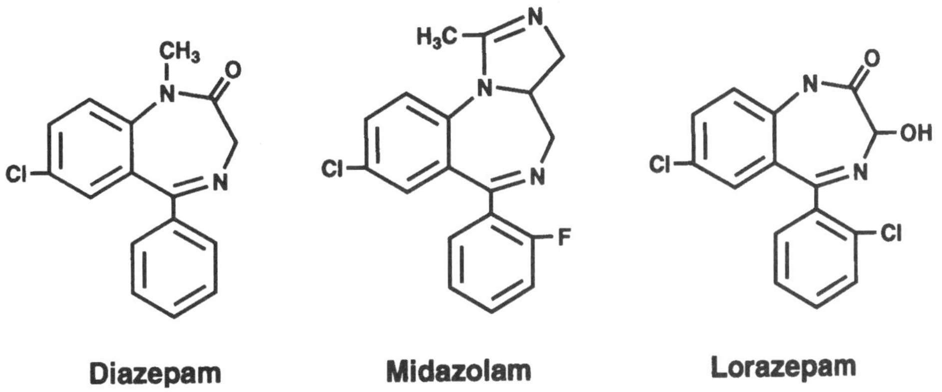

Diazepam Midazolam Lorazepam

Figure 5-4. Chemical structures of benzodiazepines commonly administered in the perioperative period.

General Pharmacology

Mechanism of Action

Benzodiazepines exert their pharmacologic effects by enhancing the chloride channel gating function of the inhibitory neurotransmitter GABA (Fig. 5-5).[4] The resulting enhanced opening of the chloride channel leads to hyperpolarization of cell membranes, making them more resistant to neuronal excitation. Benzodiazepine receptors occur almost exclusively on postsynaptic nerve endings in the central nervous system, with the greatest density being in the cerebral cortex. This anatomic distribution of receptors is consistent with the minimal effects of these drugs outside the central nervous system (minimal circulatory effects).[5] Indeed, the incidence and magnitude of depression of ventilation and production of hypotension produced by benzodiazepines seem to be lower than that associated with barbiturates as used for induction of anesthesia. Consistent with its greater potency, midazolam has an affinity for benzodiazepine receptors that is approximately twice that of diazepam. Exposure of midazolam to the blood pH causes a change in structure, converting this water soluble drug to a highly lipid soluble drug capable of crossing the blood-brain barrier to gain access to the central nervous system.

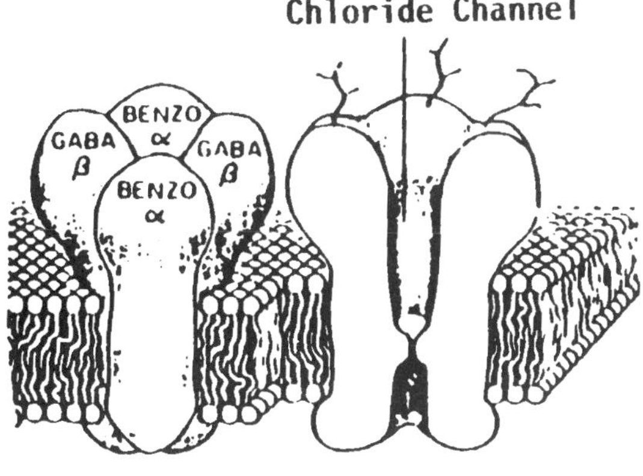

Figure 5-5. Schematic depiction of the gamma-aminobutyric acid (GABA) receptor forming a chloride channel. Benzodiazepines (BENZO) attach selectively to alpha subunits and are presumed to facilitate the action of the inhibitory neurotransmitter GABA on the alpha subunits. (From Mohler and Richards,[4] with permission.)

Pharmacokinetics

Benzodiazepines are highly lipid soluble drugs; this results in rapid entrance into the central nervous system followed by redistribution to inactive tissue sites. Diazepam undergoes hepatic metabolism to active metabolites (desmethyldiazepam and oxazepam) that may contribute to the prolonged effects of this drug. By contrast, metabolites of midazolam seem to possess little or no pharmacologic activity. The elimination half-time of diazepam greatly exceeds that of midazolam, emphasizing the likely prolonged central nervous system effects of diazepam compared with midazolam (Table 5-2).

Clinical Uses

Benzodiazepines are used for (1) preoperative medication, (2) intravenous sedation, (3) intravenous

Table 5-2. Pharmacokinetics of Benzodiazepines

	Equivalent Dose ($mg \cdot kg^{-1}$)	Elimination Half-Time (h)	Clearance ($ml \cdot kg^{-1} \cdot min^{-1}$)	Volume of Distribution ($L \cdot kg^{-1}$)
Diazepam	0.3–0.5	21–37	0.2–0.5	1–1.5
Midazolam	0.15–0.3	1–4	6–8	1–1.5
Lorazepam	0.05	10–20	0.7–1	0.8–1.3

induction of anesthesia, and (4) suppression of seizure activity. The amnesic, calming, and sedative effects of benzodiazepines are the basis for the use of these drugs in preoperative medication (see Chapter 9). Diazepam (5 to 10 mg IV) or midazolam (1 to 2.5 mg IV) is useful for sedation during regional anesthesia. Midazolam produces a more rapid onset and greater degree of amnesia than diazepam when administered for intravenous sedation. Induction of anesthesia can be produced by the administration of diazepam (0.2 to 0.3 $mg \cdot kg^{-1}$ IV) or midazolam (0.1 to 0.2 $mg \cdot kg^{-1}$ IV). Induction of anesthesia is more rapid after administration of midazolam (about 80 seconds) than after that of diazepam, but it is still slower than after administration of barbiturates (about 30 seconds).[6] Prior administration of opioids, as in the preoperative medication or intravenously immediately before injection of benzodiazepines, may facilitate the speed of induction of anesthesia produced by these drugs. The slow onset and prolonged duration of action of lorazepam limit its usefulness for preoperative medication or induction of anesthesia, especially when rapid and sustained awakening at the end of surgery is desirable. Despite the possible production of lesser circulatory effects, it is unlikely that benzodiazepines offer any advantages over barbiturates as used for rapid sequence induction of anesthesia. Delayed awakening is a potential disadvantage of administering benzodiazepines for the induction of anesthesia. Flumazenil (0.2 mg IV every 60 seconds up to a total dose of 1 mg) may be useful for treating patients experiencing delayed awakening, keeping in mind that the duration of the antagonist is brief (about 20 minutes) and resedation may occur. The efficacy of benzodiazepines, especially diazepam, as anticonvulsants is consistent with the ability of these drugs to enhance the inhibitory effects of GABA, particularly in the limbic system. Indeed, diazepam (0.1 $mg \cdot kg^{-1}$ IV) is effective in abolishing seizure activity produced by local anesthetics, alcohol withdrawal, and status epilepticus. Benzodiazepines, like barbiturates, decrease cerebral blood flow and $CMRO_2$. Allergic reactions to benzodiazepines seem to be extremely rare to nonexistent.

Pain during intravenous injection of diazepam and subsequent thrombophlebitis reflect the poor water solubility of this benzodiazepine. It is the organic solvent, propylene glycol, required to dissolve diazepam that is most likely responsible for pain during intramuscular or intravenous administration, as well as for the unpredictable absorption after intramuscular injection. Midazolam is water soluble, obviating the need for an organic solvent and decreasing the likelihood of exaggerated pain or erratic absorption after intramuscular injection or pain during intravenous administration.

OPIOIDS

Opioids include all exogenous substances that bind specifically to opioid receptors and produce at least some agonist responses. Although several opioids are available, those most often used in the perioperative period are morphine and meperidine for preoperative medication and fentanyl, sufentanil, and alfentanil for induction or maintenance of anesthesia, or both (Fig. 5-6). All opioids have a role in production of analgesia either before or after surgery. Morphine is the opioid with which all other opioids are compared.

General Pharmacology

Mechanism of Action

Opioids act as agonists at stereospecific opioid receptors in the central nervous system and other

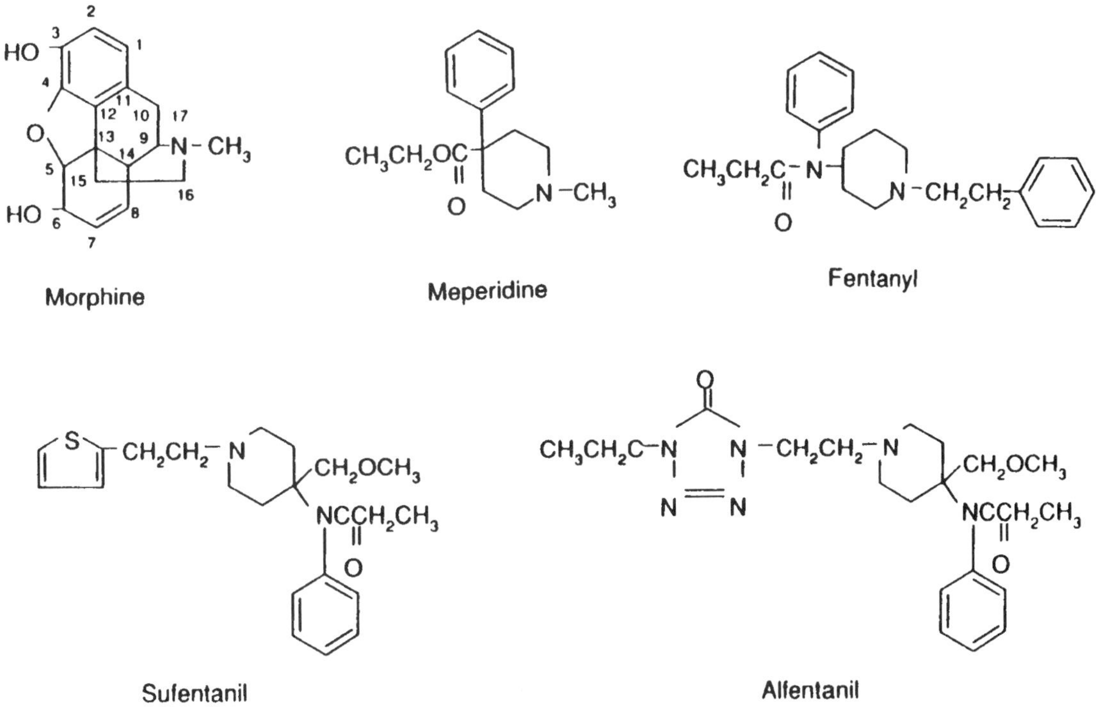

Figure 5-6. Chemical structures of opioid agonists commonly administered in the perioperative period.

tissues (Table 5-3). Analgesia is mediated through a complex interaction of mu, delta, and kappa receptors. Supraspinally, mu receptors are more important, whereas delta and kappa receptors are involved at the spinal level.[7] These opioid receptors are normally activated by endogenous ligands known as endorphins. The affinity of most opioid agonists for receptors parallels their analgesic potency. Binding of opioids to specific receptors results in inhibition of adenylate cyclase activity manifesting as hyperpolarization of the neuron, which results in suppression of spontaneous discharge and evoked responses. In addition, opioids may interfere with transmembrane transport of calcium ions and act presynaptically to interfere with the release of neurotransmitters, including acetylcholine, dopamine, norepinephrine, and substance P.

The existence of the opioid in the ionized state is important for binding to the opioid receptor. In this regard, there is a close relationship between stereochemical structure and potency of opioids, with levorotatory isomers being the most active.

Table 5-3. Opioid Receptors and Responses to Stimulation

Receptor	Response Evoked by Agonists
Mu-1	Supraspinal analgesia Euphoria Miosis Nausea and vomiting Urinary retention Pruritus
Mu-2	Depression of ventilation Sedation Bradycardia Ileus
Delta	Modulation of mu receptor activity Physical dependence
Kappa	Spinal analgesia Sedation Miosis
Sigma	Dysphoria Hypertonia Mydriasis

Cardiovascular Effects

Administration of even large doses of opioids to supine normovolemic patients is unlikely to cause significant changes in myocardial contractility (except meperidine) or decreases in blood pressure. Orthostatic hypotension may be prominent when patients change from the supine to the upright position or when hypovolemia is present, reflecting the ability of opioids to decrease sympathetic nervous system tone to peripheral veins. Morphine, but not fentanyl, sufentanil, or alfentanil, can evoke release of histamine, especially when high doses are rapidly administered intravenously (Fig. 5-7).[8] Bradycardia often accompanies opioid administration (with the exception of meperidine), presumably reflecting stimulation of the vagal nucleus in the medulla. Heart rate slowing is particularly prominent after the administration of sufentanil. Opioids do not sensitize the heart to cardiac dysrhythmic effects of catecholamines.

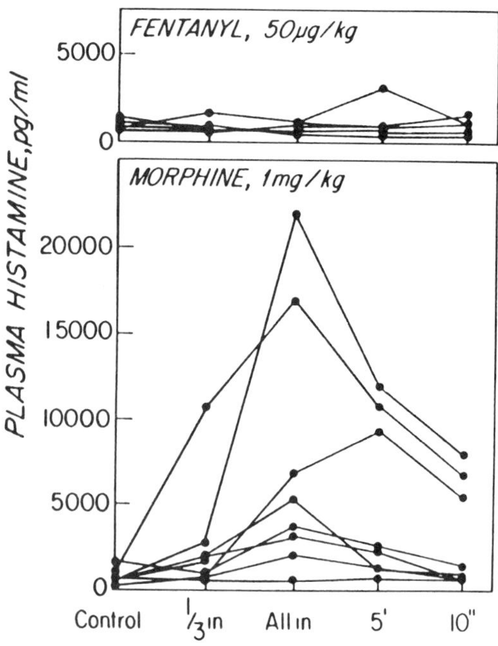

Figure 5-7. Individual data for arterial concentrations of histamine before and after intravenous administration of high doses of fentanyl or morphine. (From Rosow et al.,[8] with permission.)

Ventilation

Opioids produce rapid and sustained dose-dependent depression of ventilation characterized by increases in the resting $PaCO_2$ and decreased responsiveness to the ventilatory stimulant effects of carbon dioxide (CO_2 response curve shifted to the right). Depression of ventilation reflects effects of opioids on medullary ventilatory centers, which may include decreased release of the neurotransmitter acetylcholine. The rate of breathing is decreased while tidal volume is often increased as an incomplete compensatory response. Death due to opioid administration is almost invariably the result of depression of ventilation. Hypoventilation and arterial hypoxemia can also result from opioid-induced spasm of thoracoabdominal muscles (see the section *Skeletal and Smooth Muscle*).[9]

Central Nervous System

Opioids, even in high doses, do not reliably produce unconsciousness, especially in young patients, emphasizing that these drugs cannot be considered true anesthetics. In the absence of hypoventilation, opioids act as cerebral vasoconstrictors producing decreases in cerebral blood flow and intracranial pressure. Nevertheless, there is evidence that even modest doses of fentanyl and sufentanil can significantly increase ICP in patients with severe head trauma.[10] Miosis is a central nervous system effect of opioids.

Stimulation of dopamine receptors in the chemoreceptor trigger zone by opioids may cause nausea and vomiting. Activation of these receptors as a mechanism for opioid-induced nausea and vomiting is consistent with the antiemetic efficacy of dopamine receptor antagonists such as butyrophenones. Conversely, morphine depresses the vomiting center in the medulla. As a result, the intravenous administration of morphine produces less nausea and vomiting than the intramuscular administration of morphine, presumably because opioid administered intravenously reaches the vomiting center as rapidly as it reaches the chemoreceptor trigger zone. Nausea and vomiting are relatively uncommon in recumbent patients receiving morphine. This suggests that a vestibular component may be contributing to opioid-induced nausea and vomiting.

Table 5-4. Pharmacokinetics of Opioids

	Equivalent Potency	pK	Elimination Half-Time (min)	Clearance (ml·kg^{-1}·min^{-1})	Volume of Distribution (L·kg^{-1})
Morphine	1	7.93	114	15–23	3.2–3.4
Meperidine	0.1	8.5	180–264	10–17	2.8–4.2
Fentanyl	75–125	8.43	185–219	11–21	3.2–5.9
Sufentanil	500–1000	8.01	148–164	13	2.86
Alfentanil	25	6.5	70–98	5–7.9	0.5–1

Skeletal and Smooth Muscle

High doses of opioids rapidly administered intravenously may cause spasm of the thoracoabdominal muscles ("stiff-chest" syndrome) resulting in hypoventilation.[9] In extreme situations, skeletal muscle rigidity is sufficiently severe that it interferes with mechanical ventilation of the lungs. Administration of a muscle relaxant or an opioid antagonist such as naloxone is effective for terminating opioid-induced skeletal muscle rigidity.

Opioids may cause spasm of biliary smooth muscle, resulting in increases in intrabiliary pressure that may be associated with biliary colic. This pain, which may mimic angina pectoris, is relieved by administration of naloxone or nitroglycerin, whereas myocardial ischemia-induced pain is not altered by the opioid antagonist. During surgery, opioid-induced spasm of the sphincter of Oddi occurs in about 3% of treated patients. This spasm appears radiologically as a sharp constriction at the distal end of the common bile duct and may be misinterpreted as a common bile duct stone. It may be necessary to reverse opioid-induced biliary smooth muscle spasm with naloxone so as to correctly interpret the cholangiogram. Opioid-induced enhancement of bladder sphincter tone may make spontaneous urination difficult. Opioids, especially morphine, decrease peristaltic activity and enhance the tone of the pyloric sphincter, contributing to delayed gastric as well as intestinal emptying.

Pharmacokinetics

Clearance of opioids is principally by hepatic metabolism, but large differences in lipid solubility account for greatly different elimination half-times between these drugs (Table 5-4). Typically, metabolites of opioids possess greatly decreased pharmacologic activity. An exception is the morphine-6-glucuronide metabolite of morphine, which is pharmacologically active (analgesia, depression of ventilation) and dependent on renal clearance for its elimination.

A single dose of fentanyl administered intravenously has a more rapid onset and shorter duration of action than morphine. This reflects the greater lipid solubility of fentanyl that facilitates entrance into the central nervous system followed by prompt redistribution to inactive tissue sites, such as skeletal muscles and fat. High intravenous doses or continuous infusions of fentanyl lead to progressive saturation of these inactive tissue sites. As a result, plasma concentrations of fentanyl do not decline promptly, and pharmacologic effects, including depression of ventilation, are prolonged. Indeed, persistent or recurrent depression of ventilation owing to lingering effects of fentanyl (and presumably of other opioids too) is a potential postoperative problem[11] (see Chapter 31).

Sufentanil and alfentanil are synthetic derivatives of fentanyl. A greater affinity for opioid receptors accounts for the increased potency of sufentanil (Table 5-4). Like fentanyl, the high lipid solubility of sufentanil contributes to its prompt onset and subsequent redistribution to inactive tissue sites, (brief duration of action), as well as to the potential for cumulative effects. Alfentanil has the most rapid onset of all the listed opioids, reflecting its low pK and thus its high degree of nonionization at physiologic pH. This facilitates its passage into the central nervous system and more than offsets the impact of its lower lipid solubility. The brief duration of action of alfentanil is a result of redistribution to inactive tissue sites and hepatic metabolism. Unlike other opioids, continuous intravenous infusions of alfentanil do not seem to produce clinically significant cumulative drug effects, and postoperative awakening is prompt (rapid dissociation from opioid receptors) with minimal lingering side effects such as depression of ventilation.[12]

Clinical Uses

Clinical uses of opioids are numerous and include (1) provision of analgesia before or after surgery; (2) induction of anesthesia and maintenance of anesthesia, especially in patients with severe cardiac dysfunction; (3) inhibition of reflex sympathetic nervous system activity; and (4) supplementation of inhaled anesthetics being used for maintenance of anesthesia. Postoperative pain relief for prolonged periods (12 to 24 hours) may be produced by injection of low doses of opioids (most often morphine) into the subarachnoid or epidural space (see Chapter 32).

High doses of fentanyl (50 to 150 μg·kg^{-1} IV) or equivalent doses of sufentanil may be used as the sole anesthetic in patients who would not tolerate even modest direct cardiac depression produced by inhaled anesthetics. Compared with large doses of morphine or fentanyl, sufentanil results in more rapid induction of anesthesia, earlier emergence from anesthesia, and earlier extubation of the trachea (Fig. 5-8).[13] More often, however, opioids are administered in lower doses during maintenance of anesthesia as intermittent intravenous injections or as continuous infusions to supplement inhaled anesthetics. Alfentanil may be particularly useful for producing induction of anesthesia (150 to 300 μg·kg^{-1} IV produces unconsciousness in about 45 seconds) and for providing for anesthetic maintenance (continuous infusions of 25 to 150 μg·kg^{-1}·h^{-1} IV) in combination with inhaled anesthetics.[7] Small doses of opioids (fentanyl 1 to 2 μg·kg^{-1} IV or equivalent doses of sufentanil or alfentanil) administered 1 to 3 minutes before induction of anesthesia may attenuate blood pressure and heart rate responses evoked by direct laryngoscopy and intubation of the trachea. Conversely, opioids are frequently not useful when administered after noxious stimulation has evoked hypertension. Intraoperative tachycardia, however, may respond to small intravenous doses of opioids. Injection of an opioid, such as fentanyl, before painful surgical stimulation occurs may decrease the subsequent amount of opioid required in the postoperative period to provide analgesia (preemptive analgesia).

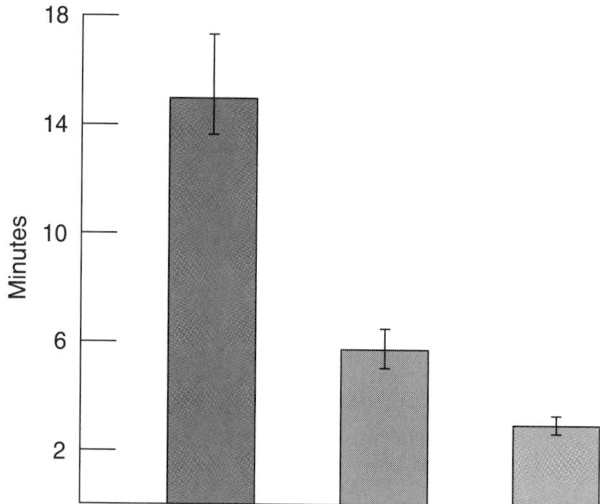

Figure 5-8. The time between the beginning of opioid administration and the patient's inability to respond to a verbal command was defined as the induction time. Sufentanil (S; light red bar) resulted in a significantly more rapid intravenous induction of anesthesia than did morphine (M; dark red bar) or fentanyl (F, gray bar). (M–S <0.05; F–S <0.05; M–F–S <0.05.) (From Sanford et al.,[13] with permission.)

Residual effects of opioids may be antagonized by a specific opioid antagonist, naloxone. Naloxone, however, is a nonselective antagonist, reversing desirable (analgesia) as well as undesirable (depression of ventilation) effects of opioids. High doses of naloxone (3 to 5 μg·kg^{-1} IV) may result in abrupt awakening associated with intense pain and activation of the sympathetic nervous system manifesting as hypertension, tachycardia, and cardiac dysrhythmias. Intermittent administration of low doses of naloxone (0.1 to 0.3 μg·kg^{-1} IV) is more likely to reverse unacceptable degrees of opioid-induced depression of ventilation while leaving intact a sufficient amount of analgesia to maintain patient comfort. Unfortunately, the duration of action of naloxone is brief (about 30 minutes), and previously antagonized undesirable effects of opioids are likely to recur unless supplemental doses of the antagonist are administered. In this regard, a continuous infusion of naloxone (3 to 5 μg·kg^{-1}·h^{-1} IV) may be considered.

Agonist-Antagonist Opioids

Opioids classified as agonist-antagonists include pentazocine, butorphanol, nalbuphine, buprenorphine, and dezocine. These drugs are often strong kappa and weak mu receptor agonists. In contrast to pure agonists, the agonist-antagonists have limited analgesic properties (ceiling effect above which increasing doses do not produce additional analgesia) and are thus unlikely to be used alone or in combination with other anesthetics for induction or maintenance of anesthesia. The antagonist properties of these drugs, however, have been used to advantage to provide postoperative analgesia with the hope that associated depression of ventilation will be minimal.

MISCELLANEOUS INDUCTION DRUGS

Ketamine, etomidate, and propofol are examples of miscellaneous drugs that are administered intravenously for the induction of anesthesia (Fig. 5-9). Occasionally, these drugs are administered as intermittent intravenous injections or continuous infusions for the maintenance of anesthesia in combination with an inhaled drug. These drugs differ from one another with respect to their pharmacokinetics and side effects (Table 5-5).

Ketamine

Ketamine is a phencyclidine derivative that produces dissociative anesthesia characterized by EEG evidence of dissociation between the thalamus and limbic system.[14] Induction of anesthesia is achieved in about 60 seconds after intravenous administration of ketamine (1 to 2 $mg \cdot kg^{-1}$) and within 2 to 4 minutes after intramuscular injection (5 to 10 $mg \cdot kg^{-1}$). Patients appear to be in cataleptic states in which the eyes remain open with a slow nystagmic gaze. Amnesia is present, and analgesia is intense. Various degrees of hypertonus and purposeful skeletal muscle movements can occur. Skeletal muscle tone helps maintain a patent upper airway, but the presence of protective upper airway reflexes should vomiting or regurgitation occur cannot be assumed.

Cardiovascular stimulation due principally to direct stimulation of sympathetic nervous system outflow from the central nervous system by ketamine is useful for induction of anesthesia and even maintenance of anesthesia in patients who are hypovolemic. These cardiac stimulant effects may be less or absent in the presence of catecholamine depletion. Furthermore, ketamine-induced cardiac stimulation may adversely increase myocardial oxygen requirements in patients with ischemic heart disease. Airway secretions are increased by ketamine, emphasizing the value of including anticholinergics in the preoperative medication when the use of this drug is planned. Decreases in airway resistance produced by sympathetic nervous system stimulation may be beneficial in patients with bronchial asthma. Ketamine is a potent cerebral vasodilator and predictably increases ICP in patients with space-occupying intracranial lesions. Allergic reactions do not seem to accompany the administration of ketamine.

Ketamine is highly lipid soluble and undergoes extensive hepatic metabolism. Redistribution to inactive tissues sites, as with barbiturates, is important in early awakening after administration of ketamine. Repeated anesthetics with ketamine, as is pop-

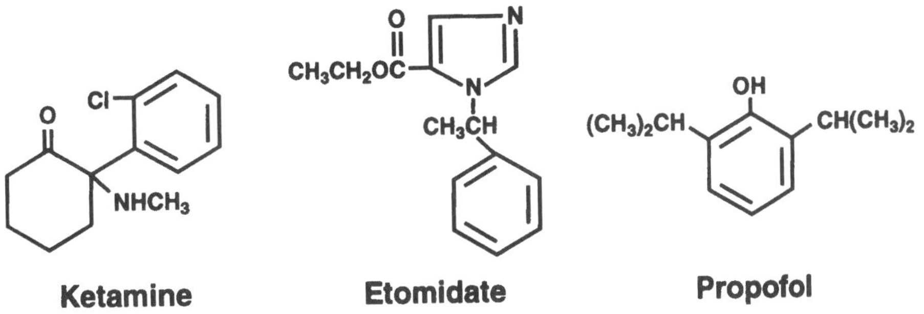

Figure 5-9. Chemical structures of miscellaneous intravenous induction drugs commonly administered in the perioperative period.

Table 5-5. Comparative Characteristics of Miscellaneous Induction Drugs

	Ketamine	Etomidate	Propofol
Elimination half-time (h)	1–2	2–5	0.5–1.5
Clearance ($ml \cdot kg^{-1} \cdot min^{-1}$)	16–18	10–20	30–60
Volume of distribution ($L \cdot kg^{-1}$)	2.5–3.5	2.2–4.5	3.5–4.5
Blood pressure	Increased	No change	Decreased
Heart rate	Increased	No change	Decreased
Analgesia	Intense	Minimal	Minimal
Emergence delirium	Yes	No	No(?)
Nausea and vomiting	No change	Increased	Decreased
Adrenocortical suppression	No	Yes	No

ular for burn dressing changes, may be associated with the development of tolerance, as manifest by progressive increases in dose requirements with each successive anesthetic.

Emergence from ketamine anesthesia may be associated with unpleasant visual, auditory, and proprioceptive illusions that may progress to delirium. The incidence of emergence delirium may approach 30%, causing many anesthesiologists to avoid the use of this drug. Administration of benzodiazepines, either preoperatively or after the induction of anesthesia, can decrease the incidence of emergence reactions associated with ketamine.

Etomidate

Etomidate is a carboxylated imidazole derivative that produces rapid intravenous induction of anesthesia (unconsciousness in less than 30 seconds) followed by awakening that is more prompt than after administration of barbiturates. Rapid awakening reflects nearly complete hydrolysis of etomidate to pharmacologically inactive metabolites. Cardiovascular stability is characteristic of patients receiving etomidate, suggesting that this drug may be useful in patients with limited cardiac reserve. Blood pressure declines are modest and reflect principally decreases in systemic vascular resistance. These blood pressure changes would likely be exaggerated in the presence of hypovolemia. Etomidate decreases cerebral blood flow, $CMRO_2$, and ICP and, like methohexital, activates seizure foci.

Disadvantages of etomidate include pain during intravenous injection, involuntary skeletal muscle movements, and an increased incidence of postoperative nausea and vomiting. More important, etomidate suppresses adrenocortical function for up to 8 hours after an induction dose.[15] During this time, the adrenal cortex is not responsive to adrenocorticotropic hormone. Theoretically, this suppression may be desirable for stress-free anesthesia or undesirable if it prevents useful protective responses against stresses that accompany the perioperative period.

Propofol

Propofol is a lipid soluble substituted isopropylphenol that produces rapid induction of anesthesia (unconsciousness in less than 30 seconds after 2 to 2.5 $mg \cdot kg^{-1}$ IV) followed by awakening in 4 to 8 minutes.[16] This awakening is more rapid and complete than following intravenous induction of anesthesia with any other anesthetic. The more rapid return to consciousness with minimal residual central nervous system effects is the most important advantage of propofol, especially for outpatient surgery or otherwise brief procedures. Hepatic metabolism to inactive metabolites is rapid, but distribution to inactive tissue sites also plays an important role in early awakening.

Maintenance of anesthesia with a continuous infusion of propofol (0.1 to 0.2 $mg \cdot kg^{-1} \cdot min^{-1}$ IV) plus an opioid or inhaled anesthetic (most often nitrous oxide) is associated with prompt awakening. Signs of light anesthesia (hypertension, tachycardia, diaphoresis, skeletal muscle movement) are used as indicators for the need to increase the intravenous infusion rate of propofol or to administer a supplemental dose (25 to 50 mg IV). The efficient clearance of propofol from the plasma minimizes the likelihood of cumulative drug effects. Sedation during regional anesthesia may also be provided with intermittent intravenous doses of propofol or a continuous infusion (0.025 to 0.05 $mg \cdot kg^{-1} \cdot min^{-1}$ IV) titrated to the desired effect.

Depressant effects of propofol on blood pressure and ventilation resemble, but may exceed, those produced by barbiturates. Awake patients are likely to experience pain at the intravenous injection site of propofol for induction of anesthesia. Prior administration of lidocaine into the vein may attenuate this pain. The solvent for propofol (Intralipid) does not contain antibacterial preservatives, emphasizing the importance of maintaining strict asepsis when handling this drug. An antiemetic effect of propofol is suggested by the low incidence of nausea and vomiting in patients receiving this drug. Life-threatening allergic reactions may follow the administration of propofol, especially to patients with a history of atopy or allergy to other drugs that, like propofol, contain a phenyl nucleus or isopropyl group.[17] The administration of propofol to patients with known seizure disorders may be avoided in view of the occasional development of seizures and opisthotonos following use of this drug.[18] Patient excitement has been observed on emergence from propofol anesthesia.

REFERENCES

1. Filner BF, Karliner JS. Alterations of normal left ventricular performance by general anesthesia. Anesthesiology 1976;45:610–20.
2. Saidman LJ. Uptake, distribution, and elimination of barbiturates. In: Eger EI, ed. Anesthetic Uptake and Action. Baltimore, Williams & Wilkins, 1974;264–84.
3. Hudson RJ, Stanski DR, Burch PG. Pharmacokinetics of methohexital and thiopental in surgical patients. Anesthesiology 1983;59:215–9.
4. Mohler H, Richards JG. The benzodiazepine receptor: A pharmacological control element of brain function. Eur J Anesthesiol 1988;2:15–24.
5. Reves JG, Fragen RJ, Vinik HR, Greenblatt DJ. Midazolam: Pharmacology and uses. Anesthesiology 1985;62:310–24.
6. Sarnquist FH, Mathers WD, Brock-Utne J, Carr B, Canup C, Brown CR. A bioassay of a water-soluble benzodiazepine against sodium thiopental. Anesthesiology 1980;52:149–53.
7. Pasternak GW. Multiple morphine and enkephalin receptors and the relief of pain. JAMA 1988;259:1362–7.
8. Rosow CE, Moss J, Philbin DM, Savarese JJ. Histamine release during morphine and fentanyl anesthesia. Anesthesiology 1982;56:93–6.
9. Benthuysen JL, Smith NT, Sanford TJ, Head N, Dec-Silver H. Physiology of alfentanil-induced rigidity. Anesthesiology 1986;64:440–6.
10. Sperry RJ, Bailey PL, Reichman MV, Peterson JC, Petersen PB, Pace NL. Fentanyl and sufentanil increase intracranial pressure in head trauma patients. Anesthesiology 1992;77:416–20.
11. Becker LD, Paulson BA, Miller RD, Severinghaus JW, Eger EI II. Biphasic respiratory depression after fentanyl-droperidol or fentanyl alone used to supplement nitrous oxide anesthesia. Anesthesiology 1976;44:291–6.
12. Nauta J, deLange S, Koopman D, Spierdijk J, vanKleff J, Stanley TH. Anesthetic induction with alfentanil: A new short-acting narcotic analgesic. Anesth Analg 1982;61:267–72.
13. Sanford TJ, Smith NT, Dec-Silver H, Harrison WK. A comparison of morphine, fentanyl and sufentanil anesthesia for cardiac surgery. Induction, emergence and extubation. Anesth Analg 1986;65:259–66.
14. Reich DL, Silvay G. Ketamine: An update on the first twenty-five years of clinical experience. Can J Anaesth 1989;36:186–97.
15. Wagner RL, White PF, Kan PB, Rosenthal MH, Feldman D. Inhibition of adrenal steroidogenesis by the anesthetic etomidate. N Engl J Med 1984;310:1415–21.
16. Sebel PS, Lowdon JD. Propofol: A new intravenous anesthetic. Anesthesiology 1989;71:260–77.
17. Laxenaire M-C, Mata-Bernejo E, Moneret-Vautrin D, Gueant J-L. Life-threatening anaphylactoid reactions to propofol (Diprivan). Anesthesiology 1992;77:275–80.
18. Finley GA, MacManus B, Simpson SE, Fernandez CV, Retallick R. Delayed seizures following sedation with propofol. Can J Anaesth 1993;40:863–5.

6
Local Anesthetics

Local anesthetics, when placed in proximity to nerve membranes, produce reversible conduction blockade of neural impulses. Progressive increases in the concentrations of local anesthetics result in interruption of transmission of autonomic, sensory, and motor neural impulses and hence produce autonomic nervous system blockade, sensory anesthesia, and skeletal muscle paralysis in the areas innervated by the affected nerves. Subsequent recovery from the effects of local anesthetics is spontaneous and complete without evidence of damage to the nerve fibers.

HISTORY

Since prehistoric times, the natives of Peru have chewed the leaves of the indigenous plant, *Erythroxylon coca,* the source of cocaine, to induce a feeling of well-being and decreased fatigue. Cocaine was introduced into clinical medicine by Koller in 1884 as a topical anesthetic for the cornea. The ability of cocaine to produce psychological dependence and its irritant properties when placed topically or around nerves led to a search for a better local anesthetic. The first synthetic local anesthetic, procaine, was introduced by Einhorn in 1905. Lidocaine, synthesized in 1943 by Lofgren, is the present-day prototype local anesthetic with which all other such drugs are compared.

GENERAL PHARMACOLOGY

Structure Activity Relationships

Local anesthetics consist of lipophilic (unsaturated benzene ring) and hydrophilic (tertiary amine and proton acceptor) portions separated by a hydrocarbon connecting chain. Linkage of the hydrocarbon chain to the lipophilic portion is by an ester (—CO—) or amide (—HNC—) bond. The nature of this bond is the basis for classifying local anesthetics as esters or amides (Fig. 6-1). Important differences between ester and amide local anesthetics relate to the site of metabolism and the potential to produce allergic reactions.

Mechanism of Action

Local anesthetics produce conduction blockade of neural impulses by preventing passage of sodium ions through ion selective sodium channels in nerve membranes. It is likely that local anesthetics stabilize and maintain sodium channels in the inactivated closed states by binding to specific receptors located in the inner portion of sodium channels.[1] Local anesthetics may also prevent changes in sodium permeability by obstructing sodium channels near their external openings. Failure of permeability to sodium ions to increase slows the rate of depolarization such that the threshold potential is not reached and an action potential is not propagated along the nerve membrane (Fig. 6-2). Local anesthetics do not alter the resting transmembrane potential or threshold potential. They are marketed as hydrochloride salts, which are water soluble. When injected into tissues, the free base form of the local anesthetic penetrates many layers of tissue to reach the nerve axon, where the cationic form acts on the sodium channel.

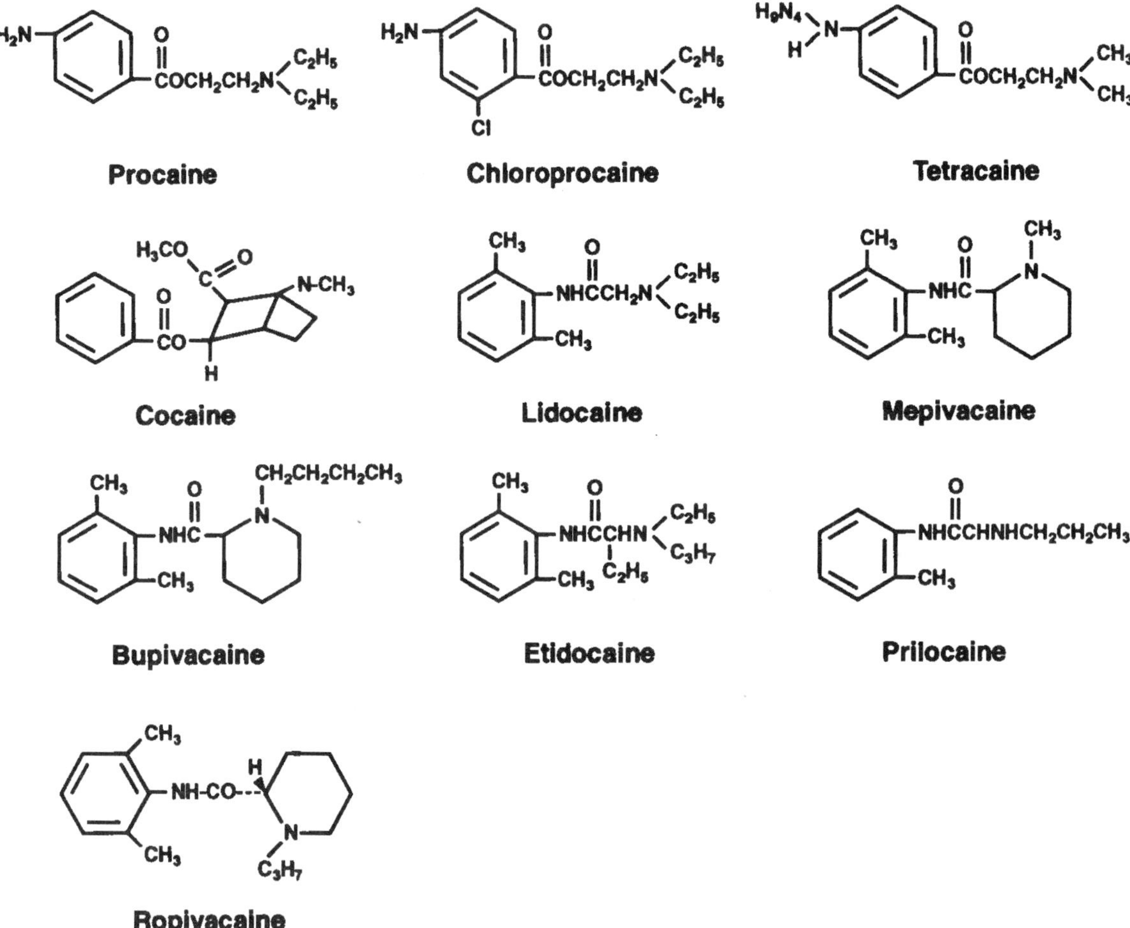

Figure 6-1. Chemical structures of ester (procaine, chloroprocaine, tetracaine, cocaine) and amide (lidocaine, mepivacaine, bupivacaine, etidocaine, prilocaine, ropivacaine) local anesthetics.

Frequency-Dependent Blockade

Frequency-dependent blockade reflects recovery from local anesthetic-induced conduction blockade between action potentials and development of additional conduction blockade each time sodium channels open during an action potential. This emphasizes that local anesthetics gain access to receptors only when sodium channels are in activated-open states (not in the inactivated-closed and rested-closed states). For this reason, selective conduction blockade of nerve fibers by local anesthetics may be related to the characteristic frequencies of activity of the nerve.

Classification of Nerves and Sensitivity to Local Anesthetics

Nerve fibers can be classified according to fiber diameter, presence (type A and B) or absence (type C) of myelin, and function (Table 6-1). Nerve fiber diameter and degree of myelination in turn determine the conduction velocity. Myelin increases conduction velocity and makes the nerve membrane more susceptible to local anesthetic-induced conduction blockade by insulating the axolemma from the surrounding media and forcing the current to flow through periodic interruptions in the myelin sheath (nodes of Ranvier). The classic concept relat-

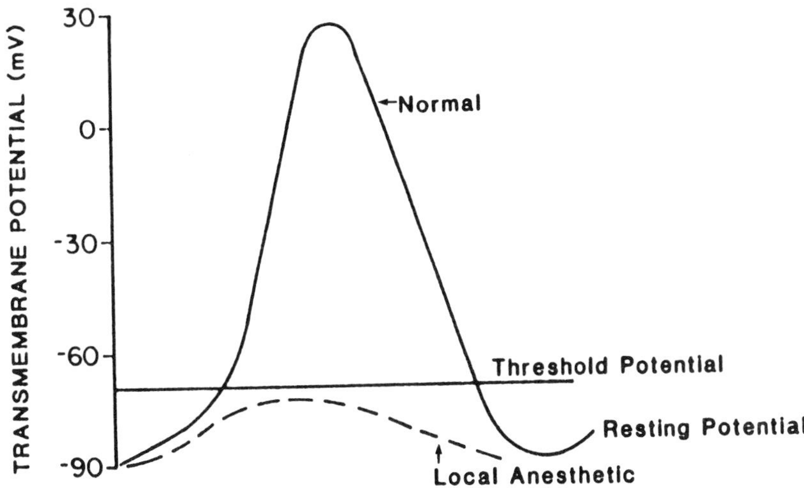

Figure 6-2. Local anesthetics slow the rate of depolarization of the nerve action potential such that the threshold potential is not reached. As a result, an action potential cannot be propagated in the presence of local anesthetics and conduction blockade occurs.

ing sensitivity to local anesthetic blockade to nerve fiber diameter (small diameter fibers are more sensitive than large diameter fibers) may be incorrect. In fact, there is evidence that large myelinated fibers are more sensitive to local anesthetic blockade than the smaller unmyelinated fibers.[2] Nevertheless, placement of a local anesthetic solution in the subarachnoid space produces conduction blockade of small diameter nerve fibers first, because the anatomy of the dorsal nerve roots is such that small diameter nerve fibers are close to the nerve root surface (which shortens the diffusion distance for the local

Table 6-1. Classification of Nerve Fibers

Fiber Type	Diameter (μm)	Conduction Velocity ($m \cdot s^{-1}$)	Sensitivity to Local Anesthetic[a] (%)	Function
A (myelinated)				
Alpha	12–20	100	1	Proprioception Large motor
Beta	5–12	[b]	1	Small motor Touch Pressure
Gamma	3–6	[b]	1	Muscle tone
Delta	2–5	5	0.5	Temperature Sharp pain
B (myelinated)	3	3–14	0.25	Preganglionic autonomic
C (unmyelinated)	0.3–1.2	1.2	0.5	Dull pain Temperature Touch

[a]Subarachnoid procaine.
[b]Conduction velocity decreases progressively from type A alpha to delta fibers.

anesthetic). The diffusion path to the large diameter nerve fibers, which are situated deep in the dorsal nerve root, is longer, making it appear that the small diameter nerve fibers are more sensitive to local anesthetic blockade than the large diameter nerve fibers. Indeed the minimum concentration of local anesthetic ([Cm] which is analogous to the MAC of inhaled anesthetics) required to block nerve conduction is greater in large diameter nerve fibers. The Cm of motor fibers is about twice that of sensory fibers, emphasizing that sensory anesthesia may not be accompanied by skeletal muscle paralysis.

There is a minimal length of myelinated nerve fiber that must be exposed to an adequate concentration of local anesthetic for conduction blockade of nerve impulses to occur. For example, if only one node of Ranvier is blocked (site of changes in sodium permeability), neural impulses can bypass this node and conduction blockade does not occur. Conduction blockade is predictably present if at least three successive nodes of Ranvier are exposed to adequate concentrations of local anesthetics. Both types of pain-conducting fibers (myelinated type A delta and nonmyelinated type C fibers) are blocked by similar concentrations of local anesthetics despite differences in diameters of these fibers. Preganglionic type B fibers are more readily blocked by local anesthetics than any fiber, even though these fibers are larger in diameter than type C fibers. Presumably, the presence of myelin and its relatively small diameter make these fibers especially susceptible to blockade by local anesthetics.

Spread of Anesthesia and Peripheral Nerve Blockade

When local anesthetics are deposited around a peripheral nerve, they diffuse from the outer surface (mantle) toward the center (core) of the nerve along a concentration gradient (Fig. 6-3).[3] As a result, nerve fibers located in the mantle of the mixed nerve are blocked first. These mantle fibers are often distributed to more proximal anatomic structures, in contrast to distal structures innervated by nerve fibers near the core of the nerve. This explains the initial development of analgesia proximally with subsequent distal spread as local anesthetics diffuse to reach more central core nerve fibers. Skeletal muscle paralysis may precede the onset of sensory blockade if motor nerve fibers are distributed peripheral to sensory fibers in the mixed peripheral nerve. Indeed, the sequence of onset and recovery from conduction blockade of sympathetic, sensory, and motor nerve fibers in a mixed peripheral nerve probably depend as much on the anatomic location of the nerve fibers within the mixed nerve as on their sensitivity to local anesthetics.

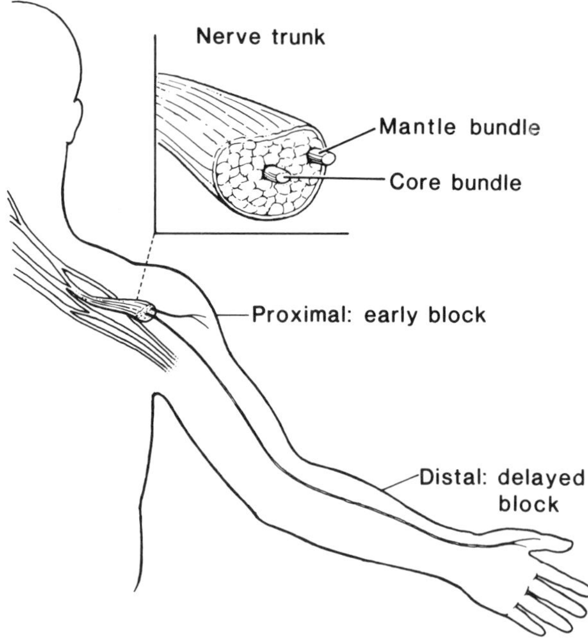

Figure 6-3. Local anesthetics deposited around a peripheral nerve diffuse along a concentration gradient to block nerve fibers on the outer surface (mantle) before more centrally located (core) fibers. This accounts for early manifestations of anesthesia in more proximal areas of the extremity.

PHARMACOKINETICS

The pKa of local anesthetics is such that less than one-half the total local anesthetic exists in a lipid soluble nonionized form at physiologic pH (Table 6-2). This is important because the nonionized form of local anesthetic is necessary to cross the lipophilic nerve sheath to gain access to sodium channels in the nerve membrane. This is consistent with the observation that local tissue acidosis as produced by infection is associated with low-quality local anesthesia, presumably reflecting an increased ionized drug fraction that limits the amount of drug available to act on sodium channels.

Lipid solubility is a primary determinant of local anesthetic potency. Peak plasma concentrations of

Table 6-2. Comparative Pharmacology of Local Anesthetics

Classification	Potency	Onset	Duration After Infiltration (min)	Maximum Single Dose for Infiltration[a] (Adult, mg)	Toxic Plasma Concentration (μg·ml⁻¹)	pKa	Nonionized (%) pH 7.2	pH 7.4	pH 7.6
Esters									
Procaine	1[b]	Rapid	45–60	500		8.9	2	3	5
Chloroprocaine	4	Rapid	30–45	600		8.7	3	5	7
Tetracaine	16	Slow	60–180	100 (topical)		8.5	5	7	11
Amides									
Lidocaine	1[c]	Rapid	60–120	300	>5	7.9	17	25	33
Mepivacaine	1	Slow	90–180	300	>5	7.6	28	39	50
Bupivacaine	4	Slow	240–480	175	~1.5	8.1	11	15	24
Etidocaine	4	Slow	240–480	300	~2	7.7	24	33	44
Prilocaine	1	Slow	60–120	400	>5	7.9	17	24	33
Ropivacaine[d]					>4	8.1			

[a]Use only as a guideline; dose may be increased if solution contains epinephrine.
[b]Standard of comparison for esters.
[c]Standard of comparison for amides.
[d]Resembles bupivacaine.

local anesthetics after their absorption from tissue injection sites are ultimately determined by the rate of tissue distribution and rate of clearance of the drug. Clearance of local anesthetics represent hydrolysis of ester drugs, whereas amide local anesthetics undergo metabolism by hepatic microsomal enzymes. The lungs are also capable of extracting local anesthetics such as lidocaine, bupivacaine, and prilocaine from the circulation. The rate of this hepatic metabolism and/or first pass pulmonary extraction influences systemic toxicity. For example, rapid metabolism prevents accumulation of local anesthetics in the plasma and systemic toxicity is unlikely (see the section *Systemic Toxicity*). In this regard, ester local anesthetics (hydrolysis of chloroprocaine is more rapid than tetracaine) may be less likely to produce sustained plasma concentrations and resultant systemic toxicity than the more slowly metabolized amide local anesthetics (lidocaine is metabolized more rapidly than bupivacaine). Patients with atypical plasma cholinesterase enzyme may be at increased risk of developing excessive plasma concentrations of ester local anesthetics due to absent or limited plasma hydrolysis. Hepatic metabolism of lidocaine is extensive, such that clearance of this local anesthetic from the plasma parallels hepatic blood flow. Liver disease or decreases in hepatic blood flow as occur during congestive heart failure or general anesthesia can decrease the rate of metabolism of lidocaine. Metabolites of lidocaine, like the parent compound, possess cardiac antidysrhythmic effects (Fig. 6-4). Low water solubility of local anesthetics limits renal excretion of unchanged drug to usually less than 5% of the injected dose.

Vasoconstrictors

Addition of epinephrine (1:200,000, 5 μg·ml⁻¹) or phenylephrine (2 mg) to local anesthetic solutions that are to be injected produces local tissue vasoconstriction, which limits systemic absorption and prolongs the duration of action of local anesthetics by keeping them in contact with nerve fibers (see Chapter 12). Decreased systemic absorption of local anesthetics produced by epinephrine increases the likelihood that the rate of metabolism will match the rate of absorption, thus decreasing the possibility of systemic toxicity. The addition of epinephrine to local anesthetic solutions has little if any effect on the rate of onset of local anesthesia, although bleeding in the area infiltrated is decreased owing to

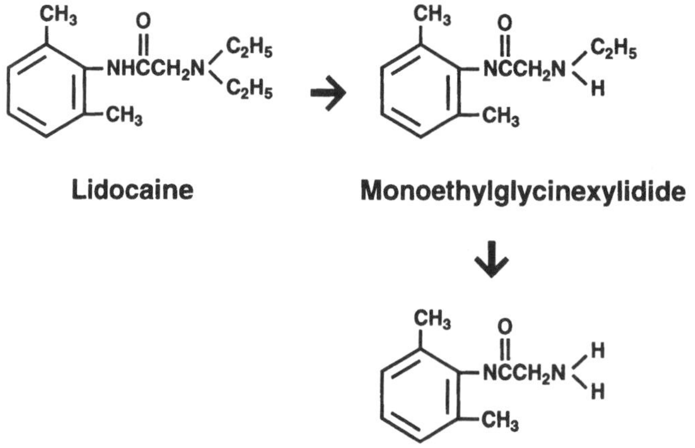

Lidocaine

Monoethylglycinexylidide

Xylidide

Figure 6-4. Metabolism of lidocaine results in metabolites with cardiac antidysrhythmic properties.

drug-induced vasoconstriction. Systemic absorption of epinephrine may contribute to cardiac dysrhythmias in the presence of volatile anesthetics or accentuate hypertension in vulnerable patients. Indeed, there are situations in which the addition of epinephrine to the local anesthetic solution is not recommended.

Addition of Epinephrine to Local Anesthetic Solutions Is Not Recommended

Unstable angina pectoris
Cardiac dysrhythmias
Uncontrolled hypertension
Uteroplacental insufficiency
Peripheral nerve block anesthesia in areas that may lack collateral blood flow (digits, penis)
Intravenous regional anesthesia

SIDE EFFECTS

Systemic toxicity, neurotoxicity, and allergic reactions represent rare but important side effects associated with use of local anesthetics.

Systemic Toxicity

Systemic toxicity of local anesthetics is due to excess plasma concentrations of these drugs, most often as a result of accidental intravascular injection of local anesthetic solutions during performance of nerve blocks. Less often, excess plasma concentrations of local anesthetics result from absorption of local anesthetics from tissue injection sites. The magnitude of this systemic absorption depends on the (1) dose injected, (2) vascularity of the injection site, and (3) inclusion of a vasoconstrictor in the local anesthetic solutions. Establishment of maximal acceptable local anesthetic doses for use during performance of regional anesthesia is an attempt to limit plasma concentrations that result from systemic absorption of these drugs (Table 6-2). Systemic absorption of local anesthetics is greatest after injection for intercostal nerve blocks and caudal anesthesia, intermediate following epidural anesthesia, and least after brachial plexus blocks (Fig. 6-5).[4]

Systemic toxicity of local anesthetics manifests most prominently as changes in the central nervous system and cardiovascular system.

Central Nervous System

Increasing plasma concentrations of local anesthetics are associated initially with restlessness, vertigo, tinnitus, and slurred speech culminating in tonic-clonic seizures. Seizures can be followed by central

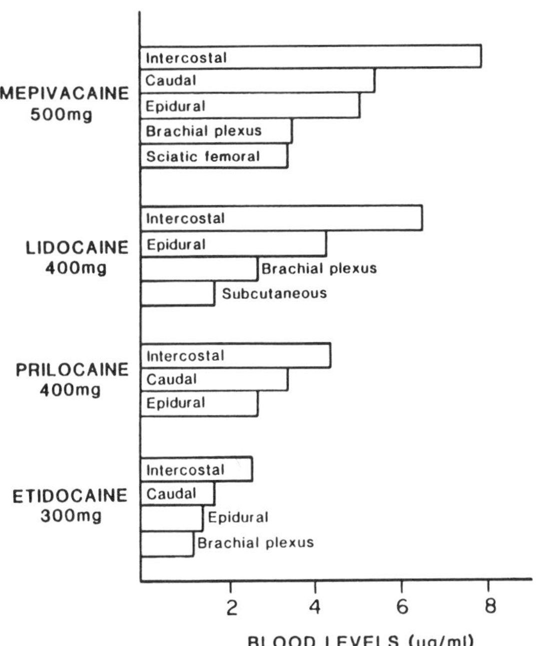

Figure 6-5. Peak plasma concentrations of local anesthetics resulting during performance of various types of regional anesthetic procedures. (From Covino and Vassallo,[4] with permission.)

nervous system depression (apnea) and death. The onset of seizures may reflect selective depression of inhibitory cortical neurons by local anesthetics, leaving excitatory pathways unopposed.

Seizures. Treatment of local anesthetic-induced seizures includes administration of drugs to stop seizures and of supplemental oxygen, as arterial hypoxemia and metabolic acidosis can occur rapidly. Hyperventilation of the lungs decreases delivery of additional local anesthetic to the brain, whereas associated respiratory alkalosis and hypokalemia result in hyperpolarization of nerve membranes and decreased local anesthetic effects. Diazepam (0.1 mg·kg^{-1} IV) is effective in stopping local anesthetic-induced seizures, most likely by exerting specific effects on the temporal lobe or amygdala. Small doses of thiopental (0.5 to 2 mg·kg^{-1} IV) also stop seizures (and have a shorter duration of action than does diazepam), but their site of action in the central nervous system is nonspecific. Paralyzing doses of rapidly acting muscle relaxants stop peripheral but not central nervous system manifestations of seizure activity. Administration of muscle relaxants followed by intubation of the trachea is indicated when benzodiazepines or barbiturates are not promptly effective in stopping seizure activity. Placement of a cuffed tracheal tube decreases the likelihood of pulmonary aspiration of gastric contents and facilitates delivery of oxygen to the lungs.

Cardiovascular System

The cardiovascular system is more resistant to toxic effects of local anesthetics than is the central nervous system. Nevertheless, high plasma concentrations of local anesthetics can produce profound hypotension due to relaxation of arteriolar vascular smooth muscle and direct myocardial depression. Part of the cardiac toxicity reflects the ability of local anesthetics to block cardiac sodium channels. As a result, cardiac automaticity and conduction of cardiac impulses are impaired, manifesting on the electrocardiogram as prolongation of the P-R interval and widening of the QRS complex. Local anesthetics differ in their ability to produce cardiotoxicity. For example, the ratio of cardiovascular to central nervous system toxicity is 4 with lidocaine and 2 with bupivacaine. Thus, bupivacaine has a greater tendency to produce cardiotoxicity than does lidocaine. The cardiotoxicity of ropivacaine (unique among local anesthetics because it is prepared as an isomer rather than a racemic mixture) is intermediate between those of lidocaine and bupivacaine.[5]

Selective Cardiac Toxicity. Accidental intravenous injection of bupivacaine may result in precipitous hypotension, cardiac dysrhythmias (including ventricular tachycardia and fibrillation), and atrioventricular heart block.[6] Pregnancy may increase sensitivity to cardiotoxic effects of bupivacaine (Fig. 6-6).[7] Bupivacaine depresses the rapid phase of depolarization in Purkinje fibers and ventricular muscle more than lidocaine does. Probably of more importance is the slow dissociation of highly lipid soluble bupivacaine from cardiac sodium channels (fast-in, slow-out local anesthetic), accounting for its exaggerated and persistent depressant effects on cardiac function. By contrast, less lipid soluble lidocaine leaves sodium channels rapidly (fast-in, fast-out local anesthetic) and cardiac toxicity is low. In an effort to minimize the potential for cardiotoxicity should accidental intravascular injection occur, the maximum recommended concentration of bupivacaine to be used for epidural anesthesia in obstetric anesthesia is 0.5%.

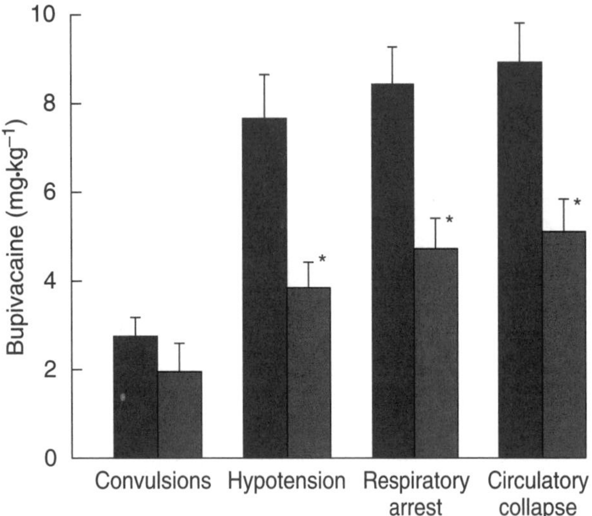

Figure 6-6. The dose of bupivacaine (mean ± SE) required to produce toxic effects is lower in pregnant (red bars) than in nonpregnant (black bars) ewes (**P* <0.05) (From Morishima et al.,[7] with permission.)

Methemoglobinemia

Prilocaine administered in large doses (higher than 600 mg) may result in accumulation of the metabolite, *ortho*-toluidine, an oxidizing compound capable of converting hemoglobin to methemoglobin. When sufficient methemoglobin is present, patients may appear cyanotic and the blood may be chocolate-colored. Methemoglobin production is readily reversed by the administration of methylene blue (1 to 2 $mg \cdot kg^{-1}$ IV). Nevertheless, the unique ability of prilocaine to cause dose-related methemoglobinemia limits the clinical usefulness of this local anesthetic.

Neurotoxicity

Local anesthetics are not neurotoxic when administered at recommended concentrations, except for chloroprocaine, which is not recommended for intravenous regional anesthesia or spinal anesthesia because of potential irritant effects. For example, accidental injection of large volumes of chloroprocaine into the subarachnoid space during the intended performance of epidural anesthesia may result in prolonged or even permanent neurologic damage. It is possible that these neurotoxic effects are due to a low pH (3.0) of the anesthetic solution and sodium bisulfite, an antioxidant in chloroprocaine, and thus are not a unique effect of the local anesthetic.[8] Newer preparations of chloroprocaine do not contain bisulfite.

Allergic Reactions

Allergic reactions to local anesthetics are rare, despite the frequent use of these drugs. Indeed, it is estimated that fewer than 1% of all adverse reactions to local anesthetics are due to allergic mechanisms. This emphasizes that the vast majority of adverse responses that are often attributed to allergic reactions are in fact manifestations of systemic toxicity due to excessive plasma concentrations of the drug.

Ester local anesthetics that produce metabolites related to *para*-aminobenzoic acid are more likely to evoke allergic reactions than are amide local anesthetics, which are not metabolized to *para*-aminobenzoic acid. Allergic reactions following use of local anesthetics may be due to methylparaben or similar substances used as preservatives in commercial preparations of ester and amide local anesthetics. These preservatives resemble *para*-aminobenzoic acid and may be responsible for stimulation of antibody production and subsequent allergic reactions independent of the local anesthetic. Cross-sensitivity does not exist between classes of local anesthetics. Therefore, patients known to be allergic to ester local anesthetics could receive amide local anesthetics. This recommendation, however, assumes that the local anesthetic and not preservatives, which may be common to both classes of drugs, was responsible for evoking the initial allergic reaction.

Documentation of allergy to local anesthetics is based on clinical history (rash, laryngeal edema, hypotension, bronchospasm) and perhaps use of intradermal testing with preservative-free solutions. Hypotension associated with syncope, tachycardia, or bradycardia when epinephrine-containing local anesthetic solutions are used is more suggestive of an accidental intravascular injection or a psychogenic-vagally mediated reaction than of an allergic reaction.

CLINICAL USES

Local anesthetics are used most often to produce regional anesthesia. Occasional unique uses of lidocaine include its intravenous administration to (1) prevent or treat cardiac ventricular dysrhythmias, (2) attenuate pressor responses associated with intu-

Table 6-3. Use of Local Anesthetics to Produce Regional Anesthesia

	Topical Anesthesia	Local Infiltration	Intravenous Regional	Peripheral Nerve Block	Epidural Anesthesia	Spinal Anesthesia
Procaine	No	Yes	No	Yes	No	Yes[a]
Chloroprocaine	No	Yes	No	Yes	Yes	No
Tetracaine	Yes	No	No	No	No	Yes[b]
Lidocaine	Yes	Yes	Yes	Yes	Yes	Yes
Mepivacaine	No	Yes	No	Yes[c]	Yes	No
Bupivacaine	No	Yes	No	Yes	Yes[d]	Yes
Etidocaine	No	Yes	No	Yes	Yes[e]	No
Prilocaine	No	Yes	Yes	Yes	Yes	No
Ropivacaine	No	?	?	Yes	Yes	?

[a]Used for differential spinal.
[b]Greater motor blockade but shorter duration of sensory anesthesia than bupivacaine.
[c]Longer sensory and greater motor blockade than lidocaine; useful when epinephrine contraindicated (Table 6-2).
[d]Sensory anesthesia greater than motor blockade.
[e]Motor blockade greater than sensory anesthesia.

bation of the trachea, (3) prevent or treat increases in intracranial pressure as are often associated with intubation of the trachea, and (4) minimize coughing during intubation or extubation of the trachea.

Regional anesthesia is classified according to the site of the local anesthetic placement as (1) topical or surface anesthesia, (2) local or subcutaneous infiltration anesthesia, (3) intravenous regional neural anesthesia (Bier block), and (4) nerve block anesthesia (Table 6-3). Nerve block anesthesia is produced by injection of local anesthetics into the epidural or subarachnoid spaces or near specific nerves (peripheral nerve anesthesia) to selectively produce anesthesia in areas innervated by the affected nerves (see Chapters 12 and 13).

Topical Anesthesia

Local anesthetics are used to produce topical anesthesia by placement on mucous membranes of areas such as the nose, mouth, or tracheobronchial tree. For example, lidocaine may be applied topically on the pharynx and trachea before intubation of the trachea. Tetracaine is an effective topical anesthetic and is commonly used to provide topical anesthesia for bronchoscopy. Procaine and chloroprocaine penetrate mucous membranes poorly and are not effective topical anesthetics.

Cocaine

Cocaine has the unique advantage of producing topical anesthesia and vasoconstriction (prevents uptake of norepinephrine back into postganglionic adrenergic nerve endings). Vasoconstriction produced by intranasal administration of cocaine is useful in decreasing the likelihood of nasal hemorrhage due to nasotracheal intubation (see Chapter 11). Administration of cocaine in doses used for topical anesthesia in rhinolaryngologic procedures may cause vasoconstriction of the coronary arteries. It is presumed that these effects would be more pronounced with the recreational use of cocaine. Cocaine-induced cardiovascular effects may manifest as myocardial ischemia, cardiac dysrhythmias, and hypertension (cerebrovascular accidents). Administration of topical cocaine plus epinephrine, or in the presence of volatile anesthetics that sensitize the myocardium, may exaggerate the cardiac stimulating effects of cocaine. Cardiovascular toxicity due to cocaine may be treated with esmolol to maintain the heart rate at less than 100 beats·min^{-1}, whereas seizures respond to diazepam.[9]

Local Infiltration Anesthesia

Local infiltration of local anesthetics is designed to produce sensory anesthesia in the injected area without any attempt to block specific nerves. For example, lidocaine is commonly injected into the area chosen for placement of an intravenous catheter.

REFERENCES

1. Butterworth JF, Strichartz GR. Molecular mechanisms of local anesthesia: A review. Anesthesiology 1990; 72:722–34.

2. Gissen AJ, Covino BG, Gregus J. Differential sensitivities of mammalian nerve fibers to local anesthetic agents. Anesthesiology 1980;53:467–73.
3. Winnie AP, Tay C-H, Patel KP, Ramamurthy S, Durrainie Z. Pharmacokinetics of local anesthetics during plexus blocks. Anesth Analg 1977;56:852–61.
4. Covino BG, Vassallo HG. Local Anesthetics: Mechanisms of Action in Clinical Use. Orlando, FL, Grune & Stratton 1976.
5. Moller R, Covino BG. Cardiac electrophysiologic properties of bupivacaine and lidocaine compared with those of ropivacaine, a new amide local anesthetic. Anesthesiology 1990;72:322–9.
6. Atlee JL, Bosnjak BJ. Mechanisms for dysrhythmias during anesthesia. Anesthesiology 1990;72:347–74.
7. Morishima HO, Pederson H, Finster M, et al. Bupivacaine toxicity in pregnant and nonpregnant ewes. Anesthesiology 1985;63:134–9.
8. Wang BC, Hillman DE, Spielholz NI, Turndorf H. Chronic neurological deficits and Nesacaine-CE: An effect of the anesthetic 2-chloroprocaine, or the antioxidant, sodium bisulfite. Anesth Analg 1984;63: 445–7.
9. Pollan S, Tadjziechy M. Esmolol in the management of epinephrine and cocaine-induced cardiovascular toxicity. Anesth Analg 1989;69:663–4.

7

Muscle Relaxants

Muscle relaxants are drugs that interrupt transmission of neural impulses at the neuromuscular junction. As such, these drugs are more accurately described as neuromuscular blockers. Nevertheless, the designation as muscle relaxants remains a commonly used and accepted term. Skeletal muscle relaxation can also be achieved by high doses of volatile anesthetics or regional anesthesia. Muscle relaxants used clinically are classified as depolarizing or nondepolarizing.

The principal uses of muscle relaxants are to provide skeletal muscle relaxation to facilitate intubation of the trachea and to provide optimal surgical working conditions. Muscle relaxants may also be administered in the intensive care setting to facilitate mechanical ventilation of the lungs. It is essential to recognize that muscle relaxants lack anesthetic or analgesic effects and must not be used to render an inadequately anesthetized patient immobile. Ventilation of the lungs must be mechanically provided whenever significant skeletal muscle weakness is produced by these drugs. Clinically, intraoperative evaluation of neuromuscular blockade is typically provided by visually monitoring the mechanical response (twitch response) produced by an electrical stimulus delivered from a peripheral nerve stimulator (see the section *Monitoring the Effects of Muscle Relaxants*).

The choice of muscle relaxant is influenced by its speed of onset, duration of action, route of elimination, and associated side effects such as drug-induced changes in arterial blood pressure and/or heart rate. A rapid onset and brief duration of skeletal muscle paralysis, as provided by succinylcholine, is useful when intubation of the trachea is the reason for administering a muscle relaxant. When longer periods of neuromuscular blockade are needed, succinylcholine can be administered as a continuous intravenous infusion or nondepolarizing muscle relaxants can be selected. When rapid onset of skeletal muscle paralysis is not necessary, it is acceptable to produce skeletal muscle relaxation by administration of nondepolarizing muscle relaxants to facilitate intubation of the trachea.

NEUROMUSCULAR JUNCTION

The neuromuscular junction consists of a prejunctional motor nerve ending separated from the highly folded postjunctional membrane of the skeletal muscle by a synaptic cleft (Fig. 7-1).[1] Neuromuscular transmission is initiated by arrival of an impulse at the motor nerve terminal with an associated influx of calcium and a resultant release of the neurotransmitter acetylcholine. Acetylcholine binds to nicotinic cholinergic receptors on postjunctional membranes, causing a change in membrane permeability to ions, principally potassium and sodium. This change in permeability and movement of ions causes a decrease in the transmembrane potential from about –90 to –45 mV (threshold potential), at which point a propagated action potential spreads over the surfaces of skeletal muscle fibers, leading to muscular contraction. Acetylcholine is rapidly hydrolyzed (within 15 ms) by the enzyme acetylcholinesterase (true cholinesterase), thus restoring membrane per-

Classification of Muscle Relaxants

Depolarizing
- Succinylcholine

Nondepolarizing
- Long-acting
  - *d*-Tubocurarine
  - Metocurine
  - Gallamine
  - Pancuronium
  - Pipecuronium
  - Doxacurium
- Intermediate-acting
  - Atracurium
  - Vecuronium
  - Rocuronium
- Short-acting
  - Mivacurium

meability (repolarization) and preventing sustained depolarization. Acetylcholinesterase is primarily located in the folds of the endplate region, placing it in close proximity to the site of action of acetylcholine.

Nicotinic Cholinergic Receptors

Nicotinic cholinergic receptors are situated on both the prejunctional and postjunctional membranes. Prejunctional receptors influence the release of acetylcholine. Postjunctional receptors are confined to the area of the endplate precisely opposite prejunctional receptors, and extrajunctional receptors are present throughout skeletal muscle. Postjunctional receptors are the most important sites of action of muscle relaxants. Extrajunctional receptor synthesis is normally suppressed by neural activity. Denervation or trauma (burn injury) to skeletal muscle may be associated with a proliferation of extrajunctional receptors. When activated, extrajunctional receptors stay open longer and permit more ions to flow, which, in part, explains the exaggerated hyperkalemic response when succinylcholine is administered to patients with denervation or burn injury.

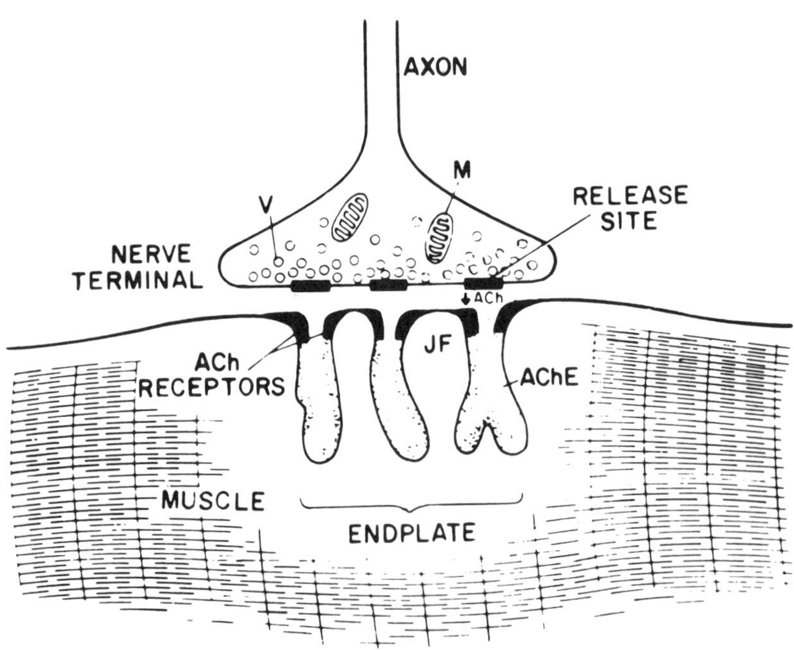

Figure 7-1. Schematic depiction of the neuromuscular junction. Acetylcholine (ACh) is present in vesicles (V) of the axon for release in response to nerve impulses. ACh diffuses across the synaptic cleft to attach to receptors that are concentrated on the junctional folds (JF) of the skeletal muscle endplate. Acetylcholinesterase (AChE) is present in the JF to facilitate rapid hydrolysis of ACh. (From Drachman,[1] with permission.)

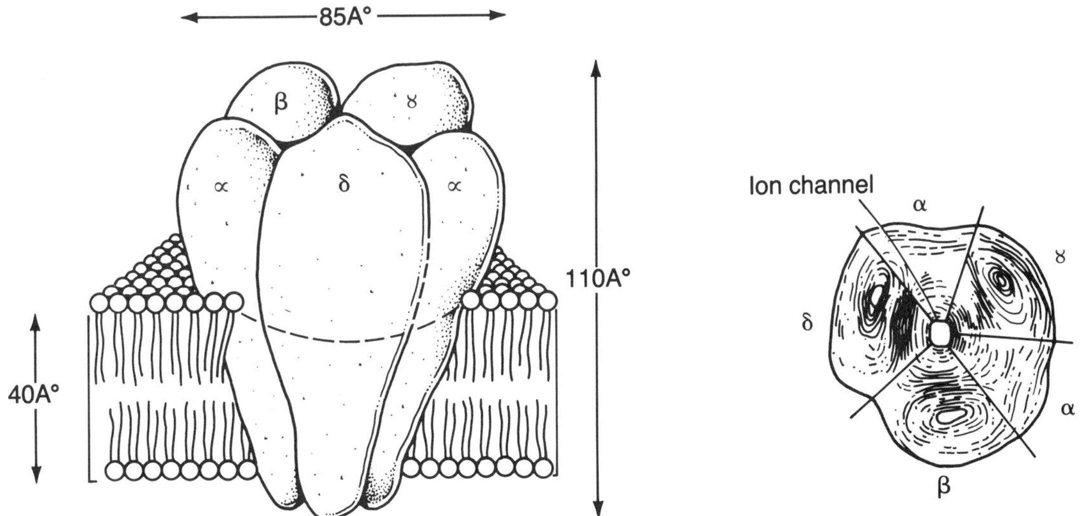

Figure 7-2. The postjunctional nicotinic cholinergic receptor consists of five subunits (two alpha, one each beta, gamma, and delta) arranged to form an ion channel. (From Taylor,[2] with permission.)

Postjunctional Receptors

Postjunctional receptors are glycoproteins consisting of five subunits designated as alpha (two subunits), beta, gamma, and delta (Fig. 7-2).[2] The subunits of the receptor are arranged such that a channel is formed that allows the flow of ions along a concentration gradient across cell membranes. This flow of ions is the basis of normal neuromuscular transmission. Extrajunctional receptors retain the two alpha subunits but may have an altered gamma or delta subunit.

The two alpha subunits are the binding sites for acetylcholine and are the sites occupied by muscle relaxants. For example, occupation of one or both alpha subunits by a nondepolarizing muscle relaxant causes the ion channel to remain closed, and ion flow to produce depolarization cannot occur. Succinylcholine attaches to alpha sites and causes the ion channel to remain open (mimics acetylcholine), resulting in prolonged depolarization. Large molecules can also act to plug the channel and in this way prevent the normal flow of ions. This is probably what happens when large overdoses of nondepolarizing muscle relaxants are administered. Unfortunately, this latter type of neuromuscular blockade cannot be readily antagonized by anticholinesterases. The lipid environment around cholinergic receptors can be altered by drugs such as volatile anesthetics, thus changing the properties of the ion channel.

STRUCTURE ACTIVITY RELATIONSHIPS

Muscle relaxants resemble the structure of acetylcholine (Fig. 7-3). For example, succinylcholine consists of two molecules of acetylcholine linked by methyl groups. Nondepolarizing muscle relaxants are bulky, rigid molecules that contain portions similar to acetylcholine. Acetylcholine and all muscle relaxants contain at least one positively charged quaternary ammonium group. This is important for attraction to the negatively charged cholinergic receptor.

DEPOLARIZING MUSCLE RELAXANTS

Succinylcholine is the only depolarizing muscle relaxant used clinically. Typically, doses of 0.5 to 1.5 $mg \cdot kg^{-1}$ IV are administered, producing a rapid onset of skeletal muscle paralysis (30 to 60 seconds) that lasts 5 to 10 minutes. These characteristics make succinylcholine useful for providing rapid skeletal muscle paralysis to facilitate intubation of the trachea during induction of anesthesia. Although a dose of 0.5 $mg \cdot kg^{-1}$ IV may be adequate, 1.0 to 1.5 $mg \cdot kg^{-1}$ IV is commonly administered. If a subparalyzing dose of a nondepolarizing muscle relaxant (pretreatment with 5% to 10% of its ED_{95} dose) is administered 2 to 4 minutes prior to injection of succinylcholine to blunt fasciculations, the dose of succinylcholine should be increased by about 70%.

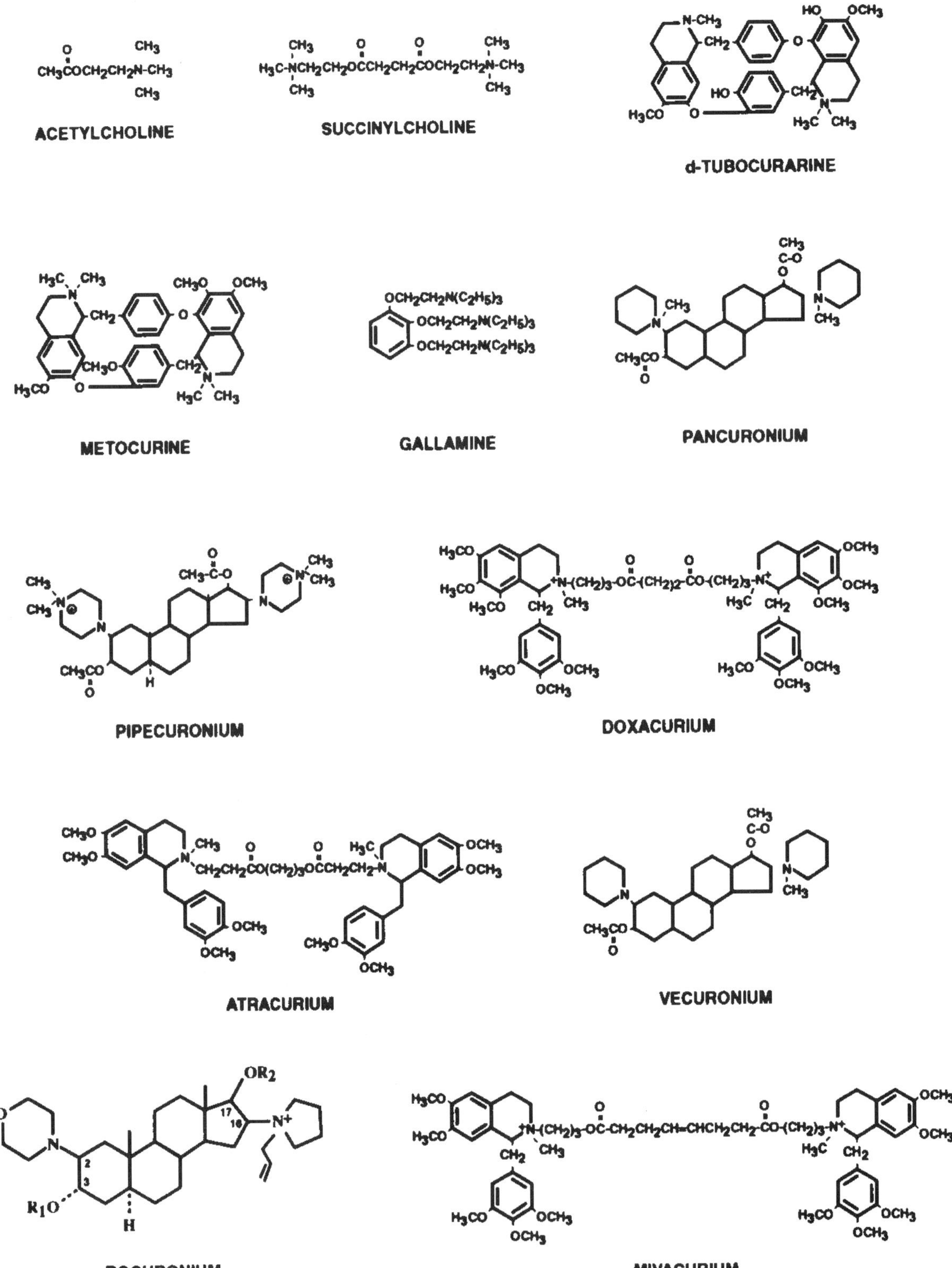

Figure 7-3. Chemical structure of acetylcholine and muscle relaxants.

Characteristics of Blockade

Succinylcholine mimics the action of acetylcholine, producing depolarization of the postjunctional membrane (Table 7-1). Compared with acetylcholine, the hydrolysis of succinylcholine is slow, resulting in sustained depolarization. Skeletal muscle paralysis occurs because a depolarized postjunctional membrane cannot respond to subsequent release of acetylcholine (hence the designation depolarizing neuromuscular blockade). Depolarizing neuromuscular blockade is also referred to as phase I blockade. Phase II blockade is present when the postjunctional membrane has become repolarized but still does not respond normally to acetylcholine (desensitization neuromuscular blockade). The mechanism of phase II blockade is unknown but may reflect development of a nonexcitable area around the endplate, which becomes repolarized but prevents spread of impulses initiated by the action of acetylcholine. Phase II blockade predominates when the dose of succinylcholine exceeds 3 to 5 $mg \cdot kg^{-1}$ IV. It resembles blockade produced by nondepolarizing muscle relaxants (Table 7-1).

The sustained depolarization produced by initial administration of succinylcholine is initially manifested by transient generalized skeletal muscle contractions known as fasciculations. Furthermore, sustained opening of ion channels produced by succinylcholine is associated with leakage of potassium from the interior of cells sufficient to increase plasma concentrations of potassium by about 0.5 $mEq \cdot L^{-1}$.

Metabolism

Hydrolysis of succinylcholine to inactive metabolites is carried out by plasma cholinesterase (pseudocholinesterase) produced in the liver (Fig. 7-4). Plasma cholinesterase has an enormous capacity to hydrolyze succinylcholine at a rapid rate such that only a small fraction of the original intravenous dose reaches the neuromuscular junction. Because plasma cholinesterase is not present at the neuromuscular junction, neuromuscular blockade produced by succinylcholine is terminated by its diffusion away from the neuromuscular junction into extracellular fluid. Therefore, plasma cholinesterase influences the duration of action of succinylcholine by controlling the amount of muscle relaxant that is hydrolyzed before reaching the neuromuscular junction. Liver disease must be severe before decreases in synthesis of plasma cholinesterase enzyme are sufficient to prolong the effects of succinylcholine. Potent anticholinesterases, as used in insecticides and in the treatment of myasthenia gravis, and certain chemotherapeutic drugs (nitrogen mustard, cyclophosphamide) may so decrease plasma cholinesterase activity that prolonged skeletal muscle paralysis follows administration of succinylcholine.

Atypical Plasma Cholinesterase

Atypical plasma cholinesterase enzyme lacks the ability to hydrolyze ester bonds in drugs such as succinylcholine and mivacurium. The presence of this atypical enzyme is often recognized only after an otherwise healthy patient experiences prolonged skeletal muscle paralysis (longer than 1 hour) after administration of a conventional dose of succinylcholine. Subsequent determination of the dibucaine number permits diagnosis of the presence of atypical plasma cholinesterase. Dibucaine is an amide local anesthetic that inhibits normal plasma

Table 7-1. Comparison of a Depolarizing (Succinylcholine) and Nondepolarizing (Pancuronium) Muscle Relaxant

	Succinylcholine		
	Phase I	Phase II	Pancuronium
Administration of pancuronium	Antagonize	Augment	Augment
Administration of succinylcholine	Augment	Augment	Antagonize
Administration of edrophonium	Augment	Antagonize	Antagonize
Fasciculations	Yes		No
Response to single electrical stimulation (single twitch)	Decreased	Decreased	Decreased
Train-of-four ratio	>0.7	<0.3	<0.3
Response to continuous (tetanus) electrical stimulation	Sustained	Unsustained	Unsustained
Post-tetanic facilitation	No	Yes	Yes

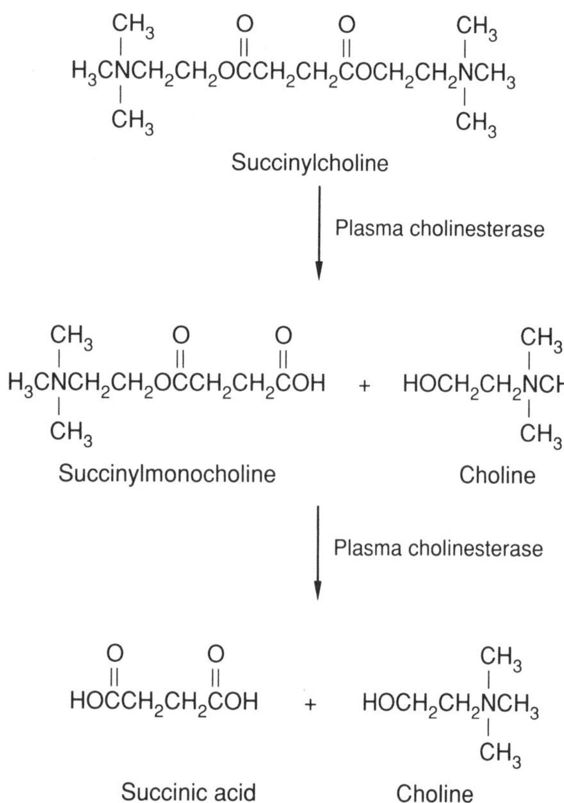

Figure 7-4. The brief duration of action of succinylcholine is principally due to its rapid hydrolysis in the plasma by cholinesterase enzyme to inactive metabolites (succinylmonocholine has 1/20 to 1/80 the activity of succinylcholine at the neuromuscular junction).

cholinesterase activity by about 80%, whereas activity of atypical enzyme is inhibited by about 20% (Table 7-2). It is important to recognize that the dibucaine number reflects the quality of plasma cholinesterase enzyme (ability to metabolize succinylcholine) and not the quantity of enzyme that is circulating in the plasma. For example, decreases in plasma cholinesterase activity owing to liver disease or anticholinesterases are associated with a normal dibucaine number.

Adverse Side Effects

Adverse side effects after administration of succinylcholine are numerous and may limit or contraindicate the use of this muscle relaxant in certain patients. Succinylcholine is contraindicated in patients after the acute phase of injury following major burns, mulitple trauma, extensive denervation of skeletal muscle, or upper motor neuron injury because succinylcholine administration to such individuals may result in severe hyperkalemia and cardiac arrest.[3] Furthermore, because of reports of cardiac arrest following administration of succinylcholine to apparently healthy children and adolescents who were subsequently found to have undiagnosed myopathies, it is now recommended that this muscle relaxant be administered to this age group only when emergency tracheal intubation or immediate securing of the airway is necessary.[4]

Adverse Side Effects of Succinylcholine

- Cardiac dysrhythmias
  - Sinus bradycardia
  - Junctional rhythm
  - Sinus arrest
- Fasciculations
- Hyperkalemia
- Myalgia
- Myoglobinuria
- Increased intraocular pressure
- Increased intragastric pressure
- Increased intracranial pressure
- Trismus
- Allergic reactions
- Trigger for malignant hyperthermia

Cardiac Dysrhythmias

Sinus bradycardia, junctional rhythm, and even sinus arrest may follow the administration of succinylcholine. These responses reflect the action of succinylcholine at cardiac postganglionic muscarinic receptors, where this drug mimics the normal effects of acetylcholine (Table 7-3). Cardiac dysrhythmias are most likely to occur when a second intravenous dose of succinylcholine is administered about 5 minutes after the first dose. Intravenous administration of atropine or subparalyzing doses of nondepolarizing muscle relaxants (pretreatment) 1 to 3 minutes before succinylcholine decreases the likelihood of these cardiac responses. Atropine administered intramuscularly with the preoperative medication does not reliably protect against suc-

Table 7-2. Variants of Plasma Cholinesterase Enzyme

	Approximate Duration of Succinylcholine-Induced Neuromuscular Blockade (min)	Dibucaine Number (Inhibition of Enzyme Activity [%])	Incidence
Homozygous	5–10	80	
Heterozygous	20	40–60	1 in 480
Homozygous atypical	60–180	20	1 in 3200

cinylcholine-induced decreases in heart rate. The effects of succinylcholine at autonomic nervous system ganglia also mimic the actions of the neurotransmitter acetylcholine, which may manifest as ganglionic stimulation with associated increases in arterial blood pressure and heart rate (Table 7-3).

Hyperkalemia

Hyperkalemia sufficient to cause cardiac arrest may follow administration of succinylcholine to patients with (1) denervation injury as caused by spinal cord transection, leading to skeletal muscle atrophy, and (2) unhealed skeletal muscle injury as produced by third-degree burns, (3) upper motor neuron injury, and (4) multiple trauma. The risk of hyperkalemia in these patients increases with time and usually peaks 7 to 10 days after the injury. There is evidence that increased release of potassium after administration of succinylcholine (doses as small as 20 mg IV) can begin within 4 days after denervation injury.[3] The duration of susceptibility to hyperkalemic effects of succinylcholine is unknown, but the risk is probably decreased 3 to 6 months after denervation injury. All factors considered, it may be prudent to avoid administration of succinylcholine to any patient more than 24 hours after spinal cord transection. Presumably, the risk of a hyperkalemic response in burn patients diminishes with healing of skeletal muscle damaged by the burn injury. Vulnerability to hyperkalemia may reflect proliferation of extrajunctional receptors (not proven to occur after burn injury), thus providing more sites for potassium to leak outward across cell membranes during depolarization.[5] Pretreatment with nondepolarizing muscle relaxants minimally influences the magnitude of potassium release evoked

Table 7-3. Autonomic Nervous System and Histamine Releasing Effects of Muscle Relaxants

Drug[a]	Nicotinic Receptors at Autonomic Ganglia	Cardiac Postganglionic Muscarinic Receptors	Histamine Release
Succinylcholine	Modest stimulation	Modest stimulation	Minimal
d-Tubocurarine	Moderate blockade[b]	None	Marked
Metocurine	Modest blockade[b]	None	Modest[b]
Gallamine	None	Moderate blockade	None
Pancuronium	None	Modest blockade	None
Pipecuronium	None	None	None
Doxacurium	None	None	None
Atracurium	None	None	Minimal[b]
Vecuronium	None	None	None
Mivacurium	None	None	Minimal[b]
Rocuronium	None	None (?)	None

[a]ED_{95} dose equivalent (see Tables 7-4 and 7-5).
[b]Occurs only with doses estimated to be two to three times the ED_{95}.

by succinylcholine and cannot be relied on as a safeguard. Patients with renal failure are not susceptible to exaggerated release of potassium, and succinylcholine can be safely administered to these patients, assuming they are normokalemic and do not have a uremic neuropathy.

Myalgia

Postoperative skeletal muscle myalgia manifesting particularly in the muscles of the neck, back, and abdomen may follow administration of succinylcholine. Myalgia localized to neck muscles may be described as a "sore throat" by the patient and incorrectly attributed to the prior presence of a tracheal tube. Young adults undergoing minor surgical procedures that permit early ambulation seem most likely to complain of myalgia. It is speculated that unsynchronized contractions of skeletal muscle fibers (fasciculations) associated with generalized depolarization lead to myalgia. Further evidence of skeletal muscle damage after the administration of succinylcholine is the appearance of myoglobinuria in some patients, especially pediatric patients during halothane anesthesia. Prevention of fasciculations by prior administration of a subparalyzing dose of a nondepolarizing muscle relaxant (pretreatment) will decrease the incidence but not totally prevent myalgia.[6]

Increased Intraocular Pressure

Succinylcholine causes a transient increase in intraocular pressure that is maximal 2 to 4 minutes after injection of the drug (see Chapter 24). The mechanism for this effect has not been clearly defined but may involve contraction of myofibrils or transient dilation of choroidal blood vessels.

For these reasons, succinylcholine given during induction of anesthesia may theoretically contribute to extrusion of intraocular contents in patients with open eye injuries, although this fear has not been realized with widespread clinical use.[7]

Increased Intragastric Pressure

Succinylcholine produces unpredictable increases in intragastric pressure. When intragastric pressure does increase, it seems to be related to the intensity of fasciculations, emphasizing the potential value of preventing this skeletal muscle activity by prior administration of subparalyzing doses of nondepolarizing muscle relaxants. An unproven assumption is that this increased intragastric pressure may cause passage of gastric fluid and contents into the esophagus and pharynx with the subsequent risk of pulmonary aspiration. Minimal to absent skeletal muscle fasciculations in children are consistent with the absence of appreciable increases in intragastric pressure that accompany administration of succinylcholine to this age group.

Increased Intracranial Pressure

Succinylcholine produces modest and transient increases in intracranial pressure that are attenuated or prevented by prior administration of subparalyzing doses of nondepolarizing muscle relaxants.[8] The clinical importance of these increases in intracranial pressure has not been ascertained.

Trismus

Various degrees of increased tension in the masseter muscles may accompany administration of succinylcholine, especially in pediatric patients. In extreme cases this response may manifest as trismus, leading to difficulty in opening the mouth for direct laryngoscopy and intubation of the trachea. Patients who develop trismus in association with the administration of a paralyzing dose of succinylcholine may be susceptible to the subsequent development of malignant hyperthermia (see Chapter 26). The occasional occurrence of trismus and malignant hyperthermia has caused some to question the wisdom of administering succinylcholine to children.

NONDEPOLARIZING MUSCLE RELAXANTS

Nondepolarizing muscle relaxants can be subdivided into long-, intermediate-, and short-acting.[8–10] Long-acting nondepolarizing muscle relaxants administered in equivalent doses produce skeletal muscle paralysis in 3 to 5 minutes that lasts 60 to 90 minutes (Table 7-4). These drugs are used most often to produce surgical muscle relaxation during maintenance of anesthesia for operations lasting 2 hours or longer.

Table 7-4. Comparative Pharmacology of Long-Acting Nondepolarizing Muscle Relaxants

	d-Tubocurarine	Metocurine	Gallamine	Pancuronium	Pipecuronium	Doxacurium
ED_{95} ($mg \cdot kg^{-1}$)	0.51	0.28	1.0[a]	0.07	0.06	0.025
Onset of maximum twitch depression (min)	3–5	3–5	3–5	3–5	3–5	4–6
Recovery to 25% of control twitch height (min)	40–70	40–70	40–70	40–70	35–70	40–70
Renal excretion (% unchanged)	45	43	95	80	70	70
Biliary excretion (% unchanged)	10–40	<2	0	5–10	20	30[a]
Hepatic degradation (%)	Insignificant	Insignificant	Insignificant	10–40	10	Insignificant
Hydrolysis in plasma	No	No	No	No	No	No

[a]Estimate.

Atracurium, vecuronium, and rocuronium are intermediate-acting nondepolarizing muscle relaxants and serve as useful alternatives to succinylcholine and long-acting nondepolarizing muscle relaxants, especially when intubation of the trachea or skeletal muscle relaxation, or both, are needed for short operations. Compared with long-acting nondepolarizing muscle relaxants, these drugs (1) have about one-third to one-half the duration of action (hence the designation intermediate-acting), (2) are relatively independent (especially atracurium) of renal function for clearance from the plasma, and (3) evoke minimal (especially vecuronium) circulatory effects (Table 7-5). While atracurium and vecuronium have an onset time similar to that of the long-acting muscle relaxants, rocuronium's onset time is 30 to 90 seconds shorter.[12] Therefore, rocuronium will probably become the nondepolarizing muscle relaxant of choice during the rapid sequence induction of anesthesia.

Mivacurium is a short-acting nondepolarizing muscle relaxant that serves as a useful alternative to succinylcholine and intermediate-acting nondepolarizing muscle relaxants (Table 7-6). The onset of blockade resembles that of other nondepolarizing muscle relaxants (delayed compared with succinylcholine and rocuronium), but its duration of action is 30% to 40% shorter than that of intermediate-acting muscle relaxants. The rapid spontaneous recovery from the neuromuscular blocking effects of mivacurium is particularly useful in brief outpatient surgical procedures in which facilitation of tracheal intubation with a muscle relaxant is desired but the anesthesiologist wishes to avoid the side effects

Table 7-5. Comparative Pharmacology of Intermediate-Acting Nondepolarizing Muscle Relaxants

	Atracurium	Vecuronium	Rocuronium
ED_{95} ($mg \cdot kg^{-1}$)	0.20	0.05	0.3
Onset of maximum twitch depression (min)	3–5	3–5	1–2
Recovery to 25% of control twitch height (min)	20–35	20–35	20–35
Dose for tracheal intubation ($mg \cdot kg^{-1}$)	0.4–0.5	0.08–0.1	0.6–0.12
Dose for continuous infusion ($\mu g \cdot kg^{-1} \cdot min^{-1}$)	6–8	1	6–10
Renal excretion (% unchanged)	Insignificant	15–25	10–25
Biliary excretion (% unchanged)	Insignificant	40–60	50–70
Hepatic degradation (%)	?	20–30	10–20
Hydrolysis in plasma	Spontaneous Enzymatic		

Table 7-6. Comparative Pharmacology of a Short-Acting Nondepolarizing Muscle Relaxant

	Mivacurium
ED_{95} (mg·kg^{-1})	0.07
Onset of maximum twitch depression (min)	2.5–4
Recovery to 25% of control twitch height (min)	12–20
Dose for tracheal intubation (mg·kg^{-1})	0.15–0.25
Dose for continuous infusion (μg·kg^{-1}·min^{-1})	5–6
Renal excretion (% unchanged)[a]	Insignificant
Biliary excretion (% unchanged)	Insignificant
Hepatic degradation (%)	Insignificant
Hydrolysis in plasma[a]	Enzymatic

[a]Because plasma cholinesterase is decreased in patients with renal failure, an increased duration of action may occur.

(especially myalgia) associated with the use of succinylcholine.

Drugs and events that alter responses produced by long-acting nondepolarizing muscle relaxants produce similar directional changes after administration of intermediate- or short-acting muscle relaxants.

Characteristics of Blockade

Nondepolarizing muscle relaxants compete with acetylcholine for alpha subunits and prevent changes in permeability of the postjunctional membranes (Table 7-1). As a result, depolarization cannot occur (hence, the designation nondepolarizing neuromuscular blockade) and skeletal muscle paralysis develops. Skeletal muscle fasciculations do not accompany the onset of nondepolarizing neuromuscular blockade.

Pharmacokinetics

Nondepolarizing muscle relaxants are highly ionized at physiologic pH and possess limited lipid solubility. As a result, the volume of distribution of these muscle relaxants is small, being limited principally to the extracellular fluid. In addition, these muscle relaxants cannot easily cross lipid membrane barriers, such as the blood-brain barrier, renal tubular epithelium, gastrointestinal epithelium, and placenta. Therefore, these muscle relaxants do not produce central nervous system effects (unless given in large doses for several days to facilitate controlled ventilation of the lungs), renal tubular reabsorption is minimal, oral administration is not effective, and maternal administration does not affect the fetus.

The duration of action of nondepolarizing muscle relaxants depends on their redistribution to inactive tissue sites plus their metabolism and clearance from the body (Tables 7-4 to 7-6). By virtue of their hydrophilic characteristics, all nondepolarizing muscle relaxants may be eliminated by glomerular filtration. This is the principal route of clearance for long-acting nondepolarizing muscle relaxants (pancuronium, pipecuronium, doxacurium) that undergo minimal to no metabolism. Addition of alternate pathways of drug clearance such as biodegradation in the liver (vecuronium) or chemodegradation (Hofmann elimination) as for atracurium result in an intermediate duration of action. When these additional routes of metabolism become even more efficient as reflected by ester hydrolysis in the plasma (atracurium, mivacurium) an even shorter duration of action is possible. The rapid clearance of atracurium, vecuronium, rocuronium, and mivacurium from the plasma allows adjustment of the dose to parallel clearance of the drug. As a result, continuous intravenous infusion of these drugs enhances the ability of maintaining an optimal and unchanging degree of neuromuscular blockade without a risk of significant drug accumulation.

Long-Acting Nondepolarizing Muscle Relaxants

The rate of disappearance of long-acting nondepolarizing muscle relaxants from the plasma is characterized by an initial rapid decrease followed by a slower decrease. Distribution of drug to tissues is the major cause of the initial rapid decrease in the plasma concentration, and the slower decrease is due principally to renal clearance mechanisms. Although pancuronium is excreted mainly via the kidneys, it is also metabolized in the liver to 3- and 17-hydroxy metabolites, which possess limited muscle relaxant properties. The route of excretion for the portion of the muscle relaxant dose that cannot be accounted for by known clearance mechanisms may reflect storage in mucopolysaccharides of connective tissues for prolonged periods.

Renal disease can greatly affect the pharmacokinetics of all long-acting nondepolarizing muscle relaxants. The rate at which the plasma concentration of pancuronium decreases is more influenced by renal failure than is the rate of decrease in the plasma concentration of *d*-tubocurarine or metocurine. The new long-acting nondepolarizing muscle relaxants, pipecuronium and doxacurium, are highly dependent on the kidneys for their elimination. Patients with biliary obstruction and cirrhosis of the liver manifest decreased plasma clearance and prolonged elimination half-times of pancuronium and possibly pipecuronium and doxacurium.

Intermediate-Acting Nondepolarizing Muscle Relaxants

Atracurium undergoes extensive metabolism (Hofmann elimination and ester hydrolysis), accounting for its independence from the kidneys for its clearance. It is estimated that two-thirds of the dose of atracurium undergoes ester hydrolysis, with the remainder undergoing spontaneous (Hofmann elimination) chemodegradation. Hofmann elimination is a pH and temperature-dependent breakdown that occurs spontaneously. Ester hydrolysis uses different enzymes from plasma cholinesterase, and patients with atypical cholinesterase will not experience prolonged responses after administration of atracurium. The principal metabolite of atracurium is laudanosine, which is inactive at the neuromuscular junction but in high concentrations may act as a central nervous system stimulant. Doses of atracurium administered during surgery result in low plasma concentrations of laudanosine that are unlikely to produce central nervous system effects. Continuous infusions of atracurium for several days to patients in the intensive care unit may result in higher plasma concentrations of laudanosine, especially if clearance mechanisms (hepatic elimination more important than renal elimination) for laudanosine are impaired.

Vecuronium is a monoquaternary analog of pancuronium that, unlike its analog, lacks vagolytic effects or substantial dependence on renal function for its clearance from the plasma. Metabolism is by deacetylation in the liver to 3, 17 and 3, 17-hydroxy metabolites. In addition, both unchanged vecuronium and its metabolites (up to 60% of an injected dose) are excreted predominantly in the bile. Only the 3-hydroxy metabolites have significant neuromuscular blocking properties that are equal to or slightly less than that of vecuronium. Administration of vecuronium for several days to critically ill patients with renal failure and sepsis has resulted in persistent plasma concentrations of this metabolite and prolonged neuromuscular blockade.[13] Despite its rapid onset time, rocuronium has pharmacokinetic values similar to those of vecuronium. Rocuronium, however, may be less influenced by renal failure than is vecuronium.[14]

Short-Acting Nondepolarizing Muscle Relaxants

Mivacurium (a mixture of three isomers) is primarily metabolized by plasma cholinesterase in a manner similar to that of succinylcholine.[9] Although this drug is not dependent on the kidneys or liver for its elimination, its required intravenous infusion rate is decreased and the duration of action is modestly longer in patients with renal failure.[15] This is probably because patients with renal failure often develop modest decreases in the plasma concentration of cholinesterase enzyme, thus resulting in a slowed rate of mivacurium's metabolism. Dependence of mivacurium on hydrolysis by plasma cholinesterase will predictably result in a longer duration of action should this drug be administered to patients with atypical cholinesterase or decreases in the plasma concentration of cholinesterase enzyme. Despite the ability of anticholinesterase drugs to inhibit activity of both plasma and true cholinesterase, antagonism of mivacurium-induced neuromuscular blockade with drugs such as neostigmine is usually rapid.

Cardiovascular Effects

Nondepolarizing muscle relaxants may exert cardiovascular effects by virtue of (1) drug-induced histamine release, (2) effects at cardiac postganglionic muscarinic receptors, or (3) effects on nicotinic receptors at autonomic ganglia (Table 7-3). *d*-Tubocurarine, and to a lesser extent, metocurine, atracurium, and mivacurium produce decreases in arterial blood pressure principally as a result of the release of histamine. Histamine release evoked by these muscle relaxants is dose-related, occurring with 1 time ED_{95} of *d*-tubocurarine, 2 times ED_{95} of metocurine, and 3 times ED_{95} of atracurium or mivacurium (Table 7-3). Pancuronium produces modest (10% to 15%) increases in heart rate and arterial blood pressure. These cardiovascular effects are due principally to selective cardiac vagal blockade (atropine-like effect) and, to a lesser extent, to activation of the sympathetic nervous system.

Cardiovascular effects likely to be evoked by muscle relaxants are often considered in selection of these drugs. For example, muscle relaxants that cause decreases in arterial blood pressure or increases in heart rate may be avoided in patients who are hypovolemic or considered to be at risk of the development of myocardial ischemia. In this regard, drugs with few or no cardiovascular effects (rocuronium, vecuronium, pipecuronium, doxacurium) may be selected (Table 7-3). Nevertheless, cardiovascular effects of muscle relaxants are usually transient and may be influenced by other drugs administered during anesthesia. In this regard, opioids may blunt the increase in heart rate produced by pancuronium. Conversely, pancuronium may be selected in an attempt to blunt opioid-induced heart rate slowing. Administration of even large doses of atracurium or mivacurium over 30 to 45 seconds rather than as a rapid intravenous injection minimizes the likelihood of drug-induced histamine release and associated decreases in blood pressure.

Causes of Altered Responses to Nondepolarizing Muscle Relaxants

Drugs administered in the perioperative period (volatile anesthetics, aminoglycoside antibiotics, magnesium, local anesthetics, cardiac antidysrhythmics, calcium entry blockers) may enhance effects of nondepolarizing muscle relaxants. Hypothermia prolongs neuromuscular blockade produced by muscle relaxants, especially the intermediate-acting drugs. Decreases in pH may prolong the action of nondepolarizing muscle relaxants, especially atracurium, by inhibiting Hofmann elimination, although this effect may be offset by enhanced ester hydrolysis at the lower pH. Hypokalemia, as produced by chronic treatment with diuretics, may be associated with enhanced effects of muscle relaxants. Nevertheless, the changes produced by chronic hypokalemia at the neuromuscular junction are complex and often unpredictable. Third-degree burns that involve more than 30% of the body surface area are associated with resistance to the neuromuscular blocking effects of nondepolarizing muscle relaxants. This resistance peaks about 40 days after injury and declines after about 60 days, although resistance has been documented for as long as 463 days (Fig. 7-5).[16] The mechanism of this resistance is a pharmacodynamic rather pharmacokinetic change, as the plasma concentrations of muscle relaxants required to produce the same degree of neuromuscular blockade are greater in burn than in normal patients. Allergic reactions rarely accompany administration of muscle relaxants. When allergy is present, cross-sensitivity is likely to exist among all drugs, including succinylcholine. This cross-sensitivity reflects the common antigenic group, the quaternary ammonium nitrogen molecule, that is present in all muscle relaxants.

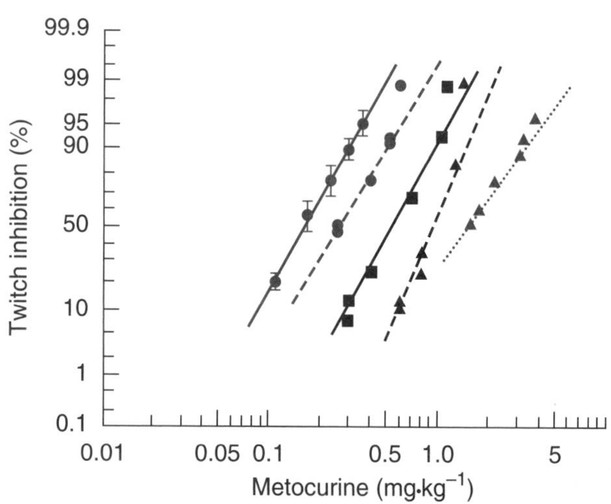

Figure 7-5. The dose-response curves for metocurine following burn injury continue to show resistance to the effects of the muscle relaxant even 463 days postburn (dashed red line and red circles). Solid red line, control; solid black line and black squares, 72 days postburn; dashed black line and black triangles, 65 days postburn; dotted red line and red triangles, 50 days postburn. (From Martyn et al.,[11] with permission.)

Volatile Anesthetics

Volatile anesthetics produce dose-dependent and drug-specific (greatest with isoflurane, enflurane, and desflurane) enhancement of the magnitude and duration of neuromuscular blockade produced by nondepolarizing muscle relaxants. This enhancement is partly due to anesthetic-induced depression of the central nervous system, which decreases the tone of skeletal muscles. In addition, volatile anesthetics may alter the sensitivity of postjunctional membranes to depolarization. This may reflect an anesthetic drug-induced alteration in the lipid environment around cholinergic receptors, thus changing the properties of the ion channel. Release of acetylcholine from the motor nerve ending of the cholinergic receptor is not altered by volatile anesthetics.

Aminoglycoside Antibiotics and Magnesium

Enhancement of neuromuscular blockade by certain antibiotics and magnesium, as is used in the treatment of pregnancy-induced hypertension, reflects complex changes at prejunctional (decreased release of acetylcholine) and postjunctional (stabilization) membranes. Inhibition of the prejunctional release of acetylcholine may reflect competition of these drugs with calcium. Indeed, calcium has been used to reverse antibiotic-enhanced neuromuscular blockade. Nevertheless, the response to calcium is unpredictable, and the usual recommendation is to mechanically support ventilation of the lungs until the blockade dissipates spontaneously. Antibiotics that do not enhance neuromuscular blockade produced by muscle relaxants include the penicillins and cephalosporins.

Local Anesthetics and Cardiac Antidysrhythmics

Lidocaine and quinidine, as administered intravenously to treat cardiac dysrhythmias, may augment co-existing neuromuscular blockade. This potential drug interaction should be considered when administering these drugs to patients recovering from general anesthesia that includes use of nondepolarizing muscle relaxants. Depending on the dose, local anesthetics and cardiac antidysrhythmics interfere with the prejunctional release of acetylcholine, stabilize postjunctional membranes, and directly depress skeletal muscle fibers. Verapamil potentiates the effects of depolarizing and nondepolarizing muscle relaxants.

ONSET TIME

The onset time of a nondepolarizing muscle relaxant can be shortened by administering an extremely large dose (6 to 8 times the ED_{90}) of the drug. For example, vecuronium (0.4 mg·kg^{-1} IV) produces adequate skeletal muscle relaxation for tracheal intubation in 60 to 120 seconds. Alternatively, the priming principle (administration of a dose equivalent to about 10% of the ED_{95} of the nondepolarizing muscle relaxant followed in 3 to 5 minutes by 2 to 3 times the ED_{95}) may be utilized. Conceptually, the initial small dose binds "spare" receptors without any significant effect on awake patients, such that the speed of onset of neuromuscular blockade is facilitated after administration of the larger "intubating" dose. Efficacy of the priming principle has been difficult to document, but some recommend its use when the goal is to make the onset of intubating conditions following the administration of a nondepolarizing muscle relaxant similar to the onset of paralysis produced by succinylcholine. With the introduction of rocuronium, a rapid onset time is possible. For example, administration of rocuronium (0.9 to 1.2 mg·kg^{-1} IV) produces an onset time similar to succinylcholine.[12]

MONITORING THE EFFECTS OF MUSCLE RELAXANTS

Evaluation of the mechanically evoked responses produced by electrical stimulation delivered from a peripheral nerve stimulator is the most reliable method for monitoring the effects of muscle relaxants administered during general anesthesia. Use of a peripheral nerve stimulator permits titration of muscle relaxant doses to produce optimal skeletal muscle relaxation. At the conclusion of surgery, responses evoked by the peripheral nerve stimulator are used to judge recovery from neuromuscular blockade that occurs spontaneously or after administration of anticholinesterase drugs (see the section *Drug-Assisted Antagonism of Nondepolarizing Muscle Relaxants*). Most often, superficial electrodes or subcutaneous needles are placed over the ulnar nerve at the wrist or elbow and a supramaximal electrical stimulation is delivered from the peripheral nerve stimulator (Fig. 7-6).[17,18] The adductor pollicis muscle is innervated solely by the ulnar nerve, accounting for the popularity of placing stimulating electrodes from the peripheral nerve stimulator over the ulnar nerve. Facial nerve stimulation, although difficult to quantitate, may be a consideration when mechanically evoked responses to stimulation of the ulnar nerve are not visible to the anesthesiologist.

Patterns of Stimulation

Mechanically evoked responses used for monitoring the effects of muscle relaxants include single twitch response, train-of-four (TOF) ratio, double burst suppression, tetanus, and post-tetanic stimulation (Figs. 7-7 to 7-10).[17,18] These mechanically evoked responses are evaluated visually, manually by touch (tactile), or by recording. Depth of neuromuscular blockade may be defined as the percentage of inhibition of twitch response from control height and duration of muscle relaxant effect as the time from drug administration until the twitch response recovers to a percentage of control height (Tables 7-1 and 7-4 to 7-6). For example, more than 90% depression of twitch response correlates with adequate skeletal muscle relaxation for intubation of the trachea or performance of intra-abdominal surgery in the presence of an adequate concentration of volatile anesthetic.

TOF (four electrical stimulations at 2 Hz delivered every 0.5 second) is based on the concept that acetylcholine is depleted by successive stimulations. Only four twitches are necessary since subsequent stimulation fails to further alter the release of additional acetylcholine. In the presence of effects produced at the neuromuscular junction by nondepolarizing muscle relaxants, the height of the fourth twitch is lower than that of the first twitch, allowing calculation of a TOF ratio (fade) (Fig. 7-8).[18] Recovery of the TOF ratio to greater than 0.7 correlates with complete return to control height of a single twitch response. In the presence of effects produced at the neuromuscular junction by succinylcholine, the TOF ratio remains near 1.0 as the height of all four twitch responses are decreased by a similar amount (phase I blockade) (Fig. 7-8).[18] A TOF ratio less than

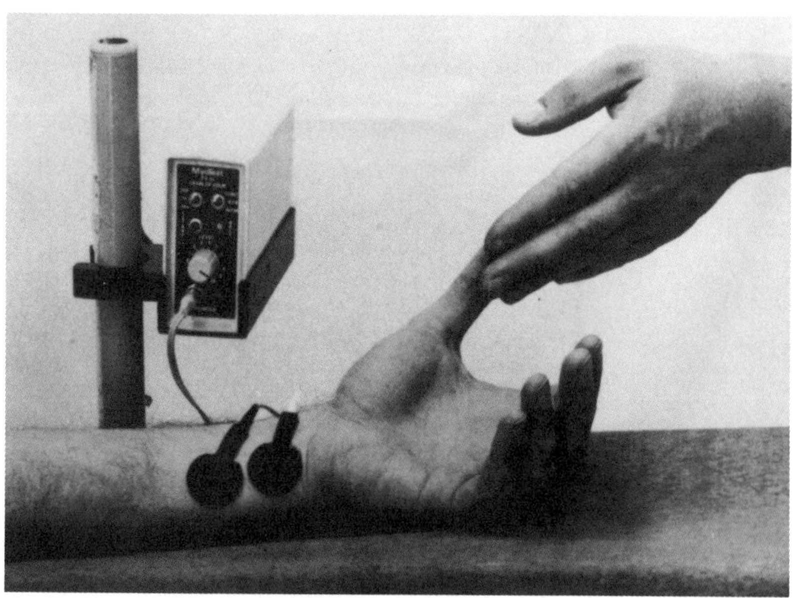

Figure 7-6. Superficial stimulating electrodes from a peripheral nerve stimulator are placed over the ulnar nerve, and the mechanical response evoked by electrical stimulation is evaluated by touch or observation. (From Viby-Mogensen,[13] with permission.)

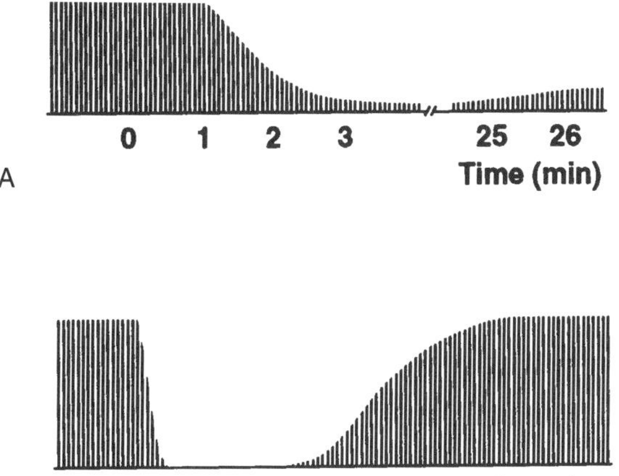

Figure 7-7. A schematic illustration of the onset and recovery from the neuromuscular blocking effects of *(A)* a nondepolarizing or *(B)* a depolarizing muscle relaxant ("0 time" indicates injection of the muscle relaxant) as depicted by the mechanically evoked single twitch response to repeated electrical stimulation of the nerve. (Modified from Viby-Mogensen,[13] with permission.)

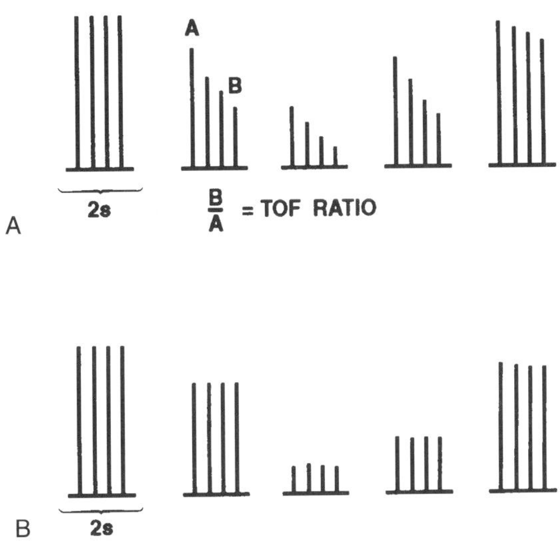

Figure 7-8. A schematic illustration of the mechanically evoked response to train-of-four (TOF) electrical stimulation of the nerve following injection of *(A)* a nondepolarizing or *(B)* a depolarizing muscle relaxant. The TOF ratio is less than 1 (fades) only in the presence of effects at the neuromuscular junction produced by a nondepolarizing muscle relaxant (Fig. A). (Modified from Viby-Mogensen,[13] with permission.)

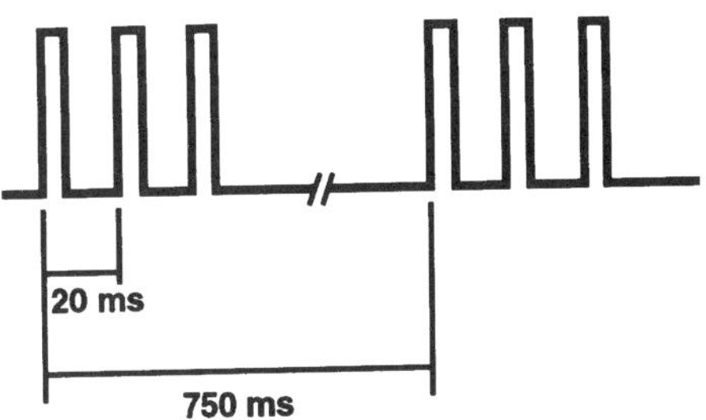

Figure 7-9. Schematic illustration of the stimulation pattern of double burst stimulation (three electrical impulses at 50 Hz separated by 750 ms). (From Bevan et al.,[14] with permission.)

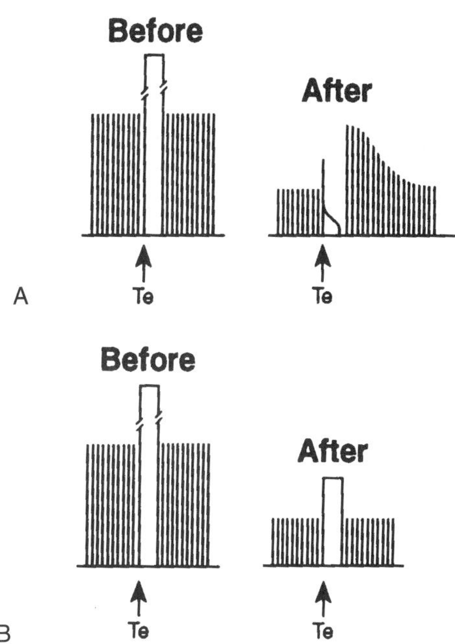

Figure 7-10. A schematic illustration of the evoked response to tetanic (Te) stimulation (50 Hz for 5 seconds) before and after the intravenous injection of *(A)* a nondepolarizing and *(B)* a depolarizing muscle relaxant. (Modified from Viby-Mogensen,[13] with permission.)

0.3 in the presence of succinylcholine reflects phase II blockade (Table 7-1).

Accurate estimation of the TOF ratio is not possible by either visual or manual assessment. Part of the difficulty in estimating the TOF ratio may be that the two middle twitch responses interfere with comparison of the first and last twitch response. In this regard, double burst suppression (two bursts of three electrical stimulations separated by 750 ms) is perceived by the clinician as two separate twitches (Fig. 7-9).[18] The clinician's ability to detect a TOF ratio less than 0.3 is improved with double burst suppression, but the ability to guarantee a TOF ratio greater than 0.7 still is not guaranteed.[17] In contrast to the difficulty in quantifying the TOF ratio, determination of the number of electrically evoked twitch responses to TOF stimulation is relatively reliable. For example, the fourth twitch can be observed when the first twitch is equivalent to 30% to 40% of control twitch height, corresponding to a TOF ratio of about 0.35. Counting the number of visible TOF responses may be helpful in predicting the ease with which neuromuscular blockade can be antagonized with an anticholinesterase drug (Table 7-7)[17] (see the section *Drug-Assisted Antagonism of Nondepolarizing Muscle Relaxants*).

Tetanus (continuous or tetanic electrical stimulation for 5 seconds at about 50 Hz) is an intense stimulus for release of acetylcholine at the neuromuscular junction. In the presence of effects produced at the neuromuscular junction by nondepolarizing muscle relaxants, the response to tetanus is not sustained (fades), whereas in the presence of succinylcholine-induced effects at the neuromuscular junction, the response to tetanus is greatly decreased but does not fade with a phase I blockade. (Fig. 7-10).[18] A sustained response to tetanus is present when the TOF ratio is greater than 0.7. At the end of tetanus, there is an increase in the immediately available store of acetylcholine such that subsequent twitch responses are transiently enhanced (post-tetanic facilitation) (Fig. 7-10).[18]

DRUG-ASSISTED ANTAGONISM OF NONDEPOLARIZING MUSCLE RELAXANTS

Drug-assisted (pharmacologic) antagonism of effects at the neuromuscular junction produced by nondepolarizing muscle relaxants is achieved by the intravenous administration of an anticholinesterase drug (edrophonium, neostigmine, or pyridostigmine). An anticholinesterase drug accelerates the already established pattern of spontaneous recovery at the neuromuscular junction by inhibiting the activity of acetylcholinesterase, leading to accumulation of acetylcholine at nicotinic (neuromuscular junction) and muscarinic sites. Increased amounts of acetylcholine in the region of the neuromuscular junction improve the chance that two acetylcholine molecules will bind to the alpha subunits of the nicotinic cholinergic receptor (Fig. 7-2). This tips the balance of the competition between acetylcholine and a nondepolarizing muscle relaxant in favor of the neurotransmitter (acetylcholine) and restores neuromuscular transmission. In addition, anticholinesterase drugs may generate antidromic action potentials and repetitive firing of the motor nerve endings (presynaptic effects).

Table 7-7. Choice of Anticholinesterase Drug

TOF Visible Twitches	Estimated TOF Fade[a]	Anticholinesterase Drug and Dose ($mg \cdot kg^{-1}$ IV)	Anticholinergic Drug and Dose[b] ($\mu g \cdot kg^{-1}$ IV)
None[c]	—	—	—
≤2	++++	Neostigmine, 0.07	Glycopyrrolate, 7 or atropine, 15
3–4	+++	Neostigmine, 0.04	Glycopyrrolate, 7 or atropine, 15
4	++	Edrophonium, 0.5	Atropine, 7
4	±	Edrophonium, 0.25	Atropine, 7

[a]The nearness of the TOF ratio to 0.7 or greater is inversely related to the intensity of fade.
[b]Administered simultaneously with anticholinesterase drug.
[c]Postpone drug-assisted antagonism until some evoked response is visible.
(Adapted from Bevan et al.,[14] with permission.)

The quaternary ammonium structure of anticholinesterase drugs greatly limits their entrance into the central nervous system such that selective antagonism of the effects of nondepolarizing muscle relaxants at the neuromuscular junction is possible. The peripheral cardiac muscarinic effects of anticholinesterase drugs (bradycardia) are attenuated by the prior or simultaneous intravenous administration of atropine or glycopyrrolate. Drug-assisted antagonism of nondepolarizing muscle relaxants is always indicated unless spontaneous recovery from the effects of the muscle relaxant are confirmed. The rapid spontaneous recovery rate from the neuromuscular blocking effects of intermediate- and short-acting nondepolarizing muscle relaxants is an advantage of these drugs compared with long-acting nondepolarizing muscle relaxants. For example, the incidence of weakness in the postoperative period despite drug-assisted antagonism is more frequent in patients receiving long-acting compared with intermediate- or short-acting nondepolarizing muscle relaxants.[17]

Choice of Anticholinesterase Drug

The choice of anticholinesterase drug is influenced by the speed of spontaneous recovery associated with the nondepolarizing muscle relaxant that is producing effects at the neuromuscular junction and the intensity of the neuromuscular blockade at the conclusion of surgery (Table 7-7).[17] Furthermore, potentiation of the neuromuscular blocking effects of nondepolarizing muscle relaxants by volatile anesthetics will wane at the conclusion of surgery, further contributing to spontaneous recovery. Antagonism of nondepolarizing neuromuscular blockade is not recommended in the absence of a twitch response as evoked by electrical stimulation; instead, mechanical ventilation of the lungs should be continued until spontaneous recovery has progressed further. Neostigmine is more effective than edrophonium or pyridostigmine in antagonizing intense neuromuscular blockade. Combining glycopyrrolate with neostigmine is logical because the slower onset of its cardiac anticholinergic effects more closely parallels the onset of muscarinic effects produced by neostigmine. The more rapid onset of edrophonium makes it a suitable choice when return of neuromuscular activity is well established. Combining atropine with edrophonium is logical because the prompt onset of its anticholinergic effects more closely parallels the onset of muscarinic effects produced by edrophonium.

Evaluation of the Adequacy of Antagonism

Adequacy of recovery (spontaneous and drug-assisted) from the neuromuscular blocking effects by nondepolarizing muscle relaxants is suggested by a TOF ratio greater than 0.7. In the absence of an accurately measured TOF ratio, a sustained response to tetanus or the ability to sustain a head lift for 5 to 10 seconds usually indicates a TOF ratio greater than 0.7. Grip strength is also a sensitive indictor of recovery from the effects of muscle relaxants. Although a TOF ratio greater than 0.7 or its equivalent provides evidence of the patient's ability to sustain adequate ventilation, a patent upper airway may not be maintained. Furthermore, a TOF ratio greater than 0.7 does not ensure comfort in an awake patient, as reflected by diplopia and difficulty swallowing that may occur in the postanesthesia care unit.[17]

When the initial response to an anticholinesterase drug seems inadequate, the following questions should be answered before additional antagonist drug is administered:

1. Has enough time elapsed for the anticholinesterase drug to antagonize the muscle relaxant (15 to 30 minutes)?
2. Is the degree of neuromuscular blockade too intense to be antagonized?
3. Is the acid-base and electrolyte status normal?
4. Is body temperature normal?
5. Is the patient receiving any drugs that may interfere with antagonism?
6. Has clearance of the muscle relaxant from the plasma been decreased by renal and/or hepatic dysfunction?

Answers to these questions will often provide the reason for failure of anticholinesterases drugs to adequately antagonize a nondepolarizing neuromuscular blockade.

REFERENCES

1. Drachman DA. Myasthenia gravis. N Engl J Med 1978;298:136–42.
2. Taylor P. Are neuromuscular blocking agents more efficacious in pairs? Anesthesiology 1985;63:1–3.

3. Gronert GA, Theye RA. Pathophysiology of hyperkalemia induced by succinylcholine. Anesthesiology 1975;43:89–99.
4. Rosenberg H, Gronert GA. Intractable cardiac arrest in children given succinylcholine. Anethesiology 1992;77:1054.
5. Marathe PH, Haschke RH, Slattery JT, Zucker JR, Pavlin EG. Acetylcholine receptor density and acetylcholinesterase activity in skeletal muscle of rats following thermal injury. Anesthesiology 1989;70:654–9.
6. Pace NL. Prevention of succinylcholine myalgias: A meta-analysis. Anesth Analg 1990;70:477–83.
7. Libonati MM, Leahy JJ, Ellison N. The use of succinylcholine in open eye surgery. Anesthesiology 1985;62: 637–40.
8. Stirt JA, Grosslight KR, Bedford RF, Vollmer D. "Defasciculation" with metocurine prevents succinylcholine-induced increases in intracranial pressure. Anesthesiology 1987;67:50–3.
9. Savarese JJ, Ali HH, Basta SJ, et al. The clinical neuromuscular pharmacology of mivacurium chloride (BW 109OU). A short-acting nondepolarizing neuromuscular blocking drug. Anesthesiology 1988;68:723–32.
10. Quill TJ, Begin M, Glass PSA, Ginsberg B, Gorback MS. Clinical responses to ORG 9426 during isoflurane anesthesia. Anesth Analg 1991;72:203–6.
11. Cook DR, Freeman JA, Lai AA, et al. Pharmacokinetics and pharmacodynamics of doxacurium in normal patients and in those with hepatic or renal failure. Anesth Analg 1991;72:145–50.
12. Magorian TT, Kelley T, Miller RD. Comparison of intubating conditions and onset times between rocuronium, succinylcholine and vecuronium. Anesthesiology 1993;79:913-80.
13. Segredo V, Caldwell JE, Matthay MA, et al. Persistent paralysis in critically ill patients after long-term administration of vecuronium. N Engl J Med 1992; 327:524–8.
14. Sze nohradszky J, Fisher DM, Segredo V, et al. Pharmacokinetics of rocuronium bromide (ORG 9426). Anesthesiology 1992;77:899–903.
15. Phillips BJ, Hunter JM. Use of mivacurium chloride by constant infusion in the anephric patient. Br J Anaesth 1992;68:492–8.
16. Martyn JAJ, Matteo RS, Szyfelbein SK, Kaplan RF. Unprecedented resistance to neuromuscular blocking effects of metocurine with persistence after complete recovery in a burned patient. Anesth Analg 1982;61: 614–7.
17. Bevan DR, Donati F, Kopman AF. Reversal of neuromuscular blockade. Anesthesiology 1992;77:785–92.
18. Viby-Mogensen J. Clinical assessment of neuromuscular transmission. Br J Anaesth 1982;54:209–23.

Section III

Preoperative Preparation and Intraoperative Management

8

Preoperative Evaluation and Choice of Anesthetic Technique

Preoperative evaluation and preparation for anesthesia begins when the anesthesiologist reviews the patient's medical record and visits with the patient, traditionally the day before elective surgery. Today, many patients undergo preoperative evaluation and planning in a preadmission anesthesia clinic or ambulatory surgical facility 1 day or more before the scheduled operation.[1] Important aspects of the preoperative evaluation include a history, review of current drug therapy, physical examination, and interpretation of laboratory data. The relevant aspects of these components of the preoperative evaluation should be available in the patient's medical record, making the chart review an integral part of the initial preparation for anesthesia. An important aspect of this preoperative visit is to inform the patient and other interested adults about events to expect on the day of surgery and to discuss the risks of anesthesia (Table 8-1). The planned management of anesthesia and methods available for relief of postoperative pain are also discussed with the patient. The patient or guardian must agree to the administration of anesthesia by signing an informed-consent statement. Informed consent does not require that the anesthesiologist describe to the patient remote risks (mortality) associated with the administration of anesthesia, as this would serve only to alarm a patient who is most likely already apprehensive. Indeed, the desire to discuss the risks of anesthesia often varies among patients and appropriately influences the detail with which the anesthesiologist pursues this topic during the preoperative evaluation. The anesthesiologist should describe, however, specific potential complications if an unusual technique or drug is to be used or if the physical condition of the patient may lead to adverse responses such as dislodgement of loose or diseased teeth during direct laryngoscopy. The apprehension-allaying effect on the patient produced by the anesthesiologist's preoperative visit is an important aspect of preoperative medication (see Chapter 9).

After the preoperative visit, a summary of pertinent findings, including details of the history, current drug therapy, physical examination, and laboratory data, should be written in the patient's medical record. A physical status classification is assigned, and the technique of anesthesia that has been discussed with the patient is detailed. Specific potential complications associated with the administration of anesthesia that have been described to the patient should be noted. The orders for the preoperative medication are written at this time (see Chapter 9).

On occasion, based on the preoperative evaluation, it may be the anesthesiologist's opinion that the patient is not in optimal medical condition (hypertension, cardiac dysrhythmia, abnormal laboratory value, upper respiratory tract infection) before elective surgery. This judgment should be discussed with the patient's primary physician and, if necessary, elective surgery deferred until the patient's medical condition improves. When

Table 8-1. Perioperative Events that Should be Discussed with the Patient Preoperatively

Risks of anesthesia (depends on patient's desire to know)
Nausea and vomiting
Myalgia
Dental injury
Peripheral neuropathy
Cardiac dysrhythmias
Myocardial infarction
Atelectasis
Aspiration
Stroke
Allergic drug reactions
Death (very unlikely)
Preoperative insomnia and medication available for its treatment
Time, route of administration, and expected effects from the preoperative medication
Time of anticipated transport to the operating room
Anticipated duration of surgery
Awakening after surgery in the postanesthesia care unit
Likely presence of catheters on awakening (tracheal, gastric, bladder, venous, arterial)
Time of expected discharge to hospital room or to home with escort after surgery
Magnitude of postoperative discomfort and methods available for its treatment

surgery is urgent, however, the benefits of immediate treatment offset the hazards introduced by less than optimal medical preparation, and the surgery is not delayed.

HISTORY

The history obtained preoperatively should include details relating to previous anesthetics experienced by the patient or relatives as well as a careful review of organ system function as altered by co-existing diseases (Table 8-2). The use of an automated health questionnaire that is completed by the patient prior to visiting with the anesthesiologist may be helpful. [2] Adverse events related to previous anesthetics should be specifically sought.

A history of chronic atopy (asthma, food sensitivities, hay fever, drug allergies) may reflect a genetic predisposition to form immunoglobulin E antibodies against antigens as possibly represented by drugs administered intravenously during the perioperative

Table 8-2. Specific Areas to Investigate in Preoperative History

Previous adverse responses related to anesthesia
Allergic reactions
Prolonged skeletal muscle paralysis
Delayed awakening
Nausea and vomiting
Hoarseness
Myalgia
Hemorrhage
Jaundice
Postspinal headache
Adverse responses in relatives
Central nervous system
Cerebrovascular insufficiency
Seizures
Cardiovascular system
Exercise tolerance
Angina pectoris
Prior myocardial infarction
Hypertension
Rheumatic fever
Claudication
Tachydysrhythmias
Lungs
Exercise tolerance
Dyspnea and orthopnea
Cough and sputum production
Bronchial asthma
Cigarette consumption
Pneumonia
Recent upper respiratory tract infection
Liver
Ethanol consumption
Hepatitis
Kidneys
Nocturia
Pyuria
Skeletal and muscular systems
Arthritis
Osteoporosis
Weakness
Endocrine system
Diabetes mellitus
Thyroid gland dysfunction
Adrenal gland dysfunction
Coagulation
Bleeding tendency
Easy bruising
Hereditary coagulopathies
Reproductive system
Menstrual history
Sexually transmitted diseases
Dentition
Dentures
Caps

period. Other than recognizing the possible increased likelihood of allergic reactions, however, there is no need to alter the drugs selected for administration during anesthesia to such patients. Certainly, a preoperative history of allergy to a specific drug mandates avoidance of that drug or the same class of drugs unless the anesthesiologist can be convinced that the symptoms described by the patient do not represent an allergic reaction. Should an unexpected allergic reaction occur during the perioperative period, it is important to document the responsible drug (often several drugs have been administered in a short time frame) for the future safety of the patient.

CURRENT DRUG THERAPY

Current drug therapy must be carefully reviewed during the preoperative evaluation because adverse interactions of these medications with drugs administered in the preoperative period must be considered (Table 8-3).[3] Potential drug interactions, however, do not dictate the need to discontinue preoperatively drugs that are producing desirable therapeutic responses. Indeed, drug therapy (antihypertensives, antianginal drugs, digitalis, diuretics, anticonvulsants, hormone replacement) should be continued throughout the perioperative period. Discontinuation of treatment with tricyclic antidepressants or monoamine oxidase inhibitors several days before elective surgery is probably not necessary, especially if the patient is suicidal or if therapy has been chronic.[4] Nevertheless, the safety of maintaining current drug therapy is based on the anesthesiologist's awareness of potential adverse drug interactions and appropriate modifications in perioperative selection of drugs and doses, as well as techniques of monitoring.

PHYSICAL EXAMINATION

The physical examination performed by the anesthesiologist is directed primarily toward the central nervous system, cardiovascular system, lungs, and upper airway (Table 8-4). In addition, the findings from the previously performed physical examination recorded on the patient's admission to the hospital are reviewed.

The presence of orthostatic hypotension may reflect previously unrecognized hypovolemia or drug-induced impairment of peripheral sympathetic nervous system activity. It is useful to listen for the murmur of aortic stenosis (systolic murmur at the right sternal border maximum in the second inter-

Table 8-3. Current Drug Usage and Potential Interactions with Drugs Administered in the Perioperative Period

Drug	Adverse Effects
Alcohol abuse	Tolerance to anesthetic drugs
Antibiotics	Prolongation of muscle relaxants
Antihypertensives	Impaired sympathetic nervous system responses
Aspirin	Bleeding tendency
Benzodiazepines	Tolerance to anesthetic drugs
Beta antagonists	Bradycardia Bronchospasm Impaired sympathetic nervous system responses Myocardial depression
Calcium channel blockers	Hypotension
Digitalis	Cardiac dysrhythmias or conduction disturbances
Diuretics	Hypokalemia Hypovolemia
Monoamine oxidase inhibitors	Exaggerated response to sympathomimetic drugs with acute treatment
Tricyclic antidepressants	Exaggerated response to sympathomimetic drugs with acute treatment

Table 8-4. Specific Areas to Investigate in the Preoperative Physical Examination

Central nervous system
Level of consciousness
Evidence of peripheral sensory or skeletal muscle dysfunction
Cardiovascular system
Auscultation of the heart (heart rate, rhythm, murmur)
Blood pressure (supine and standing)
Peripheral pulses (arterial cannulation site)
Veins (access site)
Peripheral edema
Lungs
Auscultation of the lungs (rales, wheezes)
Pattern of breathing
Anatomy of thorax (emphysema)
Upper airway (see Chapter 11)
Cervical spine mobility
Temporomandibular mobility
Prominent central incisors
Diseased or artificial teeth
Ability to visualize uvula
Thyromental distance
Coagulation
Bruising
Petechiae

costal space) because patients with this cardiac valvular abnormality may be asymptomatic but vulnerable to unexpected cardiac dysrhythmias or adverse decreases in stroke volume should blood pressure, heart rate, or systemic vascular resistance change abruptly during anesthesia and surgery. Availability of peripheral venous sites, including the external jugular veins, should be noted. The adequacy of collateral blood flow probably should be evaluated if the plan is to insert an arterial catheter for monitoring in the perioperative period (see Chapter 15). It may be important to evaluate the effect of operative position on circulation. For example, extending or turning the head may not be tolerated in the presence of carotid or vertebral artery occlusive disease. Arthritis may limit positioning of the arms and/or legs during surgery. Auscultation of the lungs for the presence or absence of wheezes is helpful if the patient has a history of asthma. Physical characteristics of the patient's upper airway that could make tracheal intubation difficult should be evaluated (see Chapter 11). If regional anesthesia is planned, it is important to inspect the site of local anesthetic injection for any anatomic abnormalities or signs of infection.

LABORATORY DATA

Many hospitals and departments of anesthesia have policies regarding which tests should be performed on all patients before anesthesia for elective surgery (Table 8-5). Ideally, however, only laboratory tests indicated on the basis of positive findings elicited during the history and physical examination of the patient should be ordered.[5] Likewise, the age of the patient and the complexity of the planned operation should be considered in determining which laboratory tests must be undertaken preoperatively. Nevertheless, because patients frequently enter the hospital the evening before or morning of surgery, it has become common to order routine laboratory screening tests before the history and physical examination and regardless of the age of the patient or complexity of the planned surgery.

Hemoglobin Concentration

Routine determination of the hemoglobin concentration (or hematocrit) is generally recommended before anesthesia for elective surgery. It is difficult to justify proceeding with an elective operation in the presence of anemia, (hemoglobin less than 10 $g \cdot dl^{-1}$) due to an unknown cause. Nevertheless, no data confirm that treatment of moderate normovolemic anemia in the preoperative period leads to a decrease in perioperative morbidity or mortality.[5]

Table 8-5. Examples of Laboratory Screening Tests that May Be Ordered Prior to Anesthesia for Elective Surgery

Hemoglobin and/or hematocrit
Blood chemistries
Glucose
Urea nitrogen and/or creatinine
Electrolytes (especially potassium)
Liver enzymes
Coagulation studies
Prothrombin time
Partial thromboplastin time
Urinalysis
Electrocardiogram
Chest radiograph
Pulmonary function studies
Forced exhaled volume in 1 second (FEV_1)
Vital capacity (VC)
FEV_1/VC
Flow volume loops
Arterial blood gases and pH

In contrast to anemia, there is evidence that the preoperative presence of polycythemia is associated with adverse perioperative events such as hemorrhage or thrombosis, or both. Furthermore, the presence of unexpected polycythemia may be a clue preoperatively to the unexpected existence of chronic arterial hypoxemia or depletion of intravascular fluid volume related to diuretic therapy.

Blood Chemistries

Routine blood chemistry screening tests in the absence of positive findings in the history or physical examination reveal unexpected abnormal findings in 2.5% to 7.5% of patients with the highest incidence in patients older than 60 years of age.[5] The most frequent abnormal findings in these otherwise asymptomatic patients are related to measurement of the blood glucose concentration and blood urea nitrogen concentration. Serum potassium concentration is generally measured before anesthesia for elective surgery if the patient has been receiving diuretic therapy.

Coagulation Studies

In the absence of positive findings in the history or physical examination suggesting the possibility of abnormal coagulation, the routine determination of prothrombin time and partial thromboplastin time before anesthesia for elective surgery is not necessary.

Urinalysis

Routine urinalysis as a screen before anesthesia for elective surgery offers little or no new information and in many respects only duplicates the blood chemistry measurements.

Electrocardiogram

In the absence of positive findings in the history and physical examination, a routine electrocardiogram (ECG) before anesthesia for elective surgery is not necessary in patients younger than 40 years of age.[5] This recommendation assumes that evaluation of the ECG will take place in the operating room before the induction of anesthesia. Indeed, most if not all the important abnormalities that might alter the management of anesthesia should be recognizable on a single lead ECG as routinely observed before the induction of anesthesia. After 40 years of age, a routine preoperative ECG before anesthesia for elective surgery is generally recommended.

Unexpected Abnormalities Detected on a Preoperative Electrocardiogram

- Atrial fibrillation
- Atrioventricular heart block
- ST-T changes suggestive of myocardial ischemia
- Atrial premature contractions
- Ventricular premature contractions
- Left or right ventricular hypertrophy
- Prolonged Q-T interval
- Tall peaked T waves
- Evidence of pre-excitation syndrome
- Evidence of a prior myocardial infarction

Chest Radiograph

There is no reason to obtain a routine preoperative chest radiograph for elective surgery in patients younger than 40 years of age with no evidence of chest disease in the history and physical examination.[5,6]

Pulmonary Function Tests

Pulmonary function tests are not necessary in the absence of positive findings in the history and physi-

Unexpected Abnormalities Detected on a Preoperative Chest Radiograph

- Tracheal deviation
- Mediastinal masses
- Pulmonary masses
- Pulmonary blebs
- Aortic aneurysm
- Pulmonary edema
- Pneumonia
- Atelectasis
- Fractures of the ribs or vertebrae
- Cardiomegaly
- Dextrocardia

Table 8-6. Physical Status Classification of the American Society of Anesthesiologists

Physical Status Classification	Description
PS-1	A normal healthy patient
PS-2	A patient with mild systemic disease that results in no functional limitation Examples: Hypertension, diabetes mellitus, chronic bronchitis, morbid obesity, extremes of age
PS-3	A patient with severe systemic disease that results in functional limitation Examples: Poorly controlled hypertension, diabetes mellitus with vascular complications, angina pectoris, prior myocardial infarction, pulmonary disease that limits activity
PS-4	A patient with severe systemic disease that is a constant threat to life Examples: Congestive heart failure, unstable angina pectoris, advanced pulmonary, renal, or hepatic dysfunction
PS-5	A moribund patient who is not expected to survive without the operation Examples: Ruptured abdominal aneurysm, pulmonary embolus, head injury with increased intracranial pressure
PS-6	A declared brain-dead patient whose organs are being removed for donor purposes
Emergency operation (E)	Any patient in whom an emergency operation is required Example: An otherwise healthy 30-year-old female who requires dilation and curettage for moderate but persistent vaginal bleeding (PS-1E)

(From information in American Society of Anesthesiologists.[7])

cal examination of patients undergoing elective surgery that does not involve the thorax. Conversely, pulmonary function tests may be useful in the preoperative preparation and subsequent intraoperative management of patients with evidence of pulmonary disease and undergoing upper abdominal or intrathoracic operations (see Chapter 19).

PHYSICAL STATUS CLASSIFICATION

Assignment of a physical status classification (class 1 through 6) is based on the physical condition of the patient independent of the planned operation (Table 8-6).[7] It is important to recognize that the physical status classification is not intended to represent an estimate of anesthetic risk. Instead, the physical status classification serves as a "common language" among different institutions for subsequent examination of anesthetic morbidity and mortality. Not surprisingly, intraoperative cardiac arrest is more frequent in the poor physical status classification, particularly if emergency surgery is necessary.

ANESTHETIC TECHNIQUE

After the preoperative evaluation, the anesthesiologist selects as the anesthetic technique either a general anesthetic, regional anesthetic (see Chapter 12), or peripheral nerve block (see Chapter 13). The anesthetic technique is determined by several considerations. In many instances, more than one anesthetic technique is acceptable. It is the responsibility of the anesthesiologist to evaluate the medical condition and unique needs of each patient and to select an appropriate anesthetic technique.

Considerations that Influence the Anesthetic Technique

- Co-existing diseases that may or may not be related to the reason for surgery
- Site of surgery
- Body position of patient during surgery
- Elective or emergency surgery
- Likelihood of increased amounts of gastric contents
- Age of patient
- Preference of patient

General Anesthetic

Induction of general anesthesia (loss of consciousness) is most often accomplished by the intravenous administration of drugs such as thiopental, propofol, or etomidate that produce the rapid onset of unconsciousness (see Chapter 5). In the absence of a known contraindication, succinylcholine is also commonly administered intravenously shortly after the induction drug to produce skeletal muscle relaxation so as to facilitate direct laryngoscopy for intubation of the trachea (see Chapter 7). The intravenous injection of drugs to produce unconsciousness followed immediately by succinylcholine is referred to as a "rapid-sequence" induction of anesthesia. Frequently the patient is breathing oxygen via a mask (preoxygenation) before a rapid sequence induction of anesthesia. Preoxygenation is intended to replace air and nitrogen (denitrogenation) in the patient's functional residual capacity (about 2500 ml of 21% oxygen) with oxygen. This practice should increase the margin of safety during periods of upper airway obstruction or apnea (drug-induced, during direct laryngoscopy for intubation of the trachea) that may accompany induction of anesthesia. In healthy awake patients the increase in arterial hemoglobin oxygen saturation achieved with four vital capacity breaths of 100% oxygen over 30 seconds is similar to that achieved during breathing 100% oxygen for 3 to 5 minutes at normal tidal volumes.[8]

Evidence of Patent Upper Airway After Induction of Anesthesia

- Upper chest expands and reservoir bag partially empties during inspiration
- Reservoir bag refills during exhalation
- Capnography reveals cyclic waveforms decreasing to zero during inhalation and plateau peak (>20 mmHg) during exhalation
- Pulse oximeter continues to read >95%

A typical rapid-sequence induction of anesthesia includes preoxygenation followed by administration of a nonparalyzing (defasciculating) dose of a nondepolarizing muscle relaxant (pancuronium 1 to 2 mg IV or its equivalent) followed 1 to 3 minutes later by thiopental (3 to 5 mg·kg^{-1} IV or its equivalent) and succinylcholine (1 to 2 mg·kg^{-1} IV). It is a common practice to administer an opioid (fentanyl 1 to 2 μg·kg^{-1} IV or its equivalent) 1 to 3 minutes before administration of the induction drug. The opioid is intended to blunt subsequent pressor and heart rate responses to direct laryngoscopy and tracheal intubation and also to initiate preemptive analgesia (see Chapter 9). With the onset of unconsciousness, the patient's head is positioned to optimize the patency of the upper airway and positive pressure inflation of the patient's lungs with oxygen is instituted. Direct laryngoscopy for intubation of the trachea is initiated only after skeletal muscle paralysis is verified by the peripheral nerve stimulator (generally 30 to 60 seconds after the administration of succinylcholine). Alternatively, a nondepolarizing muscle relaxant (most often mivacurium, atracurium, or vecuronium) can be substituted for succinylcholine, realizing that the onset of skeletal muscle paralysis necessary for facilitation of tracheal intubation may be delayed (3 to 5 minutes) compared with the rapid onset of relaxation produced by succinylcholine. Because of its rapid onset time, rocuronium may be the nondepolarizing muscle relaxant of choice to facilitate tracheal intubation. Administration of the nondepolarizing muscle relaxant in divided doses (priming principle) may be selected in an attempt to speed the onset of skeletal muscle paralysis (see Chapter 7). Monitoring of arterial hemoglobin oxygen saturation with a pulse oximeter provides early warning should arterial oxygen desaturation occur during the period of apnea required for intubation of the trachea. After intubation of the trachea, it may be prudent to insert a gastric tube through the mouth to decompress the stomach and remove any easily accessible fluid. This orogastric tube should be removed at the conclusion of anesthesia. When gastric suction is needed postoperatively, the tube should be inserted through the nares rather than the mouth.

An alternative to the rapid-sequence induction of anesthesia is the inhalation of nitrous oxide plus a volatile anesthetic (most often halothane since the other volatile anesthetics are airway irritants) with or without the prior intravenous administration of a "sleep dose" of an induction drug (see Chapter 5). This is referred to as an "inhalation or mask induction." An inhalation induction is often used in pediatric patients, particularly when prior insertion of a venous catheter is not practical. When an inhalation induction of anesthesia is selected, a depolarizing or nondepolarizing muscle relaxant is administered intravenously when it is deemed appropriate to intubate the trachea. Alternatively, skeletal muscle relaxation produced by the volatile anesthetic can be used to facilitate intubation of the trachea. It may be the decision of the anesthesiologist not to place a tube in the trachea, and anesthesia is then maintained by inhalation via a mask.

The objectives during maintenance of general anesthesia are amnesia, analgesia, skeletal muscle relaxation, and control of sympathetic nervous system responses evoked by noxious stimulation. These objectives are achieved most often by the use of a combination of drugs that may include inhaled and/or injected drugs with or without muscle relaxants. Each drug selected should be administered on the basis of a specific goal that is relevant to that drug's known pharmacologic effects at therapeutic doses. For example, it is not logical to administer high concentrations of volatile anesthetics to produce skeletal muscle relaxation when muscle relaxants are specific for achieving this goal. Likewise, it is not acceptable to obscure skeletal muscle movement due to insufficient doses of anesthetics by administering excessive amounts of muscle relaxants. The selective use of drugs for their specific effect permits the anesthesiologist to tailor the anesthetic to the patient's medical condition and any unique needs introduced by the surgery.

Despite its lack of potency, nitrous oxide is the most frequently administered inhaled anesthetic. Typically, nitrous oxide (50% to 70% inhaled concentration) is administered in combination with a volatile anesthetic or opioids. It is important to remember that it is the partial pressure of an inhaled anesthetic that produces its pharmacologic effect. For example, 60% inhaled nitrous oxide administered at sea level exerts a partial pressure of 456 mmHg (60% of the total barometric pressure of 760 mmHg). The same inhaled concentration of nitrous oxide (or a volatile anesthetic) administered at an altitude where the barometric pressure is lower than 760 mmHg exerts a decreased pharmacologic effect because the partial pressure of the anesthetic that can be achieved in the brain is lower.

Volatile anesthetics have the advantage of high potency and they can be readily controlled in terms of the concentration delivered from the anesthetic machine, allowing titration of the dose to produce a desired response. Excessive sympathetic nervous system responses evoked by noxious stimulation are predictably attenuated by volatile anesthetics. Dose-dependent cardiac depression is a major disadvantage of volatile anesthetics (see Chapter 4). Indeed, a volatile drug is seldom administered as the sole anesthetic but is more often administered in combination with nitrous oxide. Substitution of nitrous oxide for a portion of the dose of the volatile anesthetic allows a decrease in the delivered concentration of the volatile drug, which results in less cardiac depression despite the same total dose of anesthetic drugs (see Chapter 4).

In certain instances, it is acceptable to administer muscle relaxants to ensure lack of patient movement and to permit a decrease in the delivered concentration of volatile anesthetics. This use of muscle relaxants, however, must not be interpreted as an endorsement for the administration of an inadequate dose of anesthetic that is obscured by skeletal muscle paralysis. Indeed, intraoperative awareness is a constant fear and risk of light anesthesia, especially when patient movement is obscured by muscle relaxant-induced paralysis.

Opioids that generally do not depress the cardiovascular system are combined most often with nitrous oxide (see Chapter 5). In patients with normal left ventricular function, however, the lack of opioid-induced cardiovascular depression and absence of attenuation of sympathetic nervous system reflexes may manifest as hypertension. When this occurs, the addition of low concentrations of a volatile anesthetic to the delivered gases is often effective in returning the increased blood pressure to an acceptable level. Muscle relaxants are often necessary, even in the absence of the need for skeletal muscle relaxation, because adequate doses of opioids with nitrous oxide are unlikely to prevent patient movement in response to painful stimulation. Another disadvantage of injected drugs compared with inhaled anesthetics is the inability to accurately titrate and maintain a therapeutic concentration of the injected drug. This disadvantage can be offset to some extent by continuous intravenous infusion of the injected anesthetic at a rate previously determined in other patients to be associated with therapeutic concentrations in the blood.

Regional Anesthetic

A regional anesthetic (spinal, epidural, caudal) is selected when maintenance of consciousness during surgery is desirable (see Chapter 12). Skeletal muscle relaxation and contraction of the gastrointestinal tract are also produced by a regional anesthetic. Patients may have preconceived and erroneous conceptions about regional anesthesia that will require the anesthesiologist to reassure them about the safety of this technique. A regional anesthetic should not be performed against the wishes of the patient. Disadvantages of this anesthetic technique include the occasional failure to produce adequate anesthesia for the surgical stimulus and the decrease in blood pressure that may accompany the peripheral sympathetic nervous system blockade by the regional anesthetic, particularly in the presence of hypovolemia.

A regional anesthetic technique is most often selected for surgery that involves the lower abdomen or lower extremities in which the level of sensory anesthesia required is associated with minimal sympathetic nervous system blockade. This should not imply that a general anesthetic is an unacceptable technique for similar types of surgery.

Peripheral Nerve Block

A peripheral nerve block is most appropriate as a technique of anesthesia for superficial operations on the extremities (see Chapter 13). Advantages of peripheral nerve blocks include maintenance of consciousness and continued presence of protective upper airway reflexes. The isolated anesthetic effect produced by a peripheral nerve block is particularly attractive in patients with chronic pulmonary disease, severe cardiac impairment, or inadequate renal function. For example, insertion of a vascular shunt in the upper extremity for hemodialysis in a patient who may have associated pulmonary and cardiac disease is often accomplished with anesthesia provided by peripheral nerve block of the brachial plexus. Likewise, the avoidance of the need for muscle relaxants in this type of patient circumvents the possible prolonged effect produced by these drugs in the absence of renal function.

A disadvantage of peripheral nerve block as an anesthetic technique is the unpredictable attainment of adequate sensory and motor anesthesia for performance of the surgery. The success rate of a peripheral nerve block is often inversely related to the frequency with which the anesthesiologist uses this anesthetic technique. Patients must be cooperative for a peripheral nerve block to be effective. For example, acutely intoxicated and agitated patients are not ideal candidates for a peripheral nerve block.

PREPARATION FOR ANESTHESIA

Preparation for anesthesia after the preoperative medication has been administered and the patient is transported to the operating room is similar regardless of the anesthetic technique that has been selected. On arrival in the operating room, the patient is identified and the planned surgery reconfirmed. The nurse's notes are consulted by the anesthesiologist to learn of any unexpected changes in the patient's medical condition, vital signs, or body temperature and to determine that the preoperative medication and, if indicated, prophylactic antibiotics have been administered. Likewise, any laboratory data that have become available since the anesthesiologist's prior visit should be reviewed.

Initial preparation for anesthesia, regardless of the technique of anesthesia selected, usually begins with insertion of a catheter in a peripheral vein and application of a blood pressure cuff. This initial preparation may be accomplished in a holding area or in the operating room. Use of separate rooms (induction rooms) distinct from the operating room for induction of anesthesia is not recommended by some because of the questionable safety of routinely moving anesthetized patients with the necessary attached equipment from one area to another. An exception to this recommendation may be the performance of peripheral nerve blocks or institution of epidural anesthesia in a holding area, thus allowing the block to be in place when the operating

Table 8-7. Routine Preparation Before Induction of Anesthesia Independent of the Anesthetic Technique Selected

Anesthesia machine (see Table 10-4)
Attach an anesthetic breathing system with a proper-size face mask
Occlude the patient end of the anesthetic breathing system and fill with oxygen from the anesthesia machine ("flush valve") (applying manual pressure to the distended reservoir bag checks for leaks in the anesthetic breathing system and confirms the ability to provide positive pressure ventilation of the patient's lungs with oxygen)
Check anesthetic breathing system valves
Calibrate oxygen analyzer with air and oxygen and set alarm
Check soda lime for color change
Check liquid level of vaporizers
Confirm function of mechanical ventilator
Confirm availability and function of wall suction
Check final position of all flowmeter, vaporizer, and monitor (alarm) settings
Drugs
Local anesthetic (lidocaine)
Induction drug (thiopental, methohexital, etomidate, propofol)
Opioid (fentanyl, sufentanil, alfentanil)
Benzodiazepine (midazolam, diazepam)
Anticholinergic (atropine)
Sympathomimetic (ephedrine, phenylephrine)
Succinylcholine
Nondepolarizing muscle relaxant (mivacurium, rocuronium, atracurium, vecuronium, pancuronium)
Anticholinesterase (neostigmine, edrophonium)
Opioid antagonist
Benzodiazepine antagonist
Catecholamine to treat an allergic reaction (epinephrine)
Equipment
Intravenous solution and connecting tubing
Catheter for vascular cannulation
Suction catheter
Oral and/or nasal airway
Laryngoscope
Tracheal tube
Nasogastric tube

room becomes available. Likewise, an epidural catheter for postoperative pain management may be placed in the holding area prior to transport of the patient to the operating room and induction of general anesthesia. Monitors such as the pulse oximeter, ECG, and peripheral nerve stimulator are also applied while the patient is still awake. Immediately before the induction of anesthesia, baseline vital signs (blood pressure, heart rate, cardiac rhythm, arterial hemoglobin oxygen saturation, breathing rate) and the corresponding time are recorded.

Regardless of the anesthetic technique selected, the anesthesia machine is present and functional and specific drugs and equipment are always immediately available (Table 8-7). It is mandatory to always be able to suction the patient's pharynx and then ventilate the lungs with oxygen via a cuffed tube placed in the trachea.

REFERENCES

1. Conway JB, Goldberg J, Chung F. Preadmission anaesthesia consultation clinic. Can J Anaesth 1992;39: 1051–7.
2. Lutner RE, Roizen MF, Stocking CB, et al. The automated interview versus the personal interview. Do patient responses to preoperative health questions differ? Anesthesiology 1991;75:394–400.
3. Cullen BF, Miller MG. Drug interactions in anesthesia. A review. Anesth Analg 1979;58:413–23.
4. Braverman B, McCarthy RJ, Ivankovich AD. Vasopressor challenges during chronic MAOI or TCA treatment in anesthetized dogs. Life Sci 1987;40:2587–95.
5. Kaplan EB, Sheiner LB, Boeckmann AJ, et al. The usefulness of preoperative laboratory screening. JAMA 1985;253:3576–81.
6. Archer C, Levy AR, McGregor M. Value of routine preoperative chest x-rays: A meta-analysis. Can J Anaesth 1993;40:1022–7
7. American Society of Anesthesiologists. New classification of physical status. Anesthesiology 1963;24:111.
8. Gold MI. Preoxygenation. Br J Anaesth 1989;62: 241–2.

9

Preoperative Medication

Management of anesthesia begins with the preoperative psychological preparation of the patient and administration of a drug or drugs selected to elicit specific pharmacologic responses. This initial psychological and pharmacologic component of anesthetic management is referred to as preoperative medication.[1] Ideally, all patients should enter the preoperative period free from anxiety, sedated but easily arousable, and fully cooperative.

PSYCHOLOGICAL PREMEDICATION

Psychological premedication is provided by the anesthesiologist's preoperative visit and interview with the patient and family members (see Chapter 8). A thorough description of the planned anesthetic and events to anticipate in the perioperative period serves as a nonpharmacologic antidote to anxiety.[2,3] Indeed, the incidence of anxiety is decreased in patients visited by the anesthesiologist preoperatively compared with patients receiving only pharmacologic premedication and no visit (Table 9-1).[2] Likewise, a booklet designed to reassure patients about anesthesia is not as effective in decreasing anxiety as is a preoperative visit and interview by the anesthesiologist.[3] Nevertheless, a shortage of time and the fact that some patients' problems do not lend themselves to reassurance may limit the value of the preoperative interview.

PHARMACOLOGIC PREMEDICATION

Pharmacologic premedication is typically administered orally or intramuscularly 1 to 2 hours before the anticipated induction of anesthesia. For outpatient surgery, premedication may be administered intravenously in the immediate preoperative period. The goals for pharmacologic premedication are multiple and must be individualized to meet each patient's unique requirements. Some previously acceptable goals of pharmacologic premedication either are no longer valid or are better achieved by intravenous administration of drugs at a time more likely to correspond to the period when pharmacologic effects are necessary. The best drug or drug combination to achieve the desired goals of pharmacologic premedication is not known and often is influenced by the individual anesthesiologist's previous experience.

The appropriate drug(s) and doses to be used for pharmacologic premedication can be selected only after the psychological and physiologic conditions of the patient have been evaluated. Drug choice and dose must take into account multiple factors. Certain types of patients should not receive depressant pharmacologic drugs in attempts to decrease preoperative anxiety and produce sedation (Table 9-2). The patient who requests to be "asleep" before being transported to the operating room must be assured that this is neither a desired nor a safe goal of pharmacologic premedication.

DRUGS ADMINISTERED FOR PHARMACOLOGIC PREMEDICATION

Several classes of drugs are available to facilitate achievement of the desired goals for pharmacologic premedication in each individual patient (Table 9-

Table 9-1. Value of Preoperative Interview Compared with Pentobarbital

	Patients (%)			
	Interview Only	Pentobarbital[a] Only	Interview and Pentobarbital	No Interview or Pentobarbital
Feel nervous	40	61	38	58
Feel drowsy	26	30	38	18
Judged adequately sedated by anesthesiologists	65	48	71	35

[a]2 mg·kg^{-1} IM 1 hour before surgery.
(Data from Egbert et al.[2])

Primary Goals for Pharmacologic Premedication

Anxiety relief (anxiolysis)
Sedation
Analgesia
Amnesia
Antisialogogue effect
Increase in gastric fluid pH
Decrease in gastric fluid volume
Attenuation of sympathetic nervous system reflex responses
Decrease in anesthetic requirements
Prophylaxis against allergic reactions

Secondary Goals for Pharmacologic Premedication

Decrease in cardiac vagal activity—better achieved with the intravenous injection of an anticholinergic (atropine) just before the time of anticipated need
Facilitation of induction of anesthesia—not necessary in view of availability of potent intravenous induction drugs
Postoperative analgesia—better achieved with neuraxial opioids or the intravenous injection of an opioid just before the time of anticipated need (preemptive analgesia)
Prevention of postoperative nausea and vomiting—better achieved with the intravenous injection of an antiemetic (droperidol, ondansetron) just before the time of anticipated need

3). These drugs are often administered intramuscularly, but when possible, the oral route of administration should be considered to improve patient comfort. The small amount of water used to facilitate oral administration of drugs introduces no hazards related to gastric fluid volume (see the section *Fasting Before Elective Surgery*). Ultimately, the specific drugs selected are based on a consideration of desirable goals to be achieved balanced against any potential undesirable effects of these drugs.

Barbiturates

Advantages of using barbiturates for pharmacologic premedication include sedation, minimal ventilatory depressant effects, minimal circulatory depression, rarity of nausea and vomiting, and effectiveness when administered orally. Disadvantages include lack of analgesia; disorientation, especially if administered to patients in pain; and absence of a specific pharmacologic antagonist. Stimulation of hepatic microsomal enzyme activity is not a consideration with a one-time administration of barbiturates for preoperative medication. A patient with porphyria, however, should not receive barbiturates since these drugs may precipitate an acute exacerbation of this disease. Use of barbiturates for pharmacologic premedication has been largely replaced by benzodiazepines.

Determinants of Drug Choice and Dose

Patient age and weight
Physical status
Level of anxiety
Tolerance for depressant drugs
Previous adverse experience with drugs used for preoperative medication
Allergies
Elective or emergency surgery
Inpatient or outpatient surgery

Opioids

Advantages of opioids as used for pharmacologic premedication include the absence of direct myocardial depression and the production of analgesia in patients who are experiencing pain preoperatively or who will require insertion of invasive monitors before the induction of anesthesia. Discomfort associated with institution of a regional anesthetic is another possible indication for use of an opioid as pharmacologic premedication. Admini-

Table 9-2. Is Depressant Pharmacologic Premedication Indicated?

No	Yes
Newborn (<1 year)	Cardiac surgery
Elderly	Cancer surgery
Decreased level of consciousness	Co-existing pain
Intracranial pathology	Regional anesthesia
Severe pulmonary disease	
Hypovolemia	

Table 9-3. Drugs and Doses Used for Pharmacologic Premedication Before Induction of Anesthesia

Classification	Drug	Typical Adult Dose[a] (mg)	Route of Administration
Barbiturates	Secobarbital	50–150	PO, IM
	Pentobarbital	50–150	PO, IM
Opioids	Morphine	5–15	IM
	Meperidine	50–100	IM
Benzodiazepines	Midazolam	2.5–5	IM
	Diazepam	5–10	PO, IM
	Lorazepam	2–4	PO, IM
	Flurazepam	15–30	PO
	Temazepam	15–30	PO
	Triazolam	0.125–0.25	PO
Antihistamines	Diphenhydramine	25–75	PO, IM
	Promethazine	25–50	IM
	Hydroxyzine	50–100	IM
Alpha-2 agonists	Clonidine	0.3–0.4	PO
	Dexmedetomidine	0.4–0.5	IV
Anticholinergics	Atropine	0.3–0.6	IM
	Scopolamine	0.3–0.6	IM
	Glycopyrrolate	0.2–0.3	IM
H_2 antagonists	Cimetidine	300	PO, IM, IV
	Ranitidine	150	PO, IM
	Famotidine	20–40	PO
Antacids	Particulate	15–30 ml	PO
	Nonparticulate	10–20 ml	PO
Stimulants of gastric motility	Metoclopramide	10–20	PO, IM, IV

[a]Except for antacids.

stration of an opioid in the preoperative medication (preemptive analgesia) may decrease the need for parenteral analgesics in the early postoperative period (Fig. 9-1).[4,5] This is consistent with the concept that activation of afferent pain pathways, especially in lightly anesthetized patients, produces changes in the central nervous system that subsequently lead to amplification and prolongation of postoperative pain. Indeed, the dose of opioid required to prevent C-fiber-induced excitability changes in the spinal cord is lower than that required to suppress these changes once they occur. Inclusion of morphine in the preoperative medication decreases the likelihood that undesirable increases in heart rate will accompany surgical stimulation during administration of volatile anesthetics (Fig. 9-2).[6] Pharmacologic premedication with intramuscular administration of opioids may seem reasonable when a nitrous oxide-opioid anesthetic is planned. The opioid, however, may be just as logically given intravenously immediately before the induction of anesthesia.

Adverse effects of opioids as used for pharmacologic premedication include depression of the medullary ventilatory center, as evidenced by decreased responsiveness to carbon dioxide, and orthostatic hypotension due to relaxation of peripheral vascular smooth muscle. Orthostatic hypotension will be further exaggerated if opioids are administered to patients with decreased intravascular fluid volumes. Nausea and vomiting most likely reflect opioid-induced stimulation of the chemoreceptor trigger zone in the medulla. Recumbency seems to minimize nausea and vomiting after administration of opioids, suggesting that stimulation of the vestibular apparatus may also be important in production of this undesirable effect. Nevertheless, opioids may be avoided for this reason in patients undergoing outpatient surgery. Opioid-induced smooth muscle constriction may manifest as choledochoduodenal sphincter spasm, causing some anesthesiologists to question the use of opioids in patients with biliary tract disease. Pain associated with opioid-induced biliary tract spasm may be difficult to differentiate from angina pectoris. In this regard, nitroglycerin will relieve pain due to both etiologies, whereas administration of an opioid antagonist, naloxone, relieves only pain due to opioid-induced biliary tract spasm. An annoying side effect of opioids used as pharmacologic premedication is pruritus, which may be particularly prominent around the nose.

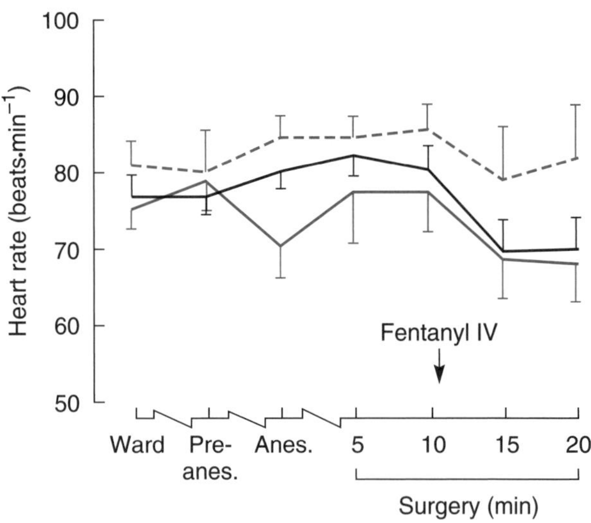

Figure 9-2. Morphine (0.1 mg·kg⁻¹ IM) administered to adult patients 30 to 60 minutes before induction of anesthesia for elective surgery may contribute to a decrease in heart rate, even during surgery. Mean ± SE. Solid red line, halothane; solid black line, isoflurane; dashed red line, enflurane. (From Cahalan et al.,[6] with permission.)

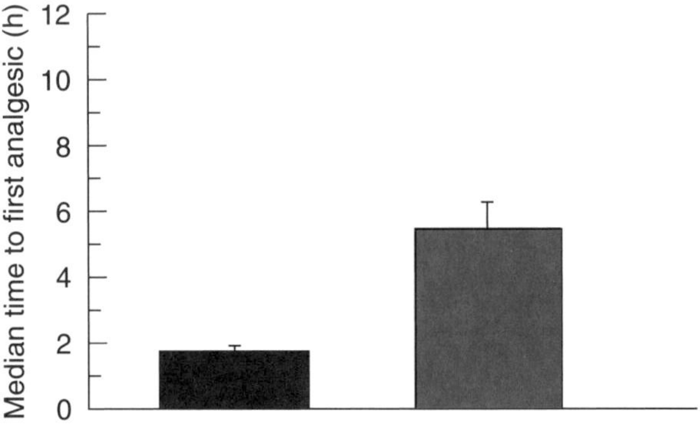

Figure 9-1. Inclusion of an opioid in the preoperative medication increases the median time in the postoperative period before an analgesic is needed. Red bar, opioid premedication (216 patients studied); black bar, no opioid premedication (514 patients studied). (Modified from McQuay et al.,[4] with permission.)

Benzodiazepines

Benzodiazepines act on specific brain receptors to produce selective anxiolytic effects at doses that do not produce excessive sedation or cardiopulmonary depression. In addition, these drugs, particularly midazolam and lorazepam, produce suppression of recall of events that occur after (anterograde amnesia) their administration (Fig. 9-3).[7] Suppression of recall for preceding events (retrograde amnesia) is less predictable. In animals, diazepam increases the seizure threshold for lidocaine, but there is no evidence that doses of benzodiazepines as used for pharmacologic premedication in humans decrease the likelihood of local anesthetic toxicity. Flurazepam, temazepam, and triazolam are examples of benzodiazepines used principally to treat insomnia that is often present the night before scheduled surgery.

Disadvantages of benzodiazepines as used for pharmacologic premedication include excessive and prolonged sedation in occasional patients. This is particularly likely in patients who receive lorazepam in doses that exceed 50 $\mu g \cdot kg^{-1}$ (the total dose administered orally should probably not exceed 4 mg). Flumazenil, a specific benzodiazepine antagonist, is effective in reversing undesirable or unacceptably persistent effects of these drugs. Pain on injection and occasional erratic absorption after intramuscular injection of diazepam reflects the presence of propylene glycol in the commercial preparation of this drug. By contrast, midazolam lacks these adverse effects since it is water soluble, obviating the need for propylene glycol.

Butyrophenones

The use of droperidol for pharmacologic premedication is limited because of the occasional production of dysphoria after its administration. These patients express a fear of death and may refuse a previously agreed to elective operative procedure. Another disadvantage of droperidol is production of dopamine receptor blockade, which may produce extrapyramidal symptoms in normal patients as well as those with co-existing paralysis agitans.

Prophylaxis Against Postoperative Nausea and Vomiting

Proponents of droperidol use cite its efficacy as a postoperative antiemetic (presumably reflecting dopamine receptor blockade) when administered intravenously most often near the end of surgery (Table 9-4 and Fig. 9-4).[8,9] The use of droperidol as a prophylactic antiemetic, however, has been associated with delayed recovery from anesthesia and an increased incidence of postoperative vertigo, anxiety, and restlessness (Table 9-5).[10] These droperidol-

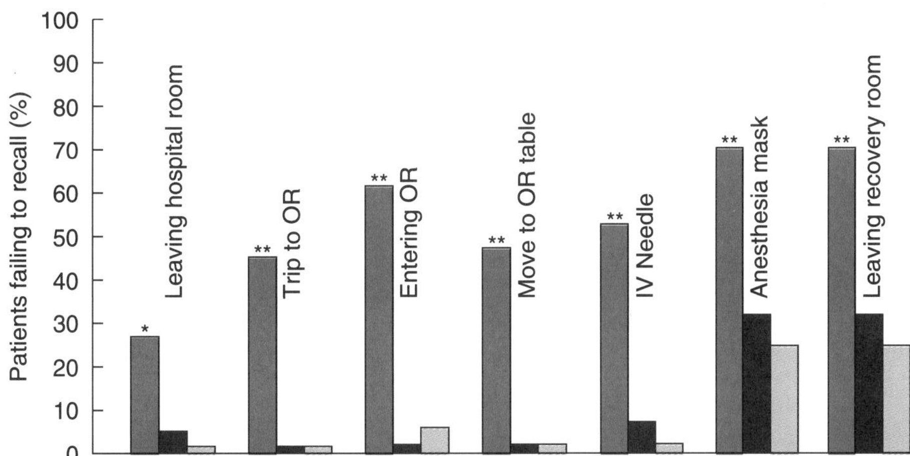

Figure 9-3. The percentage of adult patients failing to recall specific events 24 hours after intramuscular injections of lorazepam (4 mg; dark red bars), diazepam (10 mg; solid black bars), or placebo (light red bars) was significantly greater for those receiving lorazepam. *P <0.05; **P <0.01. (From Fragen and Caldwell,[7] with permission.)

Table 9-4. Frequency of Nausea and/or Vomiting in the Postanesthesia Care Unit

	Frequency of Nausea and/or Vomiting[a] (%)
Metoclopramide (5 mg)[b]	55
Metoclopramide (10 mg)	45
Droperidol (5 μg·kg^{-1})[c]	40
Droperidol (10 μg·kg^{-1})	25[d]
Droperidol (20 μg·kg^{-1})	20[d]
Metoclopramide (10 mg) plus droperidol (10 μg·kg^{-1})	25[d]
Placebo	65

[a]As a percentage of 20 patients in each group.
[b]Metoclopramide administered orally 30 minutes prior to induction of anesthesia.
[c]Droperidol administered intravenously 2 minutes prior to induction of anesthesia.
[d]P <0.05 versus placebo.
(Modified from Pandit et al.,[8] with permission.)

related side effects argue against the routine prophylactic use of this drug as an antiemetic in all patients. An alternative approach is to limit the prophylactic administration of droperidol to patients considered to be at high risk of postoperative nausea and vomiting (ophthalmologic operations, gynecologic procedures). Even with this approach, it must be recognized that droperidol does not reliably decrease the incidence of postoperative nausea and vomiting to zero.

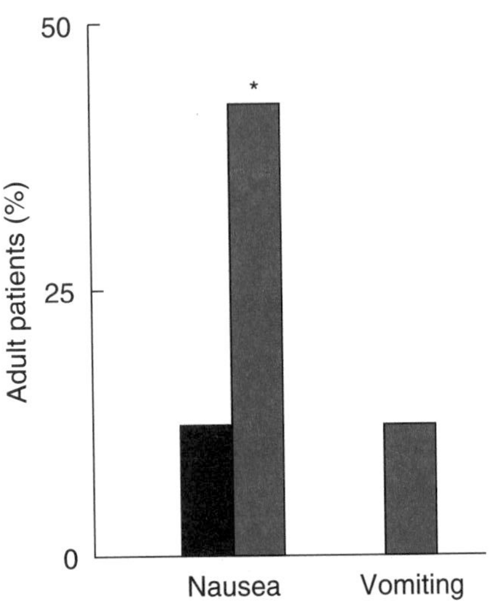

Figure 9-4. The incidence of nausea and vomiting was significantly decreased postoperatively in patients receiving droperidol (2.5 mg IV) administered near the end of surgery (group 1, black bar) compared with those treated with a placebo (group II, red bars). *P <0.05. (From Santos and Datta,[9] with permission.)

Table 9-5. Incidence of Droperidol-Induced Side Effects

Droperidol (1.25 mg IV) Administered	No. of Patients: Total	With Anxiety	With Restlessness
Yes	43	10 (23.2%)[a]	3 (7.8%)
No	46	0	0

[a]P <0.05
(Modified from Melnick et al.,[10] with permission.)

An alternative to droperidol may be ondansetron (4 to 8 mg IV), which produces its antiemetic effect by acting as a serotonin antagonist.[11] Unlike droperidol, sedation, restlessness, dysphoria, and extrapyramidal symptoms do not accompany the administration of ondansetron.

Antihistamines

Antihistamines are occasionally used for pharmacologic premedication because of their sedative and antiemetic properties. Promethazine, combined with meperidine, does not increase depression of ventilation produced by meperidine or alter the incidence of nausea and vomiting but does produce an additive sedative effect.

Prophylaxis Against Allergic Reactions

Diphenhydramine (0.5 to 1 mg·kg^{-1} PO) has been recommended as pharmacologic premedication to provide prophylaxis against intraoperative allergic reactions in patients with a history of chronic atopy or undergoing procedures (radiographic dye studies) known to be associated with allergic reactions. An H_2 antagonist such as cimetidine (4 to 6 mg·kg^{-1} PO) should be administered with diphenhydramine (see the section *H_2 Antagonists*). This combination of an H_1 antagonist (diphenhydramine) and an H_2 antagonist (cimetidine) acts to occupy peripheral receptor sites normally responsive to histamine, thus decreasing manifestations of any subsequent drug-induced release of histamine. Prednisone (50 mg PO every 6 hours for the 24 hours before surgery) may also be added to this prophylactic regimen. Even with this prophylactic regimen, drug-induced allergic reactions may still occur in highly sensitive patients.

Alpha-2 Agonists

Clonidine is a centrally acting alpha-2 agonist that acts as an antihypertensive drug. Administered as preoperative medication (5 $\mu g \cdot kg^{-1}$ PO), this drug produces sedation and attenuation of autonomic nervous system reflex responses (hypertension, tachycardia, catecholamine release) associated with preoperative anxiety and surgical stimulation.[12] Dose requirements for inhaled and injected anesthetics are also decreased in patients receiving clonidine as preoperative medication. Dexmedetomidine, a more potent and specific alpha-2 agonist than clonidine, has also been used for preoperative medication. Bradycardia and dry mouth are possible side effects of preoperative medication with alpha-2 agonists.

Anticholinergics

Routine inclusion of anticholinergics as part of the pharmacologic premedication is not necessary. The most frequent reasons for administering anticholinergics are (1) production of an antisialagogue effect, (2) production of sedative and amnesic effects, and (3) prevention of reflex bradycardia (Table 9-6). Anticholinergics are not predictably effective in increasing gastric fluid pH or decreasing gastric fluid volume.[1]

Antisialagogue Effect

The need for including an anticholinergic in the preoperative medication to produce an antisialagogue effect has been questioned, since currently used inhaled and injected (an exception is ketamine) anesthetics do not stimulate excessive upper airway secretions. Nevertheless, decreased secretions during general anesthesia, particularly when a tracheal tube is in place, are a desirable effect of an anticholinergic administered preoperatively. An antisialagogue effect is particularly important for intra-oral operations, for bronchoscopies, or when topical anesthesia is necessary, as excessive secretions may interfere with the surgery or impair production of topical anesthesia by diluting the local anesthetic. Administration of an anticholinergic for an antisialagogue effect is not necessary when regional anesthesia is planned.

Scopolamine is about three times more potent as an antisialagogue than is atropine. For this reason, scopolamine is often selected when both an antisialagogue effect and sedation are desired results of preoperative medication. Glycopyrrolate is selected when an antisialagogue effect, in the absence of sedation, is desired. As an antisialagogue, glycopyrrolate is about twice as potent as atropine and has a longer duration of action. To decrease the period of discomfort due to a dry mouth and throat, an anticholinergic can be given just before the patient is transported to the operating room. Nevertheless, anxiety, fluid deprivation before elective surgery, and other drugs used for pharmacologic premedication may produce a dry mouth and throat even in the absence of an anticholinergic.

Sedative and Amnesic Effects

Atropine and scopolamine are tertiary amines that can cross lipid barriers, including the blood-brain barrier. Resulting sedative and amnesic effects reflect penetrance of these drugs into the central nervous system. Scopolamine, more than atropine,

Table 9-6. Comparative Effects of Anticholinergics Administered Intramuscularly as Pharmacologic Premedication

	Atropine	Scopolamine	Glycopyrrolate
Antisialagogue effect	+	+++	++
Sedative and amnesic effects	+	+++	0
Increased gastric fluid pH	0	0	±
Central nervous system toxicity	+	++	0
Relaxation of lower esophageal sphincter	++	++	++
Mydriasis and cycloplegia	+	+++	0

0, none; +, mild; ++, moderate; +++, marked.

produces useful sedative effects, particularly in combination with barbiturates, opioids, or benzodiazepines as used for pharmacologic premedication. It is estimated that scopolamine is 8 to 10 times more potent than atropine in its effects on the central nervous system. Glycopyrrolate, as a quaternary ammonium compound, cannot easily cross the blood-brain barrier and thus does not produce significant sedative or amnesic effects.

Prevention of Reflex Bradycardia

Use of anticholinergics in the pharmacologic premedication for prevention of reflex bradycardia is a secondary objective since the dose and timing of intramuscular administration are not appropriate. The most logical approach, particularly in children with increased vagal activity, is to administer atropine or glycopyrrolate intravenously shortly before the anticipated need. Bradycardia has been observed following induction of anesthesia with propofol, causing some to recommend the prior intravenous injection of atropine when vagal stimulation is likely to occur in association with use of this anesthetic.

Undesirable Side Effects

Undesirable side effects of anticholinergics are multiple and must be considered in the decision to use these drugs for pharmacologic premedication.

Undesirable Side Effects of Anticholinergics

- Central nervous system toxicity
- Tachycardia
- Lower esophageal sphincter relaxation
- Mydriasis and cycloplegia
- Body temperature increase
- Drying of airway secretions
- Increased physiologic deadspace

Central Nervous System Toxicity. Central nervous system toxicity (central anticholinergic syndrome) produced by anticholinergics manifests as delirium or prolonged somnolence after anesthesia. This undesirable response is more likely to follow administration of scopolamine than atropine, but the incidence should be low with the doses used for pharmacologic premedication. Nevertheless, elderly patients may be uniquely susceptible to central nervous system toxicity secondary to atropine or scopolamine. Central nervous system toxicity is unlikely after the administration of glycopyrrolate since this drug cannot easily cross the blood-brain barrier. It must be recognized that toxicity attributed to the anticholinergic may also represent an uninhibited response to pain as the depressant effects of the anesthetic dissipate.

Central anticholinergic syndrome presumably reflects blockade of muscarinic cholinergic receptors in the central nervous system. Physostigmine, a tertiary amine anticholinesterase (15 to 60 $\mu g \cdot kg^{-1}$ IV), is a specific treatment for central nervous system toxicity due to scopolamine or atropine. Neostigmine and pyridostigmine are not effective anticholinesterase antidotes because their quaternary ammonium structure prevents these drugs from easily entering the central nervous system.

Tachycardia. Scopolamine and glycopyrrolate, which have minimal cardioaccelerator effects, may be more logical selections than atropine for pharmacologic premedication when an increased heart rate would be undesirable, as in patients with mitral stenosis and atrial fibrillation being treated with digitalis. Nevertheless, the most likely cardiac response after intramuscular administration of atropine, glycopyrrolate, or scopolamine for pharmacologic premedication is heart rate slowing, presumably reflecting a weak cholinergic agonist effect of these drugs. Previous speculation that heart rate slowing after administration of atropine reflected a central vagal action is not supported by similar heart rate changes after administration of glycopyrrolate, which cannot easily cross the blood-brain barrier.

Lower Esophageal Sphincter Relaxation. Intravenous administration of anticholinergics results in relaxation of the lower esophageal sphincter. Presumably, intramuscular administration of these drugs could also lower esophageal sphincter pressure. When barrier pressure (lower esophageal sphincter pressure minus gastric pressure) is less than 13 cmH_2O, the patient becomes vulnerable to gastroesophageal reflux and the hazards of aspiration pneumonitis. This remains a theoretical hazard of anticholinergics, however, as there is no evidence that the incidence of aspiration pneumonitis is increased in patients receiving these drugs as pharmacologic premedication.

Mydriasis and Cycloplegia. Atropine and scopolamine may produce mydriasis and cycloplegia, causing patients to experience visual impairment postoperatively. In this regard, scopolamine has a greater mydriatic effect than atropine. Conceivably, mydriasis could interfere with drainage of aqueous humor from the anterior chamber of the eye. There is no evidence, however, that the inclusion of anticholinergics in the pharmacologic premedication is contraindicated for patients with glaucoma. Nevertheless, miotic eye drops should be continued throughout the perioperative period in these patients.

Body Temperature Increase. Anticholinergics may result in increased body temperature by suppressing sweat glands that are innervated by cholinergic nerves via the sympathetic nervous system. Prevention of sweating by this mechanism may be undesirable in the presence of co-existing increases in body temperature, particularly in children.

Drying of Airway Secretions. Increased viscosity of ariway secretions may be an undesirable effect of anticholinergics, especially in patients with chronic pulmonary disease. The clinical signficance of this effect in response to a single dose of anticholinergic as adminstered for preoperative medication is unproven.

H_2 Antagonists

H_2 antagonists counter the ability of histamine to induce secretion of gastric fluid with a high concentration of hydrogen ions. Therefore, these drugs offer a pharmacologic approach for increasing gastric fluid pH before the induction of anesthesia. It is likely that 40% to 80% of adult patients undergoing elective surgery with or without an anticholinergic included in the preoperative medication have a gastric fluid pH below 2.5.[1] An increase in gastric fluid pH to higher than 2.5 is theoretically desirable since the severity of aspiration pneumonitis is likely to be accentuated by inhalation of fluid with a pH below 2.5.

Routine inclusion of H_2 antagonists in the preoperative medication of patients scheduled for elective surgery is appealing. Certainly, the use of H_2 antagonists would be particularly attractive for inclusion in the pharmacologic premedication of patients considered to be at increased risk of pulmonary aspiration of gastric contents; these patients include (1) parturients, (2) patients with symptoms of gastroesophageal reflux, (3) obese patients, and (4) patients in whom difficult airway management is anticipated. An objection to routine inclusion of H_2 antagonists in the preoperative medication is the concept that all therapies should be individualized and tailored to fit individual patients, their diseases, and specific preoperative circumstances. More important, the incidences of pulmonary aspiration and serious morbidity are sufficiently low in patients undergoing elective surgery that the cost of preventing one serious complication of pulmonary aspiration by the routine use of prophylactic medications such as H_2 antagonists would be very high.[13] Furthermore, these drugs are not 100% effective (an inherent failure rate).[1] H_2 antagonists will not alter the pH of gastric fluid that is present before administration of the drug, nor will they facilitate gastric emptying. Under no circumstances can preoperative medication with H_2 antagonists be substituted for an anesthetic technique with a cuffed tracheal tube or maintenance of consciousness to protect the lungs from inhalation of gastric fluid (see Chapter 11).

Antacids

Antacids administered 15 to 30 minutes before induction of anesthesia are nearly 100% effective in increasing the gastric fluid pH to above 2.5. The efficacy of antacids may be dependent to some extent on patient movement so as to facilitate complete mixing with gastric fluid. Inhalation of gastric fluid containing particulate antacids may initiate an inflammatory reaction that is associated with severe and persistent pulmonary dysfunction despite a high pH of the aspirated material.[1] By contrast, nonparticulate antacids, such as sodium citrate, effectively increase the gastric fluid pH to above 2.5 and do not produce significant pulmonary dysfunction should inhalation of fluid containing antacids occur.

Compared with H_2 antagonists, administration of antacids is effective in increasing the pH of gastric fluid that is present in the stomach at the time of administration (no lag time). This desirable effect, however, is predictably associated with an increased gastric fluid volume that does not occur with H_2 antagonists. Nevertheless, withholding antacids because of concern of increasing gastric fluid volume is not warranted, considering animal evidence that documents increased mortality after aspiration of low volumes of acidic gastric fluid compared with aspiration of large volumes of buffered gastric fluid (Table 9-7).[14]

Table 9-7. Gastric Fluid Volume and pH Following Unrestricted Preoperative Oral Fluid Intake

Fast (h)	Volume[a] (ml) Ingested Fluid	Residual Gastric Fluid	Gastric Fluid pH
1.3–3.0	244 (120–500)	22 (3–70)	1.5
3.1–5.0	241 (50–1200)	32 (0–130)	1.7
5.1–8	230 (50–500)	28 (2–72)	1.6
NPO		25 (0–107)	1.6

[a]Values are means; ranges are given in parentheses.
(Modified from Maltby et al.,[18] with permission.)

Metoclopramide

Metoclopramide speeds gastric emptying by selectively increasing the motility of the upper gastrointestinal tract and relaxing the pyloric sphincter. The onset of metoclopramide effect is 30 to 60 minutes after oral administration and 1 to 3 minutes after intravenous injection. This drug may be useful in preoperative medication for use in decreasing gastric fluid volume, particularly in patients with diabetes mellitus and associated gastroparesis, in parturients, and in patients who have recently ingested food and require emergency surgery for disease unrelated to the gastrointestinal tract. Nevertheless, metoclopramide does not guarantee gastric emptying, and its beneficial effects may be offset by concomitant or prior administration of anticholinergics, opioids, or antacids.[1] The ability of metoclopramide to increase lower esophageal sphincter tone may also be negated by inclusion of atropine in the preoperative medication. Metoclopramide does not predictably alter gastric fluid pH. Side effects of metoclopramide include abdominal cramping if rapidly administered intravenously and occasional neurologic dysfunction reflecting passage into the central nervous system and production of dopamine receptor blockade.[1] Any antiemetic effect produced by this drug is likely to be due to antagonism of dopamine receptors in the central nervous system. The combination of metoclopramide and droperidol has not been shown to provide an antiemetic effect superior to that of droperidol alone (Table 9-4).[8]

OUTPATIENTS

Administration of preoperative medication to outpatients must avoid introducing persistent drug effects that delay emergence from anesthesia or prevent early discharge (nausea and vomiting) after elective and usually minor surgery (see Chapter 29).

PEDIATRIC PATIENTS

Pediatric patients, like adults, benefit from attempts to tailor the preoperative medication to unique requirements of each child. Age is a particularly important aspect in considering psychological preparation of pediatric patients. In this regard, preschool children are often the most upset when separated from their family and benefit from having parents accompany them to the operating room. It becomes easier to communicate with children older than 5 years of age, allowing the anesthesiologist to explain expected events in the preoperative period and to offer reassurance. The attitude and behavior of the parents are also important in the psychological preparation of the child.

After about 1 year of age, children may benefit from pharmacologic attempts to decrease anxiety. The oral route for administration of drugs is appealing, since most children abhor intramuscular injections. In this regard, the trend in the preoperative medication of young children is the oral administration of midazolam (0.5 $mg \cdot kg^{-1}$ dissolved in a flavored syrup) to provide preinduction sedation. Atropine, administered intravenously just before the induction of anesthesia, is often recommended to attenuate increased vagal activity characteristically present in pediatric patients.

EVALUATION OF DEPRESSANT DRUGS USED FOR PHARMACOLOGIC PREMEDICATION

Precise methods to evaluate the value of depressant drugs as used for pharmacologic premedication are not available. For example, anxiety is a subjective response that may be influenced by differences in the emotional states of patients, as well as what patients expect from the preoperative medication. Sedation is a more objective measurement, but drowsiness does not always parallel relief of anxiety. Comparison of studies on pharmacologic premedication is hampered by different drug doses, sites and routes of administration, and times for measuring responses. Despite these complexities, a well-controlled study suggested that desirable (decreased anxiety, sedation) and undesirable (dry mouth, nausea, vomiting) effects of pharmacologic premedication were difficult to distinguish from placebo effects.[15] This casts doubt on the ability to measure and confirm the value of drugs used for pharmacologic premedication but should not be accepted as evidence that pharmacologic premedication fails to produce more comfortable patients in the preoperative period. Indeed, plasma concentrations of beta endorphins, as a reflection of the anterior pituitary response to stress before induction of anesthesia, are lower in patients receiving pharmacologic premedication than in patients receiving placebo injections (Fig. 9-5).[16]

FASTING BEFORE ELECTIVE SURGERY

Fasting before elective surgery (NPO after midnight) is recommended in the hope of minimizing gastric fluid volume at the time of induction of anesthesia. Nevertheless, complete gastric emptying can never be guaranteed. Furthermore, solid food passes through the stomach at variable and unpredictable rates, sometimes taking up to 12 hours. By contrast, clear liquids have a 50% emptying time of only 12 to 20 minutes. Therefore, it may be illogical to have a single guideline for solid food and clear liquid ingestion before induction of anesthesia for elective operations. Indeed, the necessity for prolonged abstinence from ingestion of clear fluids prior to the induction of anesthesia for elective surgery has been challenged.[17] Fears that ingestion of clear liquids on the morning of surgery will result in increased gastric fluid volume are unfounded (Table 9-7).[18] A consistent finding has been that gastric fluid volume and pH are independent of the duration of the fluid fast beyond 2 hours, provided that only clear liquids are ingested on the day of surgery (Fig. 9-6).[19] When longer than 2 hours has elapsed following clear liquid ingestion, endoge-

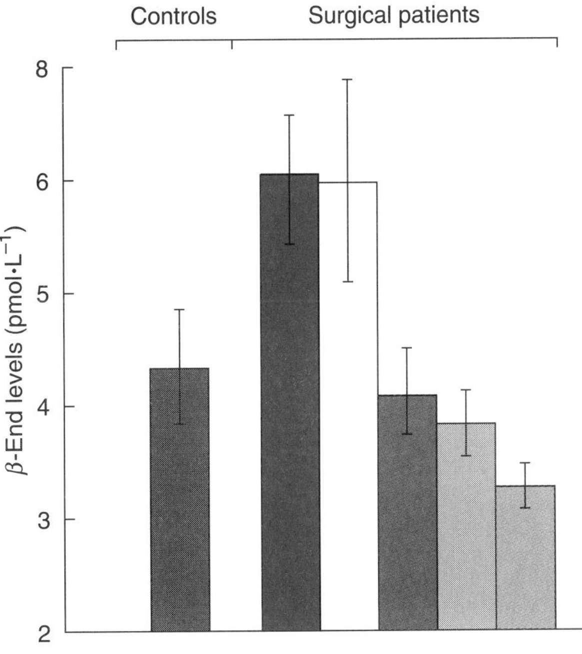

Figure 9-5. Compared with control values (dark gray bar), plasma concentrations of beta endorphins (β-End) were decreased in presurgical patients receiving preoperative medication with diazepam (10 mg PO [medium red bar]), diphenhydramine (1 mg·kg^{-1} IM [light gray bar]), or meperidine (1 mg·kg^{-1} IM [light red bar]). Plasma concentrations of β-End were increased in presurgical patients receiving a placebo injection (white bar). Mean ± SE. Measurements were made 1 hour after treatment. Dark red bar, UNP. (From Walsh et al.,[16] with permission.)

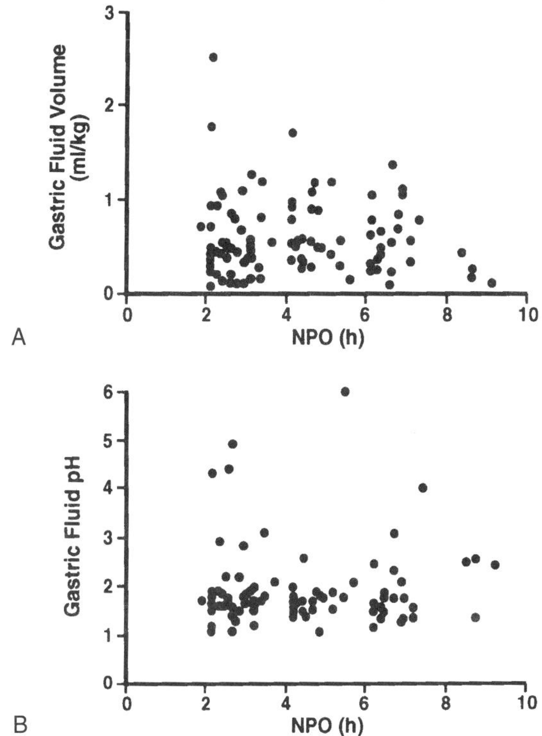

Figure 9-6. *(A & B)* Gastric fluid volume and pH do not correlate with periods of fasting ranging from 2 to 6 hours following the ingestion of water (2 ml·kg^{-1}). (Modified from Crawford et al.,[19] with permission.)

nous gastric fluid secretion is the principal determinant of the volume and pH of gastric fluid and a longer fluid fast does not improve the gastric environment. It is even possible that clear liquids stimulate gastric peristalsis and accelerate the rate of gastric emptying. Preoperative anxiety does not seem to delay gastric emptying or increase gastric fluid volume.[20] For all these reasons, it does not seem logical to (1) forbid ingestion of clear liquids up to 2 hours before elective surgery or (2) forbid the oral administration of drugs with up to 150 ml of water in the hour preceding induction of anesthesia.[21–23] This recommendation does not apply to solid food or to patients at known risk of slow gastric emptying (obese patients, parturients, patients with diabetes mellitus or gastrointestinal disease, patients in whom difficult tracheal intubation is anticipated, and patients undergoing emergency surgery). There is no evidence that opioids administered after ingestion of water adversely slow gastric emptying.[24]

RECOMMENDED PREOPERATIVE MEDICATION FOR ADULT PATIENTS UNDERGOING ELECTIVE SURGERY

Preoperative medication begins with the anesthesiologist's interview and subsequent decision as to the need for and type of pharmacologic premedication. Timing of drug administration is as important as the drugs selected for pharmacologic premedication. Drugs administered to decrease anxiety and to produce sedation are more appropriately administered 1 to 2 hours before induction of anesthesia. A benzodiazepine or an H_2 antagonist, or both, is also conveniently administered orally at this time. Metoclopramide is a logical consideration for inclusion in the pharmacologic premedication when a predictable decrease in gastric fluid volume is important. Nevertheless, there is evidence that a single oral dose of an H_2 antagonist is as effective as the combination of an H_2 antagonist, metoclopramide, and an antacid in increasing gastric fluid pH and decreasing gastric fluid volume prior to the induction anesthesia (Table 9-8).[25] Emergency surgery requiring general anesthesia in patients who have recently eaten may be an appropriate situation for intravenous administration of metoclopramide. Intramuscular administration of morphine is an alternative to benzodiazepines if analgesia is an

Suggestions for Preoperative Medication for Adults Undergoing Elective Surgery (see Table 9-3 for doses)

Patient visit and interview by anesthesiologist
Benzodiazepine (orally) to treat insomnia the night before surgery
Benzodiazepine (preferably orally) 1 to 2 hours before induction of anesthesia
Opioid (intramuscularly) instead of the benzodiazepine if analgesia is desired
Scopolamine (intramuscularly) 1 to 2 hours before induction of anesthesia if reliable sedation and amnesia are desired; alternatively, if only an antisialagogue effect is desired, glycopyrrolate intramuscularly when patient is ready for transport to the operating room (a final option is not to include an anticholinergic in the preoperative medication)
Possible use of an H_2 antagonist (orally) 1 to 2 hours before induction of anesthesia, especially in patients considered to be at increased risk of aspiration of gastric contents

Table 9-8. Gastric Fluid Volume and pH in Patients Undergoing Elective Surgery

Drug[a]	Volume[b] (ml)	pH[b]
Ranitidine (150 mg)	8 (0–40)	5.7 (1.7–8.6)
Ranitidine (150 mg) Metoclopramide (10 mg)	10 (0–80)	6.1 (1.8–8.9)
Ranitidine (150 mg) Sodium citrate (30 ml)	19 (0–58)[c]	5.8 (1.6–8.3)
Ranitidine (150 mg) Metoclopramide (10 mg) Sodium citrate (30 ml)	22 (0–68)[c]	6.3 (2.1–8.1)

[a]Ranitidine administered orally 2 to 3 hours before induction of anesthesia; metoclopramide administered orally 1 hour before induction of anesthesia; sodium citrate administered on call to the operating room.
[b]Values are means; ranges are given in parentheses.
[c]$P < 0.05$ compared with groups not receiving sodium citrate.
(Modified from Maltby et al.,[25] with permission.)

important objective of preoperative medication. Intramuscular scopolamine administered at the same time as the drug selected to decrease anxiety is indicated when it is desirable to exploit the amnesic and sedative effects of this anticholinergic. For example, the combination of intramuscular morphine with or without an oral benzodiazepine plus intramuscular scopolamine is useful for producing sedation in patients most deserving of aggressive pharmacologic premedication (Table 9-2).

An anticholinergic selected solely to produce an antisialagogue effect is most appropriately administered intramuscularly, immediately before patients are transported to the operating room. This timing minimizes the duration of the uncomfortable sensation of a dry mouth and throat experienced by patients before the induction of anesthesia. Glycopyrrolate is the most logical drug to select if an antisialagogue response without central nervous system effects is desired. Drugs that decrease vagal activity (atropine, glycopyrrolate), protect against postoperative nausea and vomiting (droperidol, ondansetron), or provide postoperative analgesia (preemptive analgesia) are most logically administered intravenously at a time just preceding that of the desired effect.

REFERENCES

1. White PF. Pharmacologic and clinical aspects of preoperative medication. Anesth Analg 1986;65:963–74.
2. Egbert LD, Battit GE, Turndorf H, Beecher HK. The value of the preoperative visit by an anesthetist. JAMA 1963;185:553–5.
3. Leigh JM, Walker J, Janaganthan P. Effect of preoperative anaesthetic visit on anxiety. Br Med J 1977; 2:987–9.
4. McQuay HJ, Carroll D, Moore RA. Postoperative orthopaedic pain—The effect of opiate premedication and local anaesthetic blocks. Pain 1988;33:291–5.
5. Katz J, Kavanagh BP, Sandler AN, et al. Preemptive analgesia. Clinical evidence of neuroplasticity contributing to postoperative pain. Anesthesiology 1992;77:439–46.
6. Cahalan MK, Lutz FW, Eger EI II, Schwartz LA, Beaupre PN, Smith JS. Narcotics decrease heart rate during inhalational anesthesia. Anesth Analg 1987;66:166–70.
7. Fragen RJ, Caldwell N. Lorazepam premedication: Lack of recall and relief of anxiety. Anesth Analg 1976;55:792–6.
8. Pandit SK, Kothary SP, Pandit UA, Randel G, Levy L. Dose-response study of droperidol and metoclopramide as antiemetics for outpatient anesthesia. Anesth Analg 1989;68:798–802.
9. Santos A, Datta S. Prophylactic use of droperidol for control of nausea and vomiting during spinal anesthesia for cesarean section. Anesth Analg 1984;63:85–7.
10. Melnick B, Sawyer R, Karambelkar D, Phitayakorn P, Uy NTL, Patel R. Delayed side effects of droperidol after ambulatory general anesthesia. Anesth Analg 1989;69:748–51.
11. McKenzie R, Kovac A, O'Connor T, et al. Comparison of ondansetron versus placebo to prevent postoperative nausea and vomiting in women undergoing ambulatory gynecologic surgery. Anesthesiology 1993;78:21–8.
12. Engelman E, Lipszyc M, Gilbart E, et al. Effects of clonidine on anesthetic drug requirements and hemodynamic response during aortic surgery. Anesthesiology 1989;71:178–87.
13. Warner MA, Warner ME, Weber JG. Clinical significance of pulmonary aspiration during the perioperative period. Anesthesiology 1993;78:56–62.
14. James CF, Modell JH, Gibbs CP, Kuck EJ, Ruiz BC. Pulmonary aspiration—Effects of volume and pH in the rat. Anesth Analg 1984;63:665–8.
15. Forrest WH, Brown CR, Brown BW. Subjective responses to six common preoperative medications. Anesthesiology 1977;47:241–7.
16. Walsh J, Puig MM, Lovitz MA, Turndorf H. Premedication abolishes the increase in plasma beta-endorphin observed in the immediate preoperative period. Anesthesiology 1987;66:402–5.
17. Coté CJ. NPO after midnight for children—A reappraisal. Anesthesiology 1990;72:589–92.
18. Maltby JR, Lewis P, Martin A, Sutherland LR. Gastric fluid volume and pH in elective patients following unrestricted oral fluid until three hours before surgery. Can J Anaesth 1991;38:425–9.
19. Crawford M, Lerman J, Christensen S, Farrow-Gillespie A. Effects of duration of fasting on gastric fluid pH and volume in healthy children. Anesth Analg 1990;71:400–3.
20. Haavik PE, Soreide E, Hofstad B, Steen PA. Does preoperative anxiety influence gastric fluid volume and acidity? Anesth Analg 1992;75:91–4.
21. Goresky GV, Maltby JR. Fasting guidelines for elective surgical patients. Can J Anaesth 1990;37:493–5.
22. Phillips S, Hutchinson S, Davidson T. Preoperative drinking does not affect gastric contents. Br J Anaesth 1993;70:6–9.
23. Søreide E, Holst-Larsen H, Reite K, Mikkelsen H, Søreide JA, Steen PA. Effects of giving water 20–450 ml with oral diazepam premedication 1–2 H before operation. Br J Anaesth 1993;71:503–6.
24. Agarwal A, Chari P, Surgh H. Fluid deprivation before operation. The effect of a small drink. Anaesthesia 1989;44:632–4.
25. Maltby JR, Elliott RH, Warnell I, Fairbrass M, Sutherland LR, Shaffer EA. Gastric fluid volume and pH in elective surgical patients: Triple prophylaxis is not superior to ranitidine alone. Can J Anaesth 1990;37:650–5.

10

Anesthesia Systems

An anesthesia system consists of the anesthesia machine and anesthetic breathing system (circuit), which permit delivery of known concentrations of inhaled anesthetics and oxygen to the patient as well as removal of the patient's exhaled carbon dioxide. Carbon dioxide can be removed either by washout (delivered gas flows higher than 5 L·min^{-1} from the anesthesia machine) or by chemical neutralization (absorption).

ANESTHESIA MACHINE

Anesthesia machines, regardless of their manufacturer, have the same basic components (700 or more individual parts integrated to perform as a single unit) (Figs. 10-1 and 10-2).[1] These components include (1) a source of compressed gases, (2) flowmeters to ensure delivery of known flows and concentrations of these gases into an anesthetic breathing system, and (3) means of vaporizing and delivering known concentrations of the vapor of liquid anesthetics. The anesthesia machine may be equipped with a mechanical ventilator and devices to monitor the electrocardiogram, blood pressure, body temperature, arterial hemoglobin saturation with oxygen, and inhaled and exhaled concentrations of oxygen, carbon dioxide, and anesthetic gases and vapors (see Chapter 15). Alarm systems to signal apnea or disconnection of the anesthetic breathing system from the patient as reflected by an oxygen supply pressure lower than 30 psi are included. Anesthesia machines are equipped with a fail-safe valve designed to prevent delivery of hypoxic gas mixtures from the machine due to failure of the oxygen supply. This valve shuts off or proportionally decreases the flow of all gases when the pressure in the oxygen delivery line decreases below 30 psi. This will protect against an unrecognized exhaustion of oxygen delivery from a cylinder attached to the anesthesia machine or from a central source. This valve, however, does not prevent the delivery of pure nitrous oxide when the oxygen flow is zero but gas-pressure in the circuit of the anesthesia machine is maintained. In this situation, an oxygen analyzer is necessary to detect the delivery of a hypoxic gas mixture. Far superior to the fail-safe valve or oxygen analyzer is the continuous presence of a vigilant anesthesiologist.

Compressed Gases

Gases used in the administration of anesthesia (oxygen, nitrous oxide, air) are most often delivered to the anesthesia machine via a central supply source located in the hospital (Fig. 10-2). Oxygen or air from a central supply source may also be used to power (pneumatic driven) the ventilator on the anesthesia machine. Gas enters the anesthesia machine through pipeline inlet connections that are gas specific (threaded noninterchangeable connections) so as to minimize the possibility of a misconnection. This gas must be delivered from the central supply source at an appropriate pressure (about 50 psi) for the flowmeters on the anesthesia machine to function properly.

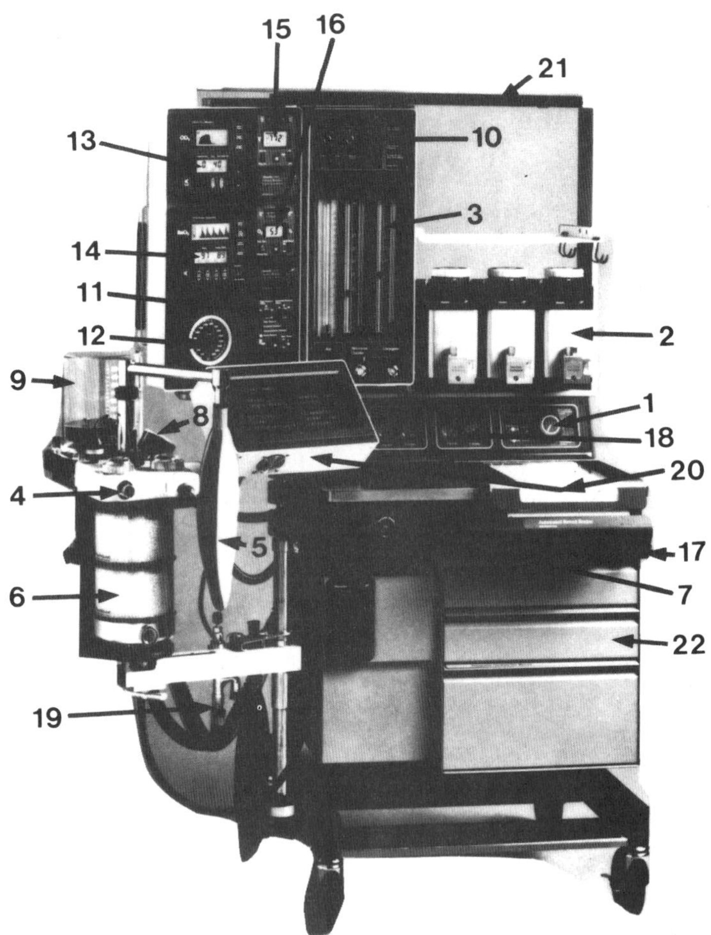

Figure 10-1. Components of an anesthesia machine include (1) on-off electrical/pneumatic switch, (2) agent specific vaporizers, (3) flowmeters, (4) connections for a circle anesthetic breathing system, (5) reservoir bag, (6) canister for granules to absorb carbon dioxide, (7) oxygen flush valve, (8) airway pressure gauge, (9) ventilator, (10) ventilator controls, (11) airway pressure monitor and alarm, (12) blood pressure gauge, (13) capnograph, (14) pulse oximeter, (15) tidal volume monitor, (16) oxygen analyzer, (17) yokes for compressed gas cylinders, (18) pressure gauges, (19) gas evacuation (scavenging) system, (20) automated anesthesia record, (21) shelf for portable equipment, and (22) drawers for storage.

Anesthesia machines are also equipped with cylinders of oxygen and nitrous oxide for use should the central gas supply fail (Fig. 10-2). Color-coded cylinders are attached to the anesthesia machine via a hanger yoke assembly, which consists of two metal pins that correspond to holes in the valve casing of the gas cylinder (pin-indexed) (Table 10-1). This design makes it impossible to attach an oxygen cylinder to any yoke other than that designed for oxygen. Otherwise, a cylinder containing nitrous oxide could be attached to the oxygen yoke, resulting in the delivery of nitrous oxide when the oxygen flowmeter was activated. Color-coded pressure gauges (green for oxygen, blue for nitrous oxide) on the anesthesia machine indicate the pressure of the gas in the corresponding gas cylinder (Table 10-1). The pressure in an oxygen cylinder is directly proportional to the volume of oxygen in the cylinder. For example, a full oxygen cylinder (E size) contains about 625 L oxygen at a pressure of 2000 psi and one-half this volume when the pressure is 1000 psi. Therefore, it is possible to calculate accurately how long a given flow rate of oxygen can be maintained before the cylinder is empty. In contrast to oxygen, the pressure gauge for nitrous oxide does not indicate the amount of gas remaining in the cylinder. This is because the pressure in the gas cylinder remains at 750 psi as long as any liquid nitrous oxide is present. When nitrous oxide as a vapor leaves the cylinder, additional liquid is vaporized to maintain an unchanging pressure in the cylinder. When all the liquid nitrous oxide is vaporized, the pressure begins to decrease and it can be assumed that about 75% of the contents of the gas cylinder have been exhausted. Because a full nitrous oxide cylinder (E size) contains about 1590 L, approximately 400 L remains when the pressure gauge begins to decrease from its previously constant value of 750 psi. Vaporization of a liquified gas (nitrous oxide), as well as expansion of a compressed gas (oxygen), absorbs heat, which is extracted from the metal cylinder and the surrounding atmosphere. For this reason, atmospheric water vapor often accumulates as frost on gas cylinders

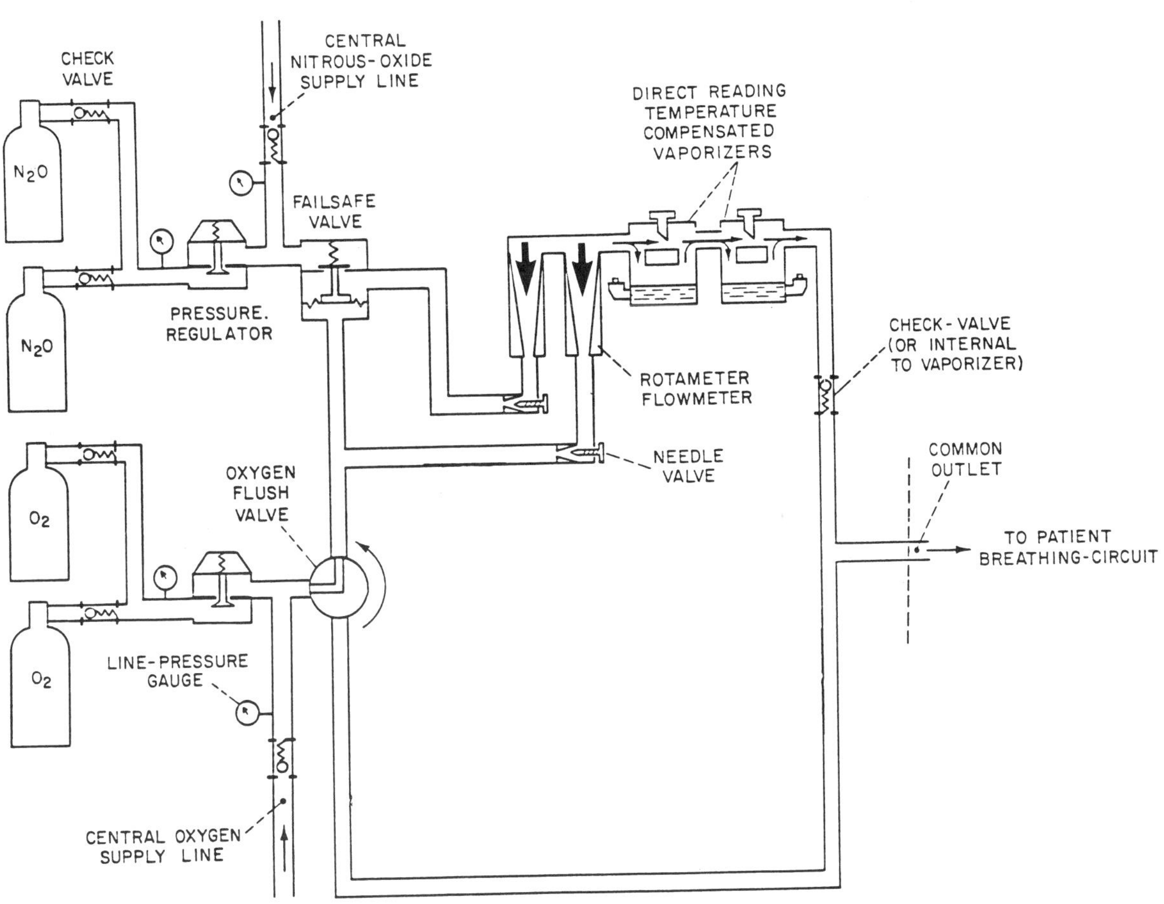

Figure 10-2. Schematic diagram of internal circuitry of an anesthesia machine. Oxygen and nitrous oxide enter the anesthesia machine via a central supply line or alternatively are provided from gas cylinders attached to pin-indexed yokes on the machine. Check valves prevent transfilling of gas cylinders or flow of gas from cylinders into the central supply line. Pressure regulators decrease pressure in the tubing from gas cylinders to about 50 psi. The fail-safe valve prevents flow of nitrous oxide if the pressure in the oxygen supply circuit decreases below about 30 psi. Needle valves control gas flows to rotameters (flowmeters). Agent-specific vaporizers provide a reliable means to deliver preselected concentrations of a volatile anesthetic. An interlock system allows only one vaporizer to be on at a time. After mixing in the manifold of the anesthesia machine, the total fresh gas flow enters the common outlet for delivery to the patient via the anesthetic breathing system (circuit). (Adapted from Check-Out,[1] with permission.)

Table 10-1. Characteristics of Compressed Gases Stored in E Size Cylinders that May Be Attached to the Anesthesia Machine

Characteristics	Oxygen	Nitrous Oxide	Carbon Dioxide	Air
Cylinder color	Green[a]	Blue	Gray	Yellow[a]
Physical state in cylinder	Gas	Liquid and gas	Liquid and gas	Gas
Cylinder contents (L)	625	1590	1590	625
Cylinder weight empty (kg)	5.90	5.90	5.90	5.90
Cylinder weight full (kg)	6.76	8.80	8.90	
Cylinder pressure full (psi)	2000	750	838	1800

[a]The World Health Organization specifies that cylinders containing oxygen for medical use be painted white but United States manufacturers use green. Likewise, the international color code for air is white and black, whereas cylinders in the United States are color-coded as yellow.

and in valves, particularly during high gas flows from these tanks. Internal icing does not occur because compressed gases are free of water vapor.

Flowmeters

Flowmeters on the anesthesia machine precisely control and measure gas flow to the common gas inlet (Fig. 10-2). Measurement of the flow of gases is based on the principle that flow past a resistance is proportional to pressure. Typically, gas flow enters the bottom of a vertically positioned and tapered (cross-sectional area increases upward from site of gas entry) glass tube. Gas flow into the flowmeter raises a bobbin- or ball-shaped float. The float comes to rest when gravity is balanced by the fall in pressure caused by the float. The upper end of the bobbin or equator of the ball indicates the gas flow in $ml \cdot min^{-1}$ or $L \cdot min^{-1}$. Proportionality between pressure and flow is determined by the shape of the tube (resistance) and physical properties (density and viscosity) of the gas. The flowmeters are initially calibrated for the indicated gas at the factory. Since few gases have the same density and viscosity, flowmeters are not interchangeable with other gases. The scale accompanying an oxygen flowmeter is green, and the scale for the nitrous oxide flowmeter is blue.

Gas flow exits the flowmeters and passes into a manifold (mixing chamber) located at the top of the flowmeters (Fig. 10-2). To ensure against accidental decreases in the delivered oxygen concentration, the oxygen flowmeter should be the last in the sequence of flowmeters and thus oxygen should be the last gas added to the manifold. This arrangement ensures that leaks in the apparatus proximal to oxygen inflow cannot diminish the delivered oxygen concentration, whereas leaks distal to that point result in loss of volume without a qualitative change in the mixture. Indeed, flowmeter leaks are a hazard reflecting the fragile construction of this component of the anesthesia machine. Subtle cracks may be overlooked, resulting in errors of delivered flows. Gases mix in the manifold and flow to an outlet port on the anesthesia machine, where they are directed into either a vaporizer or an anesthetic breathing system. For emergency purposes, provision is made for delivery to the outlet port of a large volume of oxygen (35 to 75 $L \cdot min^{-1}$) through an oxygen flush valve that bypasses the flowmeters and manifold. The oxygen flush valve allows direct communication between the oxygen high-pressure circuit and the low-pressure circuit (Fig. 10-2). Activation of the oxygen flush valve during a mechanically delivered inspiration from the anesthesia machine ventilator permits transmission of high airway pressures to the patient's lungs, with the possibility of barotrauma.

VAPORIZERS

Volatile anesthetics are liquids at room temperature and atmospheric pressure. Vaporization, which is the conversion of a liquid to a vapor, takes place in a closed container, referred to as a vaporizer. The vapor concentration resulting from vaporization of a volatile liquid anesthetic must be delivered to the patient with the same accuracy and predictability as other gases (nitrous oxide, oxygen).

Physics of Vaporization

The molecules that make up a liquid are in constant random motion. In a vaporizer containing a volatile liquid anesthetic, there is an asymmetric arrangement of intermolecular forces applied to the molecules at the liquid-oxygen interface. The result of this asymmetric arrangement is a net attractive force pulling the surface molecules into the liquid phase. This force must be overcome if surface molecules are to enter the gas phase, where their relatively sparse density constitutes a vapor. The energy necessary for molecules to escape from the liquid is supplied as heat. Heat of vaporization of a liquid is the number of calories required at a specific temperature to convert 1 g of a liquid into a vapor. The heat of vaporization necessary for molecules to leave the liquid phase is greater when the temperature of the liquid decreases.

Vaporization in the closed confines of a vaporizer ceases when equilibrium is reached between the liquid and vapor phases such that the number of molecules leaving the liquid phase is the same as the number re-entering. The molecules in the vapor phase collide with each other and the walls of the container, creating a pressure. This pressure is termed vapor pressure and is unique for each volatile anesthetic (see Table 2-1). Furthermore, vapor pressure is temperature dependent, such that a decrease in the temperature of the liquid is associated with a lower vapor pressure and fewer molecules in the vapor phase. Cooling of the liquid anesthetic reflects a loss of heat (heat of vaporization) necessary to provide energy for vaporization. This cooling is undesirable, as it lowers the vapor pressure and limits the attainable vapor concentration.

Vaporizer Classification and Design

Vaporizers (Ohemeda Tec 4, Ohemeda Tec 5, North American Drager 19.1) are classified as agent-specific, variable bypass, flow-over, temperature-compensated, out-of-circuit vaporizers (Fig. 10-3).[2,3]

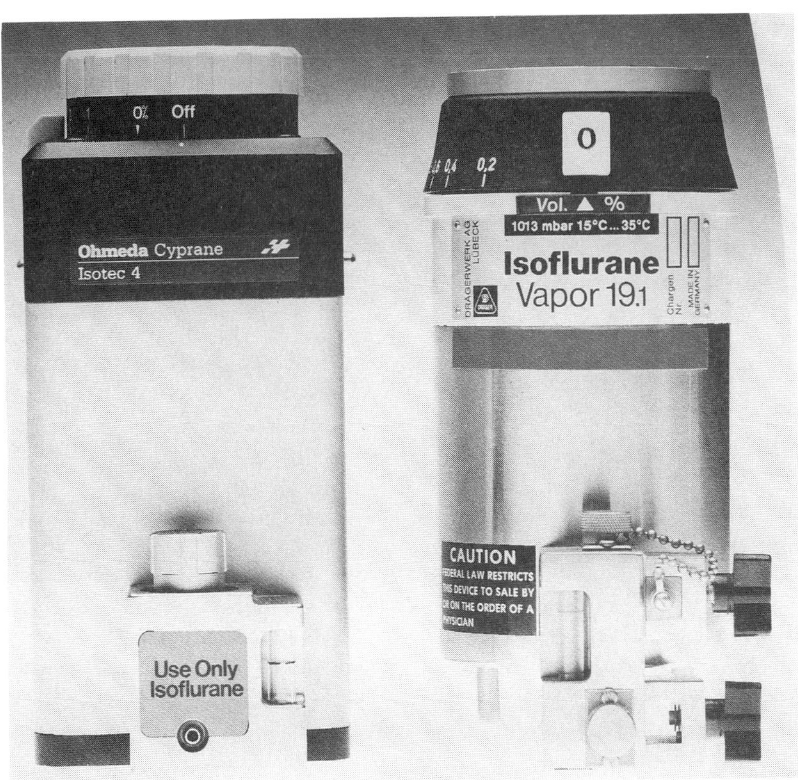

Figure 10-3. Ohmeda Tec 4 and North American Drager Vapor 19.1 are examples of agent-specific vaporizers. Note the low position of the filler port to minimize the likelihood of overfilling the vaporizer chamber and the window near the filler port to permit visual verification of the level of liquid anesthetic in the vaporizing chamber.

These contemporary vaporizers are unsuitable for the controlled vaporization of desflurane because it has a vapor pressure near 1 atm (664 mmHg) at 20°C. For this reason, the desflurane vaporizer is electrically heated (23°C to 25°C) and pressurized with a back pressure regulator (1500 mmHg) so as to create an environment in which the anesthetic has a relatively lower but predictable constant temperature volatility (Fig. 10-4).[4]

Variable bypass describes splitting of the total fresh gas flow through the vaporizer into two portions (Fig. 10-5).[5] The first portion of the fresh gas flow (20% or less) passes into the vaporizing chamber of the vaporizer, where it becomes saturated (flow-over) with the vapor of the liquid anesthetic. The second portion of the fresh gas flow passes through the bypass chamber of the vaporizer. Both portions of the fresh gas flow mix at the patient outlet side of the anesthesia machine. The proportion of fresh gas flow diverted through the vaporizing chamber, and thus the concentration of volatile anesthetic delivered to the patient, is determined by the concentration control dial. The scale on the concentration control dial is in volumes % for the specific anesthetic drug. Vaporizer output is not influenced by fresh gas flows until very low flow rates (lower than 250 ml·min^{-1}) are used. At these low fresh gas flows, vaporizer output is lower than the concentration dial setting. This reflects the relatively high specific gravity of volatile anesthetics such that insufficient pressure is generated at low flow rates in the vaporizing chamber to upwardly advance the molecules. At high fresh gas flows (higher than 15 L·min^{-1}) incomplete mixing in the vaporizing chamber also results in vaporizer output that is lower than the concentration control dial setting.

A temperature sensitive bimetallic strip or an expansion element influences proportioning of total gas flow between the vaporizing and bypass chambers as the vaporizer temperature changes (temperature compensated) (Fig. 10-5).[5] For example, as the temperature of the liquid anesthetic in the vaporizer chamber decreases, the temperature sensing elements allow increased gas inflow into this chamber to offset the effect of decreased anesthetic liquid vapor pressure. Vaporizers are often constructed of metals with high thermal conductivity (copper, bronze) to further minimize heat loss. As a result, vaporizer output is nearly linear between 20°C and 35°C.[3] Designation of vaporizers as agent-

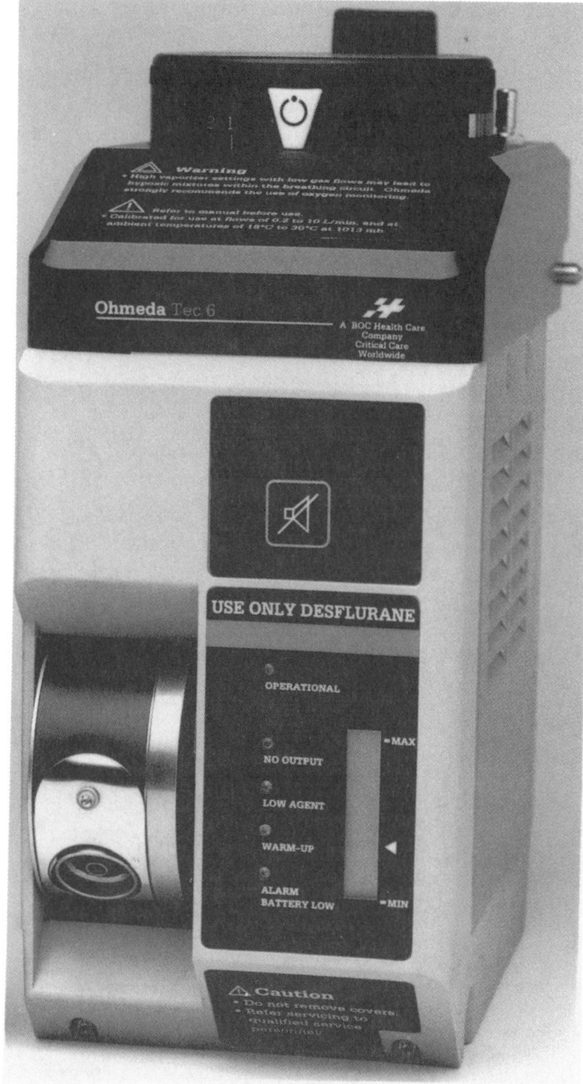

Figure 10-4. Ohmeda Tec 6 vaporizer is heated and pressurized for delivery of desflurane.

specific and out-of-circuit emphasizes that these devices are calibrated to accommodate a single volatile anesthetic and are isolated from the anesthetic breathing system (circuit).

Intermittent back pressure (pumping effect) transmitted to the vaporizing chamber as associated with positive pressure ventilation of the lungs or oxygen flush could increase vaporizer output. The design of modern agent-specific vaporizers minimize the influence of this pumping effect.[2–4] Composition of the total gas flow (presence or absence of nitrous

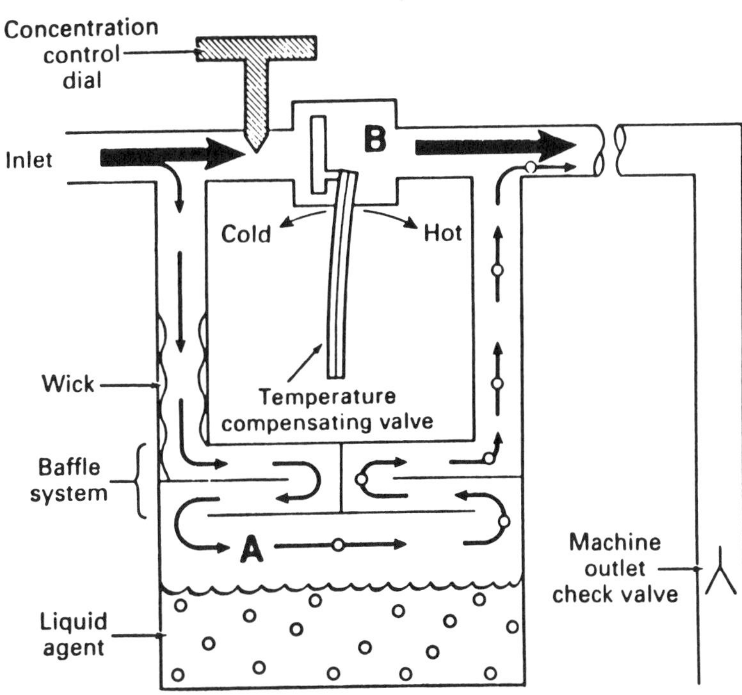

Figure 10-5. Schematic diagram of the agent-specific Ohmeda Tec 4 vaporizer. Counterclockwise rotation of the concentration control dial diverts a portion of the total fresh gas flow through the vaporizing chamber (A), where wicks saturated with liquid agent (anesthetic) ensure a large gas-liquid interface for efficient vaporization. A temperature-compensating valve diverts more or less fresh gas flow through the vaporizing chamber to offset the effect of changes in temperature on the vapor pressure of the liquid anesthetic (temperature-compensated vaporizer). Gases saturated with the vapor of the liquid anesthetic join gases that have passed through the bypass chamber (B) for delivery to the machine outlet check valve. When the concentration control dial is in the off position, no fresh gas inflow enters the vaporizing chamber. (From Andrews,[5] with permission.)

oxide) does not influence the output of these vaporizers. Tipping of vaporizers can cause liquid anesthetic to spill from the vaporizing chamber into the bypass chamber with resulting increased vapor concentrations exiting from the vaporizer. Nevertheless, the likelihood of tipping is minimized since vaporizers are secured to the anesthesia machine and there is little need to move them. Leaks associated with vaporizers are most often due to a loose filler cap.

Commonly two to three agent-specific vaporizers are present on the anesthesia machine. A safety interlock mechanism ensures that only one vaporizer can be turned on simultaneously. Turning on a vaporizer requires depression of a release button on the concentration dial followed by counterclockwise rotation of the dial. This prevents accidental movement of the dial from the off to the on position. The low location of the filler port on the vaporizer minimizes the likelihood of overfilling of the vaporizing chamber (greater than 125 ml) with anesthetic liquid. A window near the filler port permits visual verification of the level of liquid anesthetic in the vaporizing chamber. Use of an agent-specific keyed filler device prevents placement into the vaporizing chamber of a liquid anesthetic that is different from the drug for which the vaporizer was calibrated. As with anesthesia machines, periodic maintenance (usually every 12 months) is recommended by the manufacturers of vaporizers.

ANESTHETIC BREATHING SYSTEMS

Anesthetic breathing systems consist of the components necessary to deliver anesthetic gases and oxygen from the anesthesia machine to the patient.[6] Conceptually, the anesthetic breathing system is a tubular extension of the patient's upper airway. Because peak inspiratory flows as high as 60 L·min^{-1} are reached during spontaneous inspiration, anesthetic breathing systems can add considerable resistance to inhalation. The resistance imparted by an anesthetic breathing system is influenced by unidirectional valves and connectors. Minimizing resistance to breathing requires that components of the anesthetic breathing system, particularly the tracheal tube connector, have the largest possible lumen. Increased airway resistance due to sharp bends produced by right-angle connectors is minimized by replacing these devices with curved connectors. Increased resistance to breathing as a result of the anesthetic breathing system can be offset by substituting controlled ventilation of the lungs for spontaneous breathing.

Anesthetic breathing systems are classified as open, semiopen, semiclosed, and closed, according to the presence or absence of (1) a gas reservoir bag in the circuit, (2) rebreathing of exhaled gases, (3) means to chemically neutralize exhaled carbon dioxide, and (4) unidirectional valves (Table 10-2 and Figs. 10-6 to 10-8).[7–9] Depending on the characteristics of the anesthetic breathing system, there may be conservation of heat, water vapor, and exhaled anesthetics by virtue of permitting rebreathing of exhaled gases from which carbon dioxide has been removed (Fig. 10-9).[10] In this regard, description of an anesthetic breathing system includes the composition and flow rate of the inflow gases and whether ventilation is spontaneous or controlled.[11] The most commonly used anesthetic breathing systems are the (1) Mapleson F system, (2) Bain circuit, and (3) circle system.

Mapleson F System

The Mapleson F system (Jackson-Rees modification of the Mapleson D system) is an Ayre's T piece with a reservoir bag and an adjustable pressure limiting (overflow) valve on the distal end of the gas reservoir bag (Fig. 10-6).[7,12] The degree of rebreathing when using this anesthetic breathing system is influenced by the method of ventilation (spontaneous versus controlled) and adjustment of the overflow valve. A common recommendation is to deliver fresh gas inflow equal to at least twice the patient's minute ventilation so as to ensure the absence of rebreathing of exhaled gases.

The Mapleson F system is commonly used for controlled ventilation of the lungs during transport of patients whose tracheas are intubated. The popularity of this anesthetic breathing system for pediatric anesthesia is due to its minimal deadspace and low resistance to breathing. Furthermore, it can be used with a face mask or tracheal tube. Scavenging systems can be adapted to this system to decrease pollution of the atmosphere with anesthetic gases. Disadvantages include (1) the need for high fresh gas inflows to prevent rebreathing, (2) lack of humidification, and (3) possibility of high airway pressures and barotrauma should the overflow valve

Table 10-2. Classification of Anesthetic Breathing Systems

System	Gas Reservoir Bag	Rebreathing of Exhaled Gases	Chemical Neutralization of Carbon Dioxide	Unidirectional Valves	Fresh Gas Inflow Rate[a]
Open					
Insufflation	No	No	No	None	Unknown
Open drop	No	No	No	None	Unknown
Semiopen					
Mapleson A, B, C, D	Yes	No[b]	No	One	High
Bain	Yes	No[b]	No	One	High
Mapleson E	No	No[b]	No	None	High
Mapleson F (Jackson-Rees)	Yes	No[b]	No	One	High
Semiclosed					
Circle	Yes	Partial	Yes	Three	Moderate
Closed	Yes	Total	Yes	Three	Low

[a]High, greater than 6 L·min^{-1}; moderate, 3 to 6 L·min^{-1}; low, 0.3 to 0.5 L·min^{-1}.
[b]No rebreathing of exhaled gases only when fresh gas inflow is adequate.

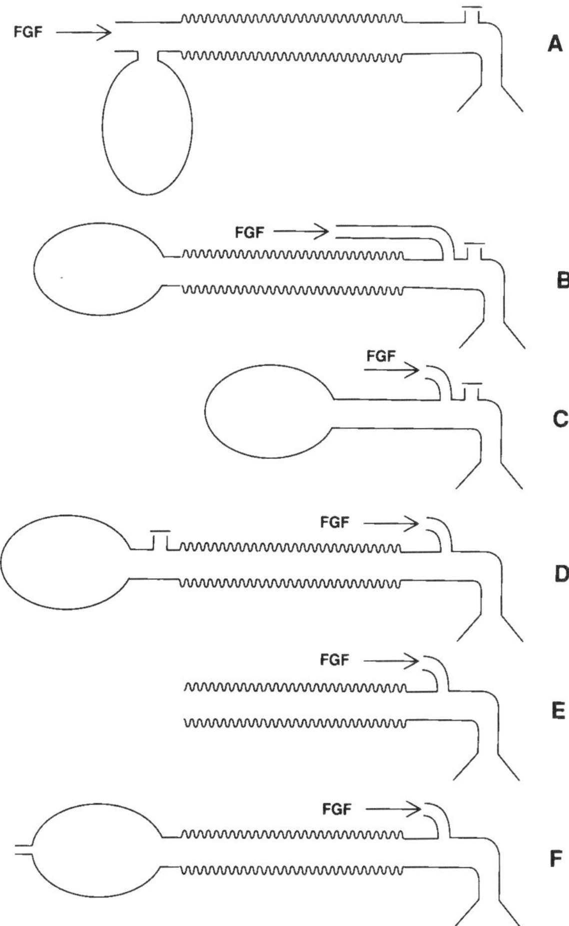

Figure 10-6. Anesthetic breathing systems classified as semiopen Mapleson A through F. (Modified from Willis et al.,[7] with permission.)

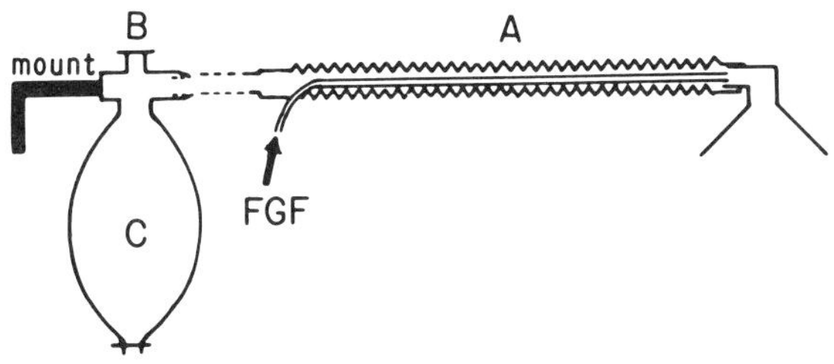

Figure 10-7. Schematic diagram of the Bain system showing fresh gas flow (FGF) entering a narrow tube within the larger corrugated expiratory limb (A). The only valve in the system (B) is an adjustable pressure-limiting (overflow) valve located near the FGF inlet and reservoir bag (C). (Modified from Bain and Spoerel,[8] with permission.)

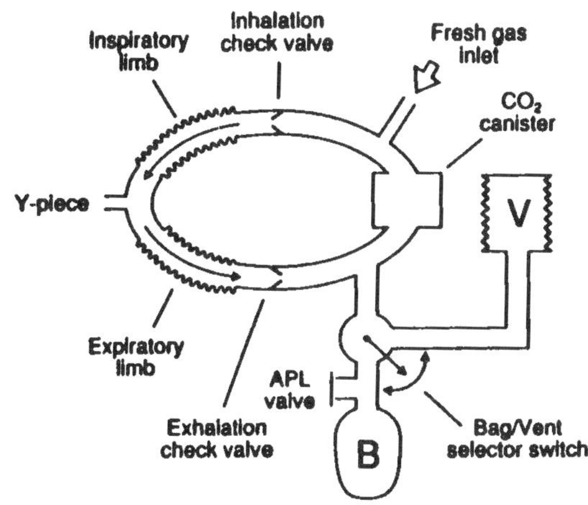

Figure 10-8. Schematic diagram of the components of a circle absorption anesthetic breathing system. Rotation of the Bag/Vent selector switch permits substitution of an anesthesia machine ventilator (V) for the reservoir bag (B). The volume of the reservoir bag is determined by fresh gas inflow and adjustment of the adjustable pressure-limiting (APL) valve. (From Andrews,[9] with permission.)

become occluded. Passage of fresh gas inflow through an in-line heated humidifier may be used to offset the lack of humidification associated with this anesthetic breathing system.

Bain Circuit

The Bain circuit is a coaxial version of the Mapleson D system in which fresh gas inflow enters through a narrow inner tube within the outer, corrugated expiratory tube (Fig. 10-7).[8] Fresh gases are delivered at the patient end of the circuit and exhaled gases are vented via the corrugated tube and through the overflow valve near the reservoir bag. Fresh gas flows necessary to prevent rebreathing are 200 to 300 $ml \cdot kg^{-1}$ during spontaneous breathing and 70 $ml \cdot kg^{-1}$ during controlled ventilation of the lungs.

Advantages cited for the Bain circuit include (1) warming of the fresh gas inflow by the surrounding exhaled gases in the corrugated expiratory limb of the system, (2) improved humidification as a result of partial rebreathing, and (3) ease of scavenging waste anesthetic gases from the overflow valve. The availability of this anesthetic breathing system as a disposable item facilitates sterility, and its light weight is particularly helpful when anesthetic equipment must be far removed from the airway, as during head and neck surgery. A hazard of the Bain cir-

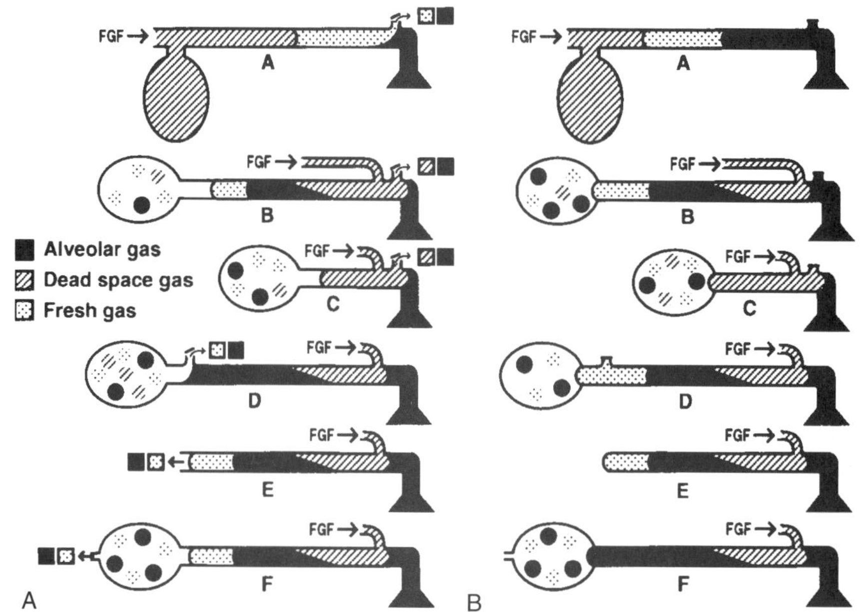

Figure 10-9. Gas disposition at end-exhalation during *(A)* spontaneous ventilation or *(B)* controlled ventilation of the lungs by using semiopen Mapleson A through F anesthetic breathing systems. (Modified from Sykes,[10] with permission.)

cuit is unrecognized disconnection or kinking of the inner fresh gas delivery tube. The outer expiratory tube is transparent to allow visual inspection of the inner tube.

Circle System

The circle system is the anesthetic breathing system that is most often selected for delivery of anesthetic gases and oxygen to children and adults. A circle system can be classified as semiopen, semiclosed, or closed depending on the amount of fresh gas inflow (Table 10-2). This system is so named because its essential components are arranged in a circular manner (Fig. 10-8).[9] Partial rebreathing of exhaled gases is acceptable because of the use of chemical neutralization (absorption) of carbon dioxide. As a result of partial rebreathing of exhaled gases, there is some conservation of airway moisture and body heat. Furthermore, the fresh gas inflow rate can be less than the patient's minute ventilation, which decreases pollution of the surrounding atmosphere with anesthetic gases. The price paid for these desirable characteristics includes increased resistance to breathing (owing to unidirectional valves and carbon dioxide canister), bulkiness with loss of portability, and enhanced opportunity for malfunction of a more complex apparatus.

The two unidirectional valves are situated so that one tube is for inhalation and the other for exhalation. This arrangement prevents the inhalation of exhaled gases until they have passed through the carbon dioxide canister (see the section *Elimination of Carbon Dioxide*) and have had their oxygen content replenished. Incompetence or absence of a unidirectional valve permits breathing back and forth in one tube, resulting in rebreathing of exhaled gases and development of hypercarbia. The two corrugated tubes serve as the conduits for delivery of anesthetic gases and oxygen to the patient. These large diameter tubes (22 mm) provide minimal resistance to breathing and are corrugated to prevent kinking. The gas reservoir bag maintains an available reserve volume of gases to satisfy inspiratory flow rates of the patient (up to 60 $L \cdot min^{-1}$), which greatly exceed conventional fresh gas flows (commonly 3 to 5 $L \cdot min^{-1}$) from the anesthesia machine. The adjustable pressure-limiting (overflow or "pop-off") valve allows the anesthesiologist to increase pressure in the anesthetic breathing system (depicted on the airway pressure gauge) so as to provide assisted or controlled ventilation of the lungs by manual compression of the gas reservoir bag. Alternatively, the anesthesiologist may provide controlled ventilation of the lungs by turning a selector valve that eliminates the gas reservoir bag and adjustable pressure-limiting valve from the circle anesthetic breathing system and substitutes intermittent positive airway pressure delivered from a mechanical ventilator (Fig. 10-8).[9]

Anesthesia machine ventilators are powered by compressed air or oxygen (pneumatic power) or by electricity, which acts to compress a bellows (equivalent of the reservoir bag) that contains anesthetic gases and oxygen. Compression of the bellows is responsible for delivery of fresh gases to the patient. A bellows that ascends during the exhalation phase is preferable to a bellows that descends, as the former will not fill if there is a leak in the anesthetic breathing system or the system becomes accidentally disconnected. The bellows of a descending bellows ventilator, however, will continue its upward and downward movement during a disconnection. This is an important consideration since accidental disconnection of the patient from the anesthetic breathing system is a leading cause of adverse events (critical incidents) in anesthesia. Most anesthesia machine ventilators are time cycled and provide ventilator support only in the control mode. Initiation of inspiration and thus the mechanically provided breathing rate are accomplished by a timing device.

Prevention of rebreathing of exhaled gases by using a circle system mandates that a unidirectional valve be placed between the patient and gas reservoir bag on both the inspiratory and expiratory limbs of the circuit.[6] The most efficient arrangement of components for both spontaneous and controlled ventilation of the lungs is placement of the (1) unidirectional valves near the patient, (2) adjustable pressure-limiting valve near the patient just distal to the exhalation valve, and (3) fresh gas inflow entry site between the carbon dioxide absorber and inhalation valve. In this arrangement, fresh gas inflow preferentially expels ("flushes") alveolar gas (as in the Mapleson A system) while conserving physiologic deadspace gas (Fig. 10-9).[10] Nevertheless, this optimal arrangement is impractical, since the bulky unidirectional valves and overflow valve are located near the patient. A more practical but less efficient arrangement is placement of the unidirectional valves and adjustable pressure-limiting valve more distal to the patient (Fig. 10-8).[9]

Rebreathing of exhaled gases using a semiclosed anesthetic breathing system influences the inhaled anesthetic concentrations of these gases. For example, when uptake of an anesthetic gas is high, as during induction of anesthesia, rebreathing of exhaled gases depleted of anesthetic greatly dilutes the concentration of anesthetic in the fresh gas inflow. This dilutional effect of uptake is offset clinically by increasing the delivered concentration of anesthetic. As uptake of anesthetic diminishes, the impact of dilution on the inspired concentration produced by rebreathing of exhaled gases is lessened.

Closed Anesthetic Breathing System

A closed anesthetic breathing system is present when the fresh gas inflow into the circle system is decreased sufficiently to permit closure of the adjustable pressure-limiting valve and all the exhaled carbon dioxide is neutralized in the carbon dioxide absorber (Table 10-2). The fresh gas inflow for a closed system (150 to 500 $ml{\cdot}min^{-1}$) satisfies the patient's metabolic oxygen requirements (150 to 250 $ml{\cdot}min^{-1}$ during anesthesia) and replaces anesthetic gases lost by virtue of tissue uptake.

Advantages of the closed circle anesthetic breathing system compared with the semiclosed circle anesthetic breathing system include (1) maximal humidification and warming of inhaled gases, (2) less pollution of the surrounding atmosphere with anesthetic gases, and (3) economy in the use of anesthetics. A disadvantage of the closed anesthetic breathing system is the inability to rapidly change the delivered concentration of anesthetic gases and oxygen due to the low fresh gas inflow. The principal dangers of a closed anesthetic breathing system are delivery of (1) unpredictable and possibly insufficient concentrations of oxygen and (2) unknown and possibly excessive concentrations of potent anesthetic gases.

Unpredictable Concentrations of Oxygen. Unpredictable and possibly insufficient concentrations of oxygen with a closed anesthetic breathing system are more likely when nitrous oxide is included in the fresh gas inflow. For example, decreased tissue uptake of nitrous oxide with time in the presence of an unchanged uptake of oxygen can result in a decreased concentration of oxygen in the alveoli (Table 10-3). Therefore, the use of an oxygen analyzer placed on the inspiratory or expiratory limb of the circle system is mandatory when nitrous oxide is delivered using a closed anesthetic breathing system.

Unknown Concentrations of Potent Anesthetic Gases. Exhaled gases, devoid of carbon dioxide, form a major part of the inhaled gases when a closed anesthetic breathing system is used. This means that the composition of the inhaled gases is influenced by the concentration present in the exhaled gases. The concentration of anesthetic in exhaled gases reflects tissue uptake of the anesthetic. Initially, tissue uptake is maximal and the concentration of anesthetic in the exhaled gases is minimal. Subsequent rebreathing of these exhaled gases dilutes the inhaled concentration of anesthetic delivered to the patient. Therefore, high inflow concentrations of anesthetic are necessary to offset maximal tissue uptake. Conversely, only small amounts of anesthetic need to be added to the inflow gases when tissue uptake is decreased. The unknown impact of tissue uptake on the concentration of anesthetic in the exhaled gases makes it difficult to estimate the inhaled concentration delivered to the patient using a closed anesthetic breathing system. This disadvantage can be partially offset by administering higher fresh gas inflows (3 $L \cdot min^{-1}$) for about 15 minutes before instituting use of a closed anesthetic breathing system. This approach permits elimination of nitrogen from the lungs and corresponds to the time of greatest tissue uptake of anesthetic.

Table 10-3. Alveolar Gas Concentration Using a Closed Circle Anesthetic Breathing System

Example 1

Gas inflow is nitrous oxide 300 $ml \cdot min^{-1}$ and oxygen 300 $ml \cdot min^{-1}$ for 15 minutes. Nitrous oxide uptake by tissues at this time is 200 $ml \cdot min^{-1}$, and oxygen consumption is 250 $ml \cdot min^{-1}$. Alveolar gas after tissue uptake consists of 100 ml nitrous oxide and 50 ml oxygen. The alveolar concentration of oxygen (FAO_2) is

$$FAO_2 = \frac{50 \text{ ml oxygen}}{100 \text{ ml nitrous oxide} + 50 \text{ ml oxygen}} \times 100 = 33\%$$

Example 2

Gas inflow as in Example 1 but duration of administration is 1 hour. At this time, tissue uptake of nitrous oxide has decreased to 100 $ml \cdot min^{-1}$ but oxygen consumption remains unchanged at 250 $ml \cdot min^{-1}$. Alveolar gas after tissue uptake consists of 200 ml nitrous oxide and 50 ml oxygen. The alveolar concentration of oxygen (FAO_2) is

$$FAO_2 = \frac{50 \text{ ml oxygen}}{200 \text{ ml nitrous oxide} + 50 \text{ ml oxygen}} \times 100 = 20\%$$

Circle System Test

The circle system test is performed prior to the induction of anesthesia to confirm the (1) absence of leaks in the system and (2) proper functioning of the inspiratory and expiratory valves. The leak test is performed by closing the adjustable pressure-limiting valve, occluding the Y-piece, and pressurizing the circuit to 30 cmH_2O with the oxygen flush. The valve on the airway pressure gauge should not decline noticeably over 10 seconds if the circle system is leak-free. Integrity of the unidirectional valves is confirmed if the anesthesiologist is able to breathe through the anesthetic breathing circuit. In addition to checking the circle system, it is recommended that a complete anesthesia machine checkout procedure be performed each day before the first case plus an abbreviated version before each subsequent case (Table 10-4 and see Table 8-7).[13]

ELIMINATION OF CARBON DIOXIDE

Carbon dioxide can be eliminated from an anesthetic breathing system by venting all exhaled gases to the atmosphere, as occurs during the use of an open or semiopen anesthetic breathing system. More often, however, partial (semiclosed anesthetic breathing system) or total (closed anesthetic breathing system) rebreathing of exhaled gases is permitted and carbon dioxide is eliminated by chemical neutralization. Chemical neutralization of carbon dioxide is achieved by directing exhaled gases through a container (canister) containing a carbon dioxide absorbent such as soda lime or baralyme.

Soda Lime

Soda lime granules consist of calcium hydroxide plus smaller amounts of sodium hydroxide and potassium hydroxide that are present as activators (Table 10-5). A specific water content of soda lime is necessary to ensure optimal activity. Silica is added to the granules to give hardness and thus minimize the formation of alkaline dust. Formation of this

Table 10-4. Anesthesia Apparatus Checkout Recommendations, 1992

This checkout, or a reasonable equivalent, should be conducted before administration of anesthesia. These recommendations are only valid for an anesthesia system that conforms to current and relevant standards and includes an ascending bellows ventilator and at least the following monitors: capnograph, pulse oximeter, oxygen analyzer, respiratory volume monitor (spirometer), and breathing system pressure monitor with high and low pressure alarms. This is a guideline that users are encouraged to modify to accommodate differences in equipment design and variations in local clinical practice. Such local modifications should have appropriate peer review. Users should refer to the operators manual for specific procedures and precautions.

Emergency Ventilation Equipment

1. Verify backup ventilation equipment is available and functioning[a]

High Pressure System

2. Check oxygen cylinder supply[a]
   a. Open O_2 cylinder and verify at least half full (about 1000 psi).
   b. Close cylinder.
3. Check central pipeline supplies[a]
   a. Check that hoses are connected and pipeline gauges read 45–55 psi.

Low Pressure System

4. Check initial status of low pressure system[a]
   a. Close flow control valves and turn vaporizers off.
   b. Check fill level and tighten vaporizers' filler caps.
   c. Remove O_2 monitor sensor from circuit.
5. Perform leak check of machine low pressure system[a]
   a. Verify that the machine master switch and flow control valves are OFF.
   b. Attach "Suction Bulb" to common (fresh) gas outlet.
   c. Squeeze bulb repeatedly until fully collapsed.
   d. Verify bulb stays *fully* collapsed for at least 10 seconds.
   e. Open one vaporizer at a time and repeat 'c' and 'd' as above.
   f. Remove suction bulb, and reconnect fresh gas hose.
6. Turn on machine master switch[a] and all other necessary electrical equipment.
7. Test flowmeters
   a. Adjust flow of all gases through their full range, checking for smooth operations of floats and undamaged flowtubes.
   b. Attempt to create a hypoxic O_2/N_2O mixture and verify correct changes in flow and/or alarm.

Breathing System

8. Calibrate O_2 monitor[a]
   a. Calibrate to read 21% in room air.
   b. Reinstall sensor in circuit and flush breathing system with O_2.
   c. Verify that monitor now reads greater than 90%.
9. Check initial status of breathing system
   a. Set selector switch in "Bag" mode.
   b. Check that breathing circuit is complete, undamaged, and unobstructed.
   c. Verify that CO_2 absorbent is adequate.
   d. Install breathing circuit accessory equipment to be used during the case.
10. Perform leak check of the breathing system
   a. Set all gas flows to zero (or minimum).
   b. Close adjustable pressure-limiting (APL) valve and occlude Y-piece.
   c. Pressurize breathing system to 30 cmH_2O with O_2 flush.
   d. Ensure that pressure remains at 30 cmH_2O for at least 10 seconds.

Scavenging System

11. Check APL valve and scavenging system
   a. Pressurize breathing system to 50 cmH_2O and ensure its integrity.
   b. Open APL valve and ensure that pressure decreases.
   c. Ensure proper scavenging connections and waste gas vacuum.
   d. Fully open APL valve and occlude Y-piece.
   e. Ensure absorber pressure gauge reads zero when
      Minimum O_2 is flowing
      O_2 flush is activated

Manual and Automatic Ventilation Systems

12. Test ventilation systems and unidirectional valves
   a. Place a second breathing bag on Y-piece.
   b. Set appropriate ventilator parameters for next patient.
   c. Set O_2 flow to 250 $ml{\cdot}min^{-1}$ and other gas flows to zero.
   d. Switch to automatic ventilation (ventilator) mode.
   e. Turn ventilator ON and fill bellows and breathing bag with O_2 flush.
   f. Verify that during inspiration bellows delivers correct tidal volume and that during expiration bellows fills completely.
   g. Check that volume monitor is consistent with ventilator parameters.
   h. *Check for proper action of unidirectional valves.*
   i. Exercise breathing circuit accessories to ensure proper function.
   j. Turn ventilator OFF and switch to manual ventilation (bag/APL) mode.
   k. Ventilate manually and ensure inflation and deflation of artificial lungs and appropriate feel of system resistance and compliance.
   l. Remove second breathing bag from Y-piece.

Monitors

13. Check, calibrate, and/or set alarm limits of all monitors

Capnometer	Oxygen analyzer
Pulse oximeter	Respiratory volume monitor (spirometer)
Pressure monitor with high and low airway pressure alarms	

Final Position

14. Check final status of machine

a. Vaporizers off.	e. Patient suction level adequate.
b. APL valve open.	f. Breathing system ready to use.
c. Selector switch to "Bag."	
d. All flowmeters to zero (or minimum)	

[a]If an anesthesioligist uses the same machine in successive cases, these steps need not be repeated or may be abbreviated after the initial checkout.

(From Anesthesia Apparatus Checkout Recommendations,[13] with permission.)

alkaline dust must be prevented because its inhalation can produce irritation of the airways, manifesting as bronchospasm.

Neutralization of carbon dioxide begins with the reaction of this gas with the water present in soda lime granules and exhaled gases to form carbonic acid. Carbonic acid then reacts with the hydroxides present in soda lime granules to form carbonates, water, and heat. The water formed by the neutralization of carbon dioxide is useful for humidifying the inhaled gases and for dissipating some of the heat generated in the exothermic neutralization reaction. Accumulation of this highly alkaline water in the bottom of the canister can produce burns on contact with the skin. The heat generated during neutralization of carbon dioxide can be detected by warmness of the canister. Failure of the canister to become warm to external touch should alert the anesthesiologist to the possibility that chemical neutralization of carbon dioxide is not taking place.

Chemical Neutralization of Carbon Dioxide

Soda lime

$$CO_2 + H_2O \rightarrow H_2CO_3$$
$$H_2CO_3 + 2NaOH \rightarrow Na_2CO_3 \text{ (rapid)} + 2H_2O + \text{heat}$$
$$H_2CO_3 + Ca(OH)_2 \rightarrow CaCO_3 \text{ (slow)} + 2H_2O + \text{heat}$$

Baralyme

$$CO_2 + H_2O \rightarrow H_2CO_3$$
$$H_2CO_3 + Ba(OH)_2 \rightarrow BaCO_3 \text{ (rapid)} + 2H_2O + \text{heat}$$
$$H_2CO_3 + Ca(OH)_2 \rightarrow CaCO_3 \text{ (slow)}$$

Baralyme

Baralyme consists of barium hydroxide and calcium hydroxide (Table 10-5). Unlike soda lime, the addition of silica to baralyme granules is not necessary to ensure hardness. This inherent hardness of baralyme granules reflects the presence of bound water of crystallization in the octahydrate salt of barium hydroxide. This bound water also accounts for the more reliable performance of baralyme than soda lime in dry environments. As with soda lime, the neutralization of carbon dioxide by baralyme results in the formation of carbonates, water, and heat.

Table 10-5. Composition of Carbon Dioxide Absorbents

Soda Lime (% of Wet Weight)	Baralyme (% of Wet Weight)
Sodium hydroxide (4)	Barium hydroxide (20)
Potassium hydroxide (1)	Calcium hydroxide (80)
Water (14–19)	Water, bound water of crystallization in the octahydrate salt of barium hydroxide
Silica (0.2)	Silica (none)
Calcium hydroxide (balance)	

Efficiency of Carbon Dioxide Neutralization

Efficiency of carbon dioxide neutralization is influenced by the size of the carbon dioxide absorbent granules and presence or absence of channeling in the canister containing the carbon dioxide absorbent. In addition, optimal absorptive conditions provide that the equivalent of the patient's tidal volume be accommodated entirely within the void space of the canister. Therefore, about one-half the volume of a properly packed canister should consist of intergranular spaces.

A pH-sensitive dye is added to soda lime or baralyme by the manufacturer. A change in color of the absorbent granules is produced when this dye is activated by carbonic acid that accumulates owing to exhaustion of the activity of absorbent granules. If the exhausted absorbent granules are not replaced with fresh granules, the color change often disappears during disuse. Minimal regeneration of absorbent granule activity, however, will have occurred, and, on re-use, the dye quickly produces the color change again. The maximum volume of carbon dioxide that can be absorbed is approximately 26 $L \cdot 100\ g^{-1}$ of absorbent granules. Usually, considerably less carbon dioxide is absorbed because of factors such as canister design and the specific end-point used to detect exhaustion of absorbent granule activity.

Absorbent Granule Size

Absorbent granule size is designated as mesh size. For example, an absorbent granule of 8 mesh (2.5 mm) will pass through a screen having 8 or fewer wires per 2.5 cm. Empirically, the optimal absorbent granule size of soda lime or baralyme has been found to be 4 to 8 mesh. This absorbent granule size represents a compromise between absorptive activity and resistance to air flow through the canister. Absorptive activity increases as absorbent granule size decreases because total surface area increases. The smaller the absorbent granules, however, the smaller the interstices through which gases must flow, resulting in increasing resistance to flow.

Channeling

Channeling is the preferential passage of exhaled gases through the canister via pathways of low resistance such that the bulk of the carbon dioxide absorbent granules are bypassed. Loose packing of the absorbent granules in the canister is the most frequent cause of channeling. Shaking the canister gently before use to ensure firm packing of the absorbent granules decreases the likelihood of channeling without substantially increasing resistance to the flow of gases. In addition, the absorbent granules are held in place with screens and baffles to facilitate uniform dispersion of gas flow.

HUMIDIFICATION

Humidification is a form of vaporization in which water vapor (moisture) is added to the gases delivered by the anesthetic breathing system. Normally, air passing through the nose is warmed to body temperature and saturated with water vapor before reaching the carina. Administration of dry anesthetic gases and oxygen at room temperature via an anesthetic breathing system that bypasses the nose may lead to cytologic damage to the respiratory epithelium within 1 hour.[14] Breathing dry gases for several hours can result in drying of secretions and, when a tracheal tube is used, airway obstruction from inspissated secretions in the tube. In addition, breathing dry and unwarmed gases is associated with water and heat loss from the patient. More important than water loss, however, is the heat loss, which may lead to adverse decreases in body temperature, particularly in infants and children who are rendered poikilothermic by general anesthesia. Indeed, the most important reason to provide heated humidification during general anesthesia is to decrease heat loss and associated decreases in body temperature (Fig. 10-10).[15]

The simplest method of increasing the water content of inhaled gases is to pass these gases through the canister used for carbon dioxide absorption. Heating due to the exothermic reaction produced by the neutralization of carbon dioxide enables the inhaled gases to hold more water. The most reliable way to warm and humidify anesthetic gases and oxygen is to use specially designed humidifiers placed in the anesthetic breathing circuit (Fig. 10-8).[9]

BACTERIAL CONTAMINATION OF ANESTHESIA EQUIPMENT

The role of bacterial contamination of the anesthesia machine and equipment and the subsequent development of pulmonary infection and cross-infection between patients is controversial.[16] Nevertheless, it is assumed that equipment used to deliver anesthesia is a potential source of bacterial contamination to patients. On the basis of this

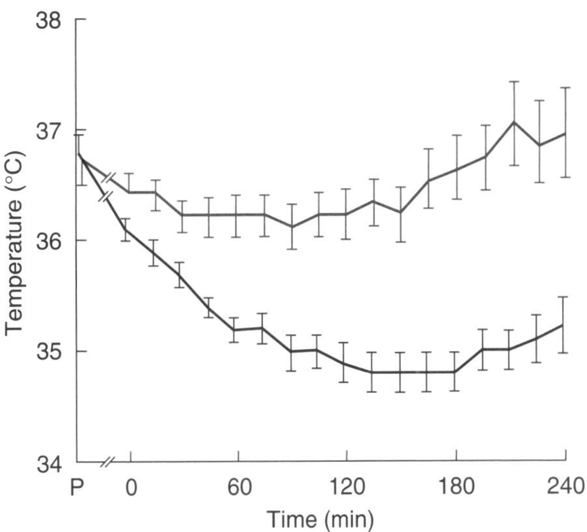

Figure 10-10. Nasopharyngeal temperature was better maintained in patients breathing humidified gases heated to 37°C (red line) than in patients breathing gases delivered at room temperature (black line). Mean ± 1 SEM.

assumption, the use of disposable anesthetic breathing systems has become popular. The incidence, however, of postoperative pulmonary infection is not altered by the use of a sterile disposable anesthetic breathing system as compared with the use of a reusable system that is cleaned by basic hygienic techniques but not sterilized between uses. Likewise, the incidence of postoperative pulmonary infection is not altered by inclusion of a bacterial filter in the anesthetic breathing system.

The reason anesthesia equipment has not been implicated as a cause of infection, in contrast to the undeniable role of respiratory therapy equipment (particularly nebulizers), involves the low likelihood of airborne transmission of bacteria from the host. Furthermore, the environment presented to organisms that may be present in the anesthesia machine and anesthetic breathing system is not conducive to bacterial survival.

Airborne Transmission

During anesthesia and quiet breathing, only a small number of bacteria are likely to be liberated from the host. Indeed, the administration of anesthesia to patients with known colonization of gram-negative bacteria does not result in contamination of the anesthetic breathing system. Bacteria that are released from the airway during violent forms of exhalation originate almost exclusively from the anterior portion of the oropharynx and rarely from the nose or pharynx, which harbors respiratory pathogens. Furthermore, even low concentrations of oxygen are often lethal to airborne bacteria.

Environment Presented to Bacteria

Airborne bacteria released into a circle anesthetic breathing system are exposed to shifts in humidity and temperature. Bacteria, particularly gram-negative organisms, are sensitive to both these changes. In fact, shifts in humidity and temperature are probably the most important factors responsible for bacterial killing that occurs within the anesthetic breathing system.

Most studies have shown that clinical concentrations of general anesthetics have little influence on the survival of bacteria in the anesthetic breathing system. However, bacteria placed in vaporizers containing liquid anesthetics do not survive. The role of anesthesia equipment in transmitting viral illnesses is not known. If patients with known viral infections, such as acquired immunodeficiency syndrome, require anesthesia, it would seem prudent to use a disposable anesthetic breathing system, including the soda lime canister and ventilator bellows. Nondisposable equipment, including laryngoscope blades, is disinfected with sodium hypochlorite (bleach), which destroys the human immunodeficiency virus.

Metallic ions of metals (copper, zinc, chromium, brass) present in the anesthesia machine and other equipment have a highly lethal effect on bacteria. A practical use of this effect has been the insertion of copper mesh or sponges into the expiratory limb of ventilators to prevent infection from contaminated respiratory therapy equipment.

Transmission of Tuberculosis

There has been no documented transmission of tuberculosis from a contaminated anesthesia machine or anesthetic breathing system to a patient.[16] Nevertheless, of all bacterial forms, acid-fast bacilli are the most adaptable and resistant to destruction. Therefore, a greater degree of vigilance should be observed in dealing with patients with pulmonary disease conceivably due to tuberculosis. This vigilance should include use of a disposable anesthetic breathing system and disinfection of nondisposable equipment with an appropriate chemical such as glutaraldehyde (Cidex). The incidence of tuberculosis is increased in immunosuppressed patients, including those with acquired immunodeficiency syndrome.

POLLUTION OF THE ATMOSPHERE WITH ANESTHETIC GASES

Chronic exposure to low concentrations of anesthetics that result from spillage of these gases into the atmosphere from the anesthesia machine and anesthetic breathing system may constitute a health hazard to operating room personnel.[17] For this reason, removal (scavenging) of trace concentrations of anesthetic gases present in the atmosphere of the operating rooms is recommended. In addition, dental and veterinary settings should be provided with gas scavenging capabilities. The National Institute of Occupational Safety and Health (NIOSH) has proposed that nitrous oxide concentrations in the atmosphere should be lower than 22 ppm and lower than 5 ppm for volatile anesthetics. It must be recognized, however, that there is no evidence that these proposed levels are either desirable or less hazardous than higher concentrations. Nevertheless, nitrous oxide concentrations higher than 200 ppm as determined by gas chromatography or infrared analysis should alert personnel to search for leaks and/or consider alterations in anesthetic techniques.

Source of Anesthetic Gases in the Environment

High pressure system leakage of anesthetic gases into the atmosphere occurs when a gas, such as nitrous oxide, escapes from tanks attached to the anesthesia machine (faulty yokes) or from tubing or connectors necessary for the delivery of nitrous oxide to the anesthesia machine from a central gas supply (faulty quick-coupler connector). Low pressure leakage is characterized by escape of anesthetic gases from sites located between the flowmeters of the anesthesia machine and the patient, including spillage from the anesthetic breathing system.

Control of Gas Leakage

Control of gas spillage into the environment requires (1) periodic maintenance of anesthesia equipment, (2) removal of excess gases vented from the anesthetic breathing system by scavenging, (3) attention to the anesthetic technique, and (4) adequate ventilation of the operating rooms.[18]

Periodic Maintenance

Periodic maintenance of the anesthesia machine by a qualified service representative is the best protection against persistence of leaks in the high or low pressure system of the anesthesia machine and anesthetic breathing system. Correction of leakage often involves simple steps such as replacing a worn canister gasket or removing a deformed washer on a yoke.

Scavenging

Scavenging is the term applied to collection and removal of excess gases that normally exit via the adjustable pressure-limiting valve of the anesthetic breathing system. These excess gases are removed by attaching a gas capturing device that includes suction to the anesthetic breathing system. Captured gases are most often delivered to the central vacuum system of the hospital for disposal. Attachment of this device to the anesthetic breathing system introduces the risk of removal of excessive volumes of gas from the system unless the fresh gas inflow is greater than the suction rate. The presence of an excessive rate of suction most often manifests as collapse of the gas reservoir bag. Conversely, occlusion of the gas disposal route may allow excessive pressure increases to occur in the anesthetic breathing system and lead to barotrauma. For these reasons, a pressure-balancing capability is included in the gas capturing device to prevent the development of negative or positive pressure in the anesthetic breathing system.

Technique of Anesthesia

Poor fit of the face mask and premature flow of anesthetic gases (before placement of the mask on the patient's face or during intubation of the trachea) result in spillage of anesthetic gases into the atmosphere. Administration of oxygen at the conclusion of anesthesia serves to eliminate anesthetic gases from the patient and anesthetic breathing system and thus decrease spillage into the atmosphere. The use of low flow or closed system techniques diminishes but does not eliminate operating room pollution with waste anesthetic gases. Care should be exercised in filling vaporizers, since spillage of liquid anesthetic results in substantial pollution.

Room Ventilation

The efficiency of operating room ventilation in terms of room air turnovers per hour should be determined and ventilation filters checked at periodic intervals by the hospital engineer.

REFERENCES

1. Check-Out. A Guide for Preoperative Inspection of an Anesthetic Machine. Chicago, American Society of Anesthesiologists 1987:1–14.
2. Tec 4 Continuous Flow Vaporizer. Operators Manual. Steeton, England, Ohmeda, the BOC Group, Inc. 1986.
3. Vapor 19.1 Operating Manual. Lubeck, Germany, Dragerwerk 1985.
4. Desflurane Vaporizer. Operators Manual. 1993.
5. Andrews JJ. Anesthesia Systems. In: Barash PG, Cullen BF, Stoelting RK, eds. Clinical Anesthesia, Philadelphia, JB Lippincott 1992;637–84.
6. Eger EI II. Anesthetic systems: Construction and function. In: Anesthetic Uptake and Action. Baltimore, Williams & Wilkins 1974:206–7.
7. Willis BA, Pender JW, Mapleson WW. Rebreathing in a T-piece: Volunteer and theoretical studies of the

Jackson-Rees modification of Ayre's T piece during spontaneous respiration. Br J Anaesth 1975;47:1239–46.
8. Bain JA, Spoerel WE. A streamlined anaesthetic system. Can Anaesth Soc J 1972;19:426–35.
9. Andrews JJ. Inhaled anesthetic delivery systems. In: Miller RD, ed. Anesthesia. New York, Churchill Livingstone 1990;171–223.
10. Sykes MK. Rebreathing circuits: A review. Br J Anaesth 1968;40:666–74.
11. Hamilton WK. Nomenclature of inhalation anesthetic systems. Anesthesiology 1964;25:3–5.
12. Jackson-Rees G. Anaesthesia in the newborn. Br Med J 1950;2:1419–22.
13. Anesthesia Apparatus Checkout Recommendations. Food and Drug Administration, 1992.
14. Chalon J, Loew DAY, Malebranche J. Effect of dry anesthetic gases on tracheobronchial ciliated epithelium. Anesthesiology 1972;37:338–43.
15. Stone DR, Downs JB, Paul WL, Perkins HM. Adult body temperature and heated humidification of anesthetic gases during general anesthesia. Anesth Analg 1981;60:736–41.
16. duMoulin GC, Hedley-White J. Bacterial interactions between anesthesiologists, their patients, and equipment. Anesthesiology 1982;57:37–41.
17. Vessey MP. Epidemiological studies of the occupational hazards of anaesthesia—A review. Anaesthesia 1978; 33:430–8.
18. Lecky JH. Anesthetic pollution in the operating room. A notice to operating room personnel. Anesthesiology 1980;52:157–9.

11

Tracheal Intubation

Tracheal intubation (translaryngeal intubation) is a safe and common practice in patients undergoing general anesthesia. Maintenance of anesthesia by mask is an acceptable alternative to tracheal intubation in selected situations such as short noninvasive surgical procedures in otherwise healthy patients. Nevertheless, the most common approach is to perform tracheal intubation in all patients undergoing general anesthesia. Atraumatic intubation of the trachea requires a knowledge of the anatomy of the upper airway and appropriate use of equipment and drugs, particularly muscle relaxants.

PREOPERATIVE EVALUATION

Preoperative evaluation of the patient's airway determines the route (oral or nasal) and method (awake or anesthetized) for intubation of the trachea. If there is a perceived possibility that intubation of the trachea or ventilation of the patient's lungs by mask, or both, will be difficult, the airway should be secured while the patient is still awake (see the section *Alternatives to Orotracheal Intubation During General Anesthesia*). In this regard, three simple preoperative examinations are useful in predicting the ease of tracheal intubation.[1,2] In addition, a thorough preoperative dental examination is necessary as teeth and dental prostheses are vulnerable to damage or dislodgement by the laryngoscope blade during direct laryngoscopy.

Examinations for Predicting the Ease of Tracheal Intubation

Tongue versus Pharyngeal Size

The size of the tongue in relationship to the size of the oral cavity can be visually graded by how much the pharynx is obscured by the tongue. This test is performed by asking the patient to sit with the head in a neutral position, the mouth opened maximally (normal opening 50 to 60 mm) and the tongue protruded as far as possible. The observer classifies the patient's airway according to the pharyngeal structures that are visible (Fig. 11-1).[3,4] Patient phonation ("ah") during the examination falsely improves the view, whereas arching of the tongue tends to obscure the uvula. When the uvula is visible (class I airway), the laryngoscopic view is classified as grade I (tracheal intubation by direct laryngoscopy technically easy) whereas in patients in whom the soft palate is not visible (class IV airway), the laryngoscopic view is classified as grade III or IV (tracheal intubation by direct laryngoscopy technically difficult or impossible) (Fig. 11-2).[5,6]

Atlanto-Occipital Joint Extension

Preoperative evaluation of atlanto-occipital joint extension (cervical spine mobility) may be performed by having the patient sit with the head held erect facing the examiner. The patient then extends the atlanto-occipital joint as much as possible (nor-

Preoperative Evaluation of the Upper Airway

Tongue versus pharyngeal size
Atlanto-occipital joint extension
Anterior mandibular space (thyromental distance)
Dental examination

mal 35 degrees). Successful exposure of the glottic opening by using direct laryngoscopy requires alignment of the oral, pharyngeal, and laryngeal axes ("sniffing position") (Fig. 11-3) (see the section *Head Position for Orotracheal Intubation*). When the atlanto-occipital joint cannot be optimally extended, vigorous attempts to do so will cause the convexity of the cervical spine to bulge further anteriorly, which will push the larynx anteriorly and compromise the view achieved during direct laryngoscopy. A greater than two-thirds decrease of atlanto-occipital joint extension from a normal of 35 degrees is associated with a grade III to IV laryngoscopic view (Fig. 11-2).[5,6]

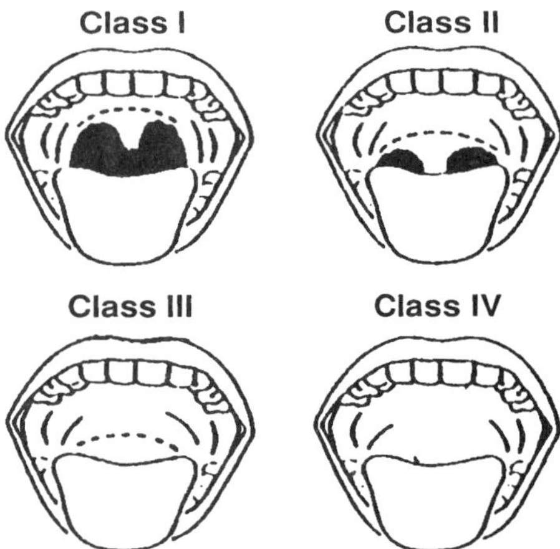

Figure 11-1. Classification of the patient's upper airway based on the size of the tongue and pharyngeal structures visible on mouth opening. Class I, soft palate, anterior and posterior tonsillar pillars, and uvula visible; class II, tonsillar pillars and base of uvula hidden by base of tongue; class III, only soft palate visible; class IV, soft palate not visible. (Modified from Frerk,[4] with permission.)

Anterior Mandibular Space

The anterior mandibular space is evaluated by asking the supine patient to maximally extend the head and measuring the distance from the notch of the thyroid cartilage to the tip of the mentum (thyromental distance) (Fig. 11-4).[4] If the thyromental distance is less than 6 cm (receding mandible, short muscular neck), the laryngeal axis will make a more acute angle with the pharyngeal axis and it will be more difficult for atlanto-occipital extension to bring these two axes into a nearly straight line (Fig. 11-5).[5] A thyromental distance greater than 6 cm and a horizontal length of the mandible greater than 9 cm are correlated with a low tongue versus pharyngeal size classification and a high likelihood that direct laryngoscopy will be relatively easy.

Dental Examination

Preoperative dental examination is intended to ascertain the presence of (1) loose teeth, (2) dental prostheses, and (3) co-existing dental abnormalities. In adults, loosening of teeth most often reflects peridontal disease and loss of bony support. Preoperative detection of the position of missing teeth and chips or fractures (especially on maxillary incisors) is important. Otherwise, subsequent discovery of these abnormalities may be incorrectly attributed to damage produced by the laryngoscope blade. It must be appreciated that prominent and/or protruberant maxillary incisors may interfere with achievement of an optimal laryngoscopic view (Fig. 11-5).[5] Furthermore, these teeth are particularly vulnerable to damage from levering effects exerted by the laryngoscope blade. The position of fixed (crowns, bridges) or removable (bridges, dentures) dental prostheses should be determined preoperatively. Removable dental prostheses may be left in place until after the induction of anesthesia so as to facilitate a mask fit to the patient's face.

INDICATIONS FOR OROTRACHEAL INTUBATION

Orotracheal intubation may be considered for every patient receiving general anesthesia. There are also specific indications for intubation of the trachea in

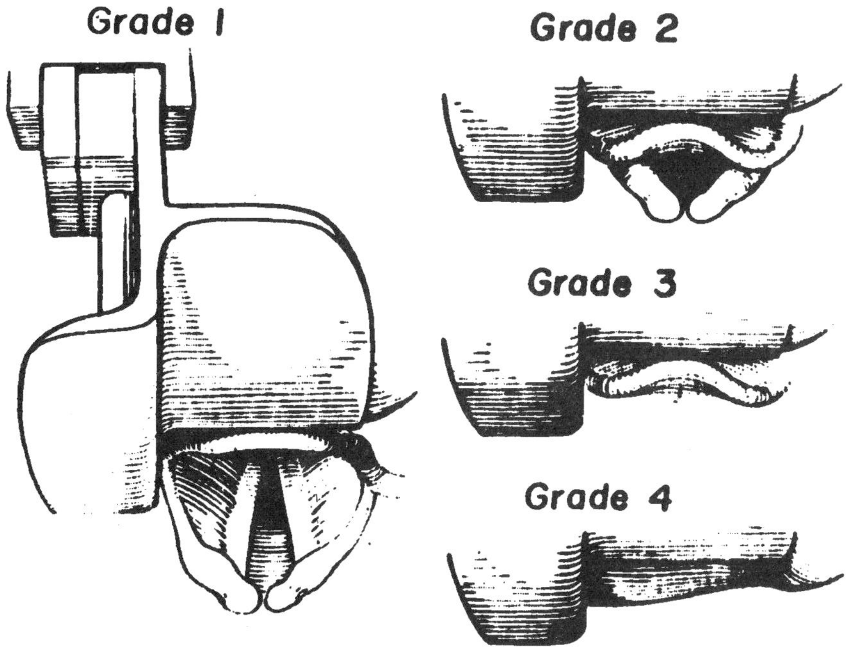

Figure 11-2. Depiction of the view of the glottic opening during direct laryngoscopy. Grade I, full view of the glottic opening; grade II, posterior portion of glottic opening is visible; grade III, only tip of epiglottis is visible; grade IV, only soft palate is visible. (Modified from Cormack and Lehane,[5] with permission.)

surgical patients. Specific indications for placement of a cuffed tracheal tube include provision of a patent airway and prevention of the inhalation (aspiration) of gastric contents, blood, or secretions into the lungs. Intubation of the trachea is mandatory in patients who have recently ingested food or in whom intestinal obstruction is present. Any patient requiring frequent tracheal suctioning is best managed with a tracheal tube in place. Patients undergoing operations in which positive pressure ventilation of the lungs is required (thoracotomy, presence of neuromuscular blockade) or in whom prolonged controlled ventilation of the lungs is necessary are most reliably managed by using a tracheal tube. Maintenance of a patent upper airway or controlled ventilation of the lungs is not reliable in the absence of a tracheal tube when operations are performed in other than the supine position (sitting, prone, lateral, lithotomy, or head-down position). Operations about the head, neck, or upper airway require a tracheal tube for both airway maintenance and removal of anesthetic equipment from the operative site. Difficult maintenance of a patent upper airway by mask may be an indication for tracheal intubation. For example, the upper airway of an edentulous patient is difficult to maintain using a face mask, but intubation of the trachea is technically easy. Disease involving the upper airway mandates placement of a tracheal tube when unconsciousness is to be produced with anesthetic drugs.

Indications for Orotracheal Intubation

- Provide patient airway
- Prevent inhalation (aspiration) of gastric contents
- Need for frequent suctioning
- Facilitate positive pressure ventilation of the lungs
- Operative position other than supine
- Operative site near or involving the upper airway
- Airway maintenance by mask difficult
- Disease involving upper airway

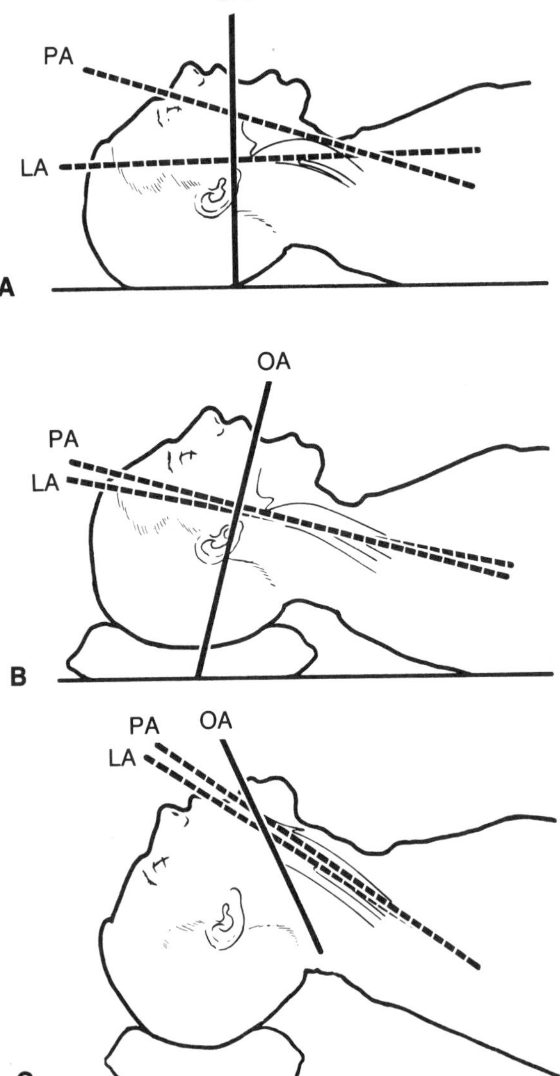

Figure 11-3. Schematic diagram demonstrating head position for intubation of the trachea. *(A)* Successful exposure of the glottic opening by direct laryngoscopy requires alignment of the oral, pharyngeal, and laryngeal axes. *(B)* Elevation of the patient's head with pads under the occiput with the shoulders remaining on the table aligns the pharyngeal and laryngeal axes. *(C)* Subsequent head extension at the atlanto-occipital joint serves to create the shortest distance and most nearly straight line from the incisor teeth to the glottic opening.

TECHNIQUE FOR OROTRACHEAL INTUBATION

Orotracheal intubation by direct laryngoscopy in anesthetized patients is routinely chosen unless specific circumstances dictate a different approach. Equipment and drugs used to intubate the trachea include a properly sized tracheal tube, laryngoscope, functioning suction catheter, appropriate anesthetic drugs, and facilities to provide positive pressure ventilation of the lungs with oxygen. If a cuffed tracheal tube is chosen, the cuff should be checked for airtightness. Techniques for induction of anesthesia before intubation of the trachea are described in Chapter 8.

Head Position for Orotracheal Intubation

Elevation of the patient's head 8 to 10 cm with pads under the occiput (shoulders remaining on the table) and extension of the head at the atlanto-occipital joint serve to align the oral, pharyngeal, and laryngeal axes such that the passage from the lips to the glottic opening is most nearly a straight line (Fig. 11-3). This posture is described as the "sniffing position." Extension of the head, without elevation of the occiput, increases the distance from the lips to the glottic opening, rotates the larynx anteriorly, and may necessitate leverage on the maxillary teeth or gums with the laryngoscope blade to expose the glottic opening. The height of the operating table should be adjusted such that the patient's face is near the level of the standing anesthesiologist's xiphoid cartilage. This table height negates the need for the anesthesiologist to bend forward and places the patient's glottic opening sufficiently distal to preserve binocular vision. If not opened by extension of the head, the patient's mouth may be manually opened by depressing the mandible with the right thumb. Simultaneously, the patient's lower lip can be rolled away with the right index finger to prevent bruising by the laryngoscope blade.

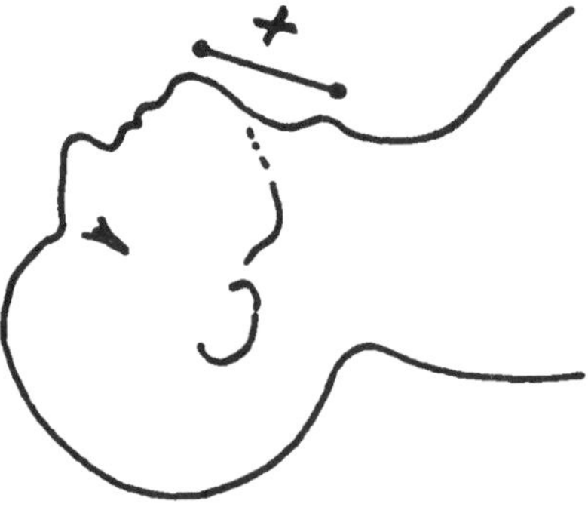

Figure 11-4. Measurement of the thyromental distance from the notch of the thyroid cartilage to the bony point of the chin (mentum) with the head maximally extended. (From Frerk,[4] with permission.)

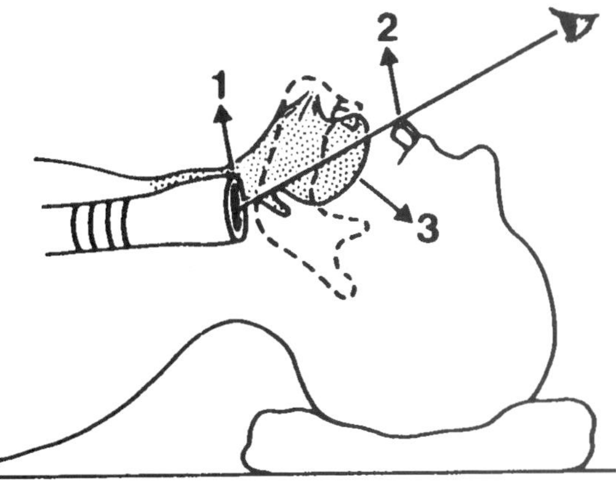

Figure 11-5. Optimal exposure of the glottic opening during direct laryngoscopy may be impaired by (1) an anterior larynx, (2) prominent upper incisors, and (3) large posteriorly located tongue. (From Cormack and Lehane,[5] with permission.)

Use of the Laryngoscope

The laryngoscope consists of a battery-containing handle to which blades with a light source may be attached and removed interchangeably (Fig. 11-6). The laryngoscope is held in the anesthesiologist's left hand near the junction between the handle and blade of the laryngoscope. The blade is then inserted on the right side of the patient's mouth so as to avoid the incisor teeth and deflect the tongue to the left, away from the lumen of the blade. Pressure on the teeth or gums must be avoided as the blade is advanced forward and centrally toward the epiglottis. A protective plastic shield placed over the upper teeth may limit the potential for damage to teeth. The wrist is held rigid to prevent using the upper teeth or gums as a fulcrum with the blade of the laryngoscope as a lever. The laryngoscope handle must never be levered toward the anesthesiologist. Once the epiglottis is visualized, the next step depends on the type of laryngoscope blade being used.

Curved (MacIntosh) Blade

The tip of the curved blade is advanced into the space between the base of the tongue and the pharyngeal surface of the epiglottis (Fig. 11-7A). Forward and upward movement of the blade exerted along the axis of the laryngoscope handle ("lift toward the patient's feet"), while avoiding any temptation to lever the blade on the teeth or gums by pulling back on the handle, serves to stretch the hypoepiglottic ligament and, in turn, to elevate the epiglottis and expose the glottic opening.

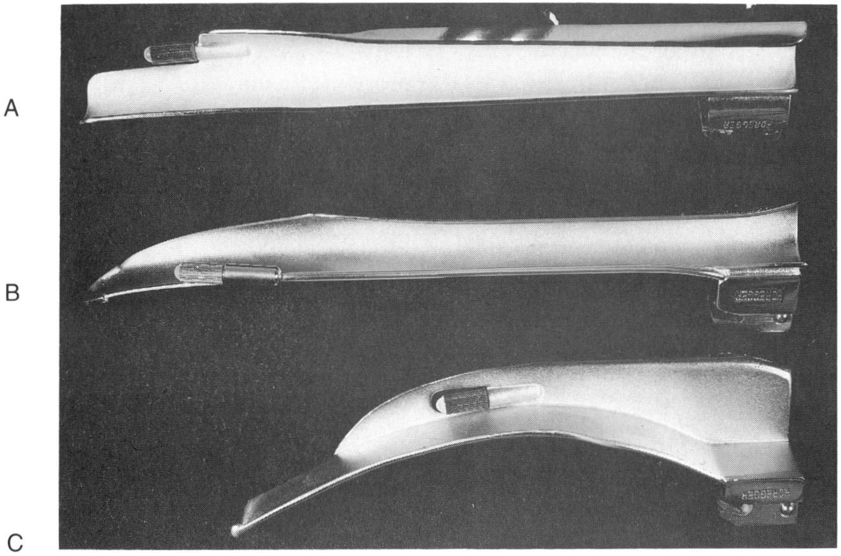

Figure 11-6. Examples of detachable laryngoscope blades, which can be used interchangeably on the same handle, include the *(A)* straight blade, *(B)* straight blade with a curved distal tip, and *(C)* curved blade.

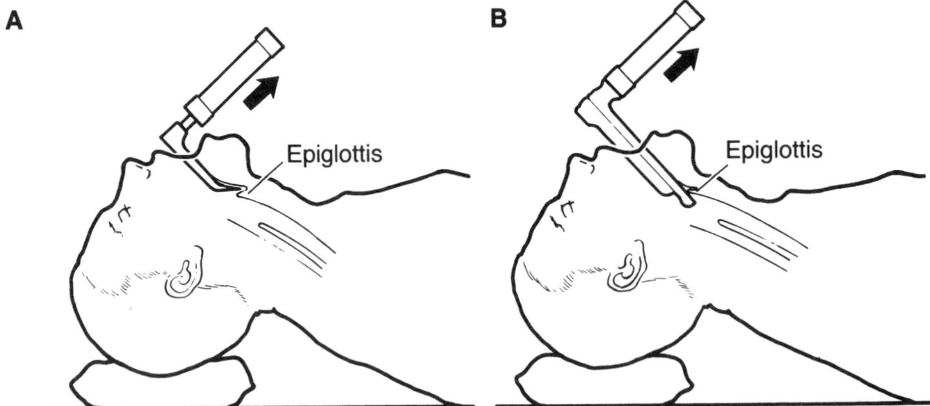

Figure 11-7. Schematic diagram depicting proper position of the laryngoscope blade for exposure of the glottic opening. *(A)* The distal end of the curved blade is advanced into the space between the base of the tongue and the pharyngeal surface of the epiglottis. *(B)* The distal end of the straight blade is advanced beneath the laryngeal surface of the epiglottis. Regardless of blade design, forward and upward movement exerted along the axis of the laryngoscope handle, as denoted by the arrows, serves to elevate the epiglottis and expose the glottic opening.

Straight (Jackson-Wisconsin) or Straight with Curved Tip (Miller) Blade

The tip of the straight blade is passed beneath the laryngeal surface of the epiglottis (Fig. 11-7B). Forward and upward movement of the blade exerted along the axis of the laryngoscope handle ("lift toward the patient's feet"), while avoiding any temptation to lever the blade on the teeth or gums by pulling back on the handle, serves to directly elevate the epiglottis and expose the glottic opening. Depression or lateral movement of the patient's thyroid cartilage externally on the neck with the anesthesiologist's right hand may facilitate exposure of the glottic opening.

Choice of Laryngoscope Blade

The choice of laryngoscope blade is often based on personal preference. Advantages cited for the curved blade include less trauma to teeth with more room for passage of the tube and less bruising of the epiglottis because the tip of the blade should not touch this structure. Advantages cited for the straight blade include better exposure of the glottic opening and less need for a stylet to direct the tube into an anterior glottic opening. Laryngoscope blades are numbered according to their length, reflecting the size of the patient. For example, a number 3 curved or straight blade is appropriate for most adult patients.

Tracheal Tube Size and Length

Tracheal tube sizes are specified according to internal diameter (ID), which is marked on each tube (Table 11-1 and Fig. 11-8). Tracheal tubes are available in 0.5-mm ID increments. Most adult tracheas (after 14 years of age) readily accept a cuffed 8- to 9-mm ID (smaller size often selected for females) tracheal tube. The tracheal tube also has lengthwise centimeter markings starting at the distal tracheal end to permit accurate determination of the tube length inserted past the lips. Tracheal tubes are most often made of clear inert polyvinyl chloride plastic that molds to the contour of the airway after softening on exposure to body temperature. Tracheal tube material should also be radiopaque to facilitate demonstration of tube position relative to the carina and transparent to permit visualization of secretions or of air flow as evidenced by condensation of water vapor in the tube lumen (breath-fogging) during exhalation. Thoracic surgery may necessitate the use of specially designed (double-lumen or built-in bronchial blocker) endobronchial tubes (see Chapter 19).

Tracheal Tube Cuff

Inflatable cuffs are built into the distal end of tracheal tubes (Fig. 11-8). The cuff is inflated with air to create a seal against the underlying tracheal mucosa. This seal facilitates positive pressure ventila-

Table 11-1. Size and Length of Tracheal Tubes Relative to Airway Anatomy

Age	Internal Diameter (mm)	Distance Inserted from Lips to Place Distal End in Midtrachea[a] (cm)	Diameter of Trachea (mm)	Length of Trachea (cm)	Distance from Lips to Carina (cm)
Premature	2.5	8			
Full term	3.0	10			
1–6 mo	3.5	11	5	6	13
6–12 mo	4.0	12			
2 y	4.5	13			
4 y	5.0	14			
6 y	5.5	15			
8 y	6.5	16	8	8	18
10 y	7.0	17–18			
12 y	7.5	18–20			
≤14 y	8.0–9.0	20–22	20[b] 15[c]	14[b] 12[c]	28[b] 24[c]

[a]Add 2–3 cm for nasal tubes.
[b]Males.
[c]Females.

tion of the lungs and decreases the likelihood of aspiration of pharyngeal or gastric secretions. When filled with air to just a no leak volume during application of positive airway pressure, low pressure large volume cuffs are intended to minimize the likelihood of mucosal ischemia resulting from prolonged pressure on the tracheal wall. Nevertheless, there is probably no period of tracheal intubation that does not produce some laryngeal tracheal damage. For example, ciliary denudation has been found to occur predominantly over the tracheal rings and underlying cuff site with only 2 hours of intubation and tracheal wall pressure maintained below 25 mmHg.[7]

Placement of a Tracheal Tube

The glottic opening is recognized by its triangular shape and pale white vocal cords (Fig. 11-9). The tracheal tube is held in the anesthesiologist's right hand like a pencil and introduced on the right side of the patient's mouth with the built-in curve directed anteriorly. Attempts to insert the tube in the midline of the mouth and then down the lumen of the laryngoscope blade usually obscure vision of the glottic opening. The tube is advanced 1 to 2 cm past the vocal cords after the cuff just disappears, which should correspond to the distance predicted to place the distal end of the tube midway between the vocal cords and carina. At this point, the laryngoscope blade is removed from the mouth. The tracheal tube cuff is next inflated with air to just a no leak volume during positive pressure ventilation of the lungs. Distension of the small pilot balloon attached to the inflation tube leading to the cuff confirms cuff inflation.

Confirmation of placement of the tube in the trachea, rather than the esophagus, is verified by several different observations.[8] Symmetric bilateral movements of the chest with manual compression of the reservoir bag combined with the presence of bilateral breath sounds on apical and/or midaxillary auscultation of the lungs are commonly established after tracheal intubation. A characteristic feel of the reservoir bag associated with normal lung compliance during manual inflation of the lungs and the presence of expiratory refilling of the bag is evaluated. Condensation of water in the tube lumen (breath-fogging) during exhalation is evidence of tracheal placement of the tube. The presence of carbon dioxide in the exhaled gases from the tracheal tube as detected by capnography or mass spectrometry (end-tidal PCO_2 higher than 30 mmHg for three to five consecutive breaths) may be the most reliable confirmatory sign of tracheal placement of the tube.[9] Carbon dioxide will not be persistently present in exhaled gases from a tube accidentally

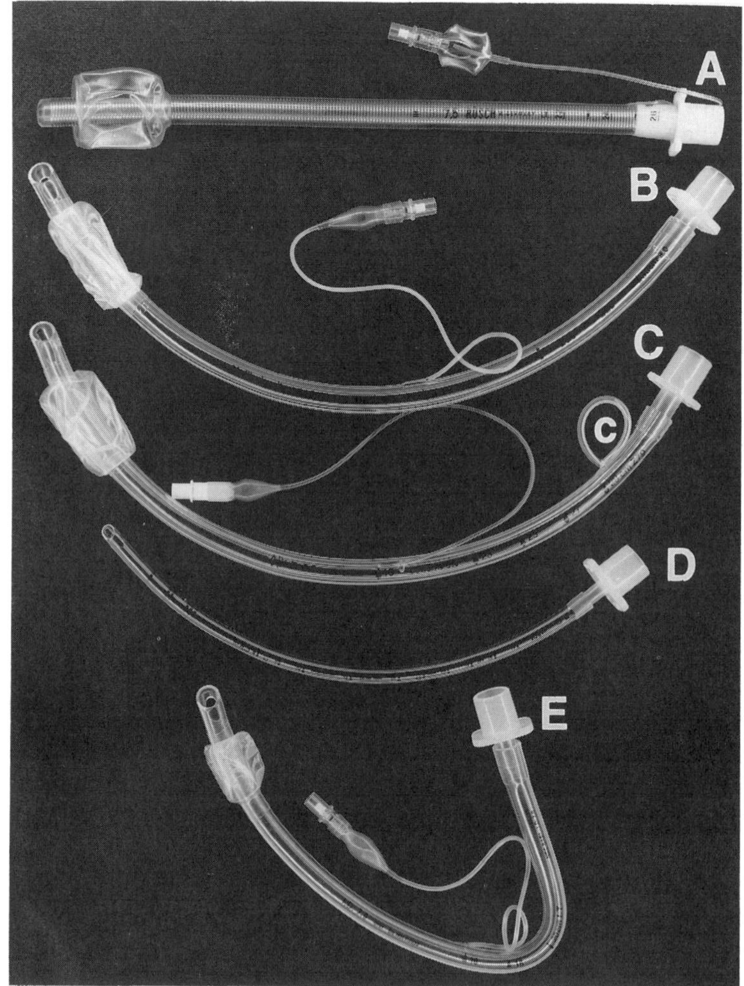

Figure 11-8. Various types of tracheal tubes. Tube A is an armored or anode tube with built-in spiral wire to minimize the opportunity of collapse or kinking. Tubes B to E are made of clear polyvinyl chloride and are recommended for single use. Tubes B and C are equipped with a built-in low pressure cuff and are appropriate sizes for adults. Tube C is unique in that it includes a tip control ring loop (c), which, when pulled, directs the distal end of the tube anteriorly. Tube D is uncuffed and is a size appropriate for children. Tube E is a preformed RAE tube that can be used to facilitate positioning of the anesthetic breathing system away from the operative site during head and neck surgery. For tubes A, B, C, and E the cuff is inflated by attaching an air-filled syringe to the small diameter tube that leads to the cuff. Distension of the small balloon near the attachment for the syringe confirms inflation of the cuff. Numbers on the tubes denote the internal diameter of the tube and the distance from the distal tracheal end of the tube.

placed in the esophagus. Declines in arterial hemoglobin oxygen saturation as evident on a pulse oximeter may alert the anesthesiologist to a previously unrecognized esophageal intubation. Noting the depth of insertion as determined by the centimeter markings on the tracheal tube at the upper incisor teeth or gums helps predict a midtrachea position of the distal end of the tube. Securing the orotracheal tube at the upper incisor teeth or gums at the 23-cm mark in adult males and the 21-cm mark in adult females should reliably place the distal end of the tube in the midtrachea and thus minimize the likelihood of accidental endobronchial intubation.[9] Furthermore, if a cuffed tube is properly placed in the midtrachea, the anesthesiologist can easily detect, by external palpation, cuff distension

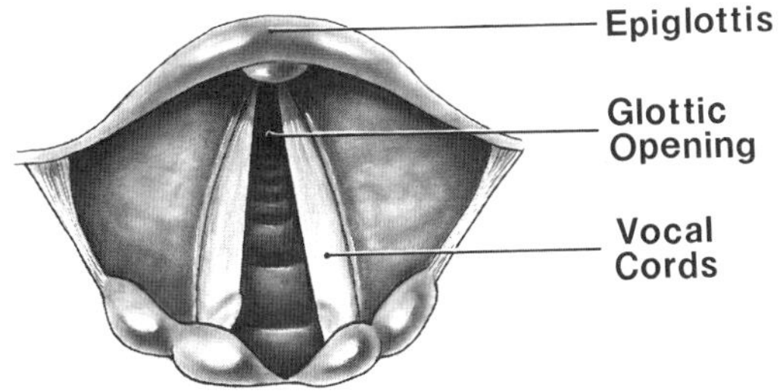

Figure 11-9. Schematic view of glottic opening as seen during direct laryngoscopy when the epiglottis is elevated with a curved or straight laryngoscope blade. The glottic opening is recognized by its triangular shape bordered by the pale white vocal cords.

in the suprasternal notch during rapid inflation of the cuff. After confirmation of correct placement, the tube is secured in position with tape placed around the tube and applied above and below the lips, extending over the cheeks.

Classification of Airway Difficulty

The technical difficulty of tracheal intubation can be classified as grade I to IV according to the laryngoscopic view of the glottic opening (Fig. 11-2).[4] Zero degree of difficulty means that a tracheal tube can be inserted into a fully visualized laryngeal aperture (grade I laryngoscopic view) with little effort. Visualization of progressively less of the laryngeal aperture (grades II and III laryngoscopic views) is associated with progressive degrees of intubation difficulty characterized by the need for increased anterior lifting force with the laryngoscope blade, optimal sniff position, and external laryngeal pressure to push the larynx more posteriorly and cephalad into better view. A grade III laryngoscopic view requiring multiple attempts and/or blades occurs in 1% to 4% of patients.[1] Failed tracheal intubation (severe grade III or grade IV laryngoscopic view) occurs in fewer than 0.35% of patients.[1] When the anesthesiologist is not able or does not expect to see the vocal cords with conventional laryngoscopy, it becomes necessary to consider alternative approaches often with the patient awake (Fig. 11-10)[1,2] (see the section *Alternatives to Orotracheal Intubation During General Anesthesia*). Indeed, difficulty in managing the airway leading to hypoventilation and arterial hypoxemia is the single most important cause of anesthesia-related morbidity and mortality.[1]

ALTERNATIVES TO OROTRACHEAL INTUBATION DURING GENERAL ANESTHESIA

Alternatives to orotracheal intubation during general anesthesia include awake orotracheal intubation, nasotracheal intubation, and intubation with a fiberoptic laryngoscope. These alternatives are considered when orotracheal intubation during general anesthesia might be unsafe (recent food ingestion, intestinal obstruction, upper airway disease) or impossible because of altered anatomy.

There are compelling reasons to advocate awake tracheal intubation when management of the airway is expected to be difficult because of either the presence of pathologic factors or a combination of anatomic factors, or both.[1] Most important is the realization that the natural airway will be better maintained when the patient remains conscious. This reflects the presence of sufficient skeletal muscle tone to keep upper airway structures (base of tongue, posterior pharyngeal wall, epiglottis, larynx) separated and much easier to identify. In the anesthetized (unconscious) or paralyzed patient, loss of skeletal muscle tone tends to cause these structures to collapse toward one another, which distorts the anatomy. Furthermore, the larynx moves to a more anterior position with induction of anesthesia and paralysis, which makes conventional tracheal intubation more difficult. Crucial to the success of an awake tracheal intubation is an informed patient (who agrees with the plan) and adequate topical and nerve block anesthesia. There is general agreement that anticipated difficult tracheal intubations are usually easier to manage than those that are unexpected, emphasizing the value of prior planning in managing the difficult airway (Fig. 11-10).[1,2]

Awake Orotracheal Intubation

Awake orotracheal intubation is often facilitated by judicious use of intravenous sedation and local anesthesia of the upper airway. Intravenous sedation (midazolam, fentanyl) can help the awake patient tolerate the institution of airway anesthesia and tracheal intubation by relieving anxiety and providing analgesia. It is important that this sedation be administered by titration to a desired effect and that the patient remain oriented and cooperative (responsive to questions and requests). Caution must be exercised if loss of protective laryngeal

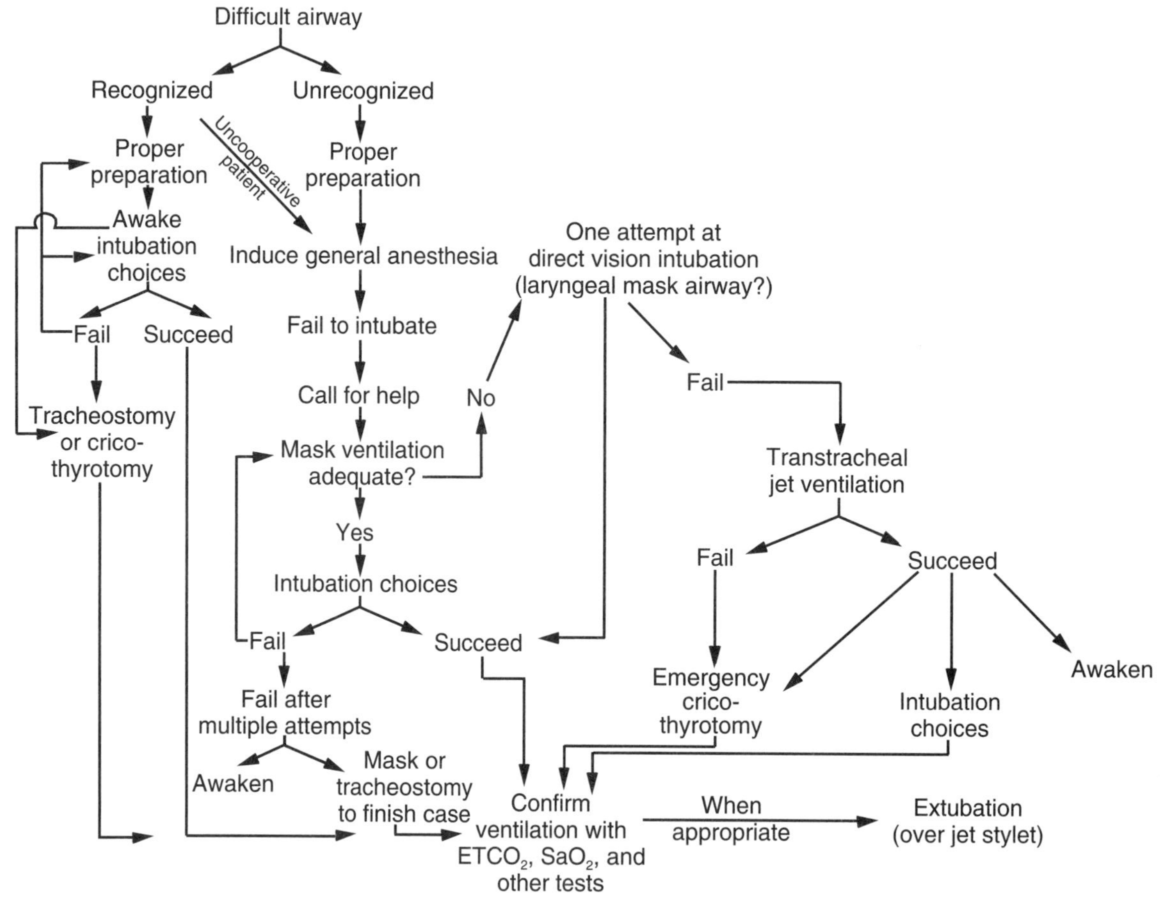

Figure 11-10. Difficult airway management algorithm. (From Benumof,[1] with permission.)

reflexes could place the patient at increased risk of pulmonary aspiration.

Airway Anesthesia

Topical anesthesia of the upper airway is often provided with pledgets or an atomizer containing 4% lidocaine (high concentration needed to penetrate mucosal membranes). When vomiting is a hazard, only topical spray is recommended, thus avoiding anesthesia of structures necessary to protect against pulmonary aspiration. Premedication with an anticholinergic serves to decrease secretions and facilitate the onset of topical anesthesia. For nasal mucosal anesthesia, a mixture of 3% to 4% lidocaine with 0.25% to 0.5% phenylephrine on cotton pledgets is an alternative to cocaine. In the past, cocaine was preferred because it provided both topical anesthesia and localized vasoconstriction that decreased the likelihood of epistaxis. The abuse potential of cocaine, however, detracts from its continued use for this purpose. The superior laryngeal nerve (branch of vagus that supplies sensory fibers to the vocal cords, epiglottis, and arytenoids) is blocked bilaterally (5 ml of 1% lidocaine) as it penetrates the thyrohyoid membrane (Fig. 11-11).[10] Tracheal anesthesia is produced by rapid injection during inspiration of 4 ml of 4% lidocaine via a needle passed through the cricothyroid membrane into the trachea (transtracheal block).

Nasotracheal Intubation

Nasotracheal intubation may be performed electively for intraoral operations, when anatomic abnormalities or disease of the upper airway make direct laryngoscopy difficult or impossible and when long-term intubation of the trachea is anticipated.

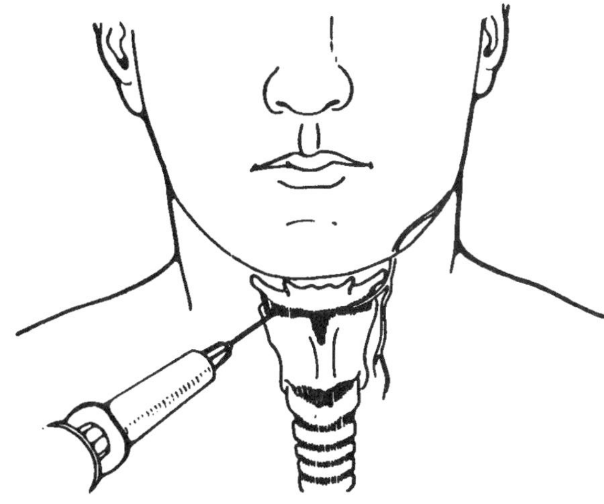

Figure 11-11. Superior laryngeal nerve block is performed by passing a needle through the thyrohyoid membrane and depositing local anesthetic solution bilaterally. (From Mulroy,[10] with permission.)

Advantages cited for nasotracheal intubation include (1) more stable tube fixation, (2) less chance for tube kinking, (3) greater comfort in awake patients, and (4) fewer oropharyngeal secretions.

Awake Blind Nasotracheal Intubation

Awake blind nasotracheal intubation is usually reserved for situations in which direct laryngoscopy or ventilation of the lungs would be impossible or induction of anesthesia before intubation of the trachea would be hazardous. To ensure maximum patient comfort and nasal patency and to minimize the chance of epistaxis, the nasal mucosa should be anesthetized (see the section *Airway Anesthesia*). Either naris may be chosen, depending on the history and physical examination, but the right naris is preferable because the bevel of most tracheal tubes when introduced through the right naris will face the flat nasal septum, decreasing the possibiity of trauma to the turbinates. Tracheal tubes can be used interchangeably for nasal or oral intubation of the trachea (Table 11-1). In adults, 7.0- to 7.5-mm ID tubes are usually adequate. After passage through the naris into the oropharynx, the tracheal tube is advanced toward the glottic opening as long as breath sounds are maximal as determined by listening to exhaled air passing from the proximal end of the tube. Ideally, the tracheal tube is swiftly passed through the glottic opening just before inspiration because the vocal cords are most open during this time and the risk of vocal cord trauma is thus minimized. Successful placement of the tube in the trachea is confirmed by continued breathing through the tube.

Nasotracheal Intubation During General Anesthesia

Nasotracheal intubation during general anesthesia is acceptable when vomiting is not a hazard and ventilation of the lungs can be maintained by a mask. General anesthesia is produced following airway anesthesia and vasoconstriction of the nasal mucosa. If blind nasotracheal intubation is to be performed, it is mandatory to maintain spontaneous ventilation in the patient so as to permit identification of the glottic opening as evidenced by passage of exhaled air from the proximal end of the tube. Alternatively, nasotracheal intubation may be accomplished by using direct laryngoscopy to expose the glottic opening. When this approach is selected, succinylcholine or a nondepolarizing muscle relaxant is administered to produce skeletal muscle relaxation and the tracheal tube is placed through the right naris into the oropharynx. The glottic opening is then visualized by direct laryngoscopy and the tracheal tube guided through the glottic opening under vision by manually advancing the tube at the proximal end. Alternatively, the tracheal tube may be grasped in the oropharynx with intubating forceps (Magill forceps) and directed so that pressure on the proximal end causes the tube to pass between the vocal cords. Technically, the right naris is preferred because a left nasotracheal tube is clumsy to advance under direct vision with the anesthesiologist's left hand holding the laryngoscope.

Complications Unique to Nasotracheal Intubation

Complications unique to nasotracheal intubation include (1) epistaxis, (2) dislodgement of pharyngeal tonsils (adenoids), (3) eustachian tube obstruction, (4) maxillary sinusitis, (5) bacteremia, and (6) gastric distension.[11] Epistaxis most likely reflects avulsion of nasal mucosa covering the turbinates. Shrinkage of nasal mucosa with cocaine or phenylephrine and use of small and generously lubricated tracheal tubes should minimize this complication. When pharyngeal tonsils are prominent, as in children, it is preferable to perform all nasotracheal intubations using direct laryngoscopy to expose the glottic opening so as to prevent unrecognized delivery into the trachea of a dislodged piece of tonsil. Patients who experience head trauma may be at particular risk of development of sinusitis as many of these patients have sinus air-fluid (blood) levels on initial computed tomography. These air-fluid levels provide an excellent culture medium for bacteria. The incidence of sinusitis appears to increase dramatically after 5 days of nasotracheal intubation. Bacteremia is not predictably associated with trauma to the nasal mucosa, nor is it reliably prevented by prior use of topical vasoconstrictors.[12] Prophylactic antibiotics are indicated when nasotracheal intubation is planned in patients with heart disease. The patient with a nasotracheal tube in place can swallow large volumes of air, leading to gastric distension in the absence of a gastric decompression tube.

Intubation with a Fiberoptic Laryngoscope

The fiberoptic laryngoscope consists of glass fibers that are bound together to provide a flexible unit for transmission of images and light (Fig. 11-12). Intubation of the trachea by a flexible fiberoptic laryngoscope is useful for patients in whom the glottic opening cannot be visualized because of anatomic abnormalities. After topical anesthesia the tracheal tube is passed through the naris into the oropharynx (see the section *Airway Anesthesia*). The lubricated fiberoptic laryngoscope (about 5-mm outer diameter) is then passed through an 8-mm ID or larger tracheal tube (a pediatric fiberoptic bronchoscope will pass through a 5-mm ID tracheal tube) until the epiglottis and glottic opening are visualized. Insertion of the adult fiberoptic laryngoscope through a tracheal tube smaller than 8-mm ID may produce the potential for autopositive end-expiratory pressure and hyperinflation of the patient's lungs. It is important, before initiating fiberoptic laryngoscopy, to focus on an external fine

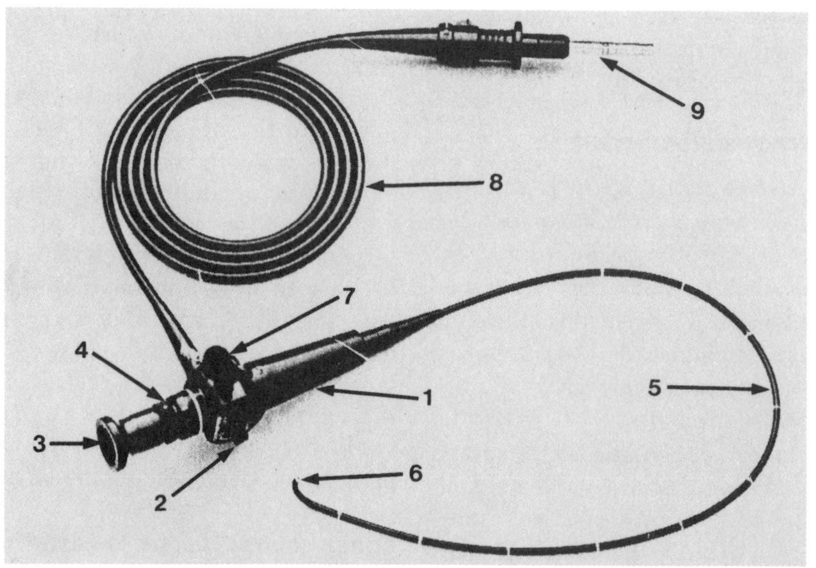

Figure 11-12. Flexible fiberoptic laryngoscope consists of (1) control unit, (2) tip deflection control lever, (3) eyepiece, (4) diopter adjustment ring, (5) flexible insertion cord, (6) bending tip responsive to the control level, (7) working channel sleeve and plug, (8) light guide cable, and (9) light guide plug. The working channel can be used to administer inhaled or topical anesthetics, deliver supplemental oxygen, and suction secretions. The length of the flexible insertion cord is 500 to 600 mm, the diameter for adult fiberoptic laryngoscopes is 4 to 6 mm, and the diameter for the pediatric bronchoscope is 3.5 mm. The diameter of the working channel is 1.2 to 2 mm. Upward and downward deflection of the bending tip in response to the control level is about 120 degrees.

> **Possible Indications for Use of a Fiberoptic Laryngoscope**
>
> Upper airway obstruction
> - Tumor
> - Abscess
> - Prior surgery
>
> Mediastinal mass
> Subglottic stenosis
> Congenital upper airway abnormalities
> - Mandibular hypoplasia
> - Craniofacial synostosis
> - Kippel-Feil syndrome
>
> Immobile cervical vertebrae
> - Arthritis
> - Traction
>
> Verify position of a double-lumen endobronchial tube

test pattern by adjusting the diopter ring on the eyepiece. Compared with the view seen when using direct laryngoscopy, the depth of the vocal cords may seem exaggerated and the true vocal cords not seen until the false vocal cords have been passed with the fiberoptic laryngoscope. The visual field often becomes limited as the fiberoptic laryngoscope nears the glottic opening, and secretions, blood, or fogging of the lens may further obscure the view. Immersion of the tip of the fiberoptic laryngoscope in warm water or application of silicone spray to the lens may decrease the likelihood of fogging or adherence of secretions. Inclusion of an anticholinergic in the preoperative medication is useful as upper airway secretions obscure visibility when the fiberoptic laryngoscope is used. It is important to keep the fiberoptic laryngoscope in the midline to avoid entering the pyriform sinus. A helpful sign that the trachea has been entered is the glow seen over the patient's anterior neck from transillumination of the larynx and trachea as the tip of the fiberoptic laryngoscope passes through the glottic opening. The tracheal tube is then advanced into the trachea using the fiberoptic laryngoscope as a guide. Oral intubation of the trachea is accomplished in a similar manner by placing the fiberoptic laryngoscope behind the base of the tongue, often with limited downward displacement of the tongue using a laryngoscope blade. Alternatively, a plastic oropharyngeal airway with a cylindric passage (Airway Intubator) that permits passage of the tracheal tube containing the fiberoptic laryngoscope may be used (Fig. 11-13).[13] This airway can be placed in awake patients following appropriate topical anesthesia, serving to keep the fiberoptic laryngoscope in the midline and at the same time producing downward displacement of the tongue. Positive pressure ventilation may be continuously maintained during fiberoptic laryngoscopy by using an anesthesia mask that has a special fiberoptic instrument port covered by a self-sealing diaphragm along with the Airway Intubator (Fig. 11-13).[13] Use of the fiberoptic laryngoscope is facilitated in awake patients, since tissue tone is maintained and the

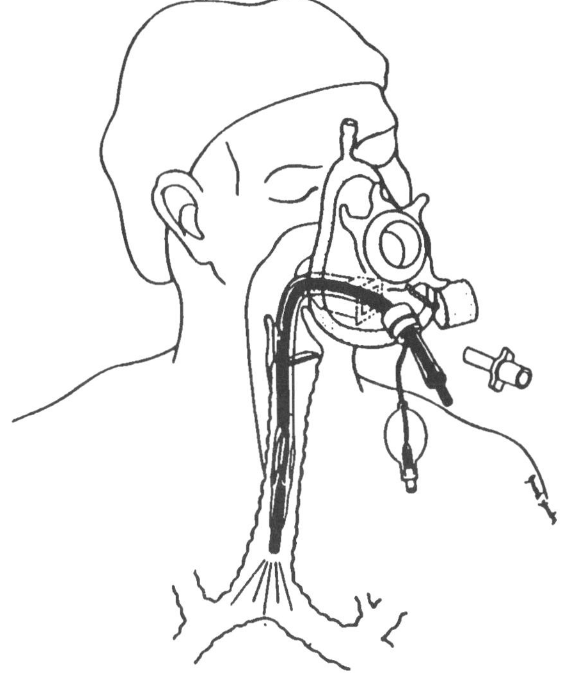

Figure 11-13. Schematic diagram showing the use of the anesthesia mask with diaphragm and oral Airway Intubator as aids to fiberoptic tracheal intubation in an anesthetized patient with or without mechanical ventilation of the lungs. The tracheal tube and the fiberoptic laryngoscope are introduced through the diaphragm in the anesthesia mask and guided via the Airway Intubator into the trachea. The fiberoptic laryngoscope and anesthesia mask are then removed over the tracheal tube, whereas removal of the oral Airway Intubator is optional. (From Rogers and Benumof,[13] with permission.)

tongue and epiglottis do not relax to obscure the vocal cords. Furthermore, the awake patient can assist by phonating or protruding the tongue. Fiberoptic nasotracheal intubation in the awake patient is often easier than the orotracheal approach because the nasopharynx is better aligned with the glottis. In addition to tracheal intubation, flexible fiberoptic endoscopy has become an essential tool for placement and repositioning of double-lumen endobronchial tubes (see Chapter 19), placement of bronchial blockers, and changing, repositioning, or checking the patency of tracheal tubes.

Bullard Intubating Laryngoscope

The Bullard intubating laryngoscope combines fiberoptic imaging and an anatomically shaped rigid blade (adult and pediatric sizes available) that facilitate rapid oral visualization of the glottic opening (Fig. 11-14). This laryngoscope may serve as an alternative to intubation with a fiberoptic laryngoscope in patients in whom tracheal intubation is difficult or impossible or in whom head or neck extension is not permissible. An oral opening of 6 mm is sufficient to allow introduction of the laryngoscope blade.

Laryngeal Mask Airway

The laryngeal mask airway (LMA) is an alternative to tracheal intubation, especially in patients in whom conventional tracheal intubation has proven to be difficult or impossible or when a less invasive alternative to tracheal intubation is desired.[14] The LMA may also serve as a guide (conduit) for a fiberoptic laryngoscope. This airway consists of a shallow mask with an inflatable cuff connected to a tube that adapts to the anesthetic delivery system (Fig. 11-15).[15] Different sizes of the LMA permit its use in children and adults.

The LMA is inserted without the use of a laryngoscope, by placing the head and neck in the usual position for tracheal intubation and inserting the deflated mask with its lumen facing backward (similar to insertion of an oropharyngeal airway) so as to facilitate negotiation of the angle behind the

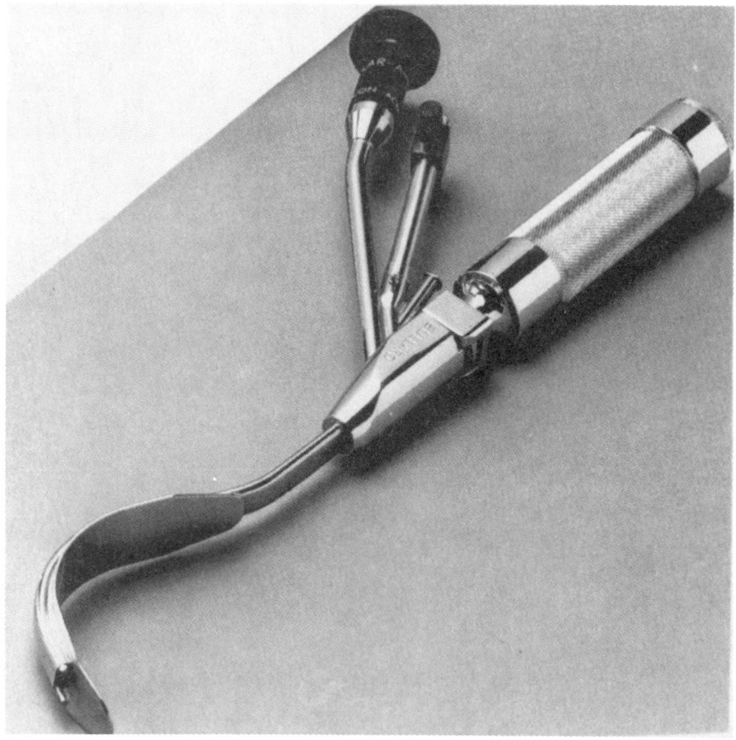

Figure 11-14. Bullard intubating laryngoscope.

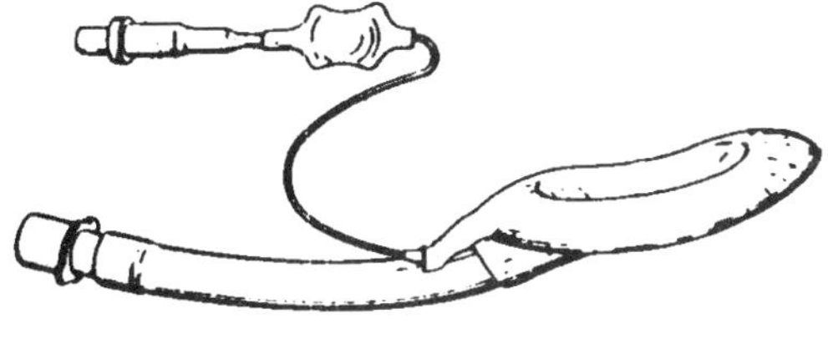

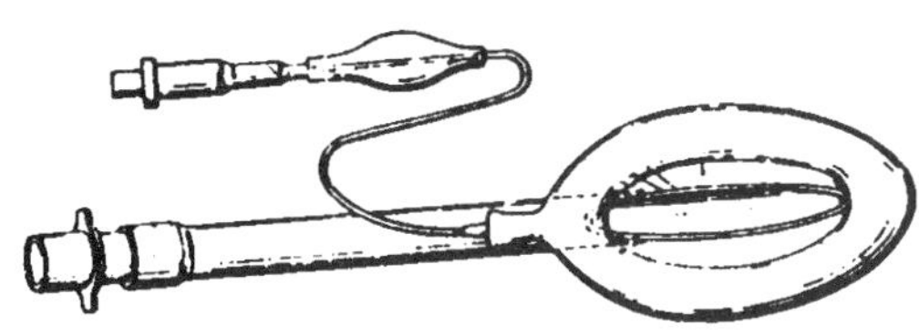

Figure 11-15. Laryngeal mask airway. (From Brain,[15] with permission.)

tongue. The LMA is advanced blindly to the base of the hypopharynx such that the mask portion of the airway is against the glottic opening. Without holding the tube, the cuff is inflated with 10 to 30 ml of air. This usually causes a characteristic outward movement of the tube of up to 1.5 cm, as the cuff centers itself around the laryngeal outlet. Furthermore, a slight bulging of tissues in the anterior neck overlying the larynx serves to indicate that the LMA is in position. It is possible to control ventilation of the lungs using an LMA, although the ability to achieve this goal is less predictable than in the presence of a cuffed tracheal tube. The principal disadvantage of the LMA is the failure of this device to reliably protect against pulmonary aspiration of gastric contents.

OROTRACHEAL INTUBATION IN CHILDREN

Orotracheal intubation in children differs from that in adults because of anatomic differences in pediatric patients, as well as the need to more carefully select the size and length of the tracheal tube inserted into these young individuals (see Chapter 26).

Anatomic Differences from Adults

The newborn head and tongue are large, and the neck is short. The larynx is more cephalad than in the adult. For example, the lower border of the cricoid cartilage is opposite the fourth cervical vertebra at birth and opposite the fifth cervical vertebra at age 6. The epiglottis is U-shaped and stiff. These anatomic differences result in difficulty aligning the oral, pharyngeal, and laryngeal axes and elevating the epiglottis to expose the glottic opening (Fig. 11-3). As such, the glottic opening of the newborn tends to be anterior compared with that of the adult. It must be remembered that the cricoid cartilage is the narrowest point in the larynx of children such that a tube that passes through the glottic opening may subsequently resist advancement at this site.

Tracheal Tube Size and Length

Selection of the appropriate tracheal tube size and length is critical in children, since the margin for error is small (Table 11-1). Excessive tube size is responsible for unnecessary laryngotracheal trauma, which may manifest as laryngeal edema when the tube is removed from the trachea. Likewise, the short glottis-to-carina distance in children necessitates careful calculation of correct tube length to ensure a midtracheal position of the distal end of the tube (Table 11-1). One must be aware that head flexion or change from the supine to head-down position may shift the carina upward, converting a midtracheal tube placement to an endobronchial intubation while head extension may place the distal end of the tube in the pharynx.

A tracheal tube one size above and below the calculated size should be available, with the final choice made when the glottic opening is visualized and the tube is inserted into the trachea. Cuffed tubes are probably not necessary in children younger than 5 years of age because the narrow subglottic tracheal diameter ensures an adequate seal between the tube and tracheal mucosa. Resistance to breathing is a consideration for the small lumen tracheal tubes and connectors necessary in children. When increased airway resistance is a concern, the best approach is placement of a properly sized (not the largest possible) tube in the trachea and controlled ventilation of the lungs to prevent excessive work of breathing.

Technique for Tracheal Intubation

Orotracheal intubation is routinely chosen for short-term intubation of the trachea in children. Awake orotracheal intubation of the newborn may be preferable. After about 2 weeks of age, infants are sufficiently strong to resist awake intubation of the trachea, and induction of anesthesia may be performed before direct laryngoscopy is attempted. A straight laryngoscope blade often provides better exposure of the glottic opening than the curved blade, especially in children younger than 3 years of age.

EXTUBATION OF THE TRACHEA

Extubation of the trachea following general anesthesia is often accomplished while the patient is still adequately anesthetized so as to diminish the likelihood of coughing or laryngospasm (reflex closure of the vocal cords). This assumes that adequate ventilation of the lungs is present or can be maintained without the tracheal tube in place and that the presence of gastric contents is not a likely hazard. Suctioning of the pharynx should be performed before extubation of the trachea so that secretions proximal to the tube cuff do not drain into the trachea when the cuff is deflated. After the cuff is deflated, the tube is removed, often with simultaneous pressure on the reservoir bag so that the lungs are inflated with oxygen and the initial gas flow is outward. This maneuver may facilitate a cough and expulsion of any aspirated material. When the presence of gastric contents is predictable at the conclusion of anesthesia, the trachea should not be extubated until protective laryngeal reflexes have returned. Vigorous reaction to the tracheal tube ("bucking") signals the return of the protective cough reflex, and at this point the trachea must be extubated or further sedation instituted to permit tolerance of the tube.

Laryngospasm and vomiting are the most serious immediate hazards after extubation of the trachea. Therefore, oxygen, succinylcholine, equipment for reintubation of the trachea, and suction must be immediately available. Supplemental oxygen usually is administered in the immediate period following tracheal extubation.

COMPLICATIONS OF TRACHEAL INTUBATION

Complications of tracheal intubation are rare and should not influence the decision to place a tracheal tube. Certainly, the benefits of a properly placed tracheal tube far exceed the risks of intubation of the trachea. Complications of tracheal intubation may be categorized as those occurring (1) during direct laryngoscopy and intubation of the trachea, (2) while the tracheal tube is in place, and (3) after extubation of the trachea either immediately or after a delay.

Complications of Tracheal Intubation

- During direct laryngoscopy and intubation of the trachea
  - Dental and oral soft tissue trauma
  - Hypertension and tachycardia
  - Cardiac dysrhythmias
  - Myocardial ischemia
  - Inhalation (aspiration) of gastric contents
- While the tracheal tube is in place
  - Tracheal tube obstruction
  - Endobronchial intubation
  - Esophageal intubation
  - Tracheal tube cuff leak
  - Barotrauma
  - Nasogastric distension
  - Accidental disconnection from breathing circuit
  - Tracheal mucosa ischemia
  - Accidental extubation
- Immediate and delayed complications after extubation of the trachea
  - Laryngospasm
  - Inhalation (aspiration) of gastric contents
  - Pharyngitis (sore throat)
  - Laryngitis
  - Laryngeal or subglottic edema
  - Laryngeal ulceration with or without granuloma formulation
  - Tracheitis
  - Tracheal stenosis
  - Vocal cord paralysis
  - Arytenoid cartilage dislocation

Complications During Direct Laryngoscopy and Intubation of the Trachea

Dental trauma is the most serious and frequent type of damage related to direct laryngoscopy. Use of a plastic shield placed over the upper teeth and avoidance of using the laryngoscope blade as a lever on the teeth will minimize the likelihood of dental trauma. Should injury occur, prompt consultation with a dentist is indicated. A dislodged tooth must be recovered, but, if the search is unsuccessful, appropriate radiographs of the chest and abdomen should be taken to ensure that the tooth has not passed through the glottic opening.

Hypertension and tachycardia frequently accompany direct laryngoscopy (regardless of the type of laryngoscope blade used) and intubation of the trachea. These responses are usually transient and innocuous. In patients with co-existing hypertension or ischemic heart disease, however, these changes may be exaggerated or may jeopardize the balance between myocardial oxygen requirements and delivery. In these patients, it is important to minimize the duration of direct laryngoscopy, if possible, to less than 15 seconds. Serious or persistent cardiac dysrhythmias during intubation of the trachea are unlikely, particularly if adequate oxygenation during the period of apnea associated with direct laryngoscopy is ensured by prior inflation of the patient's lungs with oxygen (denitrogenation produced by preoxygenation).

Direct upper airway trauma is more likely to occur with difficult tracheal intubation as application of more physical force to the patient's airway than is normally applied is likely to be used as well as the need for multiple attempts. The most common consequence is a chipped or broken tooth. Posterior pharyngeal and lip lacerations and bruises are more likely with difficult tracheal intubation. In extreme cases, interruption of oxygenation and ventilation may result in cardiac arrest and brain damage. In these rare situations, passage of a 12- to 14-gauge catheter over a needle through the cricothyroid membrane into the trachea (cricothyrotomy) may be used as a temporary measure to provide oxygen to the patient's lungs (see Fig. 35-11).

Complications While the Tracheal Tube Is in Place

Obstruction of the tracheal tube may occur as a result of accumulation of secretions in the tube and kinking of the tube. Accidental endobronchial intubation is minimized by calculating the proper tracheal tube length for every patient and then noting the centimeter marking on the tube at the point of fixation at the lips. Flexion of the head may advance the tube up to 1.9 cm, converting a tracheal placement into an endobronchial intubation.[16] Conversely, extension of the head can withdraw the tube up to 1.9 cm and result in a pharyngeal placement. Lateral rotation of the head moves the distal end of the tracheal tube about 0.7 cm from the carina.

Immediate and Delayed Complications After Extubation of the Trachea

Laryngospasm and inhalation of gastric contents are the two most serious potential immediate complications after extubation of the trachea. Laryngospasm is unlikely if the depth of anesthesia is sufficient during extubation of the trachea or the patient is allowed to awaken before extubation. The patient who is lightly anesthetized at the time of extubation of the trachea is most at risk. If laryngospasm occurs, oxygen under positive pressure via a face mask and forward displacement of the mandible using the index fingers to apply pressure at the temporomandibular joints may be sufficient treatment. Administration of intravenous (or intramuscular) succinylcholine is indicated if laryngospasm persists. Inhalation of gastric contents is most likely to occur in the debilitated patient or in the presence of recent food ingestion or intestinal obstruction. Pharyngitis (sore throat) is the most frequent complaint after extubation of the trachea, particularly in females, presumably because of the thinner mucosal covering over the posterior vocal cords compared with that in males. Skeletal muscle myalgia associated with administration of succinylcholine may manifest in the peripharyngeal muscles as postoperative sore throat, which is incorrectly attributed to prior intubation of the trachea.[17] Use of large (8.5- to 9.0-mm ID) versus small (6.5- to 7-mm ID) tracheal tubes may increase the likelihood of sore throat. Regardless of the mechanism, sore throat usually disappears spontaneously in 48 to 72 hours without any treatment. Throat lozenges may be prescribed to provide symptomatic relief until pharyngitis resolves spontaneously. Symptomatic laryngeal or subglottic edema is most likely in children because a small amount of swelling greatly decreases the lumen of the larynx. The likely causes of laryngeal edema in children include traumatic intubation of the trachea, use of an oversized tracheal tube, and the presence of an upper respiratory tract infection. Even with ideal conditions, however, laryngeal edema may still occur. The efficacy of dexamethasone administered intravenously for the prevention of laryngeal edema is unproven. Laryngeal incompetence may be present in some patients in the first 4 to 8 hours after extubation of the trachea, leading to an increased risk of pulmonary aspiration.[18]

The major complication of prolonged intubation of the trachea (longer than 48 hours) is damage to the tracheal mucosa, which may progress to destruction of cartilaginous rings and subsequent circumferential cicatrical scar formation and tracheal stenosis. Stenosis becomes symptomatic when the adult tracheal lumen is decreased to less than 5 mm.

REFERENCES

1. Benumof JL. Management of the difficult adult airway: With special emphasis on awake tracheal intubation. Anesthesiology 1991;75:1087–1110.
2. Practice guidelines for management of the difficult airway. A report by the American Society of Anesthesiologists Task Force on management of the difficult airway. Anesthesiology 1993;78:597–602.
3. Mallampati SR, Gatt SP, Gugino LD, et al. A clinical study to predict difficult tracheal intubation. A prospective study. Can J Anaesth 1985;32:429–34.
4. Frerk CM. Predicting difficult intubation. Anaesthesia 1991;46:1005–8.
5. Cormack RS, Lehane J. Difficult tracheal intubation in obstetrics. Anaesthesia 1984;39:1105–11.
6. Samsoon GTL, Young JRB. Difficult tracheal intubation: A restrospective study. Anaesthesia 1987;42: 487–90.
7. Klainer AS, Turndorf H, Wen-Hsien WU, Maewal H, Allender P. Surface alterations due to endotracheal intubation. Am J Med 1975;58:674–83.
8. Buckingham PK, Cheney FW, Ward RJ. Esophageal intubation: A review of detection techniques. Anesth Analg 1986;65:886–91.
9. Owen RL, Cheney FW. Endobronchial intubation: A preventable complication. Anesthesiology 1987; 67:255–7.
10. Mulroy M. Handbook of Regional Anesthesia. Boston, Little, Brown 1989;1–289.
11. Stone DJ, Bogdonoff DL. Airway considerations in the management of patients requiring long-term endotracheal intubation. Anesth Analg 1992;74:276–87.
12. Dinner M, Tjeuw M, Artusio JF. Bacteremia as a complication of nasotracheal intubation. Anesth Analg 1987;66:460–2.
13. Rogers SN, Benumof JL. New and easy techniques for fiberoptic endoscopy-aided tracheal intubation. Anesthesiology 1983;59:569–71.
14. Pennant JH, White PF. The laryngeal mask airway: Its uses in anesthesiology. Anesthesiology 1993;79:144–63.
15. Brain AIJ. The laryngeal mask—A new concept in airway management. Br J Anaesth 1983;55:801–4.
16. Conrardy PA, Goodman LR, Lainage F, et al. Alteration of endotracheal tube position. Flexion and extension of the neck. Crit Care Med 1976;4:8–12.
17. Capan LM, Bruce DL, Patel KP, et al. Succinylcholine-induced postoperative sore throat. Anesthesiology 1983;59:202–5.
18. Bishop MJ, Weymuller EA, Fink RB. Laryngeal effects of prolonged intubation. Anesth Analg 1984;63:335–42.

12

Spinal and Epidural Anesthesia

Spinal and epidural anesthesia are commonly referred to as regional or conduction anesthesia.[1,2] Spinal anesthesia is produced by injection of local anesthetic solutions into the lumbar subarachnoid space. Epidural anesthesia is produced by injection of local anesthetic solutions into the epidural space, most often at the lumbar level. Caudal anesthesia results when local anesthetic solutions are placed in the epidural space via a needle introduced through the sacral hiatus.

Regional anesthesia produces anesthesia selective for the surgical site, in contrast to general anesthesia, which produces total body anesthesia. Patients may remain awake or sedated by intravenous administration of drugs such as benzodiazepines (midazolam), propofol, or opioids (fentanyl or its equivalent). Skeletal muscle relaxation is profound without the need for administration of muscle relaxants. Despite these advantages, patients may be fearful of "needle sticks" or being "awake" during surgery. Alleged stories of paralysis following regional anesthesia can be effectively discounted but nevertheless remain a concern to some patients.[3] Even some surgeons are biased against regional anesthesia on the grounds that it may fail and delay the start of surgery until general anesthesia is instituted.

The efficacy of opioids introduced into the epidural or subarachnoid space for providing postoperative analgesia and chronic pain relief has been one of the most important recent advances in medicine.[4] This approach has created many new options in the area of pain relief, including the development of acute postoperative pain management services (see Chapter 32).

ANATOMY

The spinal canal extends from the foramen magnum to the sacral hiatus (Fig. 12-1).[1] The vertebral column consists of 7 cervical, 12 thoracic, and 5 lumbar vertebrae. The sacrum and coccyx are distal extensions of the vertebral column. Each vertebra consists of a vertebral body and bony arch. The vertebral body consists of two pedicles anteriorly and two laminae posteriorly. The transverse processes are formed by the junction of the pedicles and laminae, whereas the spinous process is formed by the joining of each lamina. In the lumbar regions the spinous processes are nearly horizontal, such that needles introduced at this site may be directed at right angles to the sagittal plane.

The laminae of the vertebrae are connected by the ligamentum flavum, and the posterior spinous processes are connected by the interspinous ligaments (Fig. 12-2).[1] The supraspinous ligaments connect the tips of the spinous processes. Intervertebral foramina are openings between the vertebral pedicles through which the spinal nerves pass. Each spinal nerve supplies a specific region of skin (dermatome) and skeletal muscles (Fig. 12-3). Preganglionic nerves of the peripheral sympathetic nervous system originate from the spinal cord (T1–L2) and travel with the spinal nerves before leaving to form the sympathetic chain (Fig. 12-4). The sympathetic

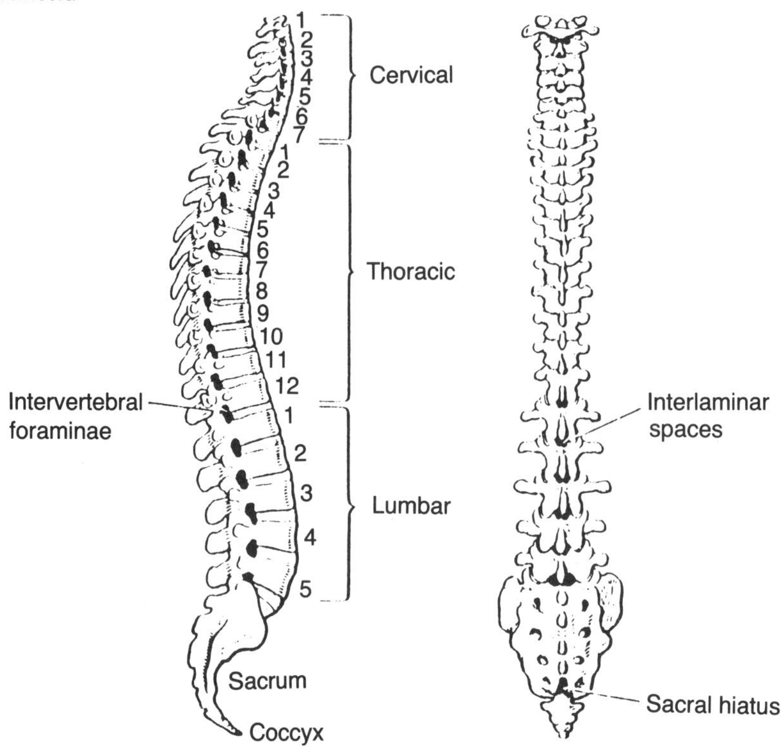

Figure 12-1. Vertebral column from a lateral (left) and a posterior (right) view, illustrating curvatures (maximum thoracic kyphosis at T6) and interlaminar spaces. The spinal cord ends at L1-L2 and the dura mater extends to S2. (From Bridenbaugh and Greene,[1] with permission.)

chain extends the entire length of the spinal column along the anterolateral aspects of the vertebral bodies, giving rise to the stellate ganglion, splanchnic nerves, and celiac plexus.

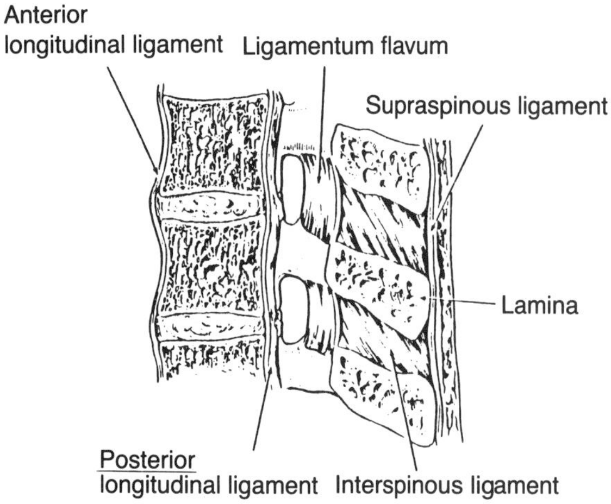

Figure 12-2. Sagittal section of the vertebral column. (From Bridenbaugh and Greene,[1] with permission.)

The spinal canal contains the spinal cord and its coverings, the pia mater, arachnoid mater, and dura mater. The spinal cord extends from the foramen magnum to L1-L2. Because the spinal cord ends at L1-L2, the lower lumbar and sacral nerves extend for some distance in the spinal canal as the cauda equina. The pia mater is adherent to the spinal cord and nerves. The space between the arachnoid mater and pia mater contains cerebrospinal fluid and is known as the subarachnoid space.

The epidural space is located between the dura mater and connective tissues covering the vertebrae and ligamentum flavum. A connective tissue band (plica mediana dorsalis) may extend from the dura mater to the ligamentum flavum and hence divide the posterior epidural space into two compartments (Fig. 12-5).[5] The epidural space is a potential space, being normally filled with connective and adipose tissue. Venous plexuses are prominent, but no free fluid exists in the epidural space.

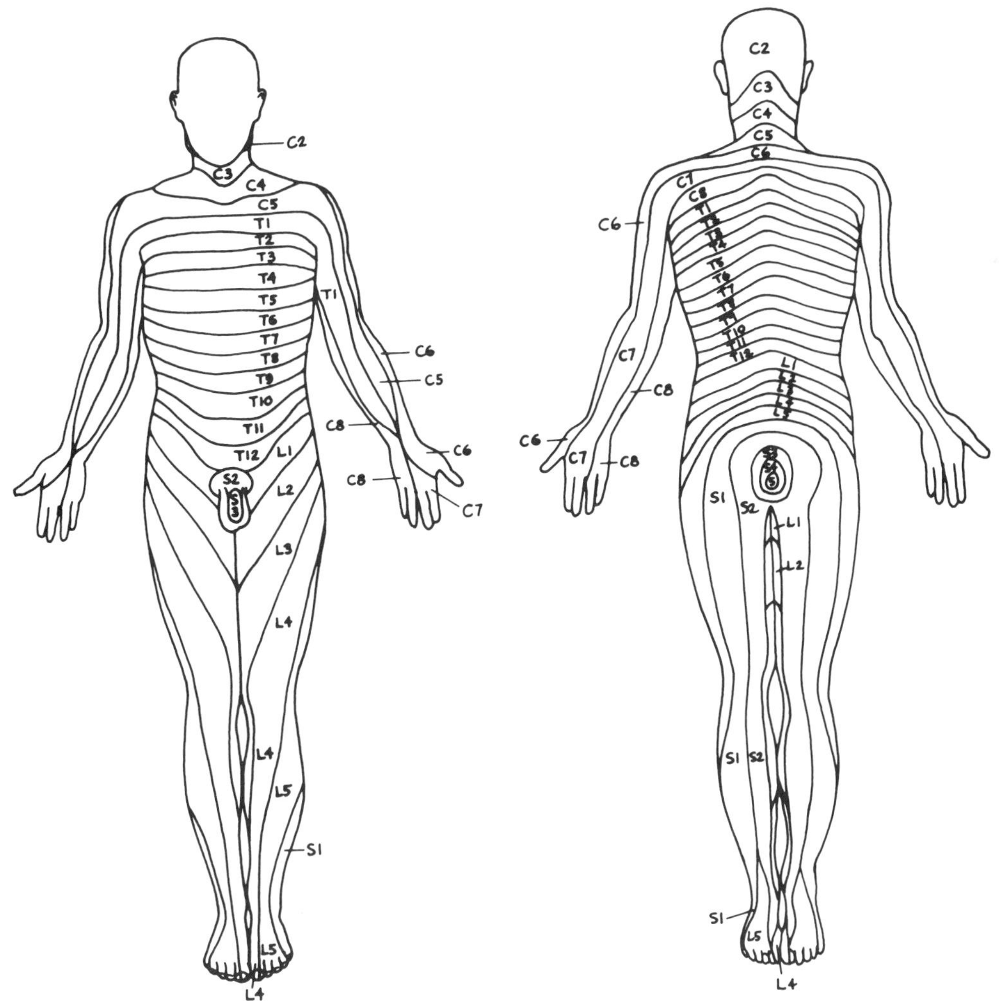

Figure 12-3. The dermatomes of the body shown in an orderly progression from the cranial to caudal aspects of the body.

PREOPERATIVE PREPARATION

Preoperative preparation for regional anesthesia does not differ from that for general anesthesia (see Chapter 8). Under no circumstances, however, should patients be encouraged against their wishes to accept the anesthesiologist's recommendation for a regional anesthetic. Examination of the back to rule out deformities or infection is uniquely important when regional anesthesia is planned. Coagulation status (determined by history and/or specific tests) should be determined, as performance of regional anesthesia in the presence of abnormal clotting is controversial. Specifically, there is concern that an epidural hematoma and neurologic symptoms may develop if a blood vessel is entered (estimated to occur in 10% of patients) during performance of the regional anesthetic. If it is elected to administer a regional anesthetic to an anticoagulated patient, it is assumed that the presumed benefits of this approach outweigh those of alternative techniques. Also unanswered is the safety of administering spinal or epidural anesthesia to a patient who will subsequently receive heparin or urokinase. It may be prudent to delay surgery (no definite time can be stated, although some recommend 24 hours) should evidence of bleeding accompany performance of a regional anesthetic

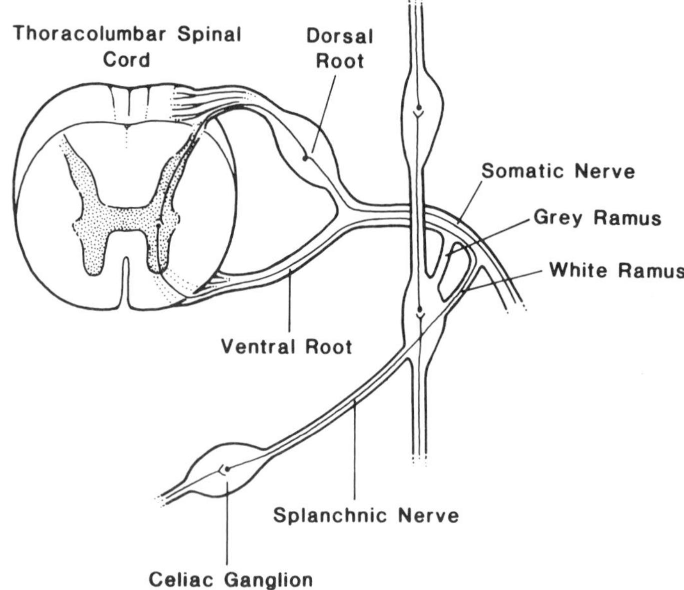

Figure 12-4. Cell bodies in the thoracolumbar portion of the spinal cord (T1–L2) give rise to the peripheral sympathetic nervous system. Efferent fibers travel in the ventral root and then via the white ramus communicans to paravertebral sympathetic ganglia or more distant sites such as the celiac ganglion. Afferent fibers from paravertebral sympathetic ganglia travel via the gray ramus communicans to join somatic nerves, which pass to the dorsal root and spinal cord.

and it is known that heparin or urokinase will be administered in the perioperative period.[6] The presence of sepsis is often considered a reason to avoid regional anesthesia for fear the needle might introduce infected blood into the subarachnoid or epidural space and cause meningitis or an epidural abscess. If regional anesthesia is selected for such a patient, it may be appropriate to institute appropriate antibiotic therapy prior to anesthesia.[7] Because of profound sympathetic nervous system blockade, regional anesthesia may not be a logical selection in patients who are hypovolemic as a result of acute hemorrhage.

Preoperative medication is dependent on each individual patient's level of anxiety (see Chapter 9). Inclusion of an opioid in the preoperative medication may be useful for decreasing pain associated with the needle insertions required to perform a regional anesthetic. Anticholinergics are probably not needed when regional anesthesia is planned, as the resulting dry mouth will be uncomfortable for awake patients. Patients must be reassured that medications will be administered intravenously as needed to ensure their comfort during the surgery. An intravenous infusion is started before performance of the anesthetic; and

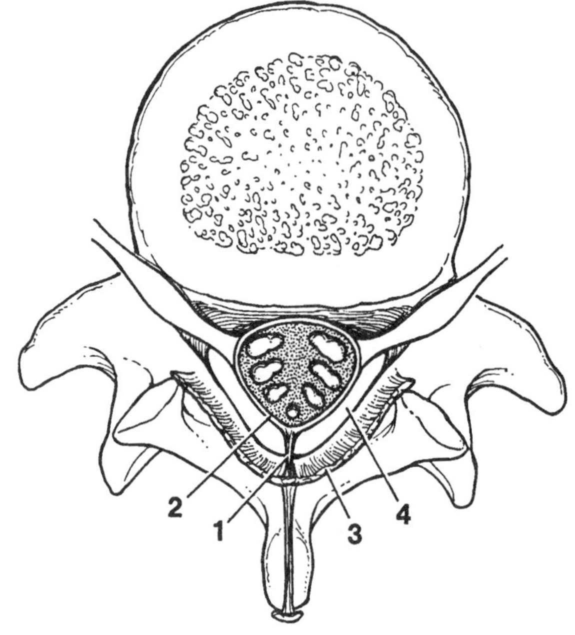

Figure 12-5. The plica mediana dorsalis (1) is a midline connective tissue band that extends from the dura mater (2) to the ligamentum flavum (3), thus dividing the posterior epidural space (4) into two compartments. (Modified from Gallart et al.,[5] with permission.)

all the equipment, drugs, and monitors normally present for a general anesthetic are also required for regional anesthesia (see Table 8-7).

SPINAL ANESTHESIA

Spinal anesthesia follows placement of local anesthetic solutions into the subarachnoid space, most often at the lumbar level. The principal landmarks for performance of spinal anesthesia are the vertebral spinous processes and the iliac crests. The spinous processes identify the midline, and a line drawn between the iliac crests usually crosses the fourth lumbar vertebrae (Fig. 12-6). The interspace above this line represents the L3-L4 interspace and the interspace below the L4-L5 interspace. These interspaces are commonly selected for insertion of the spinal needle, remembering that the spinal cord ends at the L1-L2 level.

Technique

Spinal anesthesia is typically instituted with the patient in the lateral decubitus or the sitting position (Fig. 12-6). The needle is inserted in the midline (midline approach) at an easily palpable interspace below L2 (usually L3-L4 or L4-L5). The lateral decubitus position (knees and head flexed on the chest) is useful for ill or heavily sedated patients, and the sitting position is used when there is difficulty in separating the lumbar spinous processes or a low level of spinal anesthesia is desired. The area of skin over the selected area is prepared with an antiseptic solution (1% iodine), and the anesthesiologist wears sterile gloves. A skin wheal of local anesthetic is produced, and a 22- or 25-gauge needle is inserted at this site parallel to the spinous processes. The needle is advanced with a slightly cephalad angle until it is firmly lodged in the supraspinous ligament, after which it is no longer possible to change the direction of the needle tip by bending the distal shaft of the needle. Continued needle advancement transverses the ligamentum flavum and the dura mater. A distinct "pop" is felt by the fingers of the anesthesiologist as the needle passes through the dura mater. Subarachnoid placement of the needle is confirmed by the appearance of cerebrospinal fluid at the hub. At this point, the needle is stabilized by grasping the hub of the needle between the thumb and forefinger with the dorsum of the anesthesiologist's hand resting against the patient's back. A syringe containing local anesthetic solution is attached and after aspiration of a small amount of cerebrospinal fluid into the syringe to confirm continued subarachnoid placement, the entire contents are injected over 3 to 5 seconds. Occasionally, blood-tinged cerebrospinal fluid initially appears at the hub of the needle. If blood-tinged cerebrospinal fluid continues to flow, the needle should be removed and reinserted at a different interspace. Should blood-tinged cerebrospinal fluid still persist, the attempt to produce spinal anesthesia should be terminated and the patient further evaluated. Conversely, if clear cerebrospinal fluid is obtained, the spinal anesthetic can be completed. After completion of the injection, the syringe and needle are removed as a single unit.

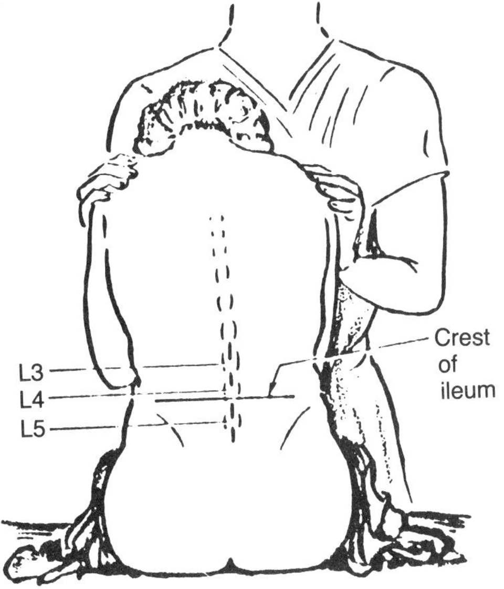

Figure 12-6. A line drawn between the iliac crests usually crosses the fourth lumbar (L4) vertebra.

The incidence of postspinal headache is lower after puncture of the dura mater with a 25-gauge needle than when a 22-gauge needle is used. For this reason, a 25-gauge needle is likely to be selected when spinal anesthesia is selected for younger patients, who are more likely than elderly patients to experience postspinal headache. Use of the flexible 25-gauge needle may be facilitated by its placement through a larger introducer needle that has been previously placed into the interspinous ligament. The larger and more rigid 22-gauge needle does not require use of an introducer needle, and cerebrospinal fluid spontaneously appears at the hub of the needle when the subarachnoid space is entered.

The small lumen of the 25-gauge needle may require syringe aspiration to confirm the presence of cerebrospinal fluid. Equipment and drugs necessary for performance of spinal anesthesia are most often provided in prepackaged and sterile kits (Fig. 12-7).

Lateral (Paramedian) Approach

The spinal needle is introduced through the skin wheal at a site 1 to 2 cm lateral to the midline opposite the center of the chosen interspace. The needle is directed medial and cephalad at an angle of 15 to 20 degrees until it passes through the ligamentum flavum into the subarachnoid space. Compared with the midline approach, the lateral approach is less dependent on patients being able to flex their backs (parturients, prone position) and circumvents calcified ligaments often encountered in the midline of elderly patients.

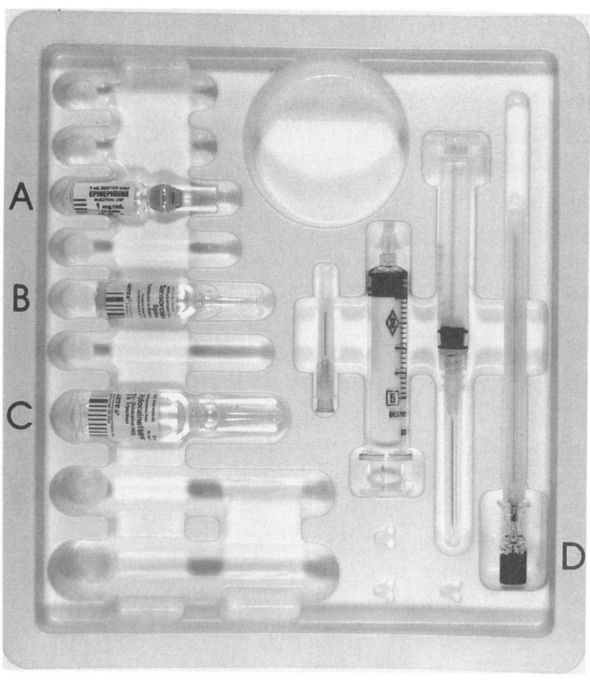

Figure 12-7. A typical prepackaged and sterile disposable kit for institution of spinal anesthesia. The contents of the glass vials are *(A)* epinephrine (1 mg·ml^{-1}), *(B)* 0.75% methylparaben-free bupivacaine (7.5 mg·ml^{-1}) in 8.25% dextrose, *(C)* 1% methylparaben-free lidocaine (10 mg·ml^{-1}), and *(D)* 22- or 25-gauge 8.9-cm long spinal needle. Other contents include paper drapes, procedural syringes, and needles.

Lumbosacral (Taylor) Approach

The largest interspace in the vertebral column is the L5-S1 interspace. To enter this space, the spinal needle is introduced through the skin wheal approximately 1 cm medial and 1 cm caudad to the posterior superior iliac spine. The spinal needle is directed in a medial and cephalad direction to enter the subarachnoid space in the midline at the L5-S1 interspace. Advantages of this approach are similar to those of the lateral approach.

Level and Duration

Distribution of local anesthetic solutions in cerebrospinal fluid is influenced principally by the (1) baricity of the solution, (2) contour of the spinal canal, and (3) position of the patient during and in the first few minutes after placement of drug into the subarachnoid space. Assuming an appropriate dose is selected, the duration of spinal anesthesia depends on the drug selected (tetracaine and bupivacaine last longer than lidocaine, which lasts longer than procaine) and the presence or absence of a vasoconstrictor (epinephrine or phenylephrine) in the local anesthetic solution (Table 12-1).

Local anesthetics produce different intensities of sensory and motor blockade. For example, sensory anesthesia below L1 seems to be more intense in the presence of bupivacaine (reduced frequency of tourniquet pain), whereas motor blockade is greatest after injection of tetracaine. Lidocaine is useful for short-duration (30 to 60 minutes) surgical and obstetric procedures. Tetracaine is commonly used for abdominal surgery lasting up to 5 hours. Bupivacaine is useful for lower extremity, vascular, and orthopaedic operations lasting up to 5 hours. During recovery, anesthesia regresses from the highest dermatome in a caudad direction.

Baricity and Patient Position

Baricity is the density of the local anesthetic solution divided by the density of cerebrospinal fluid (1.001 to 1.005) at 37°C. Local anesthetic solutions are characterized as hyperbaric, hypobaric, or isobaric relative to cerebrospinal fluid. Understanding baricity allows the anesthesiologist to "direct" the local anesthetic solution in the subarachnoid space toward the spinal nerves innervating the surgical site (Table 12-1).

Table 12-1. Local Anesthetics Used for Spinal Anesthesia

	Concentration[a] (%)	Dose[b] (mg)		Volume[b] (ml)	Onset[b] min)	Duration[b] (min)	
		T10	T4			No Epinephrine	Epinephrine (0.2mg)
Lidocaine	5	30–50	75–100	1–2	2–4	45–60	60–90
Tetracaine	0.5	6–10	12–16	1–3	4–6	60–90	120–180
Bupivacaine	0.5–0.75	6–10	12–16	1–2	4–6	90	140

[a]Mixed with glucose to render the solution hyperbaric.
[b]Dose, volume, onset, and duration are estimates for sensory anesthesia.

Hyperbaric Solutions. Hyperbaric solutions are prepared by adding glucose (dextrose) in amounts sufficient to increase the density of the local anesthetic solution above that of cerebrospinal fluid. A common hyperbaric solution is 0.5% tetracaine plus 5% glucose, obtained by the anesthesiologist mixing equal volumes of 1% tetracaine and 10% glucose. To provide a commercial hyperbaric solution, 5% lidocaine and 0.75% bupivacaine are premixed with glucose (Table 12-1). Being heavier than cerebrospinal fluid, hyperbaric local anesthetic solutions settle to the most dependent aspect of the subarachnoid space, which is determined by the position of the patient. In supine patients, hyperbaric solutions gravitate to the thoracic kyphosis (the low point is T6 in an average adult patient), ensuring an adequate level of spinal anesthesia for intra-abdominal surgery (Fig. 12-1). Conversely, injection of hyperbaric local anesthetic solutions into patients in the sitting position allows production of low levels ("saddle block anesthesia") of anesthesia as commonly used for vaginal delivery (see Chapter 25). Hyperbaric solutions are the most commonly used preparations for spinal anesthesia. This popularity reflects the belief among anesthesiologists that it is easier to control the spread of these solutions.

Hypobaric Solutions. Hypobaric solutions are prepared by adding 6 to 8 ml of sterile water to the local anesthetic solution. After injection into the subarachnoid space, the hypobaric solution "floats" up to the nerves innervating the surgical site. For example, patients undergoing hemorrhoidectomy in the jackknife prone position or hip arthroplasty in the lateral position may be positioned before production of spinal anesthesia since subsequently injected local anesthetic solutions will rise to nondependent areas in the subarachnoid space.

Isobaric Solutions. Isobaric solutions are produced by diluting local anesthetic solutions with cerebrospinal fluid. Commercially available local anesthetic solutions are commonly formulated with sodium chloride and are isobaric. Spinal anesthesia can be induced in the most convenient position for the patient and the anesthesiologist, and the patient can then be placed in the position required by the surgery. Surgery performed on areas innervated by nerves below L1 (hip surgery) is often performed using isobaric local anesthetic solutions.

Vasoconstrictors

Epinephrine (0.1 to 0.2 mg; 0.1 to 0.2 ml of a 1:1000 solution) or phenylephrine (2 to 5 mg; 0.2 to 0.5 ml of a 1% solution) is frequently added to local anesthetic solutions before their injection into the subarachnoid space (Table 12-1). Vasoconstrictors are presumed to prolong spinal anesthesia by up to 50% by localized vasoconstriction, which decreases spinal cord blood flow and subsequent vascular absorption of the local anesthetic.[8] As a result, more of the local anesthetic remains in contact with neural tissue for a longer time, creating a more intense and prolonged block. A direct antinociceptive action produced by alpha agonist effects of the vasoconstrictor on spinal cord receptors may also be contributing to prolonged spinal anesthesia.

Vasoconstrictors seem to be most useful in prolonging the duration of spinal anesthesia below L1 with all local anesthetics. This most likely reflects the high concentrations of drugs in this site because of the lumbar site of injection. For abdominal surgery, vasoconstrictors added to solutions containing lidocaine or bupivacaine may not be as efficacious in prolonging the duration of anesthesia as those added to solutions containing tetracaine.[8]

Documentation of Anesthesia

Within 30 to 60 seconds after subarachnoid injection of local anesthetic solutions, an attempt should be made to determine the developing level of spinal anesthesia. The desired level of spinal anesthesia is dependent on the type of surgery (Table 12-2). Because the sympathetic nervous system nerves are usually the first to be blocked, an early indication of the level of a spinal anesthesia can be obtained by evaluating the patient's ability to discriminate temperature changes as produced by an alcohol sponge.[9] In the area blocked by the spinal anesthetic, the alcohol sponge produces a warm or neutral sensation rather than the cold sensation perceived in the unblocked areas. It is important to remember that the level of sympathetic nervous system anesthesia usually exceeds the level of sensory blockade, which in turn exceeds the level of motor paralysis (see the section *Physiology*). The level of sensory anesthesia is often evaluated by the patient's ability to discriminate sharpness as produced by a needle touched to the abdomen or chest. Skeletal muscle power is tested by asking the patient to dorsiflex the foot (S1-S2), raise the knees (L2-L3), or tense the abdominal rectus muscles (T6–T12).

Physiology

Spinal anesthesia interrupts sensory, motor, and sympathetic nervous system innervation. According to the classic concept, local anesthetics injected into the subarachnoid space produce conduction blockade through small-diameter, unmyelinated (sympathetic) fibers before interrupting conduction via larger myelinated (sensory and motor) fibers. This reflects the anatomy of the spinal nerves in which unmyelinated small-diameter nerve fibers are close to the surface and thus are the first fibers exposed to local anesthetic solutions (see Chapter 6). Sympathetic nervous system blockade typically exceeds somatic sensory blockade by two dermatomes. This may be a conservative estimate, with sympathetic nervous system blockade sometimes exceeding somatic sensory blockade by as many as six dermatomes.[8] This explains why hypotension may accompany even low levels of a spinal anesthesia (see the section *Complications*).

Spinal anesthesia has little if any effect on resting alveolar ventilation (arterial blood gases unchanged), but high levels of motor anesthesia that produce paralysis of abdominal and intercostal muscles can lead to a decreased ability to cough and expel secretions. Patients may complain of difficulty in breathing (dyspnea) during spinal anesthesia, reflecting the lack of proprioception in abdominal and thoracic muscles. Spinal anesthesia above T5 inhibits sympathetic nervous system innervation to the gastrointestinal tract, and the resulting unopposed parasympathetic nervous system activity results in contracted intestines and relaxed sphincters. The

Table 12-2. Sensory Level of Spinal Anesthesia or Epidural Anesthesia Necessary for Certain Surgical Procedures

Level	Type of Surgery	Local Anesthetic and Dose for Spinal Anesthesia (Estimate)
S2–S5 (perineal)	Rectal surgery Hemorrhoidectomy	Lidocaine 30–50 mg
L2-L3 (knee)	Foot surgery	Tetracaine or bupivacaine 6 mg
L1 (inguinal ligament)	Lower extremity	
T10 (umbilicus)	Hip surgery Transurethral resection of prostate Vaginal delivery	Lidocaine 50–75 mg Tetracaine or bupivacaine 6–8 mg
T6 (xiphoid process)	Lower abdominal surgery	Lidocaine 75–100 mg
T4 (nipple)	Upper abdominal surgery	Tetracaine or bupivacaine 12–16 mg

ureters are contracted, and the ureterovesical orifice is relaxed. Block of afferent impulses from the surgical site by spinal anesthesia is consistent with the absence of an adrenocortical response to painful stimulation. Decreased bleeding during regional anesthesia and certain types of surgery (hip surgery, transurethral resection of the prostate) may reflect decreases in arterial blood pressure, whereas increased blood flow to lower extremities after sympathetic nervous system blockade has been proposed as an explanation for the decreased incidence of thromboembolic complications after hip surgery.[10] There is no difference in perioperative mortality between regional anesthesia or general anesthesia administered to relatively healthy patients scheduled for elective surgery.

Complications

Complications associated with spinal anesthesia are usually predictable and acceptable, considering the merits of this anesthetic technique for individual patients.[11] Neurologic complications, although a common concern among patients, are nearly nonexistent with this technique (zero incidence of paralysis in over 582,000 spinal anesthetics).[3,11]

Hypotension

Hypotension (systolic blood pressure lower than 90 mmHg) is estimated to occur in about one-third of patients receiving spinal anesthesia.[11] This hypotension results from sympathetic nervous system blockade that (1) decreases venous return to the heart and decreases cardiac output or (2) decreases systemic vascular resistance; it can also result from a combination of the two. Bradycardia (less than 50 beats·min^{-1}) due to blockade of sympathetic nervous system cardioaccelerator fibers and decreased venous return to the heart may contribute to further decreases in cardiac output. Modest decreases in blood pressure are most likely due to decreases in systemic vascular resistance, whereas large decreases in blood pressure are believed to be the result of decreases in cardiac output. The degree of hypotension often parallels the level of spinal anesthesia and the intravascular fluid volume of the patient. Indeed, the magnitude of hypotension produced by spinal anesthesia is greatly exaggerated by co-existing hypovolemia.

Treatment. Spinal anesthesia-induced hypotension is treated physiologically by restoration of venous return so as to increase cardiac output. In this regard, the internal autotransfusion produced by a modest head-down position (5 to 10 degrees) will facilitate venous return without greatly exaggerating the cephalad spread of the spinal anesthetic. Adequate hydration before institution of spinal anesthesia is important for minimizing the effects of venodilation due to sympathetic nervous system blockade. Excessive hydration in attempts to prevent or treat hypotension, however, may be undesirable in patients with ischemic heart disease if hemodilution decreases the hematocrit sufficiently to decrease myocardial oxygen delivery. Occasionally, sympathomimetics with positive inotropic and venoconstrictor effects, such as ephedrine (5 to 10 mg IV), are required to maintain perfusion pressures at acceptable levels in the first few minutes after institution of spinal anesthesia. In this regard, some anesthesiologists recommend prophylactic administration of ephedrine (25 to 50 mg IM) before institution of spinal anesthesia. Sympathomimetics, such as phenylephrine, which increase systemic vascular resistance and may decrease the cardiac output, do not specifically correct the decreased venous return responsible for spinal anesthesia-induced hypotension. Nevertheless, anesthesiologists have long used phenylephrine successfully to treat decreases in blood pressure associated with spinal anesthesia administered to nonparturients. In the rare instance when hypotension is not promptly responsive to ephedrine or phenylephrine, it is important to promptly administer epinephrine intravenously.[12]

Complications Associated with Spinal Anesthesia

Hypotension
Bradycardia
Postspinal headache
High spinal
Nausea
Urinary retention
Backache
Neurologic sequelae (very unlikely)
Hypoventilation

Postspinal Headache

Postspinal headache is characterized as frontal or occipital, made worse by the sitting position (postural component), improved by the supine position, and sometimes accompanied by diplopia. Tinnitus and decreased hearing acuity may accompany postspinal headache. A headache without a postural component is not a postspinal headache. Postspinal headache is believed to be due to decreased cerebrospinal fluid pressures and resulting tension on meningeal vessels and nerves as a result of leakage of cerebrospinal fluid through the needle hole in the dura mater created by the lumbar puncture. Diplopia is presumed to be due to traction on the abducens nerve. In support of the cerebrospinal fluid leakage theory is the observation that the incidence of postspinal headache is lower when 25-gauge needles rather than 22-gauge needles are used for spinal anesthesia. Young females, especially parturients, seem most likely to develop postspinal headache.

Treatment. Treatment of postspinal headache is initially with bed rest, analgesics, and oral or intravenous hydration (3 L or more daily). Hydration is intended to increase cerebrospinal fluid production to a level that exceeds loss through the needle hole in the dura mater. If the postspinal headache persists after 24 to 48 hours of conservative therapy, it is a common recommendation to perform a lumbar epidural "blood patch" with 10 to 20 ml of the patient's blood (obtained most often via a cubital vein with strict asepsis).[13] Prompt relief of the postspinal headache after the epidural blood patch is presumed to reflect sealing of the hole in the dura mater and re-establishment of normal pressures in the subarachnoid space. Epidural saline does not appear to be as efficacious as blood for treatment of a persistent postspinal headache. Alternatively, administration of caffeine sodium benzoate (500 mg IV) has been effective in alleviating postspinal headache in about 70% of patients.[11]

High Spinal

High spinal is the term used to describe an undesired excessive level of sensory and motor anesthesia associated with difficulty breathing (phrenic nerves are usually spared) or apnea leading to arterial hypoxemia and hypercarbia. Apnea that occurs with an excessive level of spinal anesthesia probably reflects ischemic paralysis of the medullary ventilatory centers due to profound hypotension and associated decreases in cerebral blood flow. Hypotension frequently accompanies high spinal anesthesia, and patients become nauseated and agitated. These symptoms must immediately alert the anesthesiologist to the possible presence of high spinal anesthesia.

Treatment. Treatment of high spinal anesthesia is support of breathing and circulation. Positive pressure ventilation of the patient's lungs with oxygen via an anesthetic face mask and support of circulation by the intravenous administration of fluid and sympathomimetics are indicated. Patients are placed in a head-down position to facilitate venous return. An attempt to limit the spread of local anesthetic solution in the cerebrospinal fluid by placing patients in a head-up position is not recommended as this position jeopardizes cerebral blood flow and contributes to medullary ischemia. Intubation of the trachea after induction of general anesthesia is indicated for patients at increased risk of aspiration (parturients). High spinal anesthesia typically manifests soon after injection of the local anesthetic solution into the subarachnoid space. Spread of local anesthetics to the cervical region usually produces short-lived effects because the local anesthetic concentration achieved is not high.

Nausea

Nausea occurring shortly after initiation of the spinal anesthesia must alert the anesthesiologist to the possible presence of hypotension sufficient to produce cerebral ischemia. Treatment of hypotension with sympathomimetics should eliminate nausea. Another cause of nausea during spinal anesthesia is a predominance of parasympathetic nervous system activity as a result of selective blockade of sympathetic nervous system innervation to the gastrointestinal tract. In this instance, administration of atropine (0.4 mg IV) may be effective therapy. The incidence of nausea and vomiting may be increased when a vasoconstrictor is added to the local anesthetic solution placed in the subarachnoid space.

Urinary Retention

Because spinal anesthesia interferes with innervation of the bladder, administration of large amounts of fluids intravenously can cause bladder distension, which may require catheter drainage. For this reason, it seems prudent to minimize fluid replacement to patients undergoing minor surgery with spinal anesthesia.

Backache

Backache is frequent after spinal anesthesia and may be related to the position required for the surgery. Ligament strain may be more likely when anesthesia and skeletal muscle relaxation produced by the spinal anesthetic permit positioning of patients for surgery in positions that might otherwise be uncomfortable.

Neurologic Sequelae

Neurologic sequelae are extremely rare, in part because of the use of prepackaged and sterile kits and the small doses of local anesthetics employed.[11] When a neurologic complication follows spinal anesthesia, it is important to consult a neurologist and seek to establish the cause (errantly placed spinal needle, injection of the wrong substance, exacerbation of co-existing neurologic disease, surgical retractors, pressure on peripheral nerves owing to positioning during surgery, birth trauma). In the absence of a hematoma or abscess, treatment is usually symptomatic.

Cauda equina syndrome has been reported after continuous spinal anesthesia produced by local anesthetic solutions delivered through small lumen (28-gauge) catheters.[14] It is possible that slow injection through the small lumen catheter results in nonuniform distribution of a hyperbaric local anesthetic solution and exposure of unmyelinated neural tissue to unusually high concentrations of the drug.

Hypoventilation

Exaggerated hypoventilation may accompany intravenous administration of drugs intended to produce a sleep-like state during spinal anesthesia.[12] It is conceivable that depressant effects of drugs on ventilation are enhanced in patients in whom spinal anesthesia has produced sympathetic nervous system blockade and decreases in external stimulation. Constant vigilance by the anesthesiologist that is enhanced by monitors, such as the pulse oximeter, is important to recognize dangerous hypoventilation during spinal anesthesia promptly.

EPIDURAL ANESTHESIA

Epidural anesthesia follows placement of local anesthetic solutions into the epidural space, most often at the lumbar level.

Technique

Epidural anesthesia is instituted with the patient in the sitting or lateral decubitus position, using needles and drugs from prepackaged and sterile kits (Fig. 12-8). The skin of the back is prepared with an antiseptic solution, and the needle is inserted through a local anesthetic skin wheal into a previously selected lumbar interspace using landmarks as described for midline spinal anesthesia (see the section *Spinal Anesthesia, Technique*). A 17- or 18-gauge Tuohy needle with a curved distal end is designed to decrease the likelihood of accidental puncture of the dura mater and to facilitate passage of a plastic catheter into the epidural space.

A common method for identifying the epidural space is the loss of resistance technique reflecting the presence of negative pressure in this space. The dorsum of the anesthesiologist's noninjecting hand rests on the patient's back, and the thumb and index finger grasp the hub of the needle (Fig. 12-9).[2] After the epidural needle is positioned in the interspinous ligament, a glass syringe with a freely moveable plunger is attached. If the needle is properly positioned, it will be difficult to inject air or saline and the plunger of the syringe will "spring back" to its original position. The needle is advanced in a slightly cephalad direction while continuous pressure is exerted by the anesthesiologist on the plunger of the syringe. As the needle passes through the ligamentum flavum into the epidural space, there is a sudden loss of resistance to pressure being exerted on the plunger of the syringe. A sterile plastic catheter is placed through the needle and advanced 2 to 3 cm into the epidural space to allow repeated injections of local anesthetic solutions. This allows anesthesia for operations of unpredictable duration as well as provision of postoperative analgesia. The needle is withdrawn over the catheter, taking care not to move the catheter. No attempt should be made to withdraw a catheter back through the needle, as this may result in shearing of a portion of the catheter in the epidural space. The catheter is taped to the patient's back, and a test dose of local anesthetic solution (3 ml of

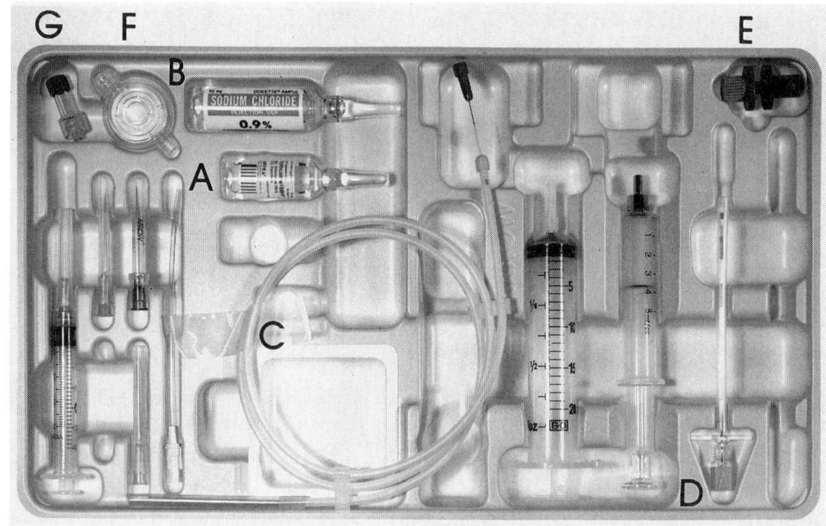

Figure 12-8. A typical prepackaged and sterile disposable kit for institution of epidural anesthesia. The contents of the glass vials are *(A)* lidocaine for infiltration anesthesia and *(B)* saline. Other contents include a *(C)* 19-gauge epidural catheter with stylet and distal centimeter markings, *(D)* 17-gauge 8.9-cm long epidural needle, *(E)* catheter/syringe adapter, *(F)* 0.2-μm-pore-size bacterial filter, and *(G)* preservative-free local anesthetic for injection into the epidural space placed in a medicine cup. Other contents include procedural syringes and needles.

1.5% lidocaine with 1:200,000 epinephrine) is injected. Failure of the test dose to produce sensory (saddle area) or motor anesthesia after 3 to 5 minutes confirms the absence of an accidental subarachnoid placement of the catheter. Absence of a heart rate increase due to epinephrine in the local anesthetic solution suggests that the drugs were not accidentally injected intravascularly. The volume and concentration (dose) of local anesthetic solution appropriate for the planned surgical procedure is then injected over 1 to 3 minutes (Table 12-3). Documentation of the level of sympathetic nervous

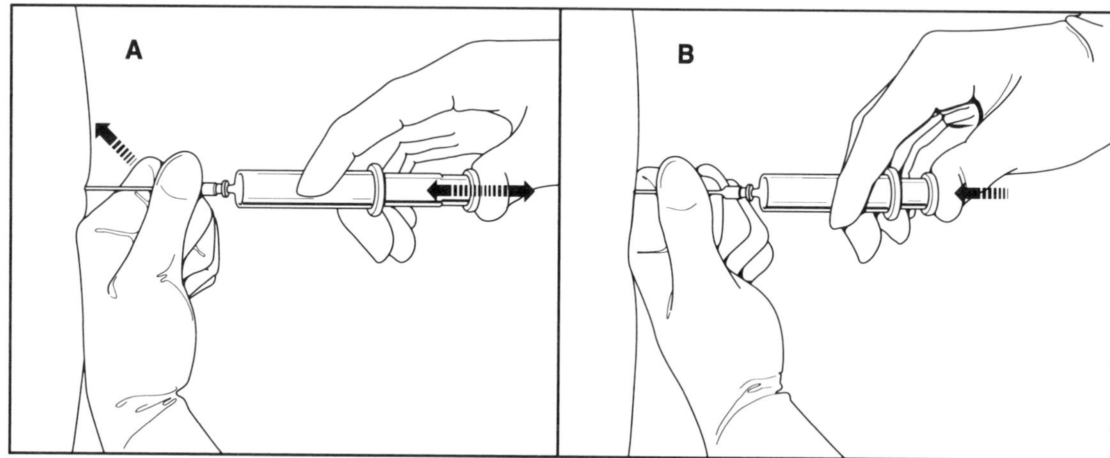

Figure 12-9. *(A)* During location of the epidural space when the needle is in the interspinous ligament, it is difficult to inject air or saline and the plunger of the syringe will "spring back" to its original position. *(B)* Entrance into the epidural space is confirmed by ease of depression of the plunger in the syringe (loss of resistance). (From Cousins and Bromage,[2] with permission.)

Table 12-3. Local Anesthetics Used for Epidural Anesthesia

	Concentration (%)	Onset[a] (min)	Duration[a] (min)
Chloroprocaine	2–3	5–15	30–90
Lidocaine	1–2	5–15	60–120
Bupivacaine	0.25–0.75[b]	10–20	120–240

[a]Onset and duration are estimates for sensory analgesia.
[b]Limit concentration to 0.5% for obstetric use.

system blockade and sensory anesthesia is determined as described for spinal anesthesia (see the section *Documentation of Anesthesia*). It is acceptable to inject local anesthetic solutions into the epidural space through the epidural needle (single-shot technique) when only a brief duration of anesthesia is required.

Level and Duration

The level and duration of epidural anesthesia depend on the (1) volume and concentration (dose) of local anesthetic and (2) presence or absence of epinephrine (1:200,000 dilution, 5 $\mu g \cdot ml^{-1}$) in the local anesthetic solution. The dose of local anesthetic seems to be more important than variations in the volume or concentration of the local anesthetic solution in determining the onset, intensity, and duration of anesthesia. Weight, height, and age of the patient and rate of injection do not seem to influence distribution of local anesthetic solutions in the epidural space.[15] In contrast to spinal anesthesia, the baricity of local anesthetic solutions does not influence the level of epidural anesthesia. Likewise, position is less important for the level of sensory anesthesia produced by an epidural anesthetic. Nevertheless, it is likely that the dependent portion of the body will manifest more intense anesthesia than the nondependent side.

Local anesthetics used for epidural anesthesia include (1) chloroprocaine (rapid onset and short duration), (2) lidocaine (intermediate onset and duration), and (3) bupivacaine (slow onset and prolonged duration of action) (Table 12-3). Procaine and tetracaine are rarely used for epidural anesthesia because of their slow onset of action. Lumbar epidural administration usually requires volumes of 15 to 25 ml to achieve sensory levels for surgery. Cephalad spread occurs more easily than caudad spread after lumbar epidural injections, in part because of transmission of negative intrathoracic pressure and the resistance to spread produced by narrowing of the epidural space at the lumbosacral junction. Free diffusion of the local anesthetic solution in the epidural space may be impaired by the plica mediana dorsalis, thus resulting in unilateral anesthesia despite proper technical performance of the procedure (Fig. 12-5).[5]

Addition of epinephrine to local anesthetic solutions decreases vascular absorption of the drug from the epidural space, thus maintaining effective anesthetic concentrations at the nerve roots for more prolonged periods. Epinephrine seems to potentiate epidural anesthesia produced by lidocaine more than that produced by bupivacaine.

Physiology

The major site of action of local anesthetic solutions placed in the epidural space appears to be the spinal nerve roots, where the dura mater is relatively thin. A spinal nerve root site of action is consistent with the often observed delay in onset or absence of anesthesia in the S1-S2 region, presumably reflecting the covering of these nerve roots with connective tissue. To a lesser extent, diffusion of local anesthetic solutions from the epidural space into the subarachnoid space produces spinal cord effects.

Sympathetic nervous system, sensory, and motor anesthesia follow injection of local anesthetic solutions into the epidural space. In contrast to spinal anesthesia, the onset of sympathetic nervous system blockade produced by epidural anesthesia is often slower, and the likelihood of abrupt hypotension is less. Furthermore, unlike spinal anesthesia, during epidural anesthesia there often is not a zone of differential sympathetic nervous system blockade, and the zone of differential motor blockade may average up to four rather than two segments below the sensory level. Relatively large volumes of local anesthetics are required for an epidural anesthetic. Vascular absorption of local anesthetic solutions may be sufficient to produce systemic toxicity (see the section *Complications*). Beta agonist effects from low plasma concentrations that result from systemic absorption of epinephrine in the local anesthetic solution produce sufficient vasodilation to accentuate blood pressure decreases compared with those produced by local anesthetics alone.[16] When epinephrine is not included in local anesthetic solutions, changes in blood pressure and calculated systemic vascular resistance are minimal. Effects of epidural anesthesia on breathing and the gastrointestinal tract resemble those produced by spinal anesthesia.

Complications

Complications of epidural anesthesia resemble those described for spinal anesthesia with the added risks of accidental dural puncture and local anesthetic toxicity. Epidural hematoma formation is a theoretical complication of epidural anesthesia, although the incidence is almost nonexistent even in the presence of bleeding abnormalities as may result from platelet dysfunction due to aspirin therapy. Patients on anticoagulants, however, may be at increased risk of this complication (see the section *Preoperative Preparation*).

Hypotension

Hypotension, as with a spinal anesthesia, parallels the degree of sympathetic nervous system blockade produced by epidural anesthesia. Because of the slower onset of sympathetic nervous system blockade, however, an excessive decrease in blood pressure does not usually accompany epidural anesthesia administered to normovolemic patients. Treatment of hypotension is as described for that produced by spinal anesthesia.

High Spinal

Accidental subarachnoid injection of the large volumes of local anesthetic solutions used for epidural anesthesia produces rapid evidence of high spinal anesthesia. Unrecognized injection of drug into the subdural space may produce a slower onset of high spinal anesthesia than that following accidental subarachnoid injection.

Accidental Dural Puncture

Accidental dural puncture is always a potential risk when performing an epidural anesthetic. Appearance of cerebrospinal fluid (warm when allowed to drop on the anesthesiologist's forearm, in contrast to saline that may be injected during determination of loss of resistance) at the hub of the epidural needle should be ample evidence of an accidental dural puncture. At this point, the anesthetic may be converted to a spinal anesthetic, or the epidural anesthetic can be attempted at a different lumbar interspace. Development of a postspinal headache is likely, considering the relatively large hole in the dura mater made by the needle used for the epidural anesthetic.

Local Anesthetic Toxicity

The high doses of local anesthetics required for epidural anesthesia plus the presence of numerous venous plexuses in the epidural space increase the likelihood of substantial blood levels of local anesthetics after an epidural anesthetic. Nevertheless, these blood levels are rarely sufficient to produce systemic toxicity, especially if epinephrine is added to the local anesthetic solution in an attempt to minimize vascular absorption. The accidental intravascular injection of local anesthetic solutions results in local anesthetic toxicity, manifesting principally as cardiovascular collapse, apnea, seizures, and unconsciousness (see Chapter 6).

CAUDAL ANESTHESIA

Caudal anesthesia is instituted with the patient in the prone position. The sacral hiatus (located about 5 cm from the tip of coccyx between the sacral cornua) is identified, and a needle is introduced perpendicular to the skin through the sacrococcygeal ligament until the sacrum is contacted (Fig. 12-10). The needle is then slightly withdrawn and the angle reduced before the needle is advanced about 2 cm into the caudal canal (Fig. 12-10). Confirmation that the needle is actually in the caudal canal and not subcutaneous can be made by injecting 5 ml of air through the needle and palpating the skin for crepitation. Although infection is rare, the nearness of this approach to the rectum suggests caution. A subarachnoid injection is a risk if the caudal needle extends

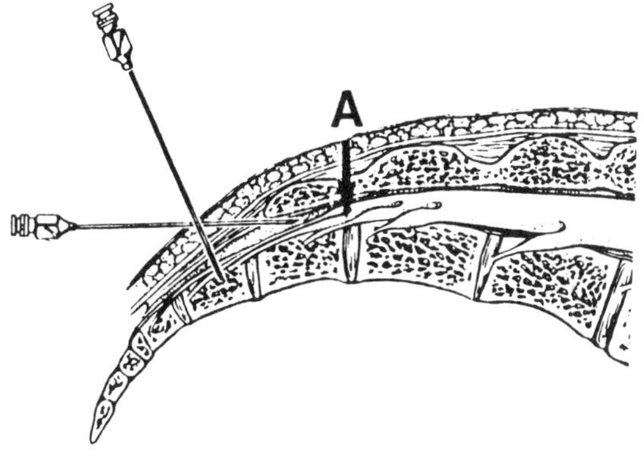

Figure 12-10. Caudal anesthesia is initiated by insertion of a needle through the sacral hiatus until the sacrum is contacted. The needle is then slightly withdrawn and the angle reduced before the needle is advanced through the sacrococcygeal membrane and into the caudal canal (A).

beyond S2, which is the termination of the dural sac. Because of abnormalities in the anatomy of the caudal canal, the failure rate with a caudal block can be as high as 10%. As a result, the lumbar rather than sacral (caudal) approach to the epidural space in adults is often preferred, since the former is more predictable and easier to perform. By contrast, location of the sacral hiatus and performance of caudal anesthesia is often technically easy in children.

REFERENCES

1. Bridenbaugh PO, Greene NM. Spinal (subarachnoid) neural blockade. In: Cousins MJ, Bridenbaugh PO, eds. Neural Blockade in Clinical Anesthesia and Management of Pain. Philadelphia, JB Lippincott 1988;213–52.
2. Cousins MJ, Bromage PR. Epidural neural blockade. In: Cousins MJ, Bridenbaugh PO, eds. Neural Blockade in Clinical Anesthesia and Management of Pain. Philadelphia, JB Lippincott 1988;253–360.
3. Lund PC. Principles and Practices of Spinal Anesthesia. Springfield, IL, Charles C Thomas 1971.
4. Cousins MJ, Mather LE. Intrathecal and epidural administration of opiates. Anesthesiology 1984;61: 276–310.
5. Gallart L, Blanco D, Samso E, Vidal F. Clinical and radiologic evidence of the epidural plica mediana dorsalis. Anesth Analg 1990;71:698–701.
6. Onishchuk JL, Carlsson C. Epidural hematoma associated with epidural anesthesia: Complications of anticoagulant therapy. Anesthesiology 1992;77:1221–3.
7. Chestnut DA. Spinal anesthesia in the febrile patient. Anesthesiology 1992;76:667–9.
8. Armstrong IR, Littlewood DG, Chambers WA. Spinal anesthesia with tetracaine-effect of added vasoconstrictor. Anesth Analg 1983;62:793–5.
9. Chamberlain DP, Chamberlain BDL. Changes in skin temperature of the trunk and their relationship to sympathetic blockade during spinal anesthesia. Anesthesiology 1986;65:139–43.
10. Modig J, Hjelmstedt A, Sahlstedt B, Maripuu E. Comparitive influences of epidural and general anesthesia on deep vein thrombosis and pulmonary embolism after total hip replacement. Acta Chir Scand 1981;147:125–8.
11. Carpenter RL, Caplan RA, Brown DL, Stephenson C, Wu R. Incidence and risk factors for side effects of spinal anesthesia. Anesthesiology 1992;76:906–16.
12. Caplan RA, Ward RJ, Posner K, Cheney FW. Unexpected cardiac arrest during spinal anesthesia: A closed claims analysis of predisposing factors. Anesthesiology 1988;68:5–11.
13. Szeinfeld M, Ihmeidan IH, Moser MM, Machado R, Klose KJ, Serafini AN. Epidural blood patch: Evaluation of the volume and spread of blood injected into the epidural space. Anesthesiology 1986;64: 820–2.
14. Lambert DH, Hurley RJ. Cauda equina syndrome and continuous spinal anesthesia. Anesth Analg 1991; 72:817–9.
15. Park WY, Massengale M, Kim S-I, Poon KC, Macnamara TE. Age and spread of local anesthetic solutions in the epidural space. Anesth Analg 1980; 59:768–71.
16. Ward RJ, Bonica JJ, Freund FG. Epidural and subarachnoid anesthesia. JAMA 1965;191:275–8.

13

Peripheral Nerve Blocks

Peripheral nerve blocks are used for (1) anesthesia, (2) postoperative analgesia, and (3) diagnosis and treatment of chronic pain syndromes (see Chapter 34). Advantages and disadvantages of peripheral nerve blocks for anesthesia must be considered when advising patients about the choice of anesthesia (see Chapter 8). Patients are often more receptive to peripheral nerve blocks when they are reassured that supplemental sedation can be administered intravenously if they become uncomfortable during surgery. During the preoperative evaluation the patient should be examined for bony landmarks, which are required to perform peripheral nerve blocks. The presence of a skin infection in the area to be used for insertion of needles must be recognized preoperatively. Confirmation of normal coagulation (by history or specific tests, or both) is generally recommended before performance of peripheral nerve blocks. The presence of a preexisting neuropathy, especially in the area involved by the proposed operation, may deter the anesthesiologist from selecting peripheral nerve block anesthesia.

PREPARATION FOR NERVE BLOCKS

Patients scheduled for peripheral nerve block anesthesia are evaluated medically in the same way as are patients scheduled for general or regional anesthesia (see Chapter 8). Preoperative medication is useful for decreasing apprehension and providing analgesia during needle insertions necessary to perform the block. A holding area for performing peripheral nerve blocks may be useful for minimizing any delay once the operating room becomes available. This area must have available appropriate monitors, equipment, and drugs should toxic reactions to local anesthetics occur. Also for this reason, an intravenous catheter should usually be in place before performance of the peripheral nerve block. Prepackaged and sterile trays are often used for performance of peripheral nerve blocks. Needles used for peripheral nerve blocks usually have a shorter angulation to the bevel (to push the nerve away) and the addition of a small bead to the shaft about 6 mm from the hub, which prevents skin from retracting over the needle in the event that the shaft separates from the hub. Paresthesias ("electric shocks") reflect successful localization of the nerve but introduce the risk of intraneural injection of the local anesthetic solution (cramping or aching pain during injection). Alternatively the nerve may be localized with a low current electrical impulse delivered from a nerve stimulator. Electrical stimulation activates motor fibers without actual needle contact with the nerve. Syringes may include control rings to facilitate delivery of the local anesthetic solution and allow the anesthesiologist to refill the syringe with one hand (Fig. 13-1).[1] Compared with epidural or spinal anesthesia, peripheral nerve block anesthesia is accomplished with lower concentrations of local anesthetics (1% lidocaine, 0.25% to 0.5% bupivacaine) because of concerns about local and systemic toxicity. Lower concentrations are also indicated because larger volumes of the local anesthetic solutions are often required to anesthetize poorly localized peripheral nerves or to block a series of nerves. Epinephrine may be added to the local anes-

Peripheral Nerve Blocks

Cervical plexus
Brachial plexus
- Interscalene
- Supraclavicular
- Axillary

Median nerve
Ulnar nerve
Radial nerve
Intercostal nerves
Sciatic nerve
Femoral nerve
Lateral femoral cutaneous nerve
Obturator nerve
Stellate ganglion
Celiac plexus
Intravenous regional neural anesthesia

thetic solution in selected patients (see Chapter 12). Organic iodide solutions are useful for skin preparation. In the operating room the anesthesiologist must be prepared to provide appropriate supplemental intravenous sedation (midazolam, continuous infusion of propofol) and analgesia (fentanyl or its equivalent) or induce general anesthesia should the peripheral nerve block anesthesia be inadequate.

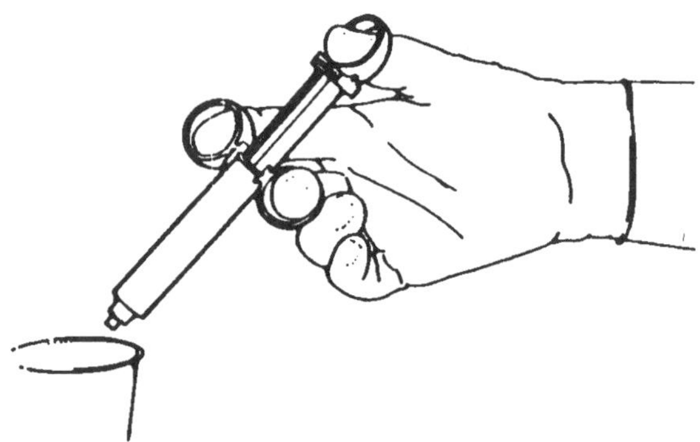

Figure 13-1. A three-ring syringe allows greater control of injection of local anesthetic solution, easier aspiration, and the ability to refill the syringe with one hand. (From Mulroy,[1] with permission.)

CERVICAL PLEXUS BLOCK

The cervical plexus is formed by the first four cervical nerves, which pass behind the vertebral artery and lie in the nerve sulci of the transverse processes of the cervical vertebrae. With the patient's head turned to the opposite side, a line connecting the tip of the mastoid process of the temporal bone and the anterior tubercle of the transverse process of the sixth cervical vertebra (Chassaignac's tubercle, which is the most prominent of the cervical transverse processes) identifies the approximate plane in which the cervical transverse processes lie (Fig. 13-2). The transverse processes of C2–C4 are palpated, and 3 to 5 ml of local anesthetic solution is injected. Blockade of the phrenic nerve is common (a reason to avoid bilateral cervical plexus block) but rarely requires treatment, as the intercostal muscles are able to compensate fully. Care must be taken to avoid intravascular injections, because this region is highly vascular and the vertebral artery is located nearby. A Horner syndrome (ptosis, miosis, enophthalmos, and anhydrosis) is possible, and hoarseness occurs when the recurrent laryngeal nerve is blocked by diffusion of local anesthetic solutions. Accidental injection of local anesthetic solution into the epidural or sub-

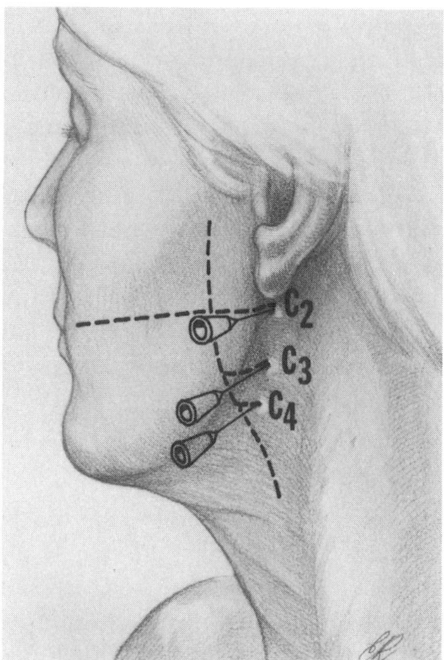

Figure 13-2. Superficial landmarks for performance of a cervical plexus block.

arachnoid space is a potential complication of cervical plexus block. Subcutaneous injection of local anesthetic solutions along the posterior lateral border of the sternocleidomastoid muscle blocks branches of the superficial cervical plexus.

Anesthesia produced by cervical plexus block includes the area from the inferior surface of the mandible to the level of the second rib. Skeletal muscles of the neck are profoundly relaxed. Cervical plexus block is used most often to provide anesthesia in an otherwise conscious patient undergoing carotid endarterectomy surgery.

BRACHIAL PLEXUS

The brachial plexus arises from the anterior rami of C5–C8 and T1. These rami unite to form three trunks in the space between the anterior and middle scalene muscles and then pass over the first rib and under the midpoint of the clavicle to enter the apex of the axilla (Fig. 13-3).[2] All of the motor and nearly all of the sensory function (skin over the shoulders supplied by the cervical plexus and posterior medical aspect of the arm supplied by the intercostobrachial branch of the second intercostal nerve) of the upper extremity is via the brachial plexus (Fig. 13-4).[1] Mepivacaine provides a greater degree of motor blockade than lidocaine for brachial plexus anesthesia and also produces a longer duration of sensory anesthesia. Bupivacaine (0.25% to 0.5%) or ropivacaine (less cardiotoxicity) is also used for brachial plexus block.[3] The three anatomic locations where local anesthetic solutions are placed to block the brachial plexus are designated as interscalene, supraclavicular, and axillary.[4]

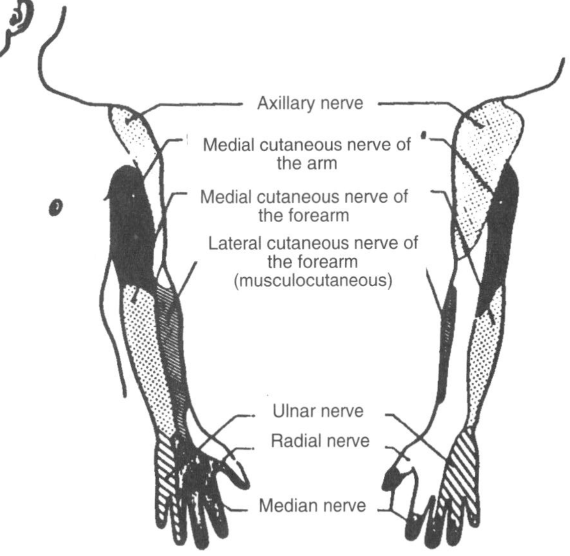

Figure 13-4. Sensory dermatomes of the arm. (From Mulroy,[1] with permission.)

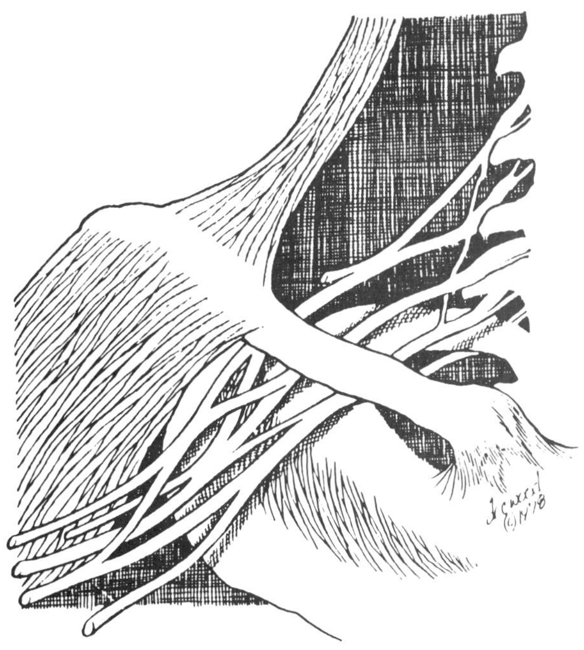

Figure 13-3. Schematic depiction of the brachial plexus in its course from the intervertebral foramina over the first rib and under the clavicle into the axilla. (From Bridenbaugh,[2] with permission.)

Interscalene Block

Interscalene block of the brachial plexus is achieved by injecting 25 to 40 ml of local anesthetic solution into the interscalene groove opposite the transverse process of C6 (the external jugular vein often overlies this area) (Fig. 13-5).[2] A line extended laterally from the cricoid cartilage intersects the interscalene groove at C6. Paresthesias must be elicited before injection of local anesthetic solutions, keeping in mind that the transverse process is superficial (1.5 to 2 cm). Although a paresthesia to the shoulder is not considered to reflect stimulation of the brachial plexus, such a paresthesia is associated with the anesthesia necessary for shoulder surgery.[5] Also, at the time a paresthesia is elicited, a catheter may be placed for continuous infusion of a local anesthetic solution, as when prolonged brachial plexus anesthesia (reanastomosis of digits, postoperative physi-

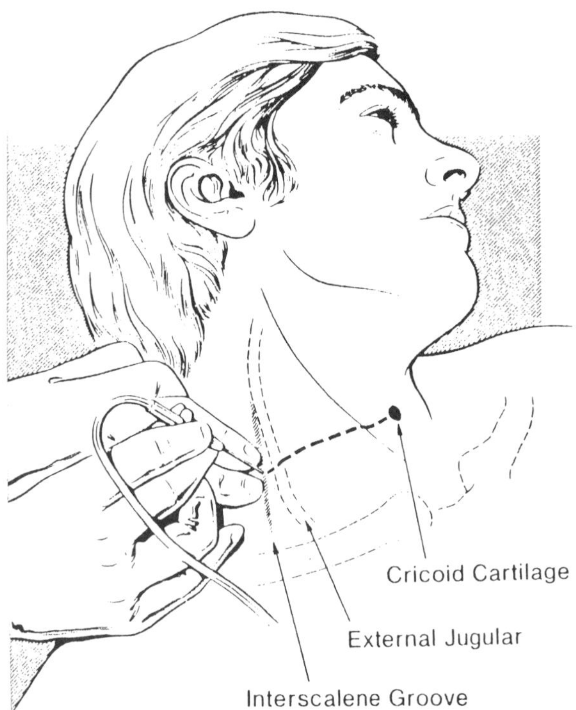

Figure 13-5. Interscalene block of the brachial plexus. A line drawn from the cricoid cartilage crosses the approximate location of the transverse process of C6. For convenience of injection and minimal displacement of the needle from its correct position, the needle can be connected with tubing to a syringe containing the local anesthetic solution. (From Bridenbaugh,[2] with permission.)

cal therapy) is desirable. Injection of 40 ml of local anesthetic solution will anesthetize the cervical plexus and brachial plexus, permitting surgery on the acromioclavicular joint, although fibers that innervate the ulnar border of the forearm (C8-T1) may be spared (Fig. 13-4).[1] Interscalene block of the brachial plexus can be performed with the arm at the patient's side, and the risk of pneumothorax is remote. On the other hand, phrenic nerve and/or laryngeal nerve block with associated ipsilateral hemiparesis of the diaphragm and laryngeal musculature are common side effects of the interscalene approach to the brachial plexus. Epidural anesthesia and spinal anesthesia are possible using this approach, and the vertebral artery is located nearby. If local anesthetics are accidentally injected into the vertebral artery, convulsions are likely to follow.

Supraclavicular Block

Supraclavicular block of the brachial plexus is achieved by injecting 25 to 40 ml of local anesthetic solution at a point just behind the midpoint of the clavicle where the nerves cross the first rib (Fig. 13-6).[2] The midpoint of the clavicle is confirmed by palpating the subclavian artery pulse or by extending an imaginary straight line from the end of the external jugular vein. Paresthesias should be elicited before injection of local anesthetic solution. Pneumothorax is the most common complication of supraclavicular block (about a 1% incidence), manifesting initially as cough, dyspnea, and pleuritic chest pain. Block of the phrenic nerve occurs frequently but generally causes no clinically significant symptoms. Bilateral supraclavicular blocks are not recommended for fear of bilateral pneumothoraces or phrenic nerve paralysis. Likewise, patients with chronic obstructive pulmonary disease may not be ideal candidates for supraclavicular block. Advantages of the supraclavicular block are the

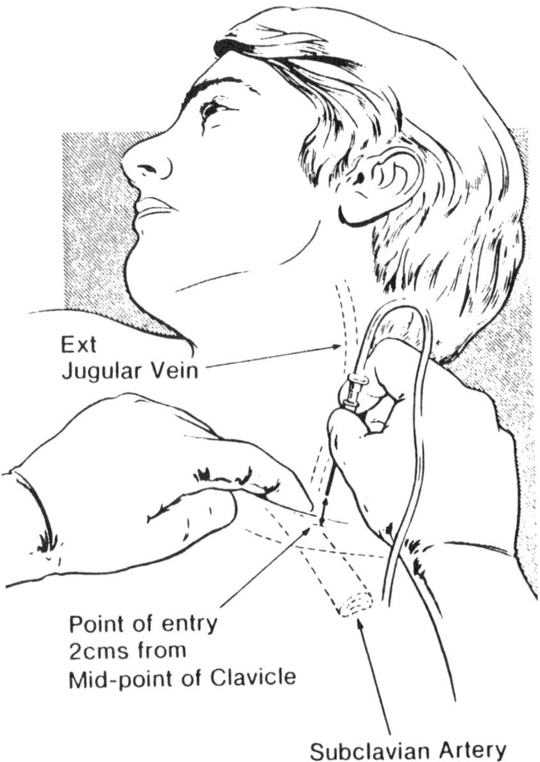

Figure 13-6. Supraclavicular block of the brachial plexus. An imaginary line from the end of the external jugular vein crosses the midpoint of the clavicle, beneath which passes the compact nerves of the brachial plexus. For convenience of injection and minimal displacement of the needle from its correct position, the needle can be connected with tubing to a syringe containing the local anesthetic solution.

rapid onset and ability to perform the block with the arm in any position.

Axillary Block

Axillary block (perivascular axillary infiltration) of the brachial plexus is achieved by injecting 25 to 40 ml of local anesthetic solution into the axillary sheath in the axilla. The nerves are anesthetized around the axillary artery (Fig. 13-7). Individual fascial septa may surround each nerve, necessitating separate injections into each compartment, in contrast to other single injection approaches.

The arm is abducted to 90 degrees and externally rotated (Fig. 13-8).[2] The axillary artery is palpated and traced as far as possible toward the axilla. As the finger of one hand palpates the artery, the needle is inserted just anterior to the vessel into the axillary sheath. Entrance of the needle into the axillary sheath transmits a "popping" sensation to the anesthesiologist's fingers, and the needle pulsates with arterial pulsations. Paresthesias are useful but not mandatory for confirming correct placement of the needle. Digital pressure applied distal to the needle during and after injection promotes proximal flow of local anesthetic solutions within the sheath toward the site where the musculocutaneous nerve exits.

An alternative approach to locating the axillary sheath is identification of the axillary artery with the exploring needle (transarterial approach). The needle is advanced until aspiration confirms that it has passed just posterior to the artery, at which point one-half the local anesthetic solution is injected. The needle is then withdrawn until aspiration confirms that it is just anterior to the artery, and the other half of the local anesthetic solution is injected.

Regardless of the approach, frequent aspiration during injection of the local anesthetic solution is essential to ensure that the needle remains outside the axillary artery. A small amount of local anesthetic solution is deposited in the subcutaneous tissue (a cuff over the proximal medial aspect of the axilla) during withdrawal of the needle to block the intercostobrachial nerve. The musculocutaneous nerve is sometimes not blocked because it leaves the sheath proximal to the point of injection. This nerve is important because of its extensive area of innervation on the radial side of the forearm extending onto the thenar eminence (Fig. 13-4).[1] Block of the musculocutaneous nerve, as it emerges from between the biceps and brachialis muscles 5 cm proximal to the elbow crease, is usually performed as a supplement to an axillary plexus block.

The axillary approach carries the least risk of pneumothorax, making it useful for outpatients undergoing surgery on the forearm and hand. Surgery on the shoulder, upper arm, or elbow is usually not possible with this block.

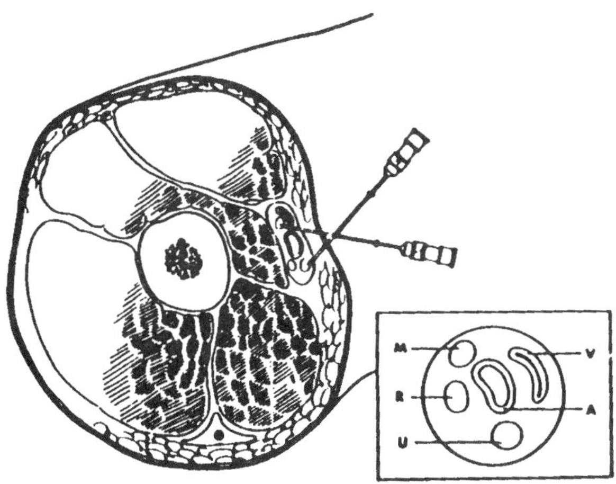

Figure 13-7. Needle positions for axillary injection of local anesthetic solution. M, median nerve; R, radial nerve; U, ulnar nerve; A, axillary artery; V, axillary vein.

DISTAL NERVE BLOCKS OF THE UPPER EXTREMITY

Reliable brachial plexus anesthesia has reduced the need for block of individual nerves distal to the axilla. Blockade at the elbow does not produce greater anesthesia than blockade at the wrist, reflecting extensive branching of the sensory nerves to the forearm, principally from the musculocutaneous nerve.

Median Nerve Block

Injection of 3 to 5 ml of local anesthetic solution 1 cm medial to the brachial artery in the flexion crease of the elbow will block the median nerve. At the wrist, the median nerve is blocked by 3 to 5 ml of local anesthetic solution injected just lateral (radial side) to the flexor palmaris longus tendon (Fig. 13-9).[1]

Ulnar Nerve Block

Injection of 1 to 4 ml of local anesthetic solution in the groove formed by the medial condyle of the humerus and the olecranon of the ulna at the elbow

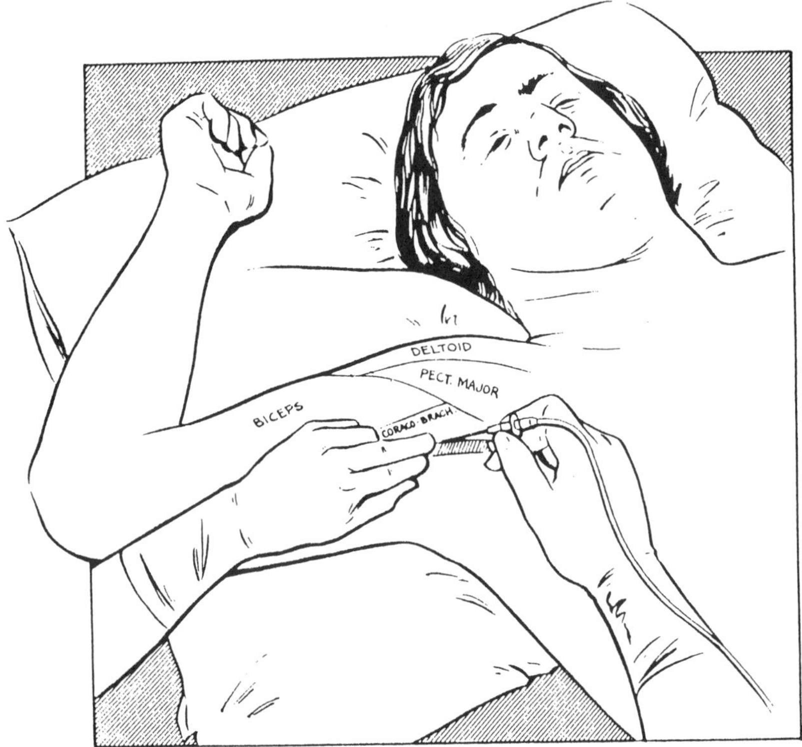

Figure 13-8. Axillary block of the brachial plexus. The needle is inserted just anterior to the axillary artery while the fingers of the other hand provide distal compression, so as to facilitate central spread of the local anesthetic solution. A distally placed tourniquet may also be used to facilitate central spread of the local anesthetic solution. For convenience of injection and minimal displacement of the needle from its correct position, the needle can be connected with tubing to a syringe containing the local anesthetic solution. (From Bridenbaugh,[2] with permission.)

will block the ulnar nerve. At the wrist, the ulnar nerve is blocked by local anesthetic solution injected medial to the ulnar artery.

Radial Nerve Block

At the wrist, the radial nerve is blocked by 2 to 3 ml of local anesthetic solution injected lateral to the radial artery (Fig. 13-9).[1] In addition, a subcutaneous cuff of anesthesia is produced on the lateral and dorsal aspects of the radial side of the wrist to anesthetize those branches of the radial nerve that have left the parent trunk in the lower third of the forearm.

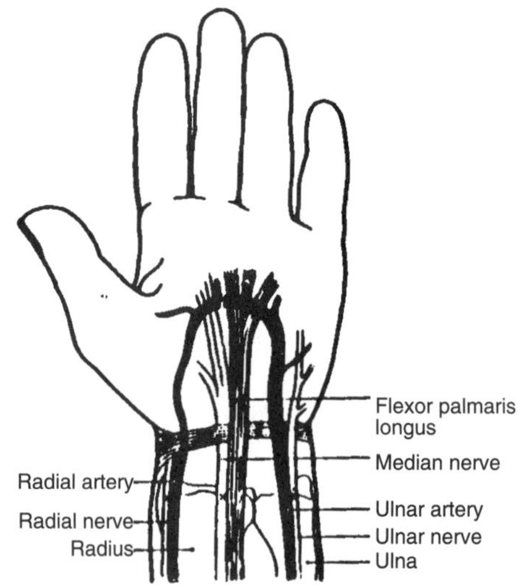

Figure 13-9. Terminal nerves at the wrist. (From Mulroy,[1] with permission.)

INTERCOSTAL NERVE BLOCKS

Intercostal nerves (12 pairs) pursue a circumferential course in the inferior groove of each rib supplying skin and abdominal wall skeletal muscles. Each nerve is accompanied by an intercostal vein and artery, which lie superior to the nerve in the inferior groove. The location of these vessels explains the frequent occurrence of high plasma concentrations of local anesthetics after performance of intercostal nerve blocks.

Intercostal nerve blocks are optimally performed with the patient prone and the needle inserted about 8 cm from the midline posteriorly where the rib can be palpated. Lateral cutaneous branches of intercostal nerves arise at the midaxillary line and may not be blocked if the needle is inserted too far laterally. The needle is advanced until the rib is contacted, at which point the needle is redirected caudad and "walked off" the inferior border of the rib (Fig. 13-10).[1] The needle is then advanced an additional 4 to 6 mm, and 5 ml of local anesthetic solution is injected with frequent aspiration to minimize the likelihood of accidental intravascular injections.

Block of the intercostal nerves provides sensory and motor anesthesia of the entire abdominal wall without associated sympathetic nervous system blockade. Multiple intercostal blocks may be performed to provide postoperative analgesia after thoracic or abdominal surgery or to relieve pain related to rib fractures. Supplementation of intercostal nerve blocks with other blocks (celiac plexus block) is usually necessary when surgical procedures are planned. The principal risks of intercostal nerve blocks are pneumothorax and accidental intravascular injection of local anesthetic solutions.

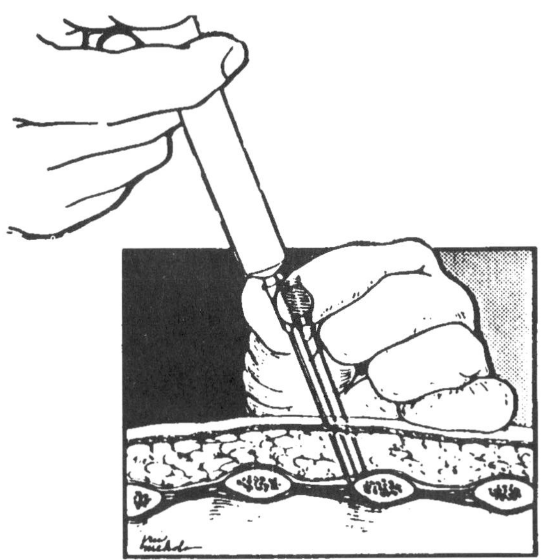

Figure 13-10. Hand and needle positions for injection of local anesthetic solution under the rib to block an intercostal nerve. The depth of the needle insertion is controlled by the anesthesiologist's hand resting on the patient's back. (From Mulroy,[1] with permission.)

BLOCKS OF THE LOWER EXTREMITY

Unlike the compactness of the brachial plexus, the lower extremity is supplied by nerves that are widely separated from each other as they enter the thigh. Major nerves to the lower extremity include the sciatic, femoral, lateral femoral cutaneous, and obturator nerves. The sciatic nerve divides in the popliteal fossa into the tibial nerve passing medially and the common peroneal nerve passing laterally. In many respects, it is easier to perform an epidural anesthetic or spinal anesthetic than to attempt to achieve the same degree of anesthesia with multiple peripheral nerve blocks.

Sciatic Nerve Block

The sacral plexus (L4-L5, S1–S3) gives rise to the sciatic nerve, which is nearly 2 cm wide as it leaves the pelvis. The classic approach to sciatic nerve block is with the patient lying on the side opposite the one to be blocked (Fig. 13-11).[1] A line is drawn from the posterior superior iliac spine and the greater trochanter of the femur. The needle is inserted about 5 cm caudad from the midpoint of this line, and about 25 ml of 1.5% lidocaine or 0.5% bupivacaine is injected after elicitation of a paresthesia. This block provides adequate anesthesia of the foot and lower leg. More often, sciatic nerve block is combined with other nerve blocks to provide more extensive anesthesia.

Femoral Nerve Block

Femoral nerve block is produced by injection of 10 to 20 ml of local anesthetic solution immediately lateral to the femoral artery just below the midpoint of the inguinal ligament. A line drawn from the anterior superior iliac spine to the symphysis pubis will approximate the inguinal ligament.

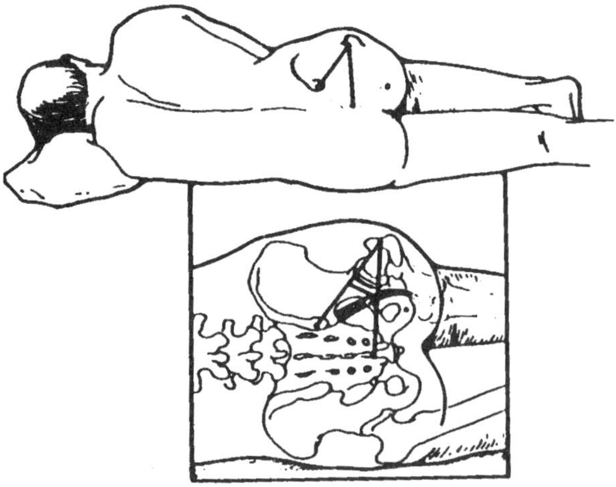

Figure 13-11. Posterior approach to sciatic nerve block. The sciatic nerve lies beneath a point 5 cm caudad along the perpendicular line that bisects the line joining the posterior superior iliac spine and the greater trochanter of the femur. This point is also usually the intersection of that perpendicular line with another line joining the greater trochanter and the sacral hiatus. (From Mulroy,[1] with permission.)

Lateral Femoral Cutaneous Nerve Block

The lateral femoral cutaneous nerve is blocked by injection of 5 to 10 ml of local anesthetic solution at a point 2 cm medial and 2 cm below the anterior superior iliac spine. This block may provide suitable anesthesia for removal of small skin grafts but is most often used to supplement sciatic, femoral, and obturator nerve blocks for surgery on or above the knee.

Obturator Nerve Block

Obturator nerve block is performed by introducing a needle 1 to 2 cm below and lateral to the pubic tubercle. When the pubic bone is reached, the needle is withdrawn and redirected cephalad to identify the obturator canal, where 10 to 15 ml of local anesthetic solution is placed. Successful obturator nerve block is evidenced by paresis of the adductor muscles. This block is useful for diagnosing painful conditions of the hip and is sometimes necessary to supplement sciatic, femoral, and lateral femoral cutaneous nerve blocks for surgery on or above the knee.

Inguinal Paravascular Technique of Lumbar Plexus Block

Blockade of the femoral, obturator, and lateral femoral cutaneous nerves is achieved with a single injection (thus the description as a "three-in-one block").[6] The lumbar plexus can be blocked because a fascial envelope surrounds the femoral nerve, which serves as a conduit for carrying local anesthetic solution injected below the inguinal ligament cephalad to the level where the lumbar plexus forms.

Ankle Block

All five nerves of the foot can be blocked at the level of the ankle (Fig. 13-12).[1] The posterior tibial nerve is the major nerve to the sole of the foot. To block

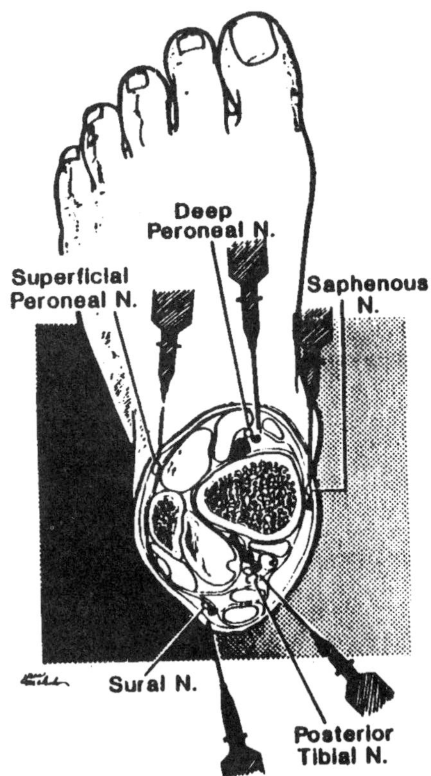

Figure 13-12. Ankle block is performed by injection of local anesthetic solution at five separate nerve locations. The superficial peroneal nerve, sural nerve, and saphenous nerve are usually blocked by subcutaneous infiltration, since they may have already branched as they cross the ankle joint. (From Mulroy,[1] with permission.)

this nerve the needle is introduced just behind the posterior tibial artery and advanced until a paresthesia to the sole of the foot is elicited, at which point 5 ml of local anesthetic solution is injected. The sural nerve is blocked by injecting 5 ml of local anesthetic solution in the groove between the lateral malleolus and calcaneus. Infiltration of 5 ml of local anesthetic solution anterior to the medial malleolus blocks the saphenous nerve. The deep peroneal nerve is the major nerve to the dorsum of the foot and is blocked by injection of 5 ml of local anesthetic solution just lateral to the anterior tibial artery. Superficial branches of the peroneal nerve are blocked by a subcutaneous ridge of local anesthetic solution injected between the anterior tibial artery and lateral malleolus.

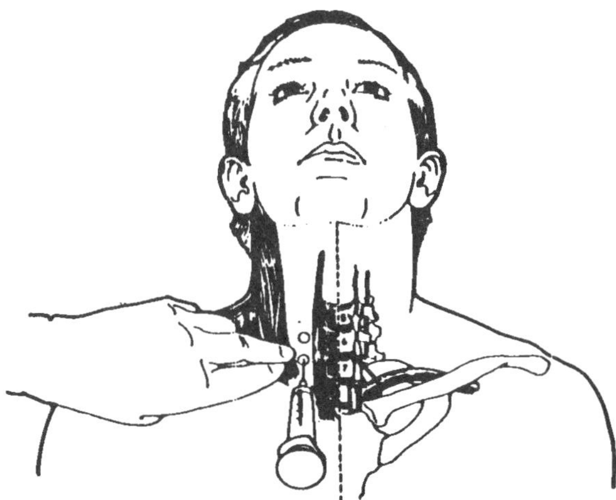

Figure 13-13. Stellate ganglion block is accomplished by retraction of the sternocleidomastoid muscle and the carotid sheath laterally and injection of local anesthetic solution through a needle positioned just medial to the transverse process of C7. (From Mulroy,[1] with permission.)

STELLATE GANGLION BLOCK

The cervical sympathetic chain consists of superior, middle, and inferior cervical ganglia. The inferior cervical ganglion and first thoracic ganglion often fuse to form the stellate ganglion. Sympathetic nervous system fibers that traverse the stellate ganglion supply the head and arm. A common approach to stellate ganglion block is the anterior or paratracheal technique. With the patient supine and the head extended on a pillow, the anesthesiologist retracts the sternocleidomastoid muscle laterally and locates the transverse process of the sixth cervical vertebra (Chassaignac's tubercle), which is typically at the level of the cricoid cartilage (Fig. 13-13).[1] The needle is inserted through the skin over this transverse process and advanced 2.5 to 4 cm until it makes contact with bone (C7), at which point the needle is withdrawn 2 to 3 mm and a 2-ml test dose is administered followed by up to 8 ml of 1% lidocaine or 0.25% bupivacaine. Onset of ipsilateral sympathetic nervous system blockade (Horner syndrome) is usually evident within 10 minutes. Increased skin temperature is the only conclusive evidence of interruption of sympathetic nervous system innervation to the upper extremity. A Horner syndrome alone does not ensure complete sympathetic denervation of the upper extremity, which may

Signs of Sympathetic Nervous System Blockade After Stellate Ganglion Block (Horner Syndrome)

Ptosis
Miosis
Anhydrosis
Nasal congestion
Vasodilation
Increased skin temperature

Complications of Stellate Ganglion Block

Pneumothorax
Intravascular injection (vertebral artery)
Block of cardioaccelerator fibers
Hoarseness from recurrent laryngeal nerve paralysis
Spinal anesthesia (diffusion of local anesthetic along dural sheath enclosing cervical nerves)

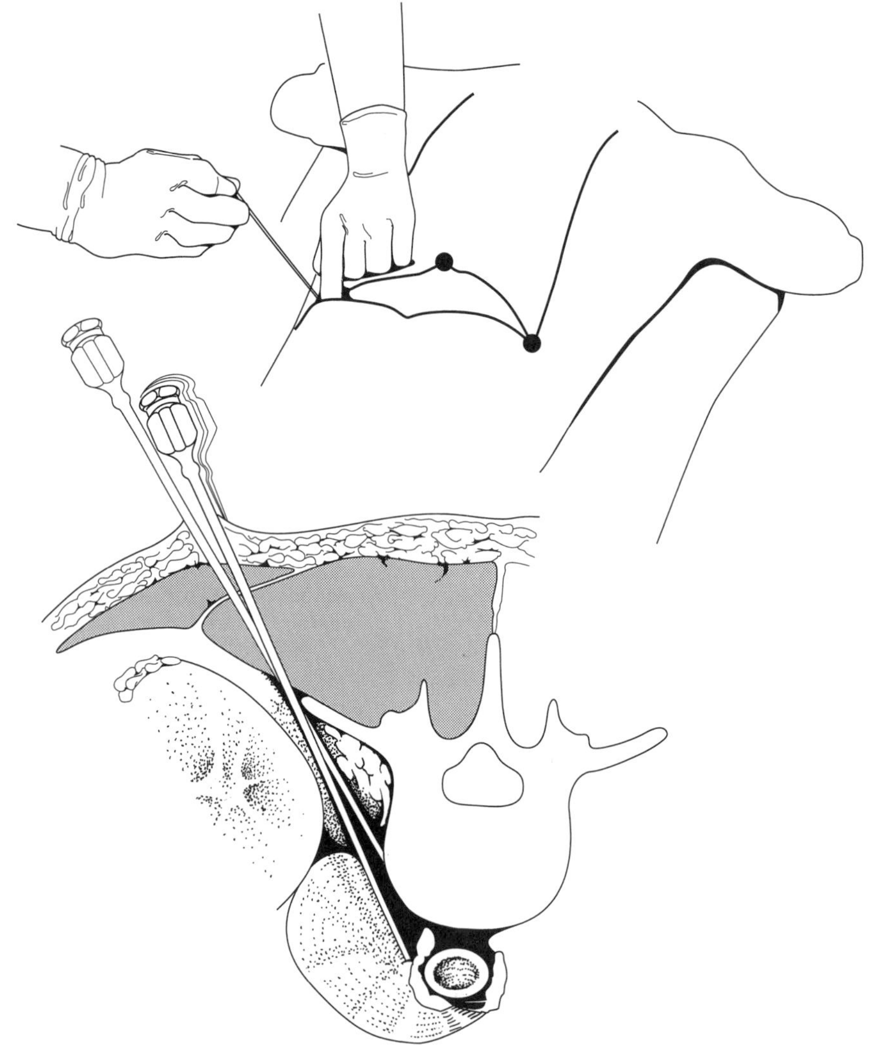

Figure 13-14. Landmarks for performance of a celiac plexus block. A needle is inserted at the inferior edge of the twelfth rib about 8 cm from the midline and advanced 10 to 12 cm until it contacts the body of the L1 vertebra. The needle is then withdrawn and redirected so that it passes to the anterior lateral side of the vertebral body. (From Thompson and Moore,[7] with permission.)

receive sympathetic fibers from as low as T9. Complications of stellate ganglion block reflect the surrounding anatomy. Common indications for stellate ganglion block are diagnosis and treatment of reflex sympathetic dystrophies (see Chapter 34) and management of circulatory insufficiency in the upper extremity.

CELIAC PLEXUS BLOCK

The celiac plexus is the largest plexus of the sympathetic nervous system, providing innervation to abdominal organs (pancreas, liver, stomach). A needle is inserted about 8 cm from the midline at the inferior edge of the twelfth rib and advanced until it contacts the lateral body of the L1 vertebra at an average depth of 10 to 12 cm (Fig. 13-14).[7] The needle is then withdrawn and redirected so that it will slide off the anterolateral side of the vertebral body. Many anesthesiologists recommend radiography or computed tomography to confirm proper needle placement before injection of a 2-ml test dose of local anesthetic solution. Assuming the absence of unexpected sensory blockade following the test dose, the remaining 25 to 35 ml of local anesthetic solution is injected. The complexity and complications of this block suggest that it should be performed only by anesthesiologists experienced in its use. Celiac plexus block with alcohol or phenol is the most effective block for treatment of pancreatic cancer pain (see Chapter 34).

Complications of Celiac Plexus Block

- Hypotension (reflects extensive sympathetic nervous system blockade)
- Intravascular injection
- Spinal or epidural anesthesia
- Visceral puncture
- Retroperitoneal hematoma (bleeding from the aorta and/or inferior vena cava)

INTRAVENOUS REGIONAL NEURAL ANESTHESIA

Intravenous regional neural anesthesia (Bier block) is a simple method of producing anesthesia of the arm or leg by injection of large volumes of local anesthetic solutions intravenously while the circulation to that extremity is occluded by a tourniquet. A venous catheter is placed in a distal portion of the involved extremity, and the arm or leg is exsanguinated by wrapping with an Esmarch bandage (Fig. 13-15).[8] The tourniquet is then inflated to about 50 mmHg above the patient's systolic blood pressure, and local anesthetic solution (25 to 50 ml for the upper extremity, and 100 to 200 ml for the lower extremity) is injected. A double tourniquet technique can be used to eliminate tourniquet pain. The proximal tourniquet is initially inflated, and when the patient subsequently experiences pain, the more distal tourniquet over anesthetized skin is inflated and the proximal cuff is then deflated.

Commonly used local anesthetic solutions for intravenous regional neural anesthesia are 0.5% lidocaine or prilocaine. Chloroprocaine is not used for intravenous regional anesthesia because of its association with thrombophlebitis, and bupivacaine is avoided because of concern of systemic toxic effects, especially on the heart, when the drug enters the circulation. Onset of anesthesia is rapid, and skeletal muscle relaxation is profound. The duration of anesthesia depends on the time the tourniquet is inflated and not on the local anesthetic selected. Technically, this block is easier to perform than a brachial plexus block or lower extremi-

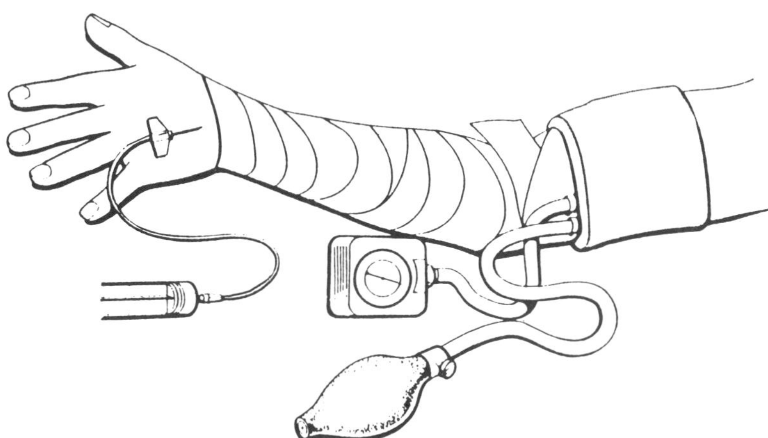

Figure 13-15. Exsanguination of the arm with an Esmarch bandage before inflation of the tourniquet and injection of the local anesthetic solution through the distally placed intravenous needle. (From Holmes,[8] with permission.)

ty block and is readily applicable to all age groups, including pediatric patients.

The principal risk of intravenous regional neural anesthesia is the potential systemic toxicity that may occur when the tourniquet is deflated and local anesthetic solutions from the previously isolated extremity enter the circulation. For this reason, slow or intermittent deflations and inflations of the tourniquet at the conclusion of surgery are recommended in an attempt to prevent excessive plasma concentrations of local anesthetics. Likewise, limitation of extremity movement after release of the tourniquet is useful for minimizing anesthetic blood levels. The rapid metabolism of prilocaine is advantageous for decreasing the likelihood of systemic toxicity following deflation of the tourniquet. Significant methemoglobinemia is unlikely to accompany metabolism of prilocaine when the total dose of this local anesthetic administered to adults is lower than 600 mg (see Chapter 6).

REFERENCES

1. Mulroy M. Handbook of Regional Anesthesia. Boston, Little, Brown, 1989;1–289.
2. Bridenbaugh LD. The upper extremity: Somatic blockade. In: Cousins MJ, Bridenbaugh PO, eds. Neural Blockade in Clinical Anesthesia and Management of Pain. Philadelphia, JB Lippincott 1988:387–416.
3. Hickey R, Hoffman J, Ramamurthy S. A comparison of ropivacaine 0.5% and bupivacaine 0.5% for brachial plexus block. Anesthesiology 1991;74:639–42.
4. Winnie AP. Plexus Anesthesia I: The Perivascular Technique of Brachial Plexus Block. Philadelphia, WB Saunders 1983.
5. Roch JJ, Sharrock NE, Neudachin L. Interscalene brachial plexus block for shoulder surgery: A proximal paresthesia is effective. Anesth Analg 1992; 75:386–8.
6. Winnie AP, Ramamurthy S, Durrani Z. The inguinal paravascular technique of lumbar plexus anesthesia. Anesth Analg 1973;52:989–96.
7. Thompson GE, Moore DR. Celiac plexus, intercostal and minor peripheral blockade. In: Cousins MJ, Bridenbaugh PO, eds. Neural Blockade in Clinical Anesthesia and Management of Pain. Philadelphia, JB Lippincott 1988:503–32.
8. Holmes CM. Intravenous regional neural blockade. In: Cousins MJ, Bridenbaugh PO, eds. Neural Blockade in Clinical Anesthesia and Management of Pain. Philadelphia, JB Lippincott 1988:443–60.

14

Positioning and Associated Risks

Following the induction of anesthesia, patients are positioned so as to offer optimal surgical exposure. From the standpoint of surgical exposure, however, these desirable positions may evoke undesirable changes, which manifest most often as impaired venous return to the heart and interference with ventilation-to-perfusion relationships in the lungs. Postural changes associated with positioning may result in hypotension, especially if the position change is abrupt or hypovolemia is present, or both. General anesthesia may blunt compensatory sympathetic nervous system reflex responses that would normally minimize blood pressure changes associated with abrupt position changes. Frequent initial measurement of blood pressure is necessary to determine whether the new position is acceptable. If hypotension occurs, further changes in position are postponed until the blood pressure is restored to an acceptable level by administration of a vasopressor, infusion of intravenous fluids, or decreasing the concentrations of inhaled anesthetics, or any combination of the above. When these interventions are not promptly effective, the position is adjusted to one that is better tolerated by the patient. Positioning problems may be anticipated from preoperative conditions such as limited joint mobility owing to arthritis. A sufficient number of trained personnel must be available to help with positioning to minimize the risk to patients and those responsible for moving the patient.

The absence of pain during general anesthesia plus the likely presence of drug-induced skeletal muscle relaxation may permit placement of patients in positions that would not be tolerated in the awake state. For example, in awake supine patients, abduction of the arm to more than 90 degrees often becomes painful in a few minutes. The same patient rendered unresponsive by anesthetic drugs could not warn the anesthesiologist about the unacceptability of this position. Likewise, sensations of nerve compression as perceived by awake patients (tingling, numbness) would not provide warning of possible developing peripheral nerve injury in the unconscious state. Indeed, peripheral nerve injuries are an ever present danger in anesthetized patients. Padding of pressure points on the extremities, especially at the elbows, is routinely performed in hopes of decreasing the likelihood of compression injury to peripheral nerves.

At the conclusion of surgery, return of the patient to a supine position or movement to a stretcher for transport may again unmask hypovolemia and attendant hypotension. Movement of lightly anesthetized patients may cause airway stimulation from the tracheal tube or pain manifesting as hypertension, requiring treatment with appropriate drugs.

Proper positioning of patients is a "team effort" and a "shared responsibility" between the anesthesiologist, surgeon, and nurses. Operations performed with patients in other than the supine position uniquely require the participation of the surgeon in placing the patient on the operating table in a way that maximizes surgical exposure without introducing the risk of peripheral nerve injury (see the section *Special Positions*). During the operation, the anesthesiologist remains vigilant to any changes in the patient's position, although the requirements of the operation and placement of drapes may limit the extent of these observations. Description of the patient's position during surgery, including position of the extremities and use of padding, is often documented in the medical record by the anesthesiologist and nurses.

SPECIAL POSITIONS

Most surgical procedures can be performed with patients in the supine or prone positions. On occasion, the needs of the surgical procedure may necessitate placement of patients in the head-down, lateral decubitus, sitting, or lithotomy positions. *Decubitus* is used to indicate the part of the patient that is in contact with the operating table.

Supine

The supine position produces minimal effects on circulation, and perfusion of the lungs tends to be homogeneous. Functional residual capacity decreases about 800 ml when changing from the standing to supine position. Subsequent administration of muscle relaxants further decreases functional residual capacity, reflecting accentuation of the cephalad displacement of the diaphragm and compression of the adjacent lung.[1] Loss of skeletal muscle tone in the chest wall decreases opposition to the inherent elastic recoil of the lungs, further contributing to decreases in lung volumes. These adverse effects on lung volumes may be offset by mechanical (controlled) ventilation of the lungs.

In the supine position, the hips and knees should be flexed slightly (lawn-chair position). This position facilitates venous drainage from the lower extremities and shortens the xiphoid-to-pubis distance, which decreases anterior abdominal wall tension during surgical closure. The legs must remain uncrossed, and the heels are padded. Pressure on the occiput of the head with the risk of focal alopecia is minimized by appropriate use of padding. Backache that manifests in the postoperative period may reflect loss of normal lumbar curvature in the supine position owing to ligamentous relaxation associated with anesthesia.

Head Down

The head-down (Trendelenburg) position does not predictably improve cardiac output in hypotensive and hypovolemic patients.[2] Presumably, displacement of abdominal viscera pushes the diaphragm against the heart, resulting in decreases in stroke volume and, in some patients, accentuation of coexisting hypotension. Furthermore, this position accentuates compression of the lung bases by abdominal viscera. In vulnerable patients, the head-down position will increase intracranial pressure by elevating venous pressures, leading to decreased venous outflow from the brain. Placement of patients in the head-down position may require use of shoulder braces to prevent cephalad movement of the entire body. Proper placement of these shoulder braces is mandatory to avoid peripheral nerve injuries (see the section *Peripheral Nerve Injuries*).

Prone

Pressure from the mattress of the surgical table on the abdominal wall of prone patients results in cephalad displacement of the diaphragm, impediment of downward descent of the diaphragm, and compression of the inferior vena cava and aorta. Mechanical ventilation of the lungs may offset undesirable effects of the prone position on breathing, but associated increases in venous pressure may further jeopardize venous return and cardiac output. Turning of the head necessitated by the prone position may obstruct jugular venous drainage and vertebral artery blood flow and may be responsible for postoperative neck pain or, in rare cases, thrombosis. In the presence of cervical arthritis or known cerebrovascular disease, it is recommended that the patient's head not be turned. This is accomplished using a horseshoe-shaped pad (Mayfield headrest) that supports the periphery of the face without pressing on the eyes. Protection of the prominent aspects of the face and eyes must be ensured when patients are placed in the prone position. The patient's arms are placed at the sides or extended alongside the head on arm boards, taking care to avoid compression of the ulnar nerves (Figs. 14-1 and 14-2). It may be preferable to place the patient's arms at the sides if the preoperative interview elicits complaints of discomfort when the arms are placed above the head. Firm rolls (bolsters) are placed under the patient's sides from the clavicle to iliac crest (Fig. 14-1). These rolls serve to relieve abdominal compression by the mattress of the surgical table, thus facilitating venous return to the heart and ease of ventilation of the lungs. The legs are often fitted with elastic stockings to minimize pooling of blood, which is particularly likely to occur

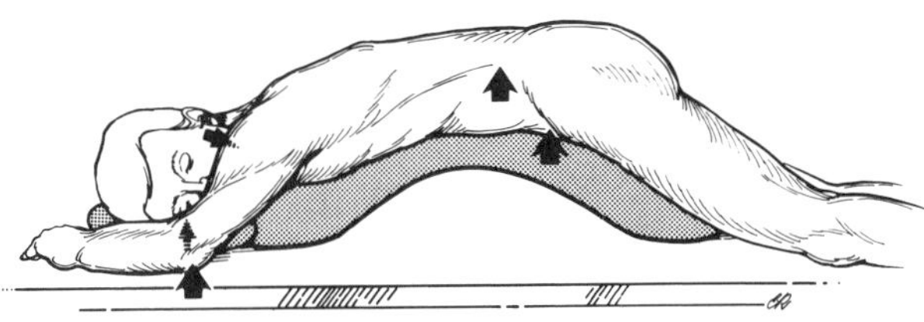

Figure 14-1. This position indicates the multiple problems that can occur with an improperly positioned patient in the flexed prone position. If excessively stretched, the brachial plexus can be damaged. The ulnar nerve can be damaged by compression of the nerve at the elbow. Inadequate padding under the head can cause eye damage or undue pressure to the face or lower eyelid. Excessive compression to the inferior vena cava can be minimized by padding under the inferior iliac spine.

when flexion as needed for laminectomy is added to the prone position. Movement of patients into and from the prone position requires assistance from multiple personnel and is accomplished slowly to allow time for compensatory sympathetic nervous system responses to minimize undesirable decreases in blood pressure. During this time, the anesthesiologist is responsible for stabilizing the patient's head and ensuring continued proper position of the tracheal tube.

There are several variations of the prone position, such as the knee-chest position, and many devices are used to achieve these positions. The principles, including padding of pressure points (knees and face), free abdominal and chest expansion, and limiting abduction of the arms to less than 90 degrees, apply to all of these variations of the prone position.

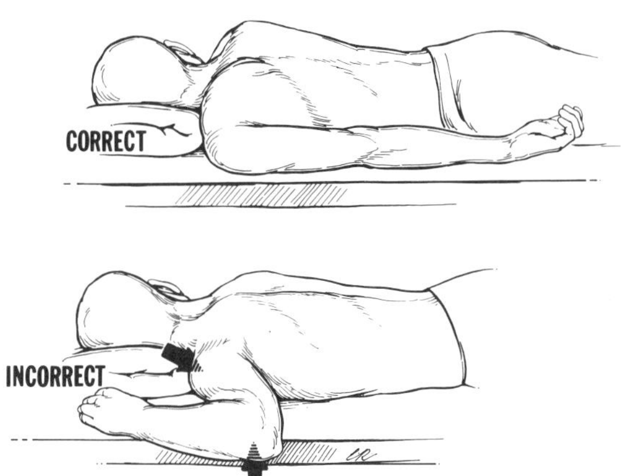

Figure 14-2. Proper padding in the prone position should minimize damage to the brachial plexus, especially the ulnar nerve.

Lateral Decubitus

The lateral decubitus position may be associated with significant circulatory and ventilatory effects during mechnical ventilation of the lungs. Compression of the inferior vena cava may occur, especially if the kidney rest (properly placed under the dependent iliac crest) is elevated. The dependent lung tends to be underventilated because it is compressed by the pressure of the abdominal contents and the weight of the mediastinum. The nondependent lung is relatively overventilated because the compliance of this lung is increased, particularly when the corresponding hemithorax is opened. At the same time, gravity favors distribution of pulmonary blood flow to the underventilated dependent lung. The accentuated mismatching of ventilation to perfusion introduced by the lateral decubitus position may manifest as unexpected arterial hypoxemia.

To avoid compression of the dependent neurovascular bundle in the axilla, a roll is often placed under the thorax just caudal to the axilla. It is useful to periodically check the radial pulse to ensure absence of neurovascular compression. A pulse oximeter can be used to ensure adequate perfusion of the dependent hand. A pillow beneath the head minimizes stretch on the dependent brachial plexus, and a pillow between the knees, with the dependent leg flexed at the knee, minimizes pressure on bony prominences and stretch on nerves of the lower extremity (Figs. 14-3 and 14-4). The nondependent arm can be positioned on an elevated board bent in front of the patient's face or suspended from a well-padded support bar with care taken to avoid stretch on the brachial plexus (Fig. 14-5).[3]

Sitting

The sitting position is most often used for posterior fossa craniotomy, as this position facilitates venous drainage from the head and improves surgical exposure. The cardiovascular effects of the sitting position are complex and may include decreases in cardiac output, cerebral perfusion pressure, and intrathoracic blood volume.[4] Venous return from dependent extremities is enhanced by placing the legs in elastic stockings. Venous air embolism is the principal hazard of the sitting position (see Chapter 23).

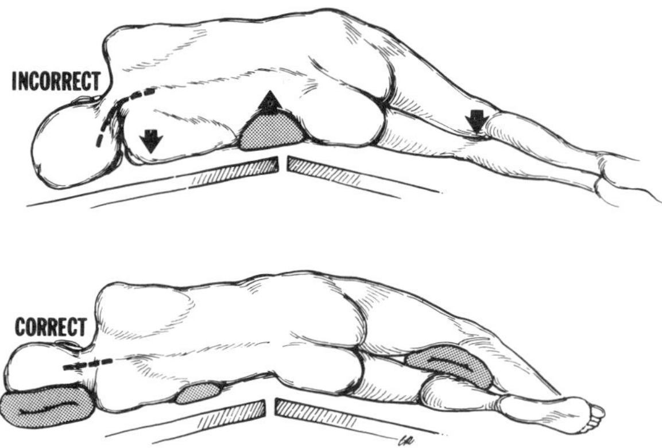

Figure 14-3. In the lateral decubitus position, pillows between the legs and elbows help distribute the weight of the extremities.

Lithotomy

Circulatory effects of the lithotomy position are not detrimental unless an abdominal mass (ascites, gravid uterus) contributes to obstruction of the inferior vena cava. The effect of this position on breathing is manifest as cephalad displacement of the diaphragm by abdominal viscera. Elevation of the legs can increase the pain of a herniated nucleus pulposis. When the lithotomy position is planned for a patient with a history of low back pain or lumbar disc disease, it may be helpful to have the awake patient assume this posture to determine whether this position can be tolerated during anesthesia.

Injury to peripheral nerves (sciatic, common peroneal, femoral, saphenous, obturator) are the principal hazards of the lithotomy position (see the section *Peripheral Nerve Injuries*). Proper padding between the metal leg braces and the patient's legs is intended to decrease the likelihood of injury to these peripheral nerves. During positioning, both of the patient's legs should be elevated and flexed simultaneously to avoid stretching of peripheral nerves. The thigh should be flexed at no greater than 90 degrees before rotating the stirrups laterally. Prolonged placement of patients in the lithotomy position (usually longer than 4 hours) may result in skeletal muscle ischemia, loss of capillary integrity, and massive edema leading to tissue necrosis (compartment syndrome). If there is a question of inadequate circulation, the legs should probably be returned to the horizontal position.

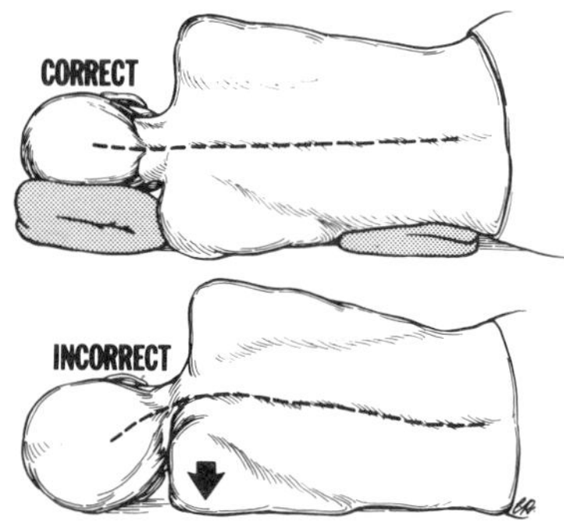

Figure 14-4. Injury to the nondependent brachial plexus can be minimized by proper padding underneath the head.

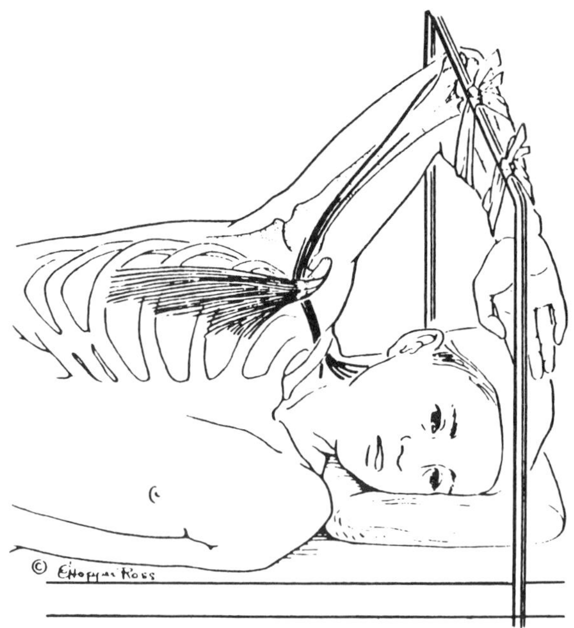

Figure 14-5. Suspension of the arm on a metal brace with extreme abduction of the arm depresses the brachial plexus posteriorly behind the tendon of the pectoralis major muscle. (From Britt and Gordon,[3] with permission.)

PERIPHERAL NERVE INJURIES

Peripheral nerve injuries are a significant source of anesthesia-related liability claims.[5] These injuries are more likely to occur in the patient who undergoes general anesthesia since discomfort that accompanies unphysiologic positions is not perceived. The traditional explanation when a postoperative neuropathy occurs is a position-related compression or stretching injury causing ischemia of the involved nerve or nerves. In this regard, it is often assumed that proper positioning and padding during surgery will decrease the risk of peripheral nerve injuries. Nevertheless, there is compelling evidence that upper extremity nerve injury, manifesting initially in the postoperative period, may have many different causes and may occur despite appropriate padding and independent of the arm position (abducted or at the side, pronated, or supinated) during surgery.[6,7] When a peripheral nerve injury manifests in the postoperative period, it is useful to seek neurologic consultation, including performance of nerve conduction velocity and electromyographic studies. If the electromyogram is performed promptly after the onset of symptoms, it is possible to determine whether the neuropathy was present preoperatively because the signs of denervation resulting from acute injury appear 18 to 21 days after the event and are limited to a specific nerve distribution. Testing of both arms is useful as it is known that patients who develop postoperative ulnar nerve neuropathy usually manifest abnormalities of nerve conduction testing in both the affected and contralateral (asymptomatic) arm.[6]

Causes of Peripheral Nerve Injuries

- Position-related compression or stretching
- Occupational trauma
- Co-existing diseases
  - Diabetes mellitus
  - Vitamin deficiency
  - Alcoholism
  - Cancer
- Congenital anomalies (cervical rib)
- Cubital tunnel entrapment
- Type of surgery (cardiac surgery)
- Anticoagulant therapy and hematomas
- Hypothermia
- Hypotension
- Prolonged (usually longer than 3 hours) application of tourniquet

Characteristic sensory and motor changes accompany many peripheral nerve injuries (Figs. 14-6 and 14-7).[8] Recovery from peripheral nerve injury is often slow, taking 3 to 12 months, and during this time the patient may experience pain and disability. Severe stretch injury that results in disruption of axons within an intact sheath of the nerve trunk may result in irreversible changes and disability.

Ulnar Nerve

Ulnar nerve injury is the most common postoperative peripheral neuropathy.[5] The ulnar nerve may be injured when it is compressed against the posterior aspect of the medial epicondyle of the humerus, as by the sharp edge of an operating room table (Fig. 14-8). Compression of the ulnar nerve in the cubital tunnel (cubital tunnel external compression syndrome) may be more likely when the elbow is fully flexed or the forearm is pronated (Fig. 14-9).[8,9] Supination of the forearm rotates the elbow such that the olecranon process of the ulna is in contact with any flat supporting surface, thus protecting the ulnar nerve from compression in the cubital tunnel (Fig. 14-9).[8,9] Despite the theoretical value of placing the supine patient's forearms in supination during surgery, there is no evidence that this practice decreases the likelihood of postoperative ulnar nerve injury.[6] Furthermore, attempted maintenance of forearm supination in an awake patient often results in discomfort (skeletal muscle spasm) and

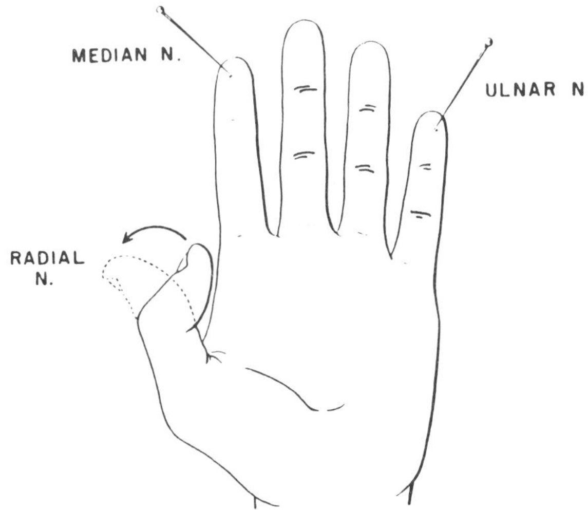

Figure 14-6. Schematic diagram for the rapid identification of peripheral nerve injuries to the upper extremity. (From Martin,[8] with permission.)

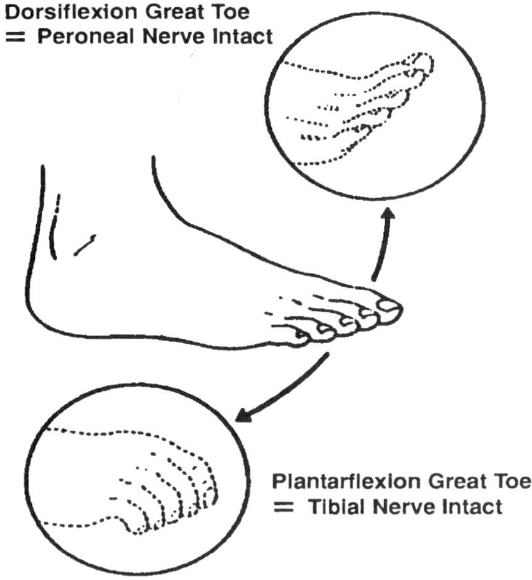

Figure 14-7. Schematic diagram for the rapid identification of peripheral nerve injuries to the lower extremity. (From Martin,[8] with permission.)

spontaneous movement of the patient's forearms to a midposition between supination and pronation.

A predominance of ulnar nerve injury in males suggests an anatomic predisposition (hypermobile nerve, shallow cubital tunnel) that renders the ulnar nerve more vulnerable to damage from external compression. Sternal retraction as required for cardiac surgery and cardiopulmonary bypass is associated with an increased incidence of postoperative ulnar nerve palsy.[6] Co-existing medical conditions (diabetes mellitus, vitamin deficiency, alcoholism, cancer) or chronic subclinical (asymptomatic) compression of the ulnar nerve in the cubital tunnel (degenerative arthritis, occupational trauma) may render the ulnar nerve of some patients uniquely vulnerable to damage from external compression. It is conceivable that unavoidable events associated with anesthesia and surgery (external pressure from positioning, changes in blood pressure) would produce additive effects on a previously damaged nerve, converting subclinical entrapment of the nerve to a recognized peripheral nerve injury.[6] Delayed appearance of ulnar nerve injury until several hours postoperatively suggests that damage may be occurring during the postoperative period rather than during anesthesia and surgery. Injury to the ulnar nerve manifests as inability to abduct or oppose the fifth finger, diminished sensation over both surfaces of the medial one and one-half fingers and adjacent hand, and eventually atrophy of the intrinsic muscles of the hand (claw hand) (Fig. 14-6).[8]

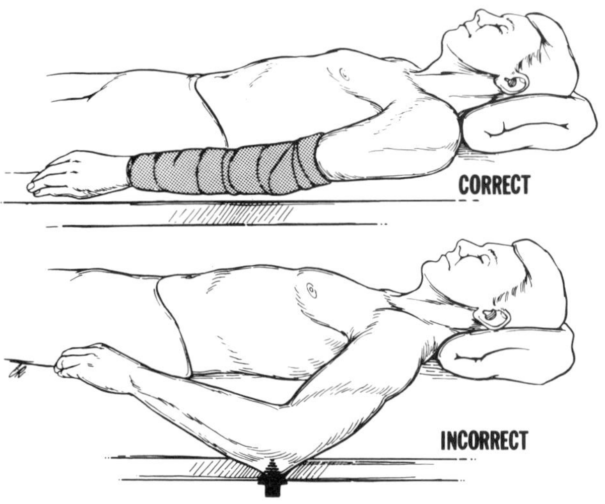

Figure 14-8. If the arm is allowed to hang over the edge of the operating table when the patient is in the supine position, an ulnar nerve injury may occur.

Brachial Plexus

After the ulnar nerve, the brachial plexus is the next most common postoperative neurologic injury.[5] The brachial plexus, because of its long superficial course in the axilla between two points of fixation (vertebra above and axillary fascia below) and proximity to freely movable bony structures (clavicle and humerus), is susceptible to damage from compression and stretching. Stretching of the brachial plexus may occur when the neck is extended, the head is turned to the opposite side, or the arm is abducted to greater than 90 degrees (Fig. 14-10).[3] The brachial plexus may be compressed between the clavicle and first rib when shoulder braces are not placed properly over the acromioclavicular joint. Spreading of the sternum as necessary for cardiac surgery requiring cardiopulmonary bypass may result in stretching of the brachial plexus or damage to the plexus from first-rib fractures.[6]

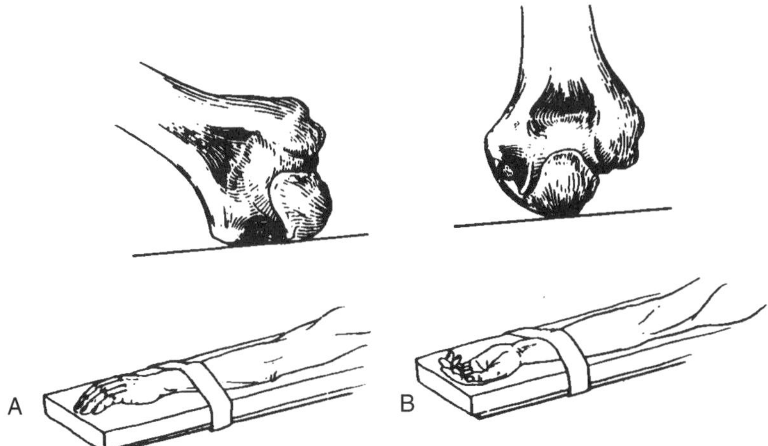

Figure 14-9. In a supine patient, pronation of the forearm rotates the elbow such that *(A)* the cubital tunnel is in contact with any flat supporting surface, presumably placing the ulnar nerve at risk of external compression. *(B)* Conversely, supination of the forearm rotates the elbow such that the cubital tunnel is no longer in contact with any flat support surface. (Modified from Martin,[8] with permission.)

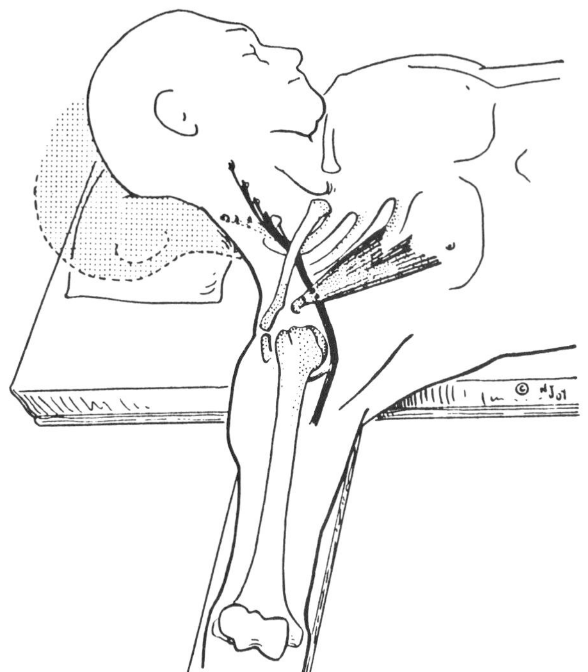

Figure 14-10. Dorsal extension and lateral flexion of the head to the opposite side may produce an undesirable amount of stretch on the brachial plexus. (From Britt and Gordon,[3] with permission.)

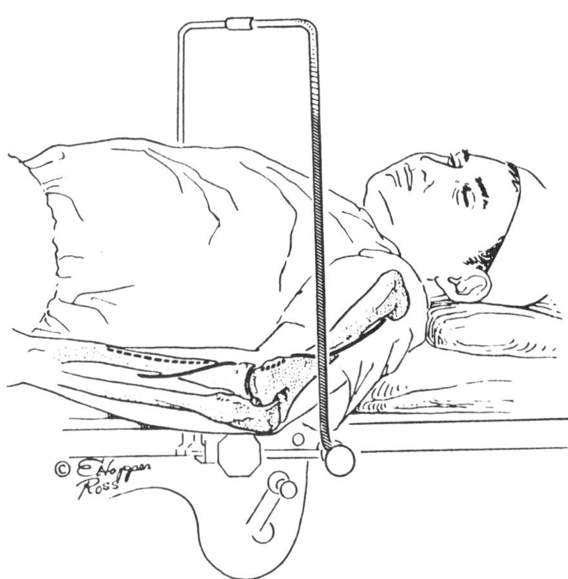

Figure 14-11. The radial nerve may be compressed against the humerus and the metal brace at the patient's head. (From Britt and Gordon,[3] with permission.)

Radial Nerve

The radial nerve may be injured if the arm slips off the side of the surgical table or if pressure is applied to the nerve as it traverses the spiral groove of the humerus (Fig. 14-11).[3] For example, the mechanical effects of differential pressure exerted at the distal edge of the inflatable cuff of an automated blood pressure monitor may be a rare cause of injury to the radial nerve. Clinically, radial nerve injury is manifested by wrist drop, inability to extend the metacarpophalangeal joints, and weakness of abduction of the thumb (Fig. 14-6).[8] There is also decreased sensation over the dorsal surface of the lateral three and one-half fingers and adjacent hand.

Median Nerve

Injury to the median nerve from positioning is unlikely. Rather, the median nerve, which runs adjacent to the medial cubital and basilic veins in the antecubital fossa, may be injured during intravenous injection of drugs such as thiopental, either by the needle itself or by extravasation of the drug. Injury to the median nerve manifests as inability to oppose the first and fifth digits and decreased sensation on the palmar surface of the lateral three and one-half fingers and adjacent hand (Fig. 14-6).[8]

Sciatic Nerve

The sciatic nerve may be injured by compression as the nerve passes under the piriformis muscle or by stretching, since the distance between points of fixation of the nerve (sciatic notch and fibula) is increased by external rotation of the leg or extension of the knee. Stretch of the sciatic nerve is most likely to occur when patients are placed improperly into the lithotomy position (see the section *Lithotomy*). To minimize stretch of the sciatic nerve, the patient should be positioned such that external rotation of the legs is minimal and the knees should be flexed. Intramuscular injections into the buttock may damage the sciatic nerve, especially when needle placement is not in the recommended upper outer quadrant of the buttock. For this reason, intramuscular injections into the lateral aspect of the thigh may be the preferred approach. Injury to the sciatic nerve manifests as weakness of all the skeletal muscles below the knee and diminished sensation over the lateral half of the leg and almost all of the foot, with the exception of the inner border of the arch.

Common Peroneal Nerve

The common peroneal nerve, which is a branch of the sciatic nerve, is the most frequently damaged nerve in the lower extremity. Most often this damage reflects compression of the nerve between the head of the fibula and the metal brace used in the lithotomy position. Proper padding greatly decreases the likelihood of this complication. Injury to the common peroneal nerve manifests as foot drop, loss of dorsal extension of the toes, and inability to evert the foot (Fig. 14-7).[8]

Anterior Tibial Nerve

Foot drop may manifest postoperatively if the feet are plantar flexed for extended periods during anesthesia (Fig. 14-7).[8] Patients in the sitting position should have a foot support under their feet, and patients in the prone position should have a roll placed under the anterior aspect of the ankle to maintain the extended position.

Femoral Nerve

The femoral nerve may be compressed at the pelvic brim by the blade of a self-retaining retractor as used during a laparotomy (abdominal hysterectomy) or by excessive angulation of the thigh when the patient is placed in the lithotomy position (vaginal hysterectomy). On examination, there is a decreased or absent knee jerk and loss of flexion of the hip and extension of the knee as a result of quadriceps femoris injury. Sensation is absent to decreased over the superior aspect of the thigh and medial and anteromedial side of the leg. Diabetes mellitus is present in most patients who develop femoral neuropathy. The possibility of femoral nerve injury due to these mechanisms must be considered when neurologic deficits in the postoperative period are attributed to a prior regional anesthetic.

Saphenous Nerve

The saphenous nerve is a branch of the femoral nerve and can be damaged by compression against the medial tibial condyle if the foot is suspended lateral to a vertical brace (Fig. 14-12).[3] This complication is minimized by appropriate padding between the legs and metal leg brace.

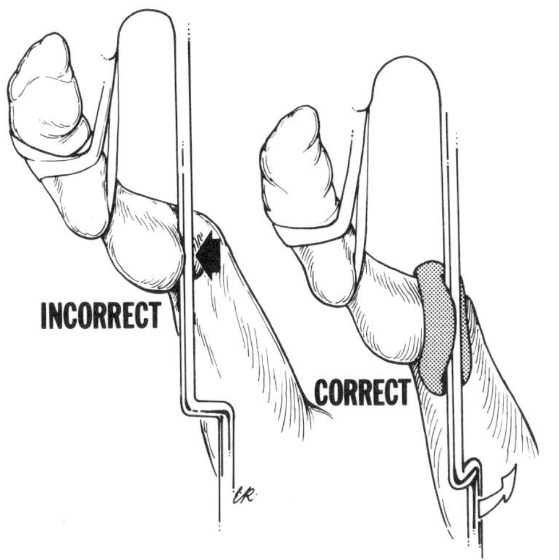

Figure 14-12. In the lithotomy position, the saphenous nerve can be compressed by the stirrups used to elevate the legs when padding is inadequate. (From Britt and Gordon,[3] with permission.)

Obturator Nerve

Damage to the obturator nerve manifests as inability to adduct the leg and diminished sensation over the medial side of the thigh. This nerve may be damaged during difficult forceps delivery or by excessive flexion of the thigh to the groin.

NON-NEURAL INJURY

Injury to the skin, eyes, and appendages are examples of non-neural damage related to positioning during anesthesia.

Skin

Excessive pressure over an area of skin may result in ischemia and localized ulceration. In severe cases, a skin graft may be required. Any area of skin on which excessive pressure has been exerted, as over bony prominences (medial malleoli, heels, supraorbital ridge), is vulnerable to ischemic damage. Ulceration of skin at the corner of the mouth may result from pressure of a tracheal tube at this site. Care must be taken to ensure that orthopaedic frames used to support patients during hip procedures are well padded to prevent pressure necrosis, especially in the groin.

Eyes

Pressure on the eyes, as may occur from headrests used in the prone position, may cause thrombosis of the central retinal artery with permanent blindness. The likelihood of this complication is increased when deliberate or accidental hypotension accompanies the anesthetic. Care must be exercised by the anesthesiologist to ensure that the orbit of the eye can be felt in its entirety so as to ensure absence of pressure on the eye.

Appendages

Whenever parts of a surgical table are being moved, the possibility of a finger or toe being damaged in a progressively narrowing gap between the main portion and the part of the table being moved must be appreciated. The most likely problem is trauma to the fingers when the foot of the adjustable surgical table is returned to the horizontal position from the lithotomy position. The ear may be damaged if it is forcibly folded between the patient's head and the mattress of the surgical table.

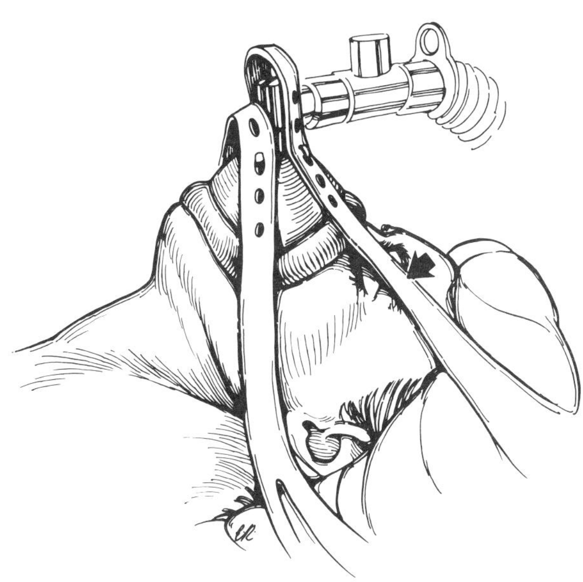

Figure 14-13. Several complications can occur from excessive pressure with application of an anesthetic face mask and mask strap. The outer third of the eyebrow can disappear with excessive compression from the strap. The buccal branch of the facial nerve can be injured from the mask strap; also, necrosis of the bridge of the nose can occur from excessive pressure by the anesthetic mask.

DAMAGE RELATED TO THE ANESTHETIC FACE MASK

Improper application of the anesthetic face mask may result in several complications. For example, loss of hair of the outer third of the eyebrow (which does not grow back) may reflect pressure from the face mask strap (Fig. 14-13). The likelihood of this complication is decreased by placing a gauze pad beneath the face mask strap to avoid discrete pressure on the outer third of the eyebrow. Another complication from the face mask strap is pressure on the buccal branch of the facial nerve, resulting in paresis of the orbicularis oris muscle. Pressure from the anesthetic face mask may cause necrosis of the bridge of the nose. The likelihood of this complication is minimized by removing the mask from the face periodically and massaging the bridge of the nose to restore circulation to the compressed area.

Compression of the supraorbital nerve by the tracheal tube connector manifests as decreased sensation over the forehead and pain in the eye (Fig. 14-14). The facial nerve may be damaged by compression between the anesthesiologist's fingers and the ascending ramus of the patient's mandible if extreme and prolonged manual forward pressure is required to maintain a patent upper airway.

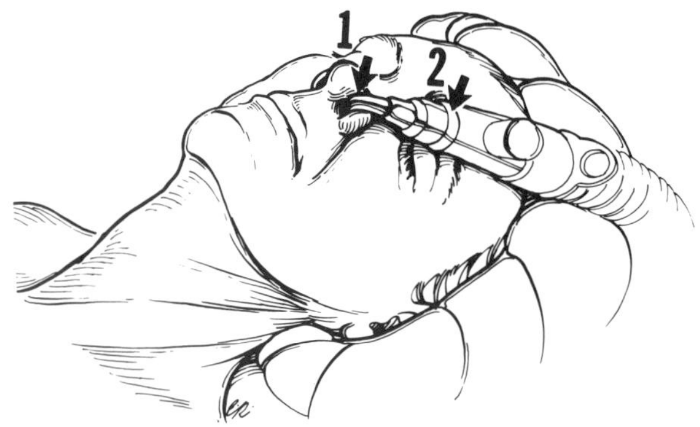

Figure 14-14. Pressure on the nasal opening by the connector can result in tissue ischemia and damage (1). The supraorbital nerve can be compressed by a tracheal tube connector, especially when padding is insufficient (2).

REFERENCES

1. Froese AB, Bryan AC. Effects of anesthesia and paralysis on diaphragmatic mechanisms in man. Anesthesiology 1974;41:242–7.
2. Wilcox S, Vandam LD. Alas, poor Trendelenburg and his position! A critique of its uses and effectiveness. Anesth Analg 1988;67:574–8.
3. Britt BA, Gordon RA. Peripheral nerve injuries associated with anaesthesia. Can Anaesth Soc J 1964; 11:514–36.
4. Dalrymple DG, MacGowan SW. Cardiorespiratory effects of the sitting position in neurosurgery. Br J Anaesth 1979;51:1079–82.
5. Kroll DA, Caplan RA, Posner K, Ward RJ, Cheney FW. Nerve injury associated with anesthesia. Anesthesiology 1990;73:202-7.
6. Stoelting RK. Postoperative ulnar nerve palsy—Is it a preventable complication? Anesth Analg 1993;76:7–9.
7. Britt BA, Joy N, Mackay MB. Positioning trauma. In: Orkin FK, Cooperman LH, eds. Complications of Anesthesia. Philadelphia, JB Lippincott 1983;646–70.
8. Martin JT (ed). Positioning in Anesthesia and Surgery. 2nd Ed. Philadelphia, WB Saunders 1987;1–347
9. Wadsworth TG. The cubital tunnel and the external compression syndrome. Anesth Analg 1974;53:303–8.

15 Monitoring

Monitoring of anesthetized patients is designed to collect data that reflect (1) physiologic homeostasis, allowing prompt recognition of adverse changes; (2) responses to therapeutic interventions; and (3) proper functioning of anesthetic equipment. Monitoring as such provides an early warning of adverse changes or trends before irreversible damage occurs. The most important monitor in the operating room is the vigilant anesthesiologist, who continuously obtains subjective and objective information from the anesthetized patient. Subjective monitoring depends on the anesthesiologist's senses (visual, touching, auditory, "sixth sense") and experience. This continual vigilance (awareness) on the part of the anesthesiologist is enhanced by the use of monitoring equipment designed to provide objective data relevant to the anesthetized patient's well-being. Indeed, human vigilance is not infallible, which emphasizes the importance of using monitors beyond the anesthesiologist's subjective observation.[1]

Standards for basic intraoperative monitoring have been adopted by the American Society of Anesthesiologists (see Appendix 1). For example, these standards either encourage or mandate the use of pulse oximetry, capnography, an oxygen analyzer, a disconnnect alarm, and a visual display of the electrocardiogram (ECG) in all patients undergoing anesthesia. Blood pressure and heart rate must be evaluated at least every 5 minutes. As with all such policy statements, however, the anesthesiologist must exercise medical judgments in the application of these standards as dictated by extenuating circumstances. Depending on the patient's medical condition and the complexity of surgery, intraoperative monitoring may be expanded to include more technologically sophisticated and often invasive monitors. The inherent risk in the use of all monitors, especially invasive monitors, must be weighed against the potential benefits in selecting their use for individual patients (Fig. 15-1).[2]

COMMONLY EMPLOYED NONINVASIVE MONITORS

Automated Arterial Blood Pressure Devices

Automated oscillometry has replaced auscultatory and palpatory techniques for routine intraoperative and early postoperative blood pressure monitoring. An oscillometric device such as the Dinamap automatically measures and displays systolic blood pressure, diastolic blood pressure, mean arterial pressure, and heart rate by sampling oscillations in the cuff (Fig. 15-2). After the cuff is inflated by an air pump, cuff pressure is held constant while oscillations are sampled. If no oscillations are sampled, the computer opens a deflation valve and the next level is sampled for oscillations. A variety of cuff sizes (the width should be about 40% of the circumference of the arm) make it possible to utilize oscillometry in all age groups. Too small a cuff or one that is too loosely wrapped around the arm may result in falsely increased blood pressure readings. Frequent blood pressure measurements can result in edema of the extremity distal to the cuff, emphasizing the importance of cycling the device only as often as deemed necessary but at least every 5 minutes.

Monitoring that Requires No Instrumentation

Inspection
- Skin—color, capillary refill, rash, edema
- Nail beds—color, capillary refill
- Mucous membranes—color, moisture, edema
- Surgical field—color of tissues and blood, rate of blood loss, skeletal muscle relaxation
- Movement—purposeful or reflex
- Eyes—conjunctiva (color and edema), pupils (size, reactivity)

Palpation
- Skin—temperature and texture
- Pulse—fullness, rate, and regularity
- Skeletal muscle—tone

Percussion
- Gastric—distension
- Chest—pneumothorax

Auscultation
Chest—ventilation and cardiac sounds
Blood pressure—sphygmomanometry

Monitors Used During Anesthesia

Blood pressure	Body temperature
Precordial or esophageal stethoscope	Oxygen analyzer
Electrocardiogram	Artery blood gases and pH
Pulse oximeter	Central venous pressure catheter
Capnograph	Pulmonary artery catheter
Mass spectrometry	Echocardiography
Raman spetroscopy	Electroencephalogram
Disconnect alarm	Evoked potentials
Spirometer	
Urine output	
Peripheral nerve stimulator	

When monitoring patients with low blood pressures, oscillometric devices may display mean arterial pressure but not systolic and diastolic blood pressure.

Precordial or Esophageal Stethoscope

A weighted precordial stethoscope is commonly applied over the suprasternal notch or heart before the induction of anesthesia and is connected with tubing to a monaural earpiece worn by the anesthesiologist (Fig. 15-3). This arrangement allows continuous monitoring of heart sounds and breath sounds by the anesthesiologist and leaves the other ear available for operating room communication. After intubation of the trachea, an esophageal stethoscope is commonly inserted. This stethoscope has the advantage of being close to the heart, where both breath sounds and heart sounds are clearly audible. Routine use of an esophageal stethoscope during maintenance of anesthesia facilitates early detection of (1) changes in heart rate, (2) onset of cardiac dysrhythmias, (3) development of increased airway resistance, and (4) failure to ventilate the lungs of a paralyzed patient. A temperature sensor may be incorporated into the esophageal stethoscope.

Electrocardiogram

Continuous visual display of the anesthetized patient's ECG on an oscilloscope is the standard of care for all patients undergoing anesthesia, thus providing information for the detection of (1) cardiac dysrhythmias, (2) myocardial ischemia as reflected by ST segment depression, and (3) electrolyte changes, particularly potassium. The heart rate is often calculated from the ECG tracing. The ability to retain a portion of the ECG on the oscilloscope screen or to obtain a hard copy recording is helpful for more detailed analysis of the tracing. An audible indicator for each QRS complex allows the anesthesiologist to carry on other activities while listening for changes in heart rate or cardiac rhythm.

Lead II is commonly used for detection of cardiac dysrhythmias because it parallels the P-wave vector, resulting in maximum amplitude of the P wave on the ECG. Inferior wall myocardial ischemia of the left ventricle may be reflected by ST segment depression in lead II. More common sites of myocardial ischemia, however, are the anterior and lateral walls of the left ventricle, which are best monitored by a precordial lead in the V5 position (fifth intercostal space along

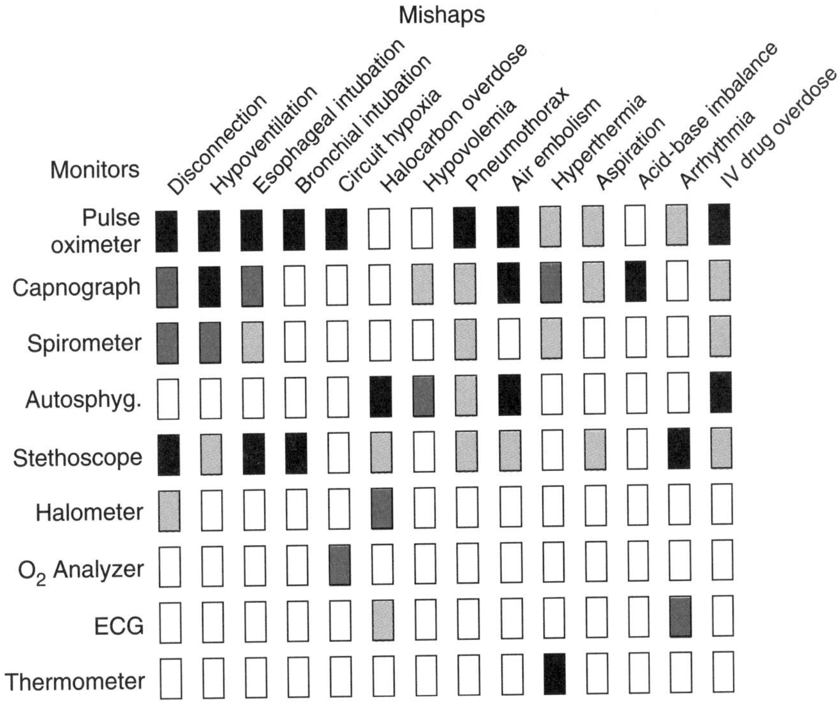

Figure 15-1. Estimate of the relative value of several monitors for detection of a variety of potential intraoperative mishaps. Most mishaps can be detected to some degree with the pulse oximeter and/or capnograph. Dark red, high value; black, moderate value; light red, low value; white, no value. (From Whitcher et al.,[2] with permission.)

the anterior axillary line). For this reason, a V5 lead is often used when the goal is to monitor the ECG for the detection of myocardial ischemia. The equivalent of a V5 lead can be obtained with three electrodes by placing the left arm electrode in the V5 position and selecting lead aVL on the monitor.

It must be recognized that the ECG reflects only the electrical activities occurring in the heart and in no way is a measure of heart function. For example, normal ECG complexes may persist on the oscilloscope in the absence of an effective cardiac output (pulseless electrical activity).

Pulse Oximetry

Pulse oximetry is the standard of care for the continuous and noninvasive monitoring of peripheral arterial hemoglobin oxygen saturation (SpO_2) as a reflection of arterial hemoglobin oxygen saturation (SaO_2) during anesthesia and the early postoperative period in all age groups. This practical, noninvasive, and reliable monitor provides an early warning of arterial hypoxemia that is often not appreciated by subjective observations.[3] The routine use of pulse

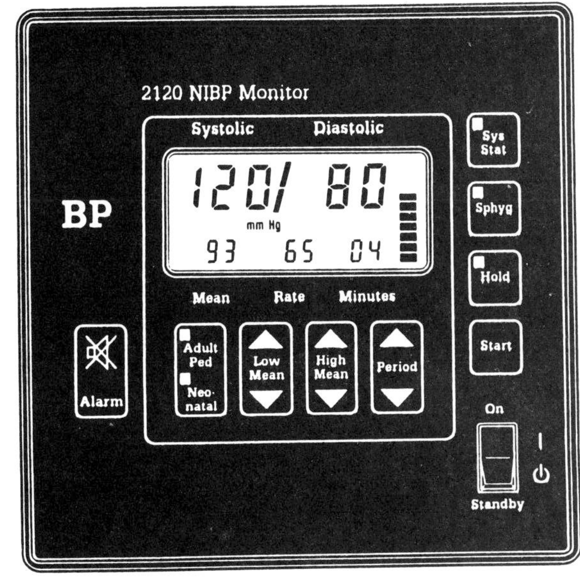

Figure 15-2. Example of a noninvasive automatic monitoring device providing digital display of blood pressure and heart rate.

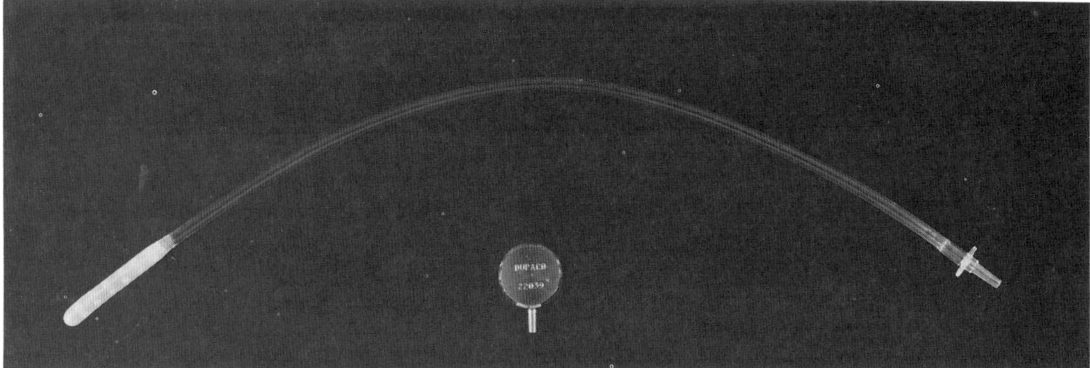

Figure 15-3. A typical weighted precordial stethoscope and esophageal stethoscope.

oximetry has decreased the need for measurement of PaO_2 to confirm the acceptability of arterial oxygenation in the perioperative period. A light-emitting diode that measures absorption of specific wavelengths of light relative to the ratio of oxyhemoglobin and reduced hemoglobin is most commonly placed on the patient's finger or ear. A computer calculates SpO_2 and displays this value along with an arterial blood pressure waveform and heart rate on a screen (Fig. 15-4). Alarms can be set for high and low values of SpO_2 and heart rate. Maintenance of SpO_2 above 90% is evidence that the PaO_2 is most likely higher than 60 mmHg. Despite the widespread clinical acceptance of the value of pulse oximetry, the relationship between the use of this monitor and enhanced patient safety remains unproven.[4]

Limitations

The appropriate use of pulse oximetry necessitates an appreciation of both physiologic and technical limitations. Because the technique uses light absorbence changes produced by arterial pulsations, any event that significantly decreases vascular pulsations (hypotension, hypothermia, vasoconstriction) will decrease the ability of the pulse oximeter to obtain and process the signal and thus calculate SpO_2. In this regard, it is often necessary to change sensor sites (finger, ear) to obtain an optimal signal. Motion artifact, as evidenced by a heart rate discrepancy between the ECG and pulse oximeter, may interfere with accurate calculation of SpO_2 in awake, agitated, or shivering patients. Ambient light as well as other light sources (radiant warmers, fluorescent bulbs) can contaminate light-emitting diode signals. Nail polish can alter the spectra of emitted light. The presence of dysfunctional hemoglobins can alter the ability of the SpO_2 to accurately reflect SaO_2. Carboxyhemoglobin is read as oxyhemoglobin by pulse oximeters, producing a falsely high SpO_2. This is the reason the SpO_2 may exceed the SaO_2 as measured by a laboratory co-oximeter. Methylene blue causes a spurious decrease in SpO_2. A high methemoglobin concentration tends to result in an SpO_2 reading of 85% regardless of the actual PaO_2 or SaO_2. Fetal hemoglobin has limited influences on the accuracy of the SpO_2 measurement. Complications from the use of pulse oximetry are most commonly caused by errors in data interpretation. Use of pulse oximetry during magnetic resonance imaging has been associated with skin burns.

Factors that Influence Accuracy of Pulse Oximetry

Low flow conditions
Motion
Ambient light
Dysfunctional hemoglobins (carboxyhemoglobin, methemoglobin)
Methylene blue
Altered relationship between PaO_2 and SaO_2 (shift in oxyhemoglobin dissociation curve)

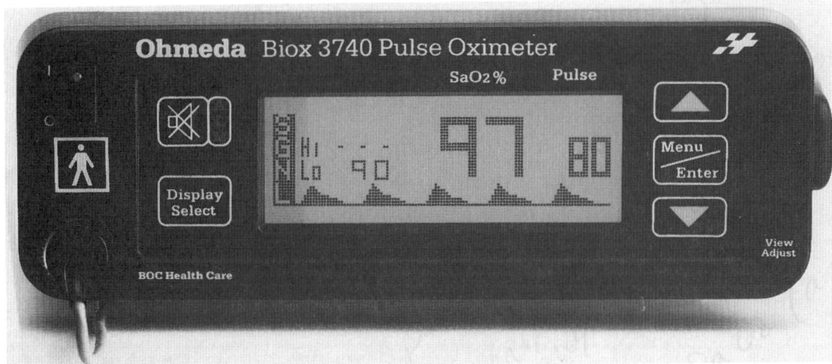

Figure 15-4. Example of a pulse oximeter providing a visual display of the arterial pulse waveform and a digital display of peripheral arterial hemoglobin oxygen saturation and heart rate.

Transcutaneous PO_2 ($PtcO_2$)

Transcutaneous oxygen sensors use polarographic oxygen electrodes to measure oxygen that diffuses to the skin surface (heated to 43°C) from the dermal capillaries beneath the electrode. The $PtcO_2$ is flow dependent such that changes in cardiac output (decreased tissue perfusion) influence the measurement. In hemodynamically stable infants the $PtcO_2$ closely estimates the PaO_2, thus permitting control of arterial oxygenation when retinopathy of prematurity is a risk.[3] Skin burns are the most common complications associated with $PtcO_2$ monitoring; the sensor site should be changed every 2 hours in neonates.

Capnography

Capnography is the continuous measurement of the patient's inhaled and exhaled concentrations of carbon dioxide (Table 15-1).[5] Display of the waveform is preferable to a digital readout of the values (Fig. 15-5). When an endotracheal tube is inserted, its presence in the trachea must be verified by clinical assessment and identification of carbon dioxide in the exhaled gases. In addition to accidental esophageal intubation, the absence of carbon dioxide in the patient's exhaled gases alerts the anesthesiologist to accidental disconnection of a paralyzed patient from the anesthetic breathing system (also detected by a disconnnect alarm) or the sudden cessation of pulmonary blood flow (cardiac arrest). A gradual decrease in exhaled carbon dioxide concentrations over several breaths may reflect a partial leak in the anesthetic breathing system or decreased

Table 15-1. Causes of Changes in the Exhaled Concentrations of Carbon Dioxide

Increase	Decrease
Hypoventilation	Hyperventilation
Malignant hyperthermia	Hypothermia
Sepsis	Low cardiac output
Rebreathing	Pulmonary embolism
Administration of bicarbonate	Accidental disconnection or tracheal extubation
Insufflation of carbon dioxide during laparoscopy	Cardiac arrest

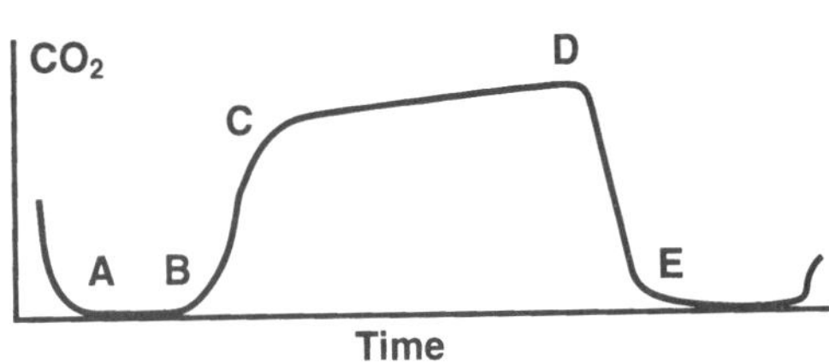

Figure 15-5. The capnogram is divided into four distinct phases. Phase A–B represents exhalation of anatomic deadspace gases and is normally devoid of carbon dioxide. Phase B–C is present on the capnogram as a sharp upstroke that is determined by the evenness of ventilation and alveolar emptying. A slow rate of rise in this phase may reflect chronic obstructive pulmonary disease or acute airway obstruction, including bronchospasm. Phase C–D reflects exhalation of alveolar gas, with point D being designated the end-tidal carbon dioxide concentration (see Table 15-1). Periodic oscillations are produced in the expiratory plateau by spontaneous breathing efforts. Phase D–E reflects the beginning of inspiration and entrainment of gases lacking carbon dioxide. Normally, unless rebreathing of carbon dioxide occurs, the baseline approaches zero.

pulmonary blood flow as may accompany hypotension or pulmonary embolism. Hypoventilation or unexpected increases in carbon dioxide production as associated with malignant hyperthermia or thyroid storm will be promptly reflected by increases in the exhaled concentrations of carbon dioxide. Rebreathing of carbon dioxide due to an exhausted carbon dioxide absorber or malfunctioning inspiratory or expiratory valves will manifest as increased inspired and exhaled concentrations of carbon dioxide. The presence of exhaled carbon dioxide during cardiopulmonary resuscitation is evidence that external cardiac compressions are generating pulmonary blood flow and presumably blood flow to major organs such as the brain and heart. The end-tidal carbon dioxide concentration often underestimates the $PaCO_2$, reflecting an alveolar-to-arterial difference for carbon dioxide due to deadspace ventilation. By contrast, transcutaneous carbon dioxide measurements have been shown to correlate with $PaCO_2$, presumably because the values are not influenced by the presence of deadspace ventilation. When precise knowledge and control of the $PaCO_2$ are indicated, as in patients with increased intracranial pressure, the possible value of transcutaneous carbon dioxide measurements may be a consideration.

Multiple Gas Analysis

Techniques to permit monitoring of the inhaled and exhaled concentrations of respiratory (oxygen, carbon dioxide, nitrogen) and anesthetic (volatile anesthetics, nitrous oxide) gases include infrared absorption, mass spectrometry, and Raman spectroscopy.

Infrared Absorption

Infrared absorption provides a rapid response time that is particularly useful for measuring real time exhaled carbon dioxide waveforms (capnography). The infrared wavelengths for carbon dioxide and nitrous oxide overlap. As a result, capnometers that use infrared absorption must measure the concentrations of both carbon dioxide and nitrous oxide so they may correct for the overlapping absorption. For a molecule to absorb infrared light, it must be asymmetric, which means infrared absorption will not be useful in detecting symmetric molecules such as oxygen and nitrogen.

Mass Spectrometry

Mass spectrometry permits intermittent or continuous measurement of airway gas composition, including inhaled anesthetics, during inhalation and exhalation. The use of mass spectrometry, particularly if continuous measurement is possible, decreases or eliminates the need for oxygen analyzers and capnography as these monitors would only duplicate information already provided. Nitrogen measurement detects air embolism and air entrainment into the anesthetic breathing system. The inspired-to-exhaled differences for anesthetic gases reflect principally the blood solubility of these drugs, whereas the exhaled concentration parallels the anesthetic depth (brain partial pressure), assuming that time for equilibration has occurred (see Chapter 2).

Raman Spectroscopy

Raman spectroscopy allows independent analysis of each respiratory and anesthetic gas. Unlike mass spectrometry, Raman spectroscopy does not alter the gas molecules, which can then be returned to the anesthetic delivery system. An instrument using Raman technology (Rascal) is commercially available and has an accuracy similar to that of mass spectrometry (Fig. 15-6).

Tidal Volume

A ventimeter or respirometer placed in the anesthetic breathing system (commonly on the exhalation limb) measures tidal volume and permits calculation of minute ventilation (frequency of breathing times tidal volume). All leaks in the anesthetic breathing system must be eliminated for accurate measurement of tidal volume.

Airway Pressure

Airway pressure created by mechanical ventilation of the lungs is measured by a gauge on the anesthesia machine (see Fig. 10-1). When the maximum inspiratory pressure does not reach predetermined levels, a low pressure disconnect alarm sounds that warns the anesthesiologist that a large leak or disconnect is present. Excessive airway pressures measured on this gauge reflect low pulmonary compliance or obstruction in the anesthetic breathing system (closed adjustable pressure-limiting valve). The gas reservoir bag is designed to expand into a

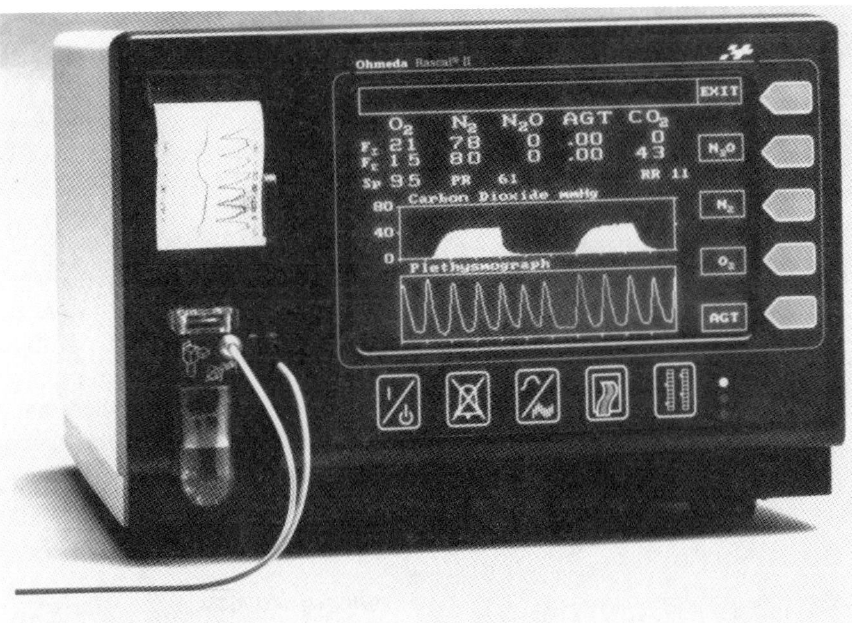

Figure 15-6. Example of a multiple respiratory and anesthetic gas analyzer (Rascal), including a built-in pulse oximeter.

sphere when pressures exceed about 50 cmH_2O, preventing transmission of higher pressures to the patient's airways. When a mechanical ventilator is used, the gas reservoir bag is excluded from the anesthetic breathing system, making it possible to deliver pressures higher than 50 cmH_2O to the airways.

Clinical Monitoring of Breathing

When patients breathe spontaneously during general anesthesia, the pattern of breathing (frequency, depth, regularity) should be continuously monitored by the anesthesiologist. This is accomplished by visual and tactile (hand on the bag) monitoring of the movements of the reservoir bag on the anesthetic breathing system, by observation of chest movement, and by auscultation of the chest via either a precordial or esophageal stethoscope. The character of respiratory movements is helpful in assessing the depth of anesthesia. Also, by correlating chest movements to movements of the reservoir bag, a judgment can be made regarding the presence or absence of upper airway obstruction. Breathing is often rapid and shallow in the presence of inhaled anesthetics, whereas opioids usually decrease breathing frequency while tidal volume may be increased.

Renal Function

In selected patients, measurement of urine output can be a useful guide to intravascular fluid volume (see Chapter 21). Monitoring urine output also permits early detection of hemoglobinuria, an initial sign of hemolytic transfusion reactions.

Peripheral Nerve Stimulator

It is desirable to monitor the status of the neuromuscular junction with a peripheral nerve stimulator when using muscle relaxants during anesthesia (see Chapter 7). This monitor facilitates the assessment of both the adequacy of neuromuscular blockade and spontaneous and/or drug-enhanced recovery.

Body Temperature

Appropriate equipment to continuously measure the patient's body temperature must be available and used when significant changes in body temperature are likely to occur. Body temperature often decreases 1°C to 4°C during anesthesia and surgery performed in cold operating rooms. Although this decrease in body temperature is usually not serious, postoperative awakening may be delayed, and shivering, when it occurs, may increase oxygen requirements by as much as 400%.

Sites for monitoring body temperature are the esophagus, nasopharynx, rectum, bladder, and tympanic membrane. A temperature probe in the lower third of the esophagus (often placed via an esophageal stethoscope) accurately reflects blood temperature. Nasopharyngeal temperature is accurate when a cuffed tube in the trachea prevents artificial cooling of the nasopharynx by respiratory gases. Epistaxis is a risk when a temperature probe is inserted into the nasopharynx. Tympanic membrane temperature reflects the temperature of blood perfusing the brain. Risks of tympanic membrane temperature probes are external auditory canal bleeding and perforation of the tympanic membrane.

Oxygen Analyzers

During every administration of general anesthesia, the inspired concentration of oxygen in the anesthetic delivery system must be measured by an oxygen analyzer with a low oxygen concentration limit alarm. The oxygen analyzer is calibrated with room air and oxygen, with the alarm usually set to sound when the inspired oxygen concentration decreases below 30%.

INVASIVE MONITORING OF THE CARDIOVASCULAR SYSTEM

Invasive monitoring of the cardiovascular system is reserved for complex and sometimes prolonged operations often in patients with significant co-existing medical diseases (Table 15-2). Intra-arterial, central venous pressure, and pulmonary artery catheters (Swan-Ganz) are examples of invasive monitors placed and used by anesthesiologists. The risk-to-benefit ratio and cost are important considerations in the selection of these monitors for individual patients. It is recommended that the anesthesiologist responsible for inserting invasive monitors wear gloves and protective eyeglasses to minimize the risk of transmission of blood-borne diseases from the patient.

Intra-arterial Blood Pressure

Continuous recording of blood pressure from a catheter placed in a peripheral artery allows beat-to-beat monitoring and provides a reliable access site to obtain samples for analyses of arterial blood gases, pH, and electrolytes. Although several peripheral arteries are available for cannulation (radial, brachial, femoral, dorsalis pedis, superficial temporal), the radial artery is most commonly selected.

Table 15-2. Measured and Calculated Hemodynamic Variables

	Normal Value	Range
Systemic blood pressure (mmHg)	120/80	90–140/70–90
Mean arterial pressure (mmHg)	93	77–97
Heart rate (beats·min^{-1})	72	60–80
Mean right atrial (central venous) pressure (mmHg)	5	0–10
Right ventricular pressure (mmHg)	25/5	15–30/0–10
Pulmonary artery pressure (mmHg)	23/10	15–30/5–15
Mean pulmonary artery pressure (mmHg)	15	10–20
Pulmonary artery occlusion (wedge) pressure (mmHg)	10	5–15
Mean left atrial pressure (mmHg)	8	4–12
Cardiac output (L·min^{-1})	5	4–6
Stroke volume (ml·beat^{-1})	70	60–90
Systemic vascular resistance (dynes·s·cm^{-5})	1200	900–1500
Pulmonary vascular resistance (dynes·s·cm^{-5})	100	50–150

Before cannulation, an Allen test may be performed to determine the adequacy of collateral flow from the ulnar artery. The Allen test is performed by simultaneously occluding the radial and ulnar arteries and asking the patient to make a tight fist, which forces blood from the hand such that the palmar surface becomes blanched and appears pale. Pressure over the ulnar artery only is then released, and the patient is instructed to open the hand, avoiding hyperextension of the fingers. Return of color to the palmar surface of the hand within 5 to 15 seconds is considered to represent adequate collateral blood flow in the hand. Alternatively, a pulse oximeter placed on the thumb can be used instead of skin color to judge the adequacy of perfusion. Traditionally, inadequate collateral ulnar arterial blood flow, as suggested by the Allen test, has been considered a relative contraindication to insertion of a catheter into the corresponding radial artery. Nevertheless, there is evidence that adverse events do not follow cannulation of the radial artery in the presence of an abnormal Allen test.[6] Furthermore, decreased or absent radial arterial blood flow after removal of the catheter (presumably as a result of emboli) is of little or no clinical significance. The inescapable conclusion is that radial artery cannulation is a low-risk, high-benefit monitoring technique that deserves frequent use.

Cannulation of the radial artery is performed with the wrist dorsiflexed 40 to 60 degrees over a towel or gauze sponges (Fig. 15-7). Tape is used to immobilize the hand, and the course of the radial artery is palpated. The selected needle entry site is prepared with an antiseptic solution such as 70% alcohol, and if the patient is awake, this site is infiltrated with a small amount of local anesthetic solution. Sometimes it is helpful to make a superficial incision to avoid damaging the tip of the catheter as it is introduced through the skin. Typically, small-gauge (20 gauge in adults, 22 to 24 gauge in children) Teflon catheters are selected. The catheter is inserted at a 15- to 30-degree angle and advanced slowly until the lumen of the artery is entered as evidenced by the appearance of blood at the distal end (hub) of the catheter (Fig. 15-7). After successful placement, the catheter should be flushed continuously with a solution containing 1 to 2 units·ml^{-1} of heparin in saline at a rate of 1 to 3 ml·h^{-1}. This continuous flush is important in minimizing thrombus formation and for maintaining adequate arterial blood pressure waveforms.

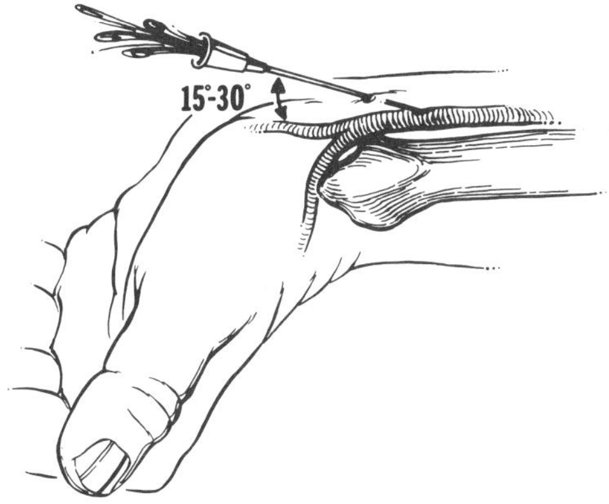

Figure 15-7. A schematic depiction of cannulation of the radial artery.

Central Venous Pressure

Catheterization of the central veins has become an important maneuver both for measuring central venous pressure and for providing long-term intravenous feedings, especially hyperalimentation. Furthermore, in an emergency, such as after acute hemorrhage with peripheral vasoconstriction, it may be impossible to catheterize a peripheral vein percutaneously and only a central vein may be available to infuse fluids for rapid restoration of blood volume. Specific central venous cannulation sites are associated with unique advantages and disadvantages (Table 15-3). The internal jugular vein is often preferred to the subclavian vein because there is a lower incidence of major complications. The nursing management of neck catheters, however, may be difficult. The right internal jugular vein is generally selected since it provides a shorter, more direct route than the left internal jugular vein to the superior vena cava. The subclavian vein has a wide caliber and is held open by surrounding tissue even in the presence of profound hypotension. The use of the subclavian vein allows the catheter to be securely fixed on the chest wall with sterile dressings. The external jugular vein is usually visible and thus easy to cannulate, serving as an alternative to arm veins.

Despite the use of a J-wire, it is not always possible to pass the catheter from the external jugular vein into the central venous circulation.

Cannulation of the internal jugular vein is initiated by placement of the patient in a head-down position (minimizes the risk of venous air embolism) with the head turned away from the site of venipuncture. The carotid artery is palpated before venipuncture to confirm that it is medial to the intended puncture site. A 22-gauge locator ("seeker") needle is often initially inserted along the anticipated course of the vein at the level of the cricoid cartilage and advanced until the return of desaturated venous blood confirms entry into the internal jugular vein. A 17- to 18-gauge thin wall needle (alternatively a catheter over needle) is advanced in the same direction as the locator needle until return of desaturated venous blood (verify venous location with a transduced pressure if any doubt) confirms entry into the internal jugular vein. At this point, a J-wire is inserted through the needle, the needle is removed, and a large catheter (sheath over dilator if a pulmonary artery catheter is to be inserted) is threaded over the wire into the vein. Accidental cannulation of the carotid artery with the sheath over dilator may necessitate surgical exploration and repair of the artery.

Cannulation of the subclavian vein is initiated by placement of the patient in a head-down position with the head turned away from the site of venipuncture. Placing a roll between the shoulder blades opens the space between the clavicle and first rib. Using an infraclavicular approach, a 17- to 18-gauge needle (alternatively a catheter over needle) is inserted 1 cm below the midpoint of the clavicle (Fig. 15-8). The needle is advanced toward the anesthesiologist's finger in the suprasternal notch, keeping close to bone. After return of desaturated venous blood confirms entry into the vein, a J-wire is inserted through the needle, the needle is removed, and a large catheter (sheath over dilator if a pulmonary artery catheter is to be inserted) is threaded over the wire into the vein. Pneumothorax occurs in about 1% of patients and is the reason for recommending a chest radiograph after catheter placement in the subclavian vein or before attempting insertion on the opposite side after a failed attempt at the first site.

Central venous pressure parallels right atrial pressure, and the normal waveform consists of three peaks and two descents (Fig. 15-9). From a clinical point of view, the right atrial pressure is influenced by the right ventricular volume. If the right ventricle fails to empty because of pulmonary hypertension or, more often, left ventricular failure, the central venous pressure will be increased and may incorrectly suggest that the patient's blood volume is expanded. If left ventricular failure is suspected, additional

Table 15-3. Central Venous Catheter Placement Sites

	Advantages	Disadvantages
Right internal jugular vein	Good landmarks Predictable anatomy Accessible from head of operating room table	Carotid artery puncture Trauma to brachial plexus
Left internal jugular vein	Same as above	Same as above Thoracic duct damage
Subclavian	Good landmarks Patent despite hypovolemia Patient comfort when awake	Pneumothorax
External jugular vein	Superficial location	Often difficult to thread catheter into the central circulation
Antecubital vein	Safety	Often difficult to thread catheter into the central circulation

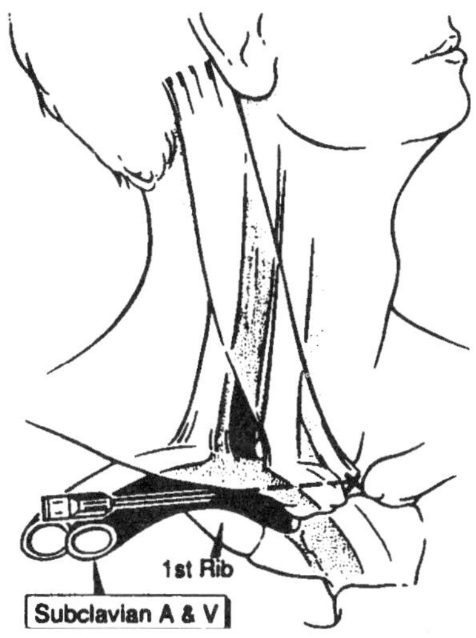

Figure 15-8. Infraclavicular approach for cannulation of the subclavian vein.

monitoring, such as a pulmonary artery catheter, may be helpful.

Pulmonary Artery Catheter

A flow-directed, balloon-tipped pulmonary artery catheter enables catheterization of the right heart for measurement of pressures without requiring the manipulative and radiologic control demanded by other methods of cardiac catheterization. The pulmonary artery occlusion (wedge) pressure reflects left atrial pressure because, at no flow, the pressures can equilibrate between the distal end of the pulmonary artery catheter and the left atrium. The flow-directed pulmonary artery catheter measures cardiac output by the thermodilution technique. Specifically, a thermistor in the distal end of the pulmonary artery catheter senses the change in blood temperature produced by the rapid injection of iced (or room temperature) solution administered through the proximal (central venous pressure) port of the catheter. Cardiac output is inversely proportional to the area under the time-temperature curve (calculated by the cardiac output computer and expressed as L·min^{-1}) because blood flow is the source of the thermal dilution. The output of only the right ventricle is measured by this technique. Specially designed pulmonary artery catheters are capable of providing cardiac pacing or fiberoptic oximetry with the ability to constantly monitor mixed venous hemoglobin oxygen saturation. When metabolic oxygen requirements are unchanging, the mixed venous hemoglobin oxygen saturation is directly proportional to the cardiac output.

Pulmonary artery catheters are often inserted percutaneously via the right internal jugular vein. Insertion of the catheter requires continuous displays of pressures and recognition of characteristic waveforms (Fig. 15-10). The balloon on the distal end of the catheter is inflated with 1 to 1.5 ml of air only after a right atrial tracing has been confirmed. The inflated balloon facilitates passage (flotation) of the distal end of the catheter with blood flow into the pulmonary artery. A right ventricular tracing

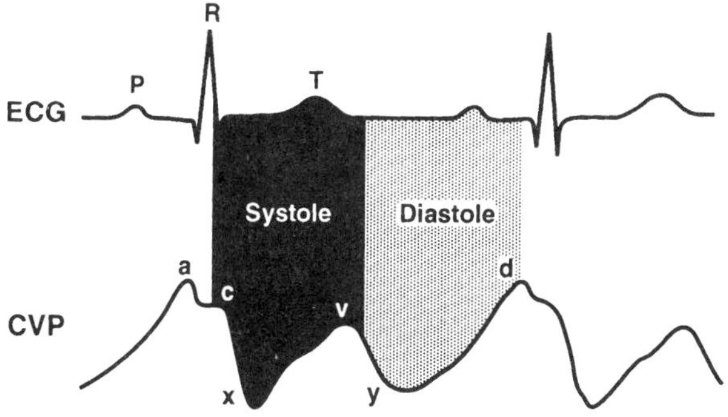

Figure 15-9. Central venous pressure (CVP) waveforms in relationship to electrical events on the electrocardiogram (ECG).

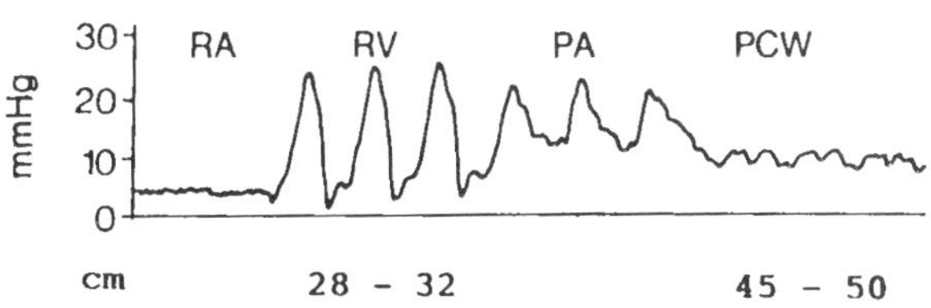

Figure 15-10. Schematic depiction of pressure waveforms as a pulmonary artery catheter passes through the right atrium (RA), right ventricle (RV), and pulmonary artery (PA). Note the narrowing of the pulse pressure ("diastolic step up") as the catheter enters the PA. Loss of a pulsatile trace as the catheter is advanced through the PA reflects the pulmonary capillary wedge (PCW) pressure (also designated pulmonary artery occlusion pressure [PAo]). Insertion of the pulmonary artery catheter through the right internal jugular vein should result in an RV tracing after the catheter has been advanced 28 to 32 cm and a PCW tracing at 45 to 50 cm.

should appear after the catheter is inserted 28 to 32 cm, and a pulmonary artery occlusion pressure tracing is evident after insertion of the catheter 45 to 50 cm. The balloon is deflated at this point, and a pulmonary artery pressure tracing should again appear. Reinflation of the balloon with about 1.0 ml of air should result in reappearance of the pulmonary artery occlusion pressure tracing. Strict adherence to these insertion distances will minimize the likelihood of catheter loops or intracardiac knot formation. The balloon should not be left in the inflated position except during actual measurement of pulmonary artery occlusion pressure so as to minimize the likelihood of pulmonary ischemia or infarction. Other risks of pulmonary artery catheter insertion include mechanically induced cardiac dysrhythmias and heart block. A rare but catastrophic complication of the use of pulmonary artery catheters is pulmonary artery perforation. Because the pulmonary artery diastolic pressure agrees well with the pulmonary artery occlusion pressure in the absence of pulmonary hypertension, it is logical to use the end-diastolic pressure as an indirect measurement of left atrial pressure.

Indications for Insertion of a Pulmonary Artery Catheter

- Poor left ventricular function (ejection fraction <0.4; cardiac index <2 $L \cdot min^{-1} \cdot m^{-2}$)
- Assessment of intravascular fluid volume
- Evaluation of response to fluid administration or administration of drugs (vasopressors, vasodilators, inotropes)
- Valvular heart disease
- Recent myocardial infarction
- Adult respiratory distress syndrome
- Massive trauma (shock, hemorrhage)
- Major vascular surgery (cross-clamping of aorta, large fluid shifts)

Indications for use of the pulmonary artery catheter are numerous and often controversial. The need for intravascular fluid volume replacement, the presence of underlying cardiac diseases, and the response to intravenous fluid infusion are commonly monitored with a pulmonary artery catheter (Table 15-4). Measurement of cardiac filling pressures and cardiac output and calculation of systemic and pulmonary vascular resistance are essential information for evaluating various disorders.

Echocardiography

Intraoperative cardiac imaging with two-dimensional transesophageal echocardiography can be used to monitor cardiac function during anesthesia and surgery in selected patients.

Information Derived from Intraoperative Echocardiography

- Regional ventricular wall motion, (myocardial ischemia)
- Ejection fraction
- Cardiac valve function (mitral, aortic)
- Intracardiac air
- Effects of anesthesia and surgery on cardiac function

MONITORING OF THE NERVOUS SYSTEM

The electroencephalogram (EEG) is used to monitor the central nervous system, and evoked potentials provide a method to evaluate the intactness of neural pathways.

Electroencephalogram

The EEG is a monitor of cerebral function that provides early evidence of cerebral ischemia, as during carotid endarterectomy or cardiopulmonary bypass. The EEG has also been advocated to monitor the depth of anesthesia. During periods of cerebral ischemia or while the patient is under general anesthesia, EEG activity generally decreases in both amplitude and frequency. The complexity of the EEG and its interpretation, plus variable and often unpredictable effects of events (changes in body temperature, alterations in $PaCO_2$) and anesthetic

Table 15-4. Use of Pulmonary Artery Catheter to Evaluate Hemodynamic Disorders

	Central Venous Pressure	Pulmonary Artery Occlusion Pressure (PAo)	Pulmonary Artery End-Diastolic Pressure (PAEDP)
Hypovolemia	Decreased	Decreased	PAEDP = PAo
Left ventricular failure	Increased	Increased	PAEDP = PAo
Right ventricular failure	Increased	No change	PAEDP = PAo
Pulmonary embolism	Increased	No change	PAEDP > PAo
Cardiac tamponade	Increased	Increased	PAEDP = PAo

drugs on the EEG tracing, detract from the frequent use of this monitor.

Evoked Potentials

Evoked potentials are the electrophysiologic responses of the nervous system to sensory stimulation (somatic, auditory, visual) that allow assessment of the functional integrity of neural pathways during anesthesia. For example, somatosensory evoked potentials are produced by application of small electrical currents that stimulate a peripheral nerve, such as the median nerve at the wrist or posterior tibial nerve at the ankle (Fig. 15-11).[7] The resulting recorded evoked potential reflects the intactness (or interruption) of neural pathways from the peripheral nerve through the spinal cord to the somatosensory cortex. This type of monitoring is particularly useful in confirming the intactness of the sensory spinal cord pathways in anesthetized patients undergoing Harrington rod procedures for treatment of scoliosis. It is important to recognize that this type of monitoring does not assess the integrity of motor spinal cord pathways. Monitoring of motor evoked potentials or a "wake-up test" to document patient movement is necessary to confirm that the Harrington rod procedure has not damaged the motor pathways of the spinal cord.

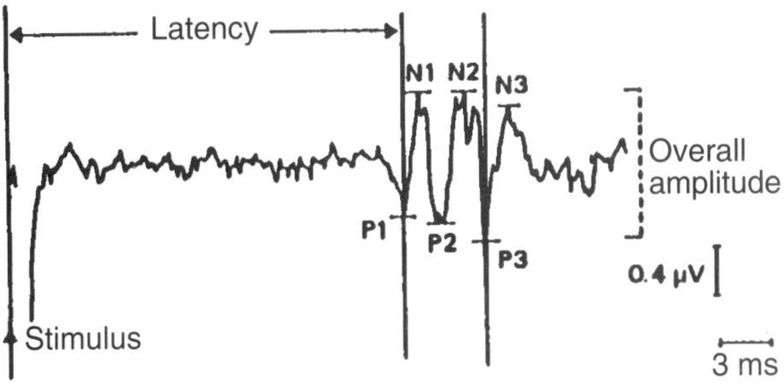

Figure 15-11. A typical somatosensory evoked potential consisting of three positive peaks (P1, P2, and P3) and three negative peaks (N1, N2, and N3). More than a 50% decrease in the amplitude of the positive peaks and/or loss of one or more of the negative peaks may indicate the effects of volatile anesthetics or interference with transmission of sensory nerve impulses. (From Loghnan and Hall,[7] with permission.)

Volatile anesthetics, especially in high concentrations, and hypothermia may produce changes in the latency period and amplitude of evoked potentials that are similar to alterations produced by neural ischemia. Opioids produce the least change in evoked potentials and may be selected for this reason to provide a portion of the anesthetic maintenance in patients undergoing operations that benefit from use of this form of monitoring. As with the EEG, the complexity and cost of evoked potential monitoring limit its frequent use.

ELECTRICAL HAZARDS

Electrical monitoring equipment that is connected to a patient may result in delivery of leakage (extraneous) currents that produce thermal injury (burns) or cardiac dysrhythmias (ventricular fibrillation). Prevention of electrical injury to patients and operating room personnel requires elimination of extraneous voltage sources, especially in the presence of connections (electrolyte-filled connecting tubing to a central venous pressure monitor) that result in complete circuits through tissues. For example, as little as 20 µA of 60 Hz applied directly to the endocardium can produce ventricular fibrillation. The high frequency current produced by the electrosurgical unit, however, does not produce cardiac dysrhythmias.

Monitors must be designed such that leakage currents are conducted to ground and not to the patient. Line isolation monitors detect leakage current and alert the anesthesiologist, by an audible alarm and the appearance of a red warning light, to discontinue use of the malfunctioning monitor until appropriate repairs are performed. Indeed, periodic preventive maintenance of electrical equipment is a recommended practice. It is important to recognize, however, that isolation transformers limit the hazard of macroshock but not microshock to the patient. An alternative to the line isolation monitor is the ground fault circuit interrupter, which monitors both sides of the circuit for the equality of current flow. If an individual contacts a faulty piece of equipment such that current flows through the individual, an imbalance is detected and the interrupter immediately stops electrical flow to the device before a significant shock occurs. The same faulty piece of equipment would evoke the line isolation monitor alarm, but the equipment, if lifesaving, could still be used until a satisfactory replacement became available.

The active electrode of the electrosurgical unit cuts or coagulates with intense heat produced by electrical current that flows through a small area. When this current exits from the body via a large

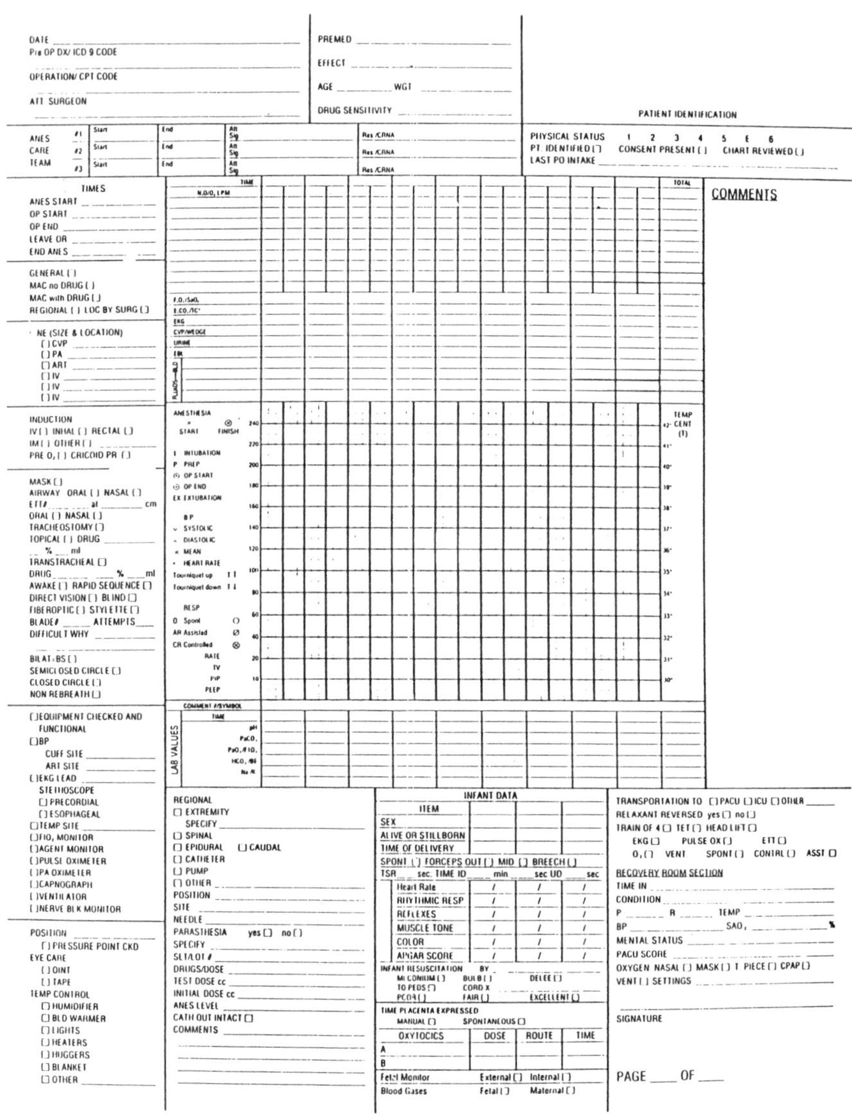
DATE
Pre OP DX/ ICD 9 CODE
OPERATION/ CPT CODE
ATT SURGEON
PREMED
EFFECT
AGE WGT
DRUG SENSITIVITY
PATIENT IDENTIFICATION

ANES CARE TEAM
#1 Start End Att Sig Res /CRNA
#2 Start End Att Sig Res /CRNA
#3 Start End Att Sig Res /CRNA

PHYSICAL STATUS 1 2 3 4 5 E 6
PT. IDENTIFIED [ ] CONSENT PRESENT [ ] CHART REVIEWED [ ]
LAST PO INTAKE

TIMES
ANES START
OP START
OP END
LEAVE OR
END ANES

GENERAL [ ]
MAC no DRUG [ ]
MAC with DRUG [ ]
REGIONAL [ ] LOC BY SURG [ ]

NE (SIZE & LOCATION)
[ ] CVP
[ ] PA
[ ] ART
[ ] IV
[ ] IV
[ ] IV

INDUCTION
IV [ ] INHAL [ ] RECTAL [ ]
IM [ ] OTHER [ ]
PRE O₂ [ ] CRICOID PR [ ]

MASK [ ]
AIRWAY ORAL [ ] NASAL [ ]
ETT# at cm
ORAL [ ] NASAL [ ]
TRACHEOSTOMY [ ]
TOPICAL [ ] DRUG
% ml
TRANSTRACHEAL [ ]
DRUG % ml
AWAKE [ ] RAPID SEQUENCE [ ]
DIRECT VISION [ ] BLIND [ ]
FIBEROPTIC [ ] STYLETTE [ ]
BLADE# ATTEMPTS
DIFFICULT WHY

BILAT=BS [ ]
SEMICLOSED CIRCLE [ ]
CLOSED CIRCLE [ ]
NON REBREATH [ ]

[ ]EQUIPMENT CHECKED AND FUNCTIONAL
[ ]BP
CUFF SITE
ART SITE
[ ]EKG LEAD
STETHOSCOPE
[ ] PRECORDIAL
[ ] ESOPHAGEAL
[ ]TEMP SITE
[ ]FIO₂ MONITOR
[ ]AGENT MONITOR
[ ]PULSE OXIMETER
[ ]PA OXIMETER
[ ]CAPNOGRAPH
[ ]VENTILATOR
[ ]NERVE BLK MONITOR

POSITION
[ ] PRESSURE POINT CKD
EYE CARE
[ ] OINT
[ ] TAPE
TEMP CONTROL
[ ] HUMIDIFIER
[ ] BLD WARMER
[ ] LIGHTS
[ ] HEATERS
[ ] HUGGERS
[ ] BLANKET
[ ] OTHER

TIME
N₂O/O₂ LPM
F₁O₂/SaO₂
E.CO₂/TC°
EKG
CVP/WEDGE
URINE
EBL
FLUIDS—BLD
TOTAL

COMMENTS

ANESTHESIA
× START ⊗ FINISH
I INTUBATION
P PREP
⊙ OP START
⊙ OP END
EX EXTUBATION
BP
∨ SYSTOLIC
∧ DIASTOLIC
× MEAN
• HEART RATE
Tourniquet up ↑↑
Tourniquet down ↓↓
RESP
O Spont ○
AR Assisted ⊘
CR Controlled ⊗
RATE
TV
PIP
PEEP
240 220 200 180 160 140 120 100 80 60 40 20 10
TEMP CENT (1) 42° 41° 40° 39° 38° 37° 36° 35° 34° 33° 32° 31° 30°

COMMENT #/SYMBOL

LAB VALUES
TIME
pH
PaCO₂
PaO₂/FIO₂
HCO₃/BE
Na/K

REGIONAL
[ ] EXTREMITY
SPECIFY
[ ] SPINAL
[ ] EPIDURAL [ ] CAUDAL
[ ] CATHETER
[ ] PUMP
[ ] OTHER
POSITION
SITE
NEEDLE
PARASTHESIA yes [ ] no [ ]
SPECIFY
SET/LOT #
DRUGS/DOSE
TEST DOSE cc
INITIAL DOSE cc
ANES LEVEL
CATH OUT INTACT [ ]
COMMENTS

INFANT DATA

ITEM			
SEX			
ALIVE OR STILLBORN			
TIME OF DELIVERY			

SPONT [ ] FORCEPS OUT [ ] MID [ ] BREECH [ ]
TSR sec. TIME ID min sec UD sec

Heart Rate	/	/	/
RHYTHMIC RESP	/	/	/
REFLEXES	/	/	/
MUSCLE TONE	/	/	/
COLOR	/	/	/
APGAR SCORE	/	/	/

INFANT RESUSCITATION BY
MECONIUM [ ] BULB [ ] DELEE [ ]
TO PEDS [ ] CORD X
POOR [ ] FAIR [ ] EXCELLENT [ ]
TIME PLACENTA EXPRESSED
MANUAL [ ] SPONTANEOUS [ ]

OXYTOCICS	DOSE	ROUTE	TIME
A			
B			

Fetal Monitor External [ ] Internal [ ]
Blood Gases Fetal [ ] Maternal [ ]

TRANSPORTATION TO [ ] PACU [ ] ICU [ ] OTHER
RELAXANT REVERSED yes [ ] no [ ]
TRAIN OF 4 [ ] TET [ ] HEAD LIFT [ ]
EKG [ ] PULSE OX [ ] ETT [ ]
O₂ [ ] VENT SPONT [ ] CONTRL [ ] ASST [ ]

RECOVERY ROOM SECTION
TIME IN
CONDITION
P R TEMP
BP SAO₂ %
MENTAL STATUS
PACU SCORE
OXYGEN NASAL [ ] MASK [ ] T PIECE [ ] CPAP [ ]
VENT [ ] SETTINGS

SIGNATURE

PAGE OF

Figure 15-12. A typical anesthesia record form.

ground plate attached to the patient, the current density is small and thermal injury does not occur. If the ground wire is broken or disconnected, the electrical current seeks alternative exit sites (electrodes for the ECG or peripheral nerve stimulator, contact sites with metal table), and therefore a high current density occurs at these small surface area sites, resulting in burns.

RECORDING OF INTRAOPERATIVE DATA (ANESTHESIA RECORD)

The anesthesia record is a required and indispensable part of anesthetic care (Fig. 15-12). As in all aspects of medicine, the anesthetic and surgical events must be documented for medical and legal purposes. The anesthesia record is the only continuous record that provides a detailed account of the intraoperative course and management of patients. It provides a mechanism by which patient responses can be analyzed and appropriate action taken. Furthermore, it can provide a reminder to the anesthesiologist that observations other than cardiopulmonary variables must be made. For example, the anesthesia record may provide spaces to record fluid and blood replacement, estimated blood loss, urinary output, body temperature, ECG findings, end-tidal PCO_2, arterial blood gases and pH, SpO_2, and central venous pressure. Also, if the anesthesiologist becomes distracted, a record exists of when the last vital signs were determined. Review of prior anesthesia records is useful in planning subsequent anesthetic management. Although patient care should take priority over creating a neat and current anesthesia record, every effort should be made to keep the anesthesia record as current as possible. There can be no doubt that information recorded on the basis of the anesthesiologist's memory will be suspect. To facilitate this process, automated anesthesia record-keeping systems are commercially available.[8]

REFERENCES

1. Cooper JB, Newbower RS, Kitz RJ. An analysis of major errors and equipment failures in anesthesia management: Considerations for prevention and detection. Anesthesiology 1984;60:34–42.
2. Whitcher C, Ream AK, Parsons D, et al. Anesthetic mishaps and the cost of monitoring: A proposed standard for monitoring equipment. J Clin Monit 1988; 4:5–15.
3. Severinghaus JW, Kelleher JF. Recent developments in pulse oximetry. Anesthesiology 1992;76:1018–38.
4. Orkin FK, Cohen MM, Duncan PG. The quest for meaningful outcomes. Anesthesiology 1993;78: 417–22.
5. Bhavani-Shankar K, Moseley H, Kumar AY, Delph Y. Capnometry and anaesthesia. Can J Anaesth 1992; 39:617–32.
6. Slogoff S, Keats AS, Arlund C. On the safety of radial artery cannulation. Anesthesiology 1983;59:42–7.
7 Loghnan BA, Hall GM. Spinal cord monitoring 1989. Br J Anaesth 1989;63:587–94.
8. Feldman JM. Computerized anesthesia recording systems. In: Stoelting RK, Barash PG, Gallagher TH, eds. Advances in Anesthesia. Chicago, Year Book Medical Publishers 1989;6:325–54.

16

Acid-Base Balance and Blood Gas Analysis

All living organisms depend on maintenance of acid-base equilibrium and oxygenation for survival. Regulation of acid-base balance is actually regulation of the hydrogen ion (H^+) and bicarbonate ion (HCO_3^-) concentrations in body fluids. Maintenance of the H^+ concentration over a narrow range is necessary to (1) ensure the optimal function of enzymes, (2) maintain the proper distribution of electrolytes, (3) optimize myocardial contractility, and (4) maintain an optimal saturation of hemoglobin with oxygen. The normal H^+ concentration in the arterial blood and extracellular fluid is 36 to 44 $nmol{\cdot}L^{-1}$, which is equivalent to an arterial pH (pHa) of 7.44 to 7.36, respectively. The normal plasma concentration of HCO_3^- is 24 ± 2 $mEq{\cdot}L^{-1}$.

MAINTENANCE OF THE HYDROGEN ION CONCENTRATION

All body fluids are provided with buffer systems, which represent the first line of defense against changes in pHa produced by excess acid or alkali. The bicarbonate buffer system is the most important and readily available buffer system, representing over 50% of the total buffering capacity of the body. The most important nonbicarbonate buffer system is hemoglobin, which is responsible for about 35% of the buffering capacity in blood. The remainder of buffering capacity is provided by phosphates and plasma proteins.

The bicarbonate buffer system depends on the hydration of carbon dioxide to carbonic acid (H_2CO_3) in the plasma and erythrocytes.

$$CO_2 + H_2O \underset{}{\overset{\text{carbonic anhydrase}}{\rightleftharpoons}} H_2CO_3 \leftrightarrows H^+ + HCO_3^-$$

Carbon dioxide (CO_2) formed from aerobic metabolism undergoes hydration to form H_2CO_3. Hydration of carbon dioxide in the plasma is a slow process, whereas in erythrocytes this reaction is greatly accelerated by the presence of the enzyme carbonic anhydrase. Dissociation of H_2CO_3 to H^+ and HCO_3^- is spontaneous. The H^+ formed by dissociation of H_2CO_3 in the erythrocytes and plasma is buffered by reduced hemoglobin. Hemoglobin can also transport carbon dioxide as carbaminohemoglobin. The HCO_3^- formed by dissociation of H_2CO_3 in erythrocytes enters the plasma, where it functions as a buffer. At the same time, chloride ions enter the erythrocytes (chloride shift) to maintain electrical neutrality.

In addition to buffers, other compensatory mechanisms necessary for maintenance of an appropriate pHa include (1) alterations in the alveolar ventilation, (2) reabsorption of HCO_3^- by renal tubule cells, and (3) secretion of H^+ by renal tubule cells (Figs. 16-1 and 16-2). Ultimately, the kidneys are the most powerful of the acid-base regulatory systems, but, in contrast to the instantaneous action of buffers and rapid adjustments via ventilation (1 to 3

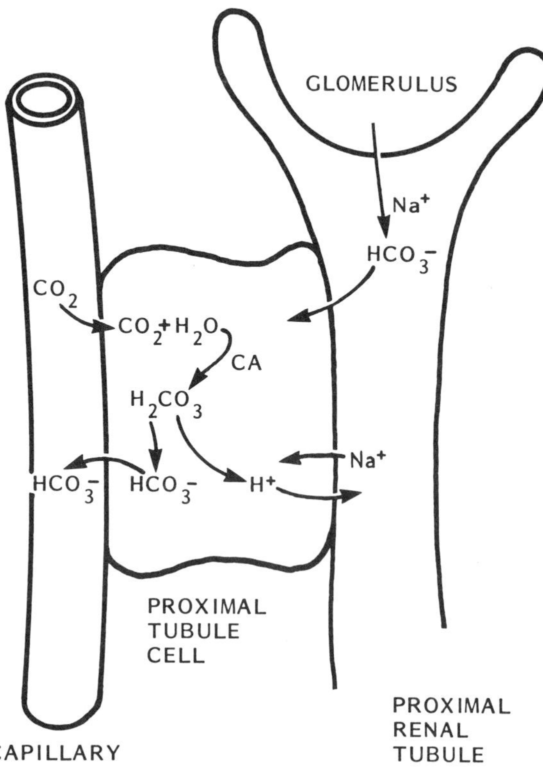

Figure 16-1. Proximal renal tubule cells can regulate acid-base equilibrium by acidifying or alkalinizing the urine via reabsorption of bicarbonate ions (HCO_3^-) and/or secretion of hydrogen ions (H^+). In addition to reabsorption of HCO_3^-, proximal renal tubule cells are able to synthesize new HCO_3^- via hydration of CO_2 and subsequent dissociation of H_2CO_3. Hydration of CO_2 in these cells is accelerated by the presence of the enzyme carbonic anhydrase (CA). Reabsorbed and newly synthesized HCO_3^- can pass from renal tubule cells into capillaries to replenish that lost due to buffering. H^+ formed by dissociation of H_2CO_3 in proximal renal tubule cells are secreted into the urine in exchange for cations, usually sodium (Na^+), so as to maintain electrical neutrality.

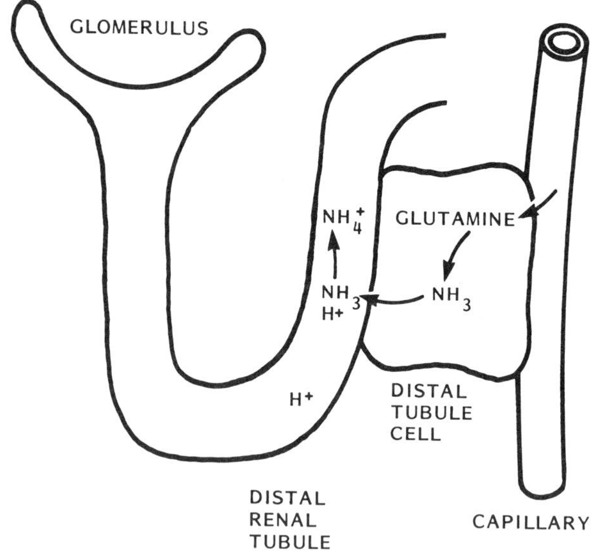

Figure 16-2. The formation of ammonia (NH_3) from glutamine in distal renal tubule cells facilitates the elimination of hydrogen ions (H^+) in the urine as ammonium (NH_4^+). Neutralization of H^+ in the urine by formation of NH_4^+ is essential because secretion of H^+ by proximal renal tubule cells (Fig. 16-1) ceases when the urine pH is lower than 4.5. Renal disease may impair the ability of distal renal tubule cells to form NH_3, resulting in decreased secretion of H^+ by renal tubule cells when the urine pH becomes more acidic.

minutes), the compensation via the kidneys requires 12 to 48 hours.

The Henderson-Hasselbalch equation emphasizes that a normal pHa depends on maintenance of an optimal 20-to-1 ratio of the concentration of HCO_3^- to carbon dioxide (Table 16-1). Acid-base disturbances characterized by changes in the plasma concentration of HCO_3^- are predictably accompanied by appropriate compensatory changes in the $PaCO_2$ secondary to alterations in alveolar ventilation. If changes in the plasma concentration of HCO_3^- and $PaCO_2$ are proportional such that a 20-to-1 ratio is maintained, the pHa will remain near or within the normal range despite disturbances of acid-base balance. For example, acid-base disturbances due to respiratory acidosis or alkalosis are compensated for by renal-induced changes in the plasma concentration of HCO_3^- such that the 20-to-1 ratio is maintained. As a result, the pHa in the presence of

Table 16-1. Henderson-Hasselbalch Equation[a]

pHa	=	$pK + \log \frac{HCO_3^-}{0.03 \times PaCO_2}$
pHa	=	negative logarithm of the arterial concentration of hydrogen ions
pK	=	6.1 at 37°C
HCO_3^-	=	concentration of bicarbonate ions
0.03	=	solubility coefficient for CO_2 in plasma
$PaCO_2$	=	arterial partial presure of CO_2

[a]Substitution of normal values for pHa (7.4) and $PaCO_2$ (40 mmHg) results in a calculated HCO_3^- concentration of 24 $mEq \cdot L^{-1}$. Maintenance of this concentration of HCO_3^- relative to the concentration of CO_2 (0.03 x 40) results in an optimal 20-to-1 ratio. Likewise, alterations in HCO_3^- or the concentration of CO_2 will not significantly change the pHa if the 20-to-1 ratio is preserved.

chronic respiratory acid-base disturbances is near normal despite persistent abnormalities of the $PaCO_2$. Likewise, acid-base disturbances due to metabolic abnormalities are compensated for by adjustments in alveolar ventilation in an effort to maintain the $PaCO_2$ in a range that preserves the 20-to-1 ratio.

DIFFERENTIAL DIAGNOSIS OF ACID-BASE DISTURBANCES

The differential diagnosis of acid-base disturbances (respiratory acidosis, respiratory alkalosis, metabolic acidosis, metabolic alkalosis) is based on the direct measurement of the pHa and $PaCO_2$ plus a derived estimate of the plasma concentration of HCO_3^- using a nomogram (Table 16-2 and Fig. 16-3).[1,2] Acidemia is present when the pHa is lower than 7.36; alkalemia is present when the pHa is higher than 7.44. A $PaCO_2$ higher than 44 mmHg is defined as hypoventilation; hyperventilation is present when the $PaCO_2$ is lower than 36 mmHg. Hypoventilation is synonymous with respiratory acidosis, and hyperventilation is synonomous with respiratory alkalosis. Acidemia and alkalemia characterized by deviations of the HCO_3^- concentration above or below 24 $mEq{\cdot}L^{-1}$ are considered to be primary metabolic disturbances. Predictable adverse responses accompany acidemia and alkalemia.

Direct effects of alkalemia on myocardial contractility are less striking than those of acidemia.[3] Although acidemia decreases myocardial contractility, little clinical effect occurs until the pHa is lower than 7.2. Because acidemia also induces the release of catecholamines, much of the direct myocardial depressant effects are mitigated in mild acidemia. When the pHa is lower than 7.1, however, myocardial responsiveness to catecholamines decreases and compensatory increases in myocardial contractility are diminished.

Respiratory acidosis may produce more rapid and profound myocardial dysfunction than does metabolic acidosis, reflecting the ability of carbon dioxide to freely diffuse across cell membranes and exacerbate intracellular acidosis to a greater extent than metabolic acids. Detrimental effects of acidemia may be accentuated in the presence of ischemic heart disease or in patients in whom sympathetic nervous system activity may be impaired, as by beta blockade or general anesthesia.

Interpretation of the plasma concentration of HCO_3^- as derived from the nomogram requires an adjustment for the level of ventilation (Fig. 16-3). For example, an increased $PaCO_2$ will lead to the hydration of carbon dioxide with a subsequent increase in the plasma concentration of HCO_3^- (see

Adverse Effects of Respiratory or Metabolic Acidosis

Increased serum potassium concentrations
Central nervous system depression
Cardiovascular depression due to direct depressant effects on the vasomotor center, arteriolar smooth muscle, and myocardial contracility (offset until severe acidosis by increased secretion of catecholamines and decreased serum concentrations of ionized calcium)
Increased incidence of cardiac dysrhythmias
Decreased precapillary and increased postcapillary sphincter tone, leading to hypovolemia

Adverse Effects of Respiratory or Metabolic Alkalosis

Decreased serum potassium concentrations
Decreased serum ionized calcium concentrations (altered neuromuscular function manifesting as tetany, decreased myocardial contractility)
Central nervous system excitation
Decreased cerebral blood flow
Coronary artery vasoconstriction
Decreased availability of oxygen to tissues owing to leftward shift of the oxyhemoglobin dissociation curve (Bohr effect)
Increased incidence of cardiac dysrhythmias
Increased airway resistance and right-to-left intrapulmonary shunting (respiratory alkalosis only)

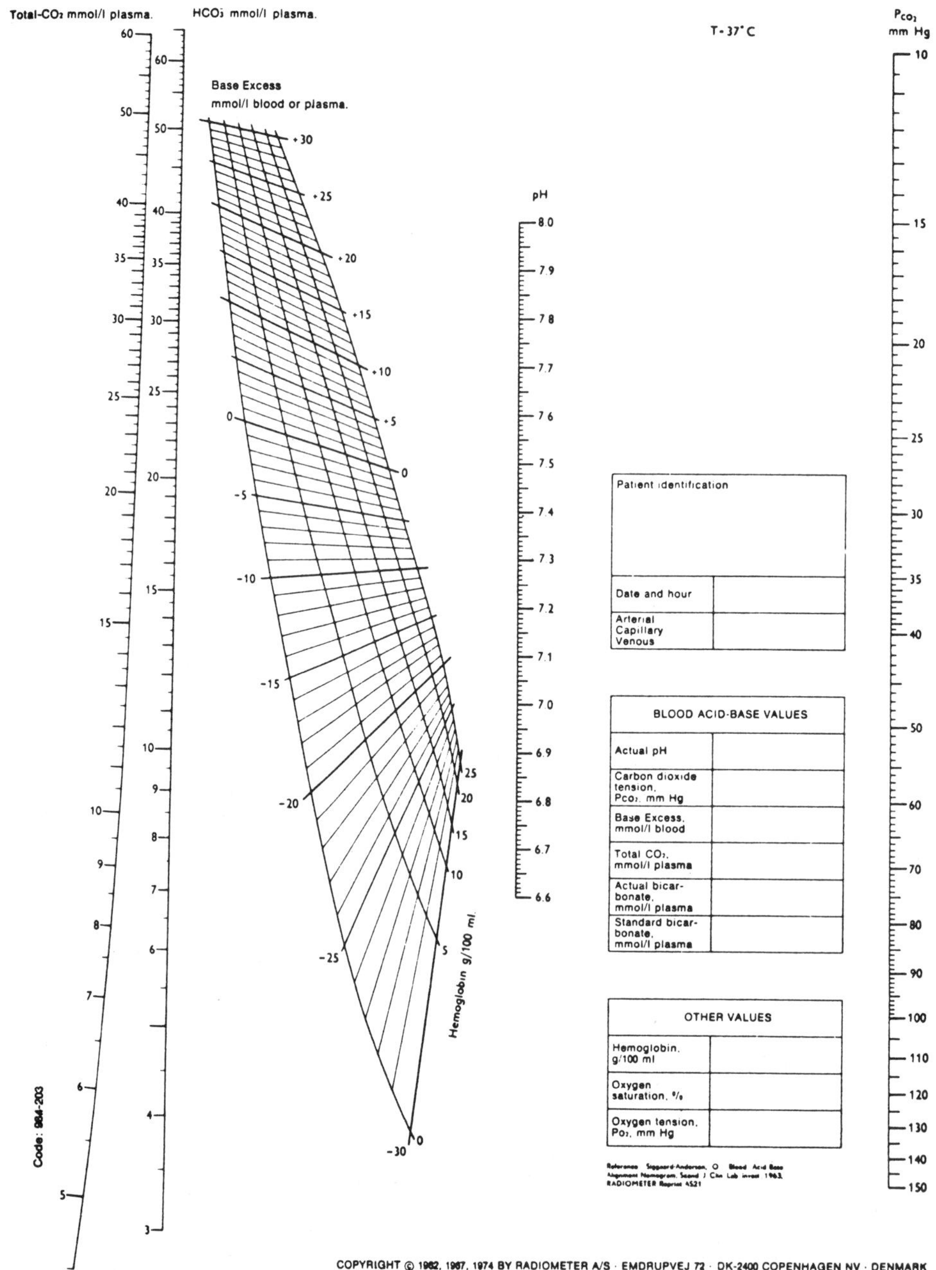

Figure 16-3. The Siggard-Andersen alignment nomogram is used to derive the estimated plasma concentration of bicarbonate ions (HCO_3^-) or, alternatively, to determine base excess. A line connecting the measured PCO_2 and pH will transect the vertical column representing the plasma concentration of HCO_3^- or base excess. (From Siggard-Andersen,[2] with permission.)

Table 16-2. Differential Diagnosis of Acid-Base Disturbances

Disturbance	pHa (7.36 to 7.44)	$PaCO_2$ (36 to 44 mmHg)	HCO_3^- (24 mEq·L^{-1})
Respiratory acidosis			
Acute	Moderate decrease	Marked increase	Slight increase
Chronic	Slight decrease to no change	Marked increase	Moderate increase
Respiratory alkalosis			
Acute	Moderate increase	Marked decrease	Slight decrease
Chronic	Slight increase to no change	Marked decrease	Moderate decrease
Metabolic acidosis			
Acute	Moderate to marked decrease	Slight decrease	Marked decrease
Chronic	Slight decrease	Moderate decrease	Marked decrease
Metabolic alkalosis			
Acute	Marked increase	Moderate increase	Marked increase
Chronic	Marked increase	Moderate increase	Marked increase

equation on p. 217). Normalization of the HCO_3^- concentration above or below 24 mEq·L^{-1} in the presence of an increased or decreased $PaCO_2$ is achieved by applying a correction factor that is dependent on the rapidity and direction of change in the $PaCO_2$ (Table 16-3).

Table 16-3. Normalization of Plasma Concentration of Bicarbonate for Alveolar Ventilation

Change in $PaCO_2$ from 40 mmHg	Change in HCO_3^- Concentration from 24 mEq·L^{-1}
Acute 10-mmHg increase	Increase 1 mEq·L^{-1}
Acute 10-mmHg decrease	Decrease 2 mEq·L^{-1}
Chronic 10-mmHg increase	Increase 3 mEq·L^{-1}
Chronic 10-mmHg decrease	Decrease 5 mEq·L^{-1}

In discussing abnormalities of acid-base balance, primary alterations should be distinguished from changes that reflect compensatory responses (Table 16-2). Compensation is the restoration of pHa toward 7.4 despite the continued presence of the primary acid-base abnormality. Indeed, compensatory responses frequently result in mixed acid-base disturbances. Ultimately, differentiation between primary respiratory and metabolic causes of acid-base disturbances is necessary to ensure proper treatment.

RESPIRATORY ACIDOSIS

Respiratory acidosis is present when the $PaCO_2$ is higher than 44 mmHg (Table 16-2). Measurement of the pHa or estimation of the plasma concentration of HCO_3^- provides evidence about the chronicity of the acid-base disturbance and gives an indication of the primary or compensatory nature of the respiratory change (Table 16-2). An increased $PaCO_2$ is due either to decreased elimination of carbon dioxide by the lungs (hypoventilation) or increased metabolic production of carbon dioxide.

The initial effect of an increase in the $PaCO_2$ is a decreased pHa owing to hydration of carbon dioxide (see equation on p. 217). The decrease in pH occurs to a similar extent in arterial blood and cerebrospinal fluid (CSF) because carbon dioxide rapid-

Causes of Respiratory Acidosis

- Decreased elimination of carbon dioxide by the lungs (hypoventilation)
  - Central nervous system depression due to drugs (anesthetics)
  - Decreased skeletal muscle strength (diseases, skeletal muscle relaxants)
  - Intrinsic pulmonary disease
  - Rebreathing of exhaled gases (exhausted soda lime, incompetent one-way valve in anesthetic breathing system)
- Increased metabolic production of carbon dioxide
  - Hyperthermia
  - Increased glucose load (hyperalimentation)

ly crosses lipid barriers such as the blood-brain barrier. The response to a decrease in pHa is stimulation of ventilation via the carotid bodies, whereas the decreased pH of the CSF stimulates medullary chemoreceptors located in the fourth cerebral ventricle. With time, stimulation of ventilation via medullary chemoreceptors is eliminated as the CSF pH is restored to normal by the active transport of HCO_3^- into the CSF.[4] Therefore, the volume of ventilation after restoration of the CSF pH to normal is lower than that present during the initial phase of respiratory acidosis. Volatile anesthetics greatly decrease the carotid body mediated responses to acidemia.

Compensatory Responses

The absolute decrease in pHa produced by respiratory acidosis depends on the degree of compensation provided by the secondary increase in the plasma concentration of HCO_3^-. It is estimated that the hydration of carbon dioxide increases the plasma concentration of HCO_3^- about 1 $mEq{\cdot}L^{-1}$ for every 10-mmHg increase of the $PaCO_2$ above normal (Table 16-3). This compensatory increase in the plasma concentration of HCO_3^- occurs within seconds after the increase in $PaCO_2$. In addition, hydration of carbon dioxide in proximal renal tubule cells promotes secretion of H^+ into the urine (Fig. 16-1). At the same time, sodium is exchanged for H^+, which facilitates reabsorption of HCO_3^- (Fig. 16-1). Likewise, distal renal tubule cells secrete H^+ (Fig. 16-2). This renal compensation requires 12 to 48 hours but eventually increases the plasma HCO_3^- concentration by about 2 $mEq{\cdot}L^{-1}$ for every 10-mmHg increase in the $PaCO_2$ above normal (Table 16-3). Thus, the total increase in the plasma concentration of HCO_3^- produced by hydration of carbon dioxide and renal reabsorption of HCO_3^- is about 3 $mEq{\cdot}L^{-1}$ for every 10-mmHg increase of the $PaCO_2$ above normal (Table 16-3). The net effect of this compensatory response is a return of the pHa to normal or near normal in patients with chronic increases in the $PaCO_2$. Acute respiratory acidosis is recognized by a decreased pHa and a smaller than predicted increase in the plasma concentration of HCO_3^- (Table 16-2).

Treatment

Chronic respiratory acidosis is treated by correction of the disorder responsible for decreased elimination of carbon dioxide by the lungs or increased metabolic production of carbon dioxide. Mechanical ventilation of the lungs is necessary when acute or chronic increase of the $PaCO_2$ is marked. Rapid lowering of a chronically increased $PaCO_2$, however, can result in metabolic alkalosis and central nervous system irritability because total body carbon dioxide washout occurs more rapidly than the kidneys can produce a corresponding decrease in the plasma concentration of HCO_3^-. Therefore, it is recommended to decrease a chronically increased $PaCO_2$ slowly so as to ensure that there is enough time for renal elimination of excess HCO_3^-. Hypochloremia due to augmentation of renal excretion of chloride in order to enhance proximal renal tubule cell reabsorption of HCO_3^- may require treatment in some patients.

Mixed Acid-Base Disturbance

Respiratory acidosis complicated by metabolic acidosis is evidenced by an increase in the plasma concentration of HCO_3^- that is less than 3 $mEq{\cdot}L^{-1}$ for every 10-mmHg increase of the $PaCO_2$. An increase in the plasma concentration of HCO_3^- that is more than 3 $mEq{\cdot}L^{-1}$ for every 10-mmHg increase of the $PaCO_2$ above normal suggests the presence of respiratory acidosis complicated by metabolic alkalosis. Metabolic alkalosis complicating respiratory acidosis is likely in the presence of hypochloremia or hypokalemia, or both. Metabolic alkalosis associated with respiratory acidosis is treated by intravenous administration of potassium chloride and avoidance of mechanical hyperventilation of the lungs.

RESPIRATORY ALKALOSIS

Respiratory alkalosis is present when the $PaCO_2$ is lower than 36 mmHg (Table 16-2). Measurement of the pHa or estimate of the plasma concentration of HCO_3^- provides evidence about the chronicity of the acid-base disturbance and gives an indication of the primary or compensatory nature of the respiratory change (Table 16-2). A decreased $PaCO_2$ is due either to increased elimination of carbon dioxide by the lungs (hyperventilation) or decreased metabolic production of carbon dioxide. The initial effect of a decrease in the $PaCO_2$ is an increased pHa due to decreased hydration of carbon dioxide (see equation on p. 217). The decreased $PaCO_2$ and increased pHa decrease the stimulus to breathe, normally mediat-

Causes of Respiratory Alkalosis

Increased elimination of carbon dioxide by the lungs (hyperventilation)
- Iatrogenic-mechanical or self-induced
- Pain
- Anxiety
- Decreased barometric pressure
- Central nervous system injury
- Arterial hypoxemia
- Pulmonary vascular disease
- Cirrhosis of the liver
- Sepsis
- Hyperthermia

Decreased metabolic production of carbon dioxide
- Hypothermia
- Skeletal muscle paralysis

ed by the carotid bodies and medullary chemoreceptors. Active transport of HCO_3^- out of the CSF subsequently restores the CSF pH to normal.[4] As a result, the activity of the medullary chemoreceptors becomes normal and the volume of ventilation is increased, despite persistence of a decreased $PaCO_2$. By the same mechanism, mechanical hyperventilation of the lungs during anesthesia can result in the initiation of spontaneous ventilation at a lower $PaCO_2$ than was present before hyperventilation (Fig. 16-4).[5] This initiation of ventilation reflects a normal CSF pH, which maintains ventilation via stimulation from the medullary chemoreceptors despite persistence of a decreased $PaCO_2$. Likewise, continued hyperventilation after returning to sea level from altitude reflects maintenance of ventilation by the medullary chemoreceptors exposed to a normal CSF pH.

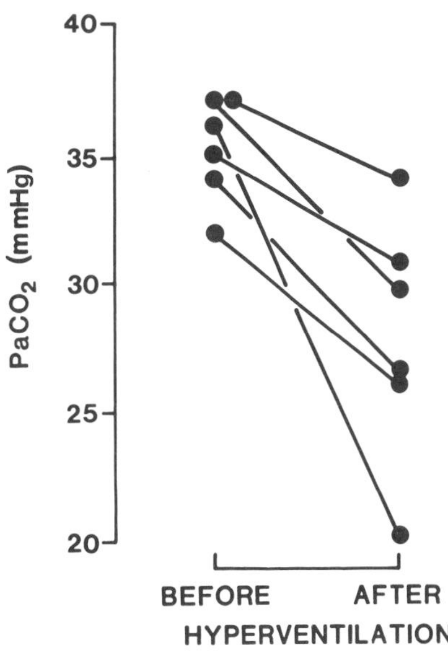

Figure 16-4. The $PaCO_2$ present during spontaneous ventilation before and after mechanical hyperventilation to a $PaCO_2$ of 20 mmHg for 2 hours was measured in six adult patients. The return of spontaneous ventilation at a lower $PaCO_2$ after mechanical hyperventilation of the lungs reflects restoration of the cerebrospinal fluid pH to normal despite persistent decreases in the $PaCO_2$. This is equivalent to resetting the threshold of the medullary chemoreceptors for carbon dioxide. (Data from Edelist and Osorio.[5])

Compensatory Responses

Three events occur simultaneously to decrease the plasma concentration of HCO_3^- and thus offset the increase in pHa that accompanies respiratory alkalosis. There is an immediate response via the bicarbonate buffer system, resulting in the production of carbon dioxide (see equation on p. 217). In addition, alkalosis stimulates the activity of phosphofructokinase enzyme, which results in glycolysis and generation of lactic acid. These two mechanisms operate rapidly to decrease the plasma concentration of HCO_3^- by about 2 $mEq \cdot L^{-1}$ for every 10-mmHg decrease in the $PaCO_2$ below normal (Table 16-3). The third compensatory mechanism is decreased renal tubule reabsorption of HCO_3^-, which becomes maximal by 12 to 48 hours (Fig. 16-1). The decrease in the plasma concentration of HCO_3^- produced by these three compensatory mechanisms is about 5 $mEq \cdot L^{-1}$ for every 10-mmHg decrease in the $PaCO_2$ below normal (Table 16-3). This degree of metabolic compensation is sufficient to return the pHa to normal or near normal in patients with chronic decreases in the $PaCO_2$ (Table 16-2).

Treatment

Treatment of chronic respiratory alkalosis is directed at correcting the underlying disorder responsible for the increased elimination of carbon dioxide by the lungs or decreased metabolic production of carbon dioxide. During anesthesia, acute respiratory alkalosis is most often treated by decreasing the breathing rate and/or tidal volume produced by the mechanical ventilator so as to decrease the alveolar ventilation. Rarely is it deemed necessary to add deadspace to the anesthetic breathing system in an attempt to increase the $PaCO_2$ by virtue of rebreathing exhaled gases.

METABOLIC ACIDOSIS

Metabolic acidosis is present when the pHa is less than 7.36 and the plasma concentration of HCO_3^- is lower than 24 $mEq \cdot L^{-1}$ (Table 16-2). Measurement of the $PaCO_2$ supplies evidence about the chronicity of the acid-base disturbance and gives an indication of the primary or compensatory nature of the metabolic change (Table 16-2). A decreased pHa, in association with a decreased plasma concentration of HCO_3^-, is due either to decreased elimination of H^+ by renal tubule cells or to increased metabolic production of H^+ relative to HCO_3^-.

Causes of Metabolic Acidosis

- Decreased renal tubule elimination of hydrogen ions
  - Renal failure
  - Cirrhosis of the liver with decreased conversion of lactate to glucose
- Increased metabolic production of hydrogen ions
  - Anaerobic glycolysis due to decreased delivery of oxygenated blood to tissues
  - Diabetic ketoacidosis
  - Metabolism of amino acids in hyperalimentation solutions
  - Idiopathic
  - Excessive loss of gastrointestinal fluids formed distal to the pylorus (diarrhea, ileostomy) leading to a relative excess of hydrogen ions
  - Renal tubular acidosis (inability of kidneys to reabsorb bicarbonate ions present in the glomerular filtrate results in a relative excess of hydrogen ions)

Compensatory Responses

Compensatory responses initiated by metabolic acidosis include renal tubule secretion of H^+ into the urine (Figs. 16-1 and 16-2) and increased alveolar ventilation due to stimulation of the carotid bodies by H^+. The decrease in $PaCO_2$ produced by increased alveolar ventilation is rapidly reflected as a corresponding decrease in the $PaCO_2$ in the CSF. As a result, the CSF pH increases, leading to an inhibition of the activity of the medullary chemoreceptors and a blunting of the increase in ventilation produced by the carotid bodies.[4] With time, however, the CSF pH normalizes, reflecting the active transport of HCO_3^- into the CSF. Therefore, inhibition of ventilation provided by the medullary chemoreceptors is removed and there is a further, although delayed, increase in alveolar ventilation. As with respiratory acidosis, volatile anesthetics blunt the carotid body mediated response to metabolic acidosis. Another compensatory mechanism is the use of buffers present in bone to neutralize nonvolatile acids present in the circulation. Indeed, chronic metabolic acidosis, as associated with chronic renal failure, is commonly associated with loss of bone mass.

Patients with lactic acidosis hyperventilate to a greater degree than do patients with other forms of metabolic acidosis such as ketoacidosis. This may reflect the brain's participation in lactic acid production, thereby directly exposing chemoreceptors to acid. In contrast to lactic acid, ketoacids produced by patients with diabetes mellitus are synthesized only in the liver and must be transported across the blood-brain barrier before stimulation of ventilation occurs.

A useful guideline is that a 1-mmHg change in $PaCO_2$ above or below 40 mmHg results in a 0.008-unit pH change in the opposite direction. Therefore, a patient with a $PaCO_2$ of 30 mmHg and a pHa of 7.38 has a "corrected" pHa of 7.30. Routine use of this rule in the initial interpretation of the $PaCO_2$ and pHa permits rapid recognition of an acid-base abnormality due to a metabolic disturbance. Another useful guideline is that $PaCO_2$ will decrease about 1 mmHg for every 1-$mEq \cdot L^{-1}$ decrease in the plasma concentration of HCO_3^-

below 24 mEq·L^{-1}. When metabolic acidosis is complicated by respiratory acidosis, the magnitude of decrease in the $PaCO_2$ is less than 1 mmHg for each 1-mEq·L^{-1} decrease in the plasma concentration.

Treatment

Metabolic acidosis is treated by removal of the cause of the accumulation of nonvolatile acids in the circulation. In addition, intravenous administration of sodium bicarbonate may be indicated if metabolic acidosis is associated with myocardial depression or cardiac dysrhythmias. Calculation of the dose of sodium bicarbonate (Table 16-4) requires use of a nomogram to determine the plasma concentration of HCO_3^- or, alternatively, the base excess (Table 16-4 and Fig. 16-3).[2] A common approach is to administer about one-half of the calculated dose of sodium bicarbonate and then perform a repeat measurement of the pHa to evaluate the impact of therapy. It is estimated that each 1 mEq of sodium bicarbonate administered intravenously will produce about 180 ml of carbon dioxide and necessitate a transient doubling of alveolar ventilation to prevent hypercarbia.[3]

METABOLIC ALKALOSIS

Metabolic alkalosis is present when the pHa is higher than 7.44 and the plasma concentration of HCO_3^- is higher than 24 mEq·L^{-1} (Table 16-2). Measurement of the $PaCO_2$ supplies evidence about the chronicity of the acid-base disturbance and gives an indication of the primary or compensatory nature of the metabolic change (Table 16-2). An increased pHa due to metabolic alkalosis reflects events that result in an excess of HCO_3^- relative to H^+. An example of an event that results in a relative excess of HCO_3^- is conversion of citrate in the liver to HCO_3^-. Indeed, metabolic alkalosis is not an infrequent finding after administration of large amounts of stored whole blood containing citrate anticoagulant.[6] Depletion of intravascular fluid volume is often the most important factor in maintenance of metabolic alkalosis. In this regard, hypovolemia should be considered in postoperative patients who develop metabolic alkalosis.

Clinically, metabolic alkalosis correlates with decreases in the total body concentrations of chloride and potassium. For example, diuretics that facilitate chloride loss via renal tubule cells are associated with increased reabsorption of HCO_3^- to main-

Table 16-4. Calculation of the Dose of Sodium Bicarbonate to Treat Metabolic Acidosis

Dose of sodium bicarbonate = body weight (kg) × deviation of HCO_3^- from 24 mEq·L^{-1}[a] × extracellular fluid volume as a fraction of body mass (0.2)

[a]The normal value for HCO_3^- (24 mEq·L^{-1}) must be adjusted for deviations in the $PaCO_2$ from 40 mmHg (see Table 16-3).

Causes of Metabolic Alkalosis

- Vomiting or nasogastric suction, resulting in excessive loss of hydrogen ions to bicarbonate ions
- Chloride and/or potassium depletion due to diuretics
- Metabolism of lactate in lactated Ringer's solution, citrate in stored whole blood, or acetate in hyperalimentation solutions to bicarbonate ions
- Depletion of intravascular fluid volume
- Hyperaldosteronism leading to increased sodium reabsorption by distal renal tubule cells that results in increased hydrogen ion secretion

Effects of Hypokalemia that Contribute to Metabolic Alkalosis

- Increased proximal renal tubule cell reabsorption of bicarbonate ions
- Increased distal renal tubule cell secretion of hydrogen ions
- Increased distal renal tubule cell synthesis of ammonia

tain electrical neutrality. Likewise, hypokalemia secondary to diuretic therapy is associated with similar renal changes that contribute to metabolic alkalosis.

Compensatory Responses

Compensatory responses initiated by metabolic alkalosis include increased reabsorption of H^+ by renal tubule cells (Fig. 16-1), decreased secretion of H^+ by renal tubule cells (Fig. 16-2), and alveolar hypoventilation. The efficiency of the renal compensatory mechanism is dependent on the presence of cations (sodium, potassium) and chloride (Figs. 16-1 and 16-2). Depletion of these ions, as occurs with vomiting, impairs the ability of the kidneys to excrete excess HCO_3^-, resulting in incomplete renal compensation for metabolic alkalosis. Hypoventilation in an attempt to compensate for metabolic alkalosis will initially stimulate the medullary chemoreceptors and thus offset the compensatory effect of decreased alveolar ventilation. With time, the CSF pH is normalized by active transport of HCO_3^- into the CSF and the volume of ventilation decreases, despite the persistence of a compensatory increase in the $PaCO_2$.[4] If the $PaCO_2$ increases again, however, the CSF pH will decrease and the same sequence will be repeated. Indeed, respiratory compensation for pure metabolic alkalosis, in contrast to metabolic acidosis, is never more than 75% complete. As a result, the pHa remains increased in patients with primary metabolic alkalosis (Table 16-2). Furthermore, a $PaCO_2$ higher than 55 mmHg is beyond the normal compensatory mechanism for metabolic alkalosis and reflects concomitant respiratory acidosis.

Treatment

Treatment of metabolic alkalosis is directed at resolution of the process responsible for the acid-base derangement plus intravenous infusion of potassium chloride, which allows the kidneys to excrete excess HCO_3^-. On occasion, intravenous infusion of H^+ in the form of ammonium chloride or 0.1 N hydrochloric acid (up to 0.2 $mEq \cdot kg^{-1} \cdot h^{-1}$) is used to facilitate the return of pHa to near normal. Administration of acid requires insertion of a central venous catheter, as peripheral injections can cause sclerosis of veins and hemolysis.

MEASUREMENT OF ARTERIAL BLOOD GASES

Technological advances that permit the analysis of arterial and mixed venous blood gases (PO_2, PCO_2), as well as pH, have contributed greatly to the management of patients during anesthesia and in the intensive care unit (see Chapter 33). The small volume of blood required for the measurement (as little as 0.1 ml) extends this technique to the care of premature infants as well as children and adults. Measurement of arterial blood gases may serve to verify the adequacy of oxygenation and alveolar ventilation as continuously monitored by pulse oximetry and capnography.

Sampling of Blood

Arterial blood is most often obtained percutaneously from the radial, brachial, or femoral artery. Arterialized venous blood may be an alternative when arterial sampling is not possible. Blood is drawn into a plastic or glass syringe that contains sufficient heparin to fill the deadspace of the syringe. Heparin is acidic, and excessive amounts of this anticoagulant in the sampling syringe could falsely lower the measured pH. Elimination of air bubbles from the syringe after obtaining the sample is important because equilibration of oxygen and carbon dioxide in the blood with the corresponding partial pressures in the air bubble could influence the measured results. Before analysis, the blood sample may be placed on ice to retard metabolism, which could consume oxygen and produce carbon dioxide.

Temperature Correction

In the past, it was recommended that blood gases and pH be corrected for temperature if the temperature of the measuring electrode (usually 37°C) differed from the patient's body temperature. This recommendation was based on the knowledge that the solubilities of oxygen and carbon dioxide in the blood are temperature dependent. Therefore, placing blood from a patient with a body temperature lower than 37°C into an electrode maintained at 37°C means that more molecules enter the gas phase to be sensed as partial pressure than would be present in vivo at the lower body temperature of the patient. Nomograms are available to correct blood gases and pH measurements for temperature; however, the need to correct PCO_2 and pH measurements for body temperature has been challenged.[7] It is argued that a normal PCO_2 and pH measured at an electrode temperature of 37°C reflect an unperturbed acid-base status of the patient, regardless of the body temperature that existed at the time the sample was drawn. The argument is based on the concept that maintenance of electrochemical neutrality (pH = pOH) requires the pH to increase with decreases in body temperature. Conversely, as body temperature increases, the neutral point falls and maintenance of electrochemical neutrality requires a decrease in pH. If this concept is accepted, it is not necessary to correct PCO_2 and pH for variations in body temperature from the temperature of the electrodes, which are usually maintained at 37°C. Temperature correction of the PO_2 remains important, however, for assessing oxygenation. As a guideline, the measured PO_2 should be decreased 6% for every 1°C the patient's body temperature is below the temperature of the electrode (37°C). The PO_2 is increased 6% for every 1°C the body temperature exceeds 37°C. Furthermore, calculation of the alveolar-to-arterial difference for oxygen (A-aDO_2) requires temperature correction of the PaO_2 (Table 16-5).

Blood Gas pH Electrodes

The oxygen electrode (Clark electrode) used to measure PO_2 is a polarographic cell consisting of a silver reference anode and a platinum cathode charged to –0.5 volts.[8] The platinum surface is covered with an oxygen-permeable membrane (polyethylene), on the other side of which is placed the unknown sample. Electrical current passing through the polarographic cell is directly proportional to the PO_2 outside the membrane.

The carbon dioxide electrode (Severinghaus electrode) used to measure PCO_2 has a carbon dioxide permeable membrane (Teflon), which permits carbon dioxide to diffuse from the unknown sample into a buffer solution containing HCO_3^- bathing a conventional glass pH electrode.[9] The measured pH

Table 16-5. Calculation of the Alveolar-to-Arterial Difference for Oxygen

$$A\text{-}aDO_2 = PAO_2 - PaO_2$$

$$PAO_2 = (P_B - P_{H_2O})FIO_2 - \frac{PaCO_2}{0.8}$$

$A\text{-}aDO_2$ = alveolar-to-arterial difference for oxygen (mmHg)
PAO_2 = alveolar partial pressure of oxygen (mmHg)
PaO_2 = arterial partial pressure of oxygen (mmHg)
P_B = barometric pressure (mmHg)
P_{H_2O} = partial pressure of water vapor (47 mmHg at 37°C)
FIO_2 = inspired concentration of oxygen
$PaCO_2$ = arterial partial pressure of carbon dioxide (mmHg)
0.8 = respiratory exchange ratio to compensate for the fact that less carbon dioxide is transferred into the alveolus than oxygen is removed from the alveolus

Example: Arterial blood gases are PaO_2 310 mmHg and $PaCO_2$ 40 mmHg breathing 100% oxygen (FIO_2 = 1.0). The P_B is 747 mmHg, and the PH_2O is 47 mmHg. The $A\text{-}aDO_2$ is

$$PAO_2 = (747 - 47)1.0 - 40/0.8$$
$$PAO_2 = 700 - 50$$
$$PAO_2 = 650 \text{ mmHg}$$

$$A\text{-}aDO_2 = 650 - 310$$
$$A\text{-}aDO_2 = 340 \text{ mmHg}^a \text{ (normal <60 mmHg)}$$

[a]Assuming each 20 mmHg $A\text{-}aDO_2$ represents venous admixture equivalent to 1% of the cardiac output, it can be estimated that 17% of the cardiac output is shunted past the lungs without exposure to ventilated alveoli.

in the bathing solution is altered in direct proportion to the PCO_2.

Measurement of pH involves a glass electrode that senses the concentration of H^+ in the unknown sample. This H^+ concentration produces a proportional change in voltage between the glass and reference electrode.

Information Provided by Blood Gases and pH

Assessment of oxygenation and ventilation includes the measurement of PaO_2 and $PaCO_2$. As an alternative to arterial samples, blood from veins on the back of the hand, which reflects primarily cutaneous blood, can be used to estimate arterial blood gases and pH. Indeed, the combination of cutaneous vasodilation and increased cutaneous blood flow associated with general anesthesia is often sufficient to arterialize peripheral venous blood.[10] As a result, the peripheral venous PCO_2 and pH measured during general anesthesia approximate arterial values closely enough to permit estimation of the adequacy of ventilation and acid-base status. For example, venous PCO_2 is only 4 to 6 mmHg higher and pH only 0.03 to 0.04 unit lower than arterial values. The calculated bicarbonate concentration in venous blood is therefore only about 2 $mEq{\cdot}L^{-1}$ higher. The peripheral venous PO_2, however, does not reliably parallel the PaO_2. Nevertheless, when the peripheral venous PO_2 is higher than 60 mmHg, the absence of arterial hypoxemia is confirmed. Additional measurements and calculations that further define the efficiency of oxygenation and ventilation include the (1) A-aDO_2, (2) arterial-to-alveolar PO_2 ratio (a/A), (3) mixed venous PO_2, (4) arterial and mixed venous content of oxygen, (5) position of the oxyhemoglobin dissociation curve, and (6) dead-space-to-tidal volume ratio (VD/VT). The anesthesiologist must be familiar with these measurements and able to rapidly adjust patient care on the basis of information derived from blood gases and pH measurements.

Oxygenation

Oxygenation is assessed by measurement of the PaO_2. Arterial hypoxemia, as reflected by a decrease in the PaO_2 to lower than 60 mmHg, may be caused by (1) a low PO_2 in the inhaled gases (altitude, accidental during anesthesia), (2) hypoventilation, and (3) venous admixture.

Hypoventilation. Decreases in PaO_2 owing to hypoventilation reflect encroachment of the $PaCO_2$ on the space available in the alveolus for oxygen. Decreases in PaO_2 are roughly equivalent to increases in alveolar PCO_2.

Venous Admixture. Venous admixture as a cause of decreased PaO_2 may reflect right-to-left intrapulmonary shunts (atelectasis, pneumonia, endobronchial intubation), intracardiac shunts (congenital heart disease), or ventilation-to-perfusion mismatching (chronic obstructive pulmonary disease). A right-to-left shunt is defined as passage of blood from the pulmonary circulation to the systemic circulation without coming into contact with alveolar gases. Arterial hypoxemia due to a right-to-left shunt represents dilution of oxygenated arterial blood with shunted and desaturated venous blood. In this instance, inhalation of 100% oxygen produces minimal, if any, effect on the PaO_2. Ventilation-to-perfusion mismatching as a cause of venous admixture and arterial hypoxemia reflects underventilation of alveoli relative to their blood flow. Inhalation of 100% oxygen eventually eliminates residual nitrogen from poorly ventilated alveoli such that blood coming from these alveoli is well oxygenated. This is the reason that even small increases in inhaled oxygen concentrations (24% to 30%) compared with room air (21%) may correct arterial hypoxemia due to the ventilation-to-perfusion mismatching characteristic of patients with chronic obstructive pulmonary disease. This therapeutic response to supplemental oxygen helps distinguish arterial hypoxemia that is due to a right-to-left shunt from that due to ventilation-to-perfusion mismatching. Diffusion limitation to the passage of oxygen from the alveoli to blood has not been documented to be a cause of arterial hypoxemia in humans.

A-aDO_2

The magnitude of venous admixture may be estimated in the clinical setting by calculation of the A-aDO_2 (Table 16-5). For example, when the PaO_2 is higher than 150 mmHg, so that hemoglobin is completely saturated with oxygen, the magnitude of venous admixture can be estimated to be equivalent to 1% of the cardiac output for every 20 mmHg of

A-aDO_2. Below a PaO_2 of 150 mmHg or when cardiac output is increased relative to metabolism, this guideline will underestimate the actual amount of venous admixture. It must be appreciated that the normal A-aDO_2 when breathing air is 5 to 10 mmHg, reflecting right-to-left intracardiac shunting of a small portion of the cardiac output via bronchial, pleural, and thebesian veins.

a/A Ratio

A disadvantage of A-aDO_2 is that the normal range changes with varying concentrations of inhaled oxygen. For this reason, the a/A ratio may be more useful because it remains relatively constant regardless of the concentration of oxygen (Table 16-6).[11] For example, a patient with an a/A ratio of 0.5 will have a PaO_2 equal to 50% of the PAO_2, regardless of the inhaled concentration of oxygen.

Mixed Venous PO_2

The mixed venous PO_2 is determined by the cardiac output and tissue oxygen consumption. In the presence of unchanging tissue oxygen consumption, the mixed venous PO_2 varies directly with changes in cardiac output. For example, when the cardiac output is decreased, less blood flow is available for tissue oxygen extraction. Therefore, the continued extraction of the same amount of oxygen from a decreased blood flow must result in a decreased mixed venous PO_2. Tissue hypoxemia is likely when the mixed venous PO_2 is lower than 30 mmHg. Disease states associated with arterial to venous admixture (sepsis, portal hypertension) may result in a high mixed venous PO_2 despite inadequate tissue oxygenation.

Arterial and Mixed Venous Content of Oxygen

The difference between the arterial and mixed venous content of oxygen is an estimate of the adequacy of cardiac output relative to tissue oxygen consumption (Table 16-7). The normal difference in oxygen content of arterial and mixed venous blood is 4 to 6 $ml \cdot dl^{-1}$ of blood. When tissue oxygen consumption is constant, a decreased cardiac output is accompanied by an increased oxygen content difference between arterial and mixed venous blood.

Table 16-6. Calculation of the Ratio of Arterial to Alveolar Oxygen Partial Pressure

$$a/A = PaO_2/PAO_2$$

Example: Arterial blood gases are PaO_2 310 mmHg and $PaCO_2$ 40 mmHg breathing 100% oxygen (FIO_2 = 1.0). The PB is 747 mmHg and the PH_2O 47 mmHg. The a/A is

$$PAO_2 = (747 - 47)1.0 - 40/0.8$$
$$PAO_2 = 700 - 50$$
$$PAO_2 = 650 \text{ mmHg}$$

$$a/A = 310/650$$
$$a/A = 0.48 \text{ (normal } >0.75)$$

Oxyhemoglobin Dissociation Curve

The oxyhemoglobin dissociation curve describes the saturation of hemoglobin with oxygen relative to the PO_2 (Fig. 16-5). Alternatively, this curve may be

Table 16-7. Calculation of Arterial and/or Venous Content of Oxygen

CaO_2	=	(Hb × 1.39)Sat + PaO_2(0.003)
CaO_2	=	oxygen content of arterial blood ($ml \cdot dl^{-1}$)
$C\bar{v}O_2$	=	oxygen content of mixed venous blood ($ml \cdot dl^{-1}$)
Hb	=	hemoglobin ($g \cdot dl^{-1}$)
1.39	=	oxygen bound to hemoglobin ($ml \cdot g^{-1}$)
Sat	=	percentage of saturation of hemoglobin with oxygen
PaO_2	=	arterial partial pressure of oxygen (mmHg)
$P\bar{v}O_2$	=	mixed venous partial pressure of oxygen (mmHg)
0.003	=	dissolved oxygen ($ml \cdot dl^{-1} \cdot mmHg^{-1}$)

Example: Hb = 15 $g \cdot dl^{-1}$ and PaO_2 100 mmHg resulting in nearly 100% saturation, $P\bar{v}O_2$ 40 mmHg resulting in 75% saturation.

$$CaO_2 = (15 \times 1.39)1.00 + 100(0.003) = 20.85 + 0.3 = 21.15 \ ml \cdot dl^{-1}$$

$$C\bar{v}O_2 = (15 \times 1.39)0.75 + 40(0.003) = 15.63 + 0.12 = 15.75 \ ml \cdot dl^{-1}$$

$$CaO_2 - C\bar{v}O_2 = 5.4 \ ml \cdot dl^{-1}$$

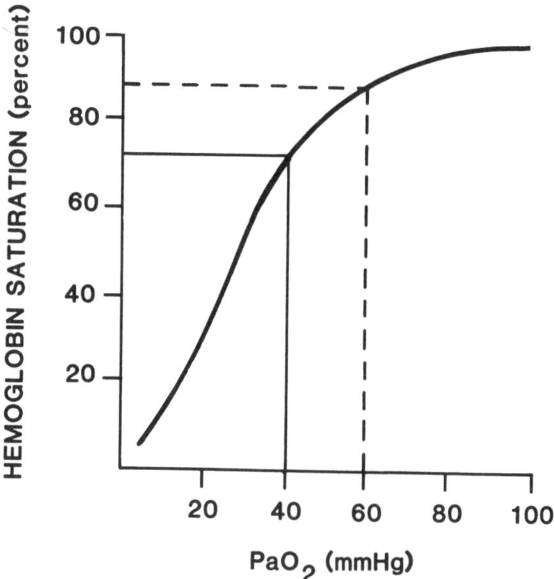

Figure 16-5. The oxyhemoglobin dissociation curve describes the relationship of the hemoglobin saturation with oxygen (%) to the PO_2. The P_{50} is the PO_2 that results in 50% saturation of hemoglobin with oxygen. In the presence of a normal pHa (7.4) and body temperature (37°C), hemoglobin is 50% saturated with oxygen at a PO_2 of 26 mmHg (P_{50}). Events that shift the oxyhemoglobin dissociation curve to the left (P_{50} lower than 26 mmHg) may jeopardize tissue oxygenation since the PaO_2 must decrease further to permit release of oxygen from hemoglobin. Conversely, a shift of the oxyhemoglobin dissociation curve to the right (P_{50} higher than 26 mmHg) permits unloading of oxygen from hemoglobin at a higher PaO_2 and thus favors tissue oxygenation. The mixed venous PO_2 is near 40 mmHg, and the associated hemoglobin saturation with oxygen is about 75%. Saturation of hemoglobin with oxygen is about 90% when the PaO_2 is 60 mmHg. The saturation of hemoglobin with oxygen can be assumed to be 100% when the PaO_2 is higher than 150 mmHg.

viewed as depicting the loading and unloading of oxygen from hemoglobin at a varying PO_2. The benefit of the sigmoid shape of the curve is ease of oxygen loading onto hemoglobin over a wide range of minimally changing PO_2 values (flat upper portion of the curve) and ease of release of oxygen from hemoglobin with small changes in PO_2 values (steep lower portion of curve). A normal oxyhemoglobin dissociation curve is characterized by 50% saturation of hemoglobin with oxygen at a PO_2 of 26 mmHg. The PO_2 that results in 50% saturation is referred to as the P_{50}. Events that shift the oxyhemoglobin dissociation curve to the left (P_{50} lower than 26 mmHg) may jeopardize tissue oxygenation since oxygen is more tightly bound to hemoglobin, and the PaO_2 must decrease to a lower than normal level before oxygen is released from hemoglobin and becomes available to tissues (Table 16-8). Events that shift the oxyhemoglobin dissociation curve to the right (P_{50} higher than 26 mmHg) facilitate tissue oxygen availability by permitting the unloading of oxygen from hemoglobin at an increased PaO_2 (Table 16-8).

Compensation for Arterial Hypoxemia

Increased cardiac output is the most important compensatory mechanism for correction of arterial hypoxemia. For example, if cardiac output increases and tissue oxygen consumption is unchanged, the result is decreased extraction of oxygen from venous blood.The effect of this decreased oxygen extraction is an increased mixed venous PO_2 that produces less dilution when arterial blood and shunted venous blood mix. A less efficient compensatory mechanism to offset arterial hypoxemia is hyperventilation. For example, the resulting decrease in alveolar PCO_2 is paralleled by a similar increase in the PaO_2. Nevertheless, an accompanying increased oxygen consumption of the respiratory muscles is likely to offset the gain in available oxygen produced by hyperventilation.

Ventilation

The $PaCO_2$ reflects the adequacy of the lungs for removing carbon dioxide from pulmonary capillary blood. In the steady state, $PaCO_2$ is directly proportional to the metabolic production of carbon dioxide and inversely proportional to alveolar ventilation. The production of carbon dioxide depends on

Table 16-8. Events that Shift the Oxyhemoglobin Dissociation Curve

Left Shift (P_{50} <26 mmHg)	Right Shift (P_{50} >26 mmHg)
Alkalosis	Acidosis
Hypothermia	Hyperthermia
Decreased 2,3-diphosphoglycerate	Increased 2,3-diphosphoglycerate (chronic arterial hypoxemia or anemia)

the metabolic state of the individual and parallels tissue oxygen consumption. Under normal conditions, only 80% as much carbon dioxide is produced as oxygen is consumed (respiratory quotient = 0.8). Assuming a tissue oxygen consumption of 250 $ml \cdot min^{-1}$, the production of carbon dioxide would be 200 $ml \cdot min^{-1}$. When the $PaCO_2$ is higher than 44 mmHg, the patient is hypoventilating relative to carbon dioxide production, whereas a $PaCO_2$ lower than 36 mmHg is defined as hyperventilation. Wasted ventilation or increased physiologic deadspace may result in an increased $PaCO_2$ even when minute ventilation is increased. The VD/VT ratio, which depicts areas in the lungs that receive adequate ventilation but inadequate or no pulmonary blood flow, should not exceed 0.3 (Table 16-9). In contrast to PaO_2, venous admixture has little to no impact on $PaCO_2$, reflecting the extreme diffusibility of carbon dioxide.

Table 16-9. Calculation of the Deadspace-to-Tidal Volume Ratio

$$V_D/V_T = \frac{PaCO_2 - P_ECO_2}{PaCO_2}$$

V_D/V_T = ratio of dead space to tidal volume
$PaCO_2$ = arterial partial pressure of carbon dioxide (mmHg)
P_ECO_2 = mixed exhaled partial pressure of carbon dioxide (mmHg)

Example: The $PaCO_2$ is 40 mmHg and P_ECO_2 20 mmHg during controlled ventilation of the lungs. The V_D/V_T is

$$V_D/V_T = \frac{40 - 20}{40}$$

$$V_D/V_T = 20/40$$

$$V_D/V_T = 0.5 \text{ (normal } <0.3)$$

REFERENCES

1. Narins RG, Emmett M. Simple and mixed acid base disorders: A practical approach. Medicine 1980; 59:161–87.
2. Siggard-Andersen O. Blood acid-base alignment nomogram. Scand J Clin Lab Invest 1963;15:211–7.
3. Hidman BJ. Sodium bicarbonate in the treatment of subtypes of acute lactic acidosis. Physiologic considerations. Anesthesiology 1990;72:1064–6.
4. Mitchell RA, Singer MM. Respiration and cerebrospinal fluid pH in metabolic acidosis. J Appl Physiol 1965;20:905–11.
5. Edelist G, Osorio A. Postanesthetic initiation of spontaneous ventilation after passive hyperventilation. Anesthesiology 1969;31:222–7.
6. Barcenas CG, Fuller TJ, Knochel JP. Metabolic alkalosis after massive blood transfusion. JAMA 1976;236:953–4.
7. Ream AK, Reitz BA, Silverberg G. Temperature correction of PCO_2 and pH in estimating acid-base status: An example of the emperor's new clothes? Anesthesiology 1982;56:41–4.
8. Clark LC. Monitor and control of blood and tissue oxygen tensions. Trans Am Soc Artif Intern Organs 1956;2:41–8.
9. Severinghaus JW, Bradley AF. Electrodes for blood PO_2 and PCO_2 determination. J Appl Physiol 1958; 13:515–20.
10. Williamson DC, Munson ES. Correlation of peripheral venous and arterial blood gas values during general anesthesia. Anesth Analg 1982;61:950–2.
11. Doyle JD. Arterial/alveolar oxygen tension ratio: A critical appraisal. Can Anaesth Soc J 1986;33:471–4.

17

Fluid and Blood Therapy

Perioperative management of a patient's fluid balance includes preoperative evaluation and intraoperative maintenance and replacement of fluid losses. Preoperative treatment of hypovolemia is helpful because circulatory changes induced by anesthesia and surgery are augmented by co-existing decreases in intravascular fluid volume. Intraoperatively, in addition to blood loss, fluids can shift into various body compartments. Knowledge of these shifts can aid in predicting fluid requirements. Maintaining normal intravascular fluid volume is dependent on knowledge of body compartmental fluid changes, quantitation of blood loss, and selection of the appropriate relacement fluid for infusion.

BODY FLUID COMPARTMENTS

Total body water can be divided into extracellular fluid (ECF) and intracellular fluid (ICF) (Fig. 17-1). The ECF is further divided into plasma volume (PV) and interstitial fluid (ISF), which are separated by the walls of the blood vessels. The PV is defined as the fluid contained within the vascular system but external to the erythrocytes, whereas ISF is confined to the compartment external to the blood vessels and cells. PV represents about 5% of body weight, and ISF constitutes about 15% of body weight. If erythrocytes are added to the PV, a total blood volume equal to approximately 7.5% of body weight results.

Total body water content varies with age, gender, and body habitus. In adult males, 55% of body weight is represented by body water, whereas 45% of body weight is represented by total body water in adult females. Because fat contains little water, obese adults have less total body water per kilogram than lean adults. Total body water constitutes about 80% of the total body weight in infants.

Preoperative Evaluation

The patient's mental status, history of intake and output, arterial blood pressure in both supine and standing positions, heart rate, skin turgor, and urinary output should be evaluated with respect to alterations in these parameters produced by changes in intravascular fluid volume and/or concentration of electrolytes. Serum electrolytes are often measured along with, in some situations, serum osmolarity. The volume, concentration, and composition of the ECF are the three steps by which the intraoperative fluid and electrolyte status are evaluated.

Volume

ECF volume should be assessed preoperatively because most anesthetic techniques and drugs can result in hypotension in patients who have a deficit of ECF volume. Tachycardia and dry mucous membranes may indicate a mild volume deficit, even though the arterial blood pressure is normal. This type of deficit can be seen in patients who have had extensive preoperative evaluation that required restricted oral intake, enemas for diagnostic radiologic procedures, and blood withdrawal for various laboratory tests.

Determining whether orthostatic hypotension is present is useful in detecting more severe forms of

Steps for Evaluation of Fluid and Electrolyte Status

Volume
- Blood pressure supine and standing
- Heart rate
- Mucous membrane moisture
- Skin turgor
- Urine output

Concentration
- Serum sodium
- Serum osmolarity

Composition
- Serum electrolytes
- Blood urea nitrogen
- Blood glucose
- Arterial blood gases and pH

intravascular fluid volume deficits. If the systolic blood pressure decreases more than 20 mmHg when the patient changes from the supine to standing position, there may be a fluid deficit of 6% to 8% of body weight. In this regard, observation of the heart rate is important in differentiating orthostatic hypotension due to antihypertensive drugs that alter autonomic nervous system activity from an intravascular fluid volume deficit. If orthostatic hypotension occurs, the heart rate should increase in a compensatory manner. If this does occur, the decrease in blood pressure is most likely due to an intravascular fluid volume deficit. If, however, the arterial blood pressure decreases and the heart rate does not increase, a defect in autonomic nervous system function, which could reflect antihypertensive drugs the patient is receiving, should be suspected (see Chapter 3). In suspected cases of severe ECF deficits, the bladder probably should be catheterized to accurately quantitate urinary output. A decrease in or absence of urinary output may indicate a severe deficit in ECF volume.

Intravascular fluid volume excess from either iatrogenic causes (excessive fluid administration) or pathologic causes (cirrhosis of the liver) may be present in surgical patients. Soft tissue edema and diuresis (more than 100 $ml \cdot h^{-1}$) are usually signs of excessive intravenous fluid administration. Arterial blood pressure will initially increase but will subsequently decrease if the intravascular fluid overload induces congestive heart failure. In severe cases, peripheral edema and even pulmonary edema will result. Congestive heart failure should be treated before elective anesthesia and surgery are performed.

Concentration

The concentration of constituents in ECF is determined to a large extent by total body water content. Although some bedside clues may be present, laboratory diagnosis is helpful for diagnosing abnormalities in body fluid concentrations. Valuable laboratory tests are the serum sodium concentration and, if available, the serum osmolarity or colloid oncotic pressure.[1] When electrolyte-free water is lost from the body, the serum sodium concentration and serum osmolarity increase. Usually, these increases are due to inadequate water intake or can occur in pathologic situations such as fever and loss of fluid from denuded tissues (burns).

When water is present in body fluids in excess of the normal ratio, the serum sodium concentration and osmolarity are decreased. Also, patients can

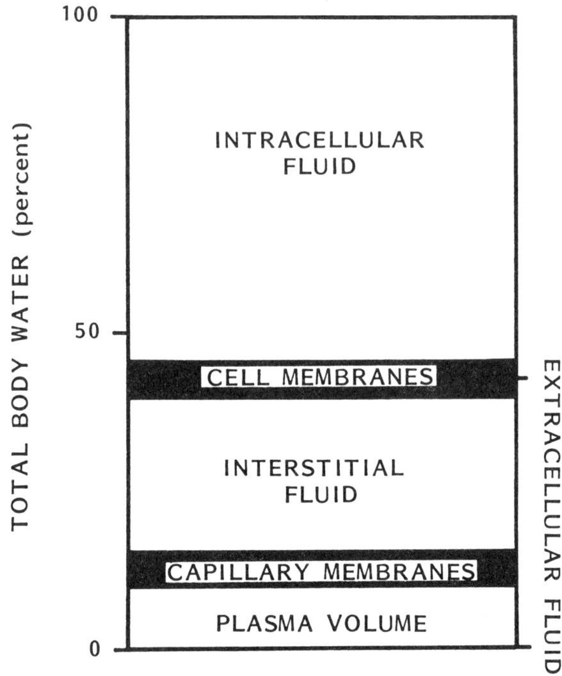

Figure 17-1. Schematic depiction of location of total body water.

develop a hypovolemic/hyponatremic condition in which electrolyte-rich fluids (such as vomitus, diarrhea, or fistula drainage) are lost and are replaced with water. Obviously, proper treatment consists of replacement with electrolyte-containing crystalloid solutions such as lactated Ringer's solution. A normovolemic/hyponatremic condition results from failure of the kidneys to conserve sodium when the intake of sodium is decreased but fluid intake has been adequate. A hypervolemic/hyponatremic condition results from excessive water intake or retention, which, during anesthesia, is most commonly seen after transurethral resection of the prostate (see Chapter 21), and when 5% dextrose in water is used to correct intravascular fluid volume deficits.

Composition

The composition of ECF is determined by the presence of various electrolytes. The distribution of electrolytes differs among the fluid compartments of the body (Table 17-1). The major cation in the blood is sodium, whereas the major cation in ICF is potassium. The electrophysiology of excitable cells depends on the intracellular and extracellular concentrations of sodium, potassium, and calcium.

Hypernatremia. Hypernatremia (serum sodium concentration higher than 145 $mEq \cdot L^{-1}$) is most often due to a deficit of total body content of water and not to an excess of total body sodium. Total body sodium can increase, however, when renal function is impaired, as occurs in patients with kidney disease, cirrhosis of the liver, or congestive heart failure. Peripheral edema is the hallmark of hypernatremia. An expanded intravascular fluid volume may manifest as hypertension. Hypernatremia due to excess total body sodium content is treated with renal tubular diuretics.

Hyponatremia. Hyponatremia (serum sodium concentration lower than 135 $mEq \cdot L^{-1}$) is most often due to an excess of total body water and not to a deficiency of total body sodium. Total body sodium can decrease, however, with vomiting, diarrhea, and third-degree burns. Hyponatremia due to sodium loss is characterized by a decreased intravascular fluid volume, which manifests as hypotension, tachycardia, oliguria, and hemoconcentration. Central nervous system signs of hyponatremia do not usually occur until the serum sodium concentration is lower than 110 $mEq \cdot L^{-1}$. Treatment of hyponatremia rarely requires the intravenous administration of hypertonic saline.

Table 17-1. Approximate Distribution of Electrolytes

	Extracellular Fluid ($mEq \cdot L^{-1}$)	Intracellular Fluid ($mEq \cdot L^{-1}$)
Sodium	140	10
Potassium	4.5	150
Calcium	5	1
Magnesium	2	40

Hyperkalemia. Hyperkalemia (serum potassium concentration higher than 5.5 $mEq \cdot L^{-1}$) can be due to an increased total body potassium content (renal failure) or altered distribution of potassium between intracellular and extracellular sites (respiratory acidosis or metabolic acidosis, succinylcholine). Adverse effects of hyperkalemia are likely to accompany acute increases in serum potassium concentrations. By contrast, chronic hyperkalemia is more likely to be associated with normal gradients between extracellular and intracellular concentrations of potassium. That patients with chronic hyperkalemia are often asymptomatic suggests that potassium gradients across cell membranes are more important than the absolute serum concentrations of potassium. The most detrimental effect of hyperkalemia is on the cardiac conduction system, manifesting on the electrocardiogram (ECG) as prolongation of the P-R interval, widening of the QRS complex, and peaking of the T wave. A frequent recommendation is that serum potassium concentrations should be lower than 5.5 $mEq \cdot L^{-1}$ before elective surgery is performed. Emergency surgery in the presence of hyperkalemia requires careful monitoring of the ECG to detect adverse effects of potassium on the heart. Avoidance of systemic acidosis due to hypoventilation or arterial hypoxemia is important, as this change would accentuate hyperkalemia.

Treatment. Treatment of acute hyperkalemia is designed to shift potassium from the serum into the cells so as to antagonize the effects of potassium on the heart (Table 17-2). The most rapidly acting therapeutic approach for reversal of cardiac effects of hyperkalemia is intravenous administration of calcium. Potassium can also be shifted into cells by production of systemic alkalosis (iatrogenic hyperventi-

Table 17-2. Treatment of Hyperkalemia

	Mechanism	Onset	Duration
Calcium gluconate 10–20 ml IV (10% solution)	Direct antagonism	Rapid	15–30 min
Hyperventilation ($PaCO_2$ 25–30 mmHg)	Shift intracellular	Rapid	
Hemodialysis	Remove	Rapid	
Sodium bicarbonate (50–100 mEq IV)	Shift intracellular	15–30 min	3–6 h
Glucose (25–50 g) plus regular insulin (10–20 units) IV	Shift intracellular	15–30 min	3–6 h

lation, intravenous administration of sodium bicarbonate) or intravenous injection of glucose combined with regular insulin. Insulin is given to ensure that glucose enters the cell and carries potassium with it. All these treatments represent temporizing measures to be taken until excess potassium can be eliminated from the body.

Hypokalemia. Hypokalemia (serum potassium concentration lower than 3.5 mEq·L^{-1}) can be due to a decreased total body potassium content (diuretic therapy, vomiting, diarrhea, nasogastric suction) or an alteration in the distribution of potassium between intracellular and extracellular sites (respiratory alkalosis, metabolic alkalosis, sympathetic nervous system stimulation). It has been observed that the plasma potassium concentration measured in a blood sample obtained immediately before the induction of anesthesia is often lower than that measured in a blood sample obtained 1 to 3 days preoperatively (Fig. 17-2).[2] The most likely explanation for this finding is stress-induced catecholamine release in the immediate preoperative period, leading to a beta-2 mediated translocation of potassium into intracellular sites. The role of acute stress-induced hypokalemia should be considered when interpreting the serum potassium concentration as measured in the immediate preoperative period. Hypokalemia is also a hazard of treating asthma or premature labor with a beta-2 agonist.

Adverse effects of chronic hypokalemia may include decreased myocardial contractility, skeletal muscle weakness, and increased automaticity of the atria and ventricles, manifesting as cardiac dysrhythmias. Alterations in cardiac conduction manifest on the ECG as prolongation of the P-R interval and Q-T interval and flattening of the T wave.

Treatment. There is evidence that treatment of chronic hypokalemia with oral potassium supplementation is ineffective and unnecessary.[3] For exam-

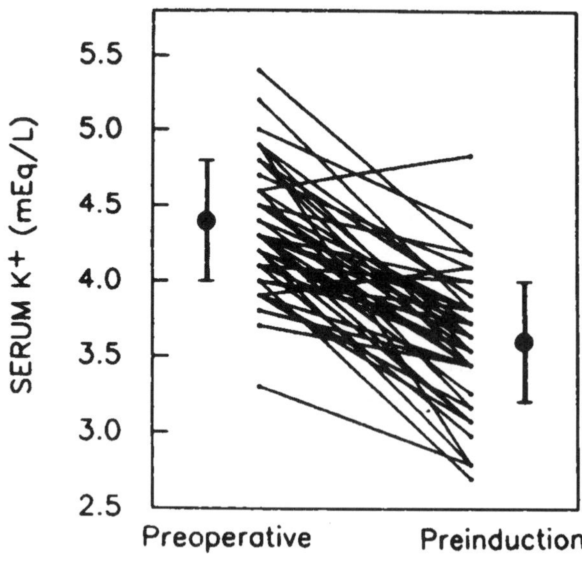

Figure 17-2. Serum potassium concentration measured 1 to 3 days preoperatively (4.4 ± 0.4 mEq·L^{-1}) is significantly higher (P <0.001) than that measured immediately before the induction of anesthesia (3.6 ± 0.4 mEq·L^{-1}). (From Kharasch and Bowdle,[2] with permission.)

ple, about 50% of patients with diuretic-induced hypokalemia fail to attain a normal serum potassium concentration despite oral supplementation. Indeed, in many treated patients, most of the oral potassium is excreted in the urine despite persistence of hypokalemia. Administration of potassium chloride (0.2 mEq·kg^{-1}·h^{-1} IV during constant monitoring of the ECG) is recommended when hypokalemia is associated with the appearance of abnormalities on the ECG.

Management of Anesthesia. The advisability of proceeding with elective surgery in the presence of chronic serum potassium concentrations lower than 3.5 mEq·L^{-1} is controversial. There is an undocumented concern that chronically hypokalemic patients are at increased risk of developing cardiac dysrhythmias intraoperatively, especially if plasma potassium concentrations are lower than 3.0 mEq·L^{-1}. Nevertheless, the incidence of intraoperative cardiac dysrhythmias is not increased in asymptomatic patients with chronic hypokalemia (2.6 to 3.5 mEq·L^{-1}) undergoing elective operations.[4] Adverse effects of hypokalemia are most likely when acute decreases in the serum potassium concentration are superimposed on co-existing chronic hypokalemia. It would seem logical to repeat the serum potassium measurement and obtain an ECG for evaluation of cardiac rhythm before the induction of anesthesia in a patient considered to be at risk of hypokalemia. In this regard, it is important to recognize that the serum potassium concentration measured just before the induction of anesthesia may be decreased due to sympathetic nervous system stimulation (anxiety) (Fig. 17-2).[2] During surgery, intravenous fluids that do not contain glucose are often selected, since hyperglycemia could contribute to hypokalemia. Addition of 10 to 20 mEq of potassium chloride to every liter of intravenous fluid maintenance can be considered but must be weighed against the risks of too rapid intravenous administration should infusion rates be accidently increased during the intraoperative period. Excessive hyperventilation of the lungs must be avoided. Capnography and measurement of arterial blood gases and pH is helpful in confirming the proper management of ventilation. It is important to monitor the ECG continuously for evidence of hypokalemia in the intraoperative and postoperative period.

Hypercalcemia. Hypercalcemia (serum calcium concentration higher than 5.5 mEq·L^{-1}) is typically due to hyperparathyroidism and neoplastic disorders with bone metastases (see Chapter 22). When serum calcium is higher than 8 mEq·L^{-1}, cardiac conduction disturbances manifest on the ECG as a prolonged P-R interval, wide QRS complex, and shortened Q-T interval. During anesthesia, it is important to maintain hydration and urine output to minimize further increases in the serum calcium concentration.

Hypocalcemia. Hypocalcemia (serum concentration lower than 4.5 mEq·L^{-1}) can be due to decreased serum albumin concentrations, hypoparathyroidism, pancreatitis, and renal failure (see Chapter 22). Impaired neuromuscular function in the presence of hypocalcemia reflects decreased presynaptic release of acetylcholine. Decreased myocardial contractility with increased central venous pressure and hypotension are typical. Skeletal muscle spasm, including laryngospasm, may accompany hypocalcemia. During anesthesia, respiratory alkalosis due to iatrogenic hyperventilation can rapidly decrease the serum ionized calcium concentration.

INTRAOPERATIVE FLUID THERAPY WITHOUT BLOOD LOSS

Solutions administered intravenously are required for maintenance of normal body fluid composition. Available solutions are classified as either crystalloids or colloids (see the section *Other Intravenous Solutions*). Colloids are frequently recommended for specific situations, such as replacement of fluid loss from fistulae, oozing from raw surfaces, and ascitic fluid. Crystalloid solutions are sufficient to maintain normal body fluid composition in most patients (Table 17-3).

Independent of the type of surgery, all patients have insensible fluid losses, which include evaporation of water from the respiratory tract, sweat, feces, and urinary excretion, all of which must be replaced. This requires intravenous administration of about 2 ml·kg^{-1}·h^{-1} of crystalloid solutions. Febrile patients or children may have larger insensible losses. Since most patients have had no caloric intake for several hours, it may be useful to include some glucose in the crystalloid solutions.

In addition to replacing insensible losses, the extent to which surgery is traumatic will dictate how much additional crystalloid solution should be given

Guidelines for Intraoperative Crystalloid Therapy

Administer isotonic electrolyte-containing solutions (2 $ml \cdot kg^{-1} \cdot h^{-1}$ IV) to replace insensible fluid losses

Administer additional electrolyte-containing solutions to replace third space loss
- Minimal surgical trauma 3–4 $ml \cdot kg^{-1} \cdot h^{-1}$ IV
- Moderate surgical trauma 5–6 $ml \cdot kg^{-1} \cdot h^{-1}$ IV
- Severe surgical trauma 7–8 $ml \cdot kg^{-1} \cdot h^{-1}$ IV

Replace 1 ml of blood loss with 3 ml of crystalloid solution

Monitor vital signs and maintain urine output (0.5–1 $ml \cdot kg^{-1} \cdot h^{-1}$)

intravenously. This reflects isotonic transfer of ECF from functional body fluid compartments to nonfunctional ones termed the third space (an acute sequestered space). This loss of fluid from the functional ECF to the third space must be replaced intraoperatively.

INTRAOPERATIVE FLUID THERAPY WITH BLOOD LOSS

If blood loss is sufficiently large, erythrocytes in the form of whole blood or packed red blood cells should be administered. Whole blood is probably preferable to packed red blood cells when replacing blood losses that exceed more than one-third of the blood volume (about 1500 ml in adults). Compensatory changes in response to blood loss include vasoconstriction of the splanchnic system and the venous capacitance vessels. This vasoconstriction can conceal the signs of acute blood loss until at least 10% of the blood volume is lost. Healthy patients may lose up to 20% of their blood volume before signs occur, such as a decrease in central venous pressure, hypotension, or tachycardia. Anesthetics decrease the ability of the body to compensate for blood loss and attenuate the classic signs of hypovolemia, such as tachycardia.

With acute blood loss, ISF and extravascular protein are transferred to the intravascular space, which tends to maintain PV. For this reason, when crystalloid solutions are used to replace blood loss, they must be given in amounts equal to about three times the amount of blood loss not only to replenish intravascular fluid volume but also to replenish the fluid lost from interstitial spaces. Dextran and hetastarch are examples of artificial solutions that are

Table 17-3. Comparison of Crystalloid Solutions

	Dextrose ($mg \cdot dl^{-1}$)	Sodium ($mEq \cdot L^{-1}$)	Chloride ($mEq \cdot L^{-1}$)	Potassium ($mEq \cdot L^{-1}$)	Magnesium ($mEq \cdot L^{-1}$)	Calcium ($mEq \cdot L^{-1}$)	Lactate ($mEq \cdot L^{-1}$)	Approximate pH	$mOsm \cdot L^{-1}$ (calculated)
ECF	90–110	40	108	4.5	2.0	5.0	5.0	7.4	290
5% dextrose in water	5000							4.3	253
5% dextrose in 0.45% NaCl	5000	77	77					4.3	406
5% dextrose in 0.9% NaCl	5000	154	154					4.2	561
0.9% NaCl		154	154					5.6	308
Lactated Ringer's solution		130	109	4.0		3.0	28	6.6	273
5% dextrose in lactated Ringer's solution	5000	130	109	4.0		3.0	28	4.9	525
Normosol-R		140	98	5.0	3.0		[a]	7.4	295
5% NaCl		855	855					5.6	1171

[a]Contains acetate 27 $mEq \cdot L^{-1}$ and gluconate 23 $mEq \cdot L^{-1}$.

useful for acute expansion of the intravascular fluid volume. In contrast to crystalloid solutions, dextran and hetastarch are more likely to remain in the intravascular space for prolonged periods. These solutions avoid complications associated with blood-containing products but obviously do not improve the oxygen carrying capacity of the blood and in large volumes (more than 20 $ml \cdot kg^{-1}$) may cause coagulation defects. Allergic reactions to dextran can result.

Arterial blood pressure, heart rate, and central venous pressure may be monitored to determine whether intravascular fluid volume is being adequately maintained. Intravascular fluid volume can be maintained with crystalloid or colloid solutions. Therefore, the only indication for packed red blood cells or whole blood is inadequate oxygen carrying capacity, the presence of which is difficult to determine with the usual monitoring approaches. For example, is hypotension or metabolic acidosis due to inadequate intravascular fluid volume or inadequate oxygen carrying capacity, or both? Serial determinations of hematocrit may be useful in this regard. Even though the hematocrit is not a reliable guide for assessing the adequacy of intravascular fluid volume, it is useful for determining whether the ratio between crystalloid and blood therapy has been appropriate. To maximize oxygen carrying capacity and, conversely, to ensure that the viscosity of blood is such that capillary flow will be adequate, a hematocrit between 21% and 30% is usually adequate. Therefore, when intravascular fluid volume is replaced, the hematocrit is commonly determined to assess whether the appropriate amount of blood has been given. For example, if the hematocrit is 35% to 40%, it would be appropriate to continue replacing blood loss with crystalloid solutions alone. If the hematocrit is 25% to 30%, it would be appropriate to administer blood as part of the replacement solutions to patients who need added oxygen carrying capacity (coronary artery disease). Patients without the need for added oxygen carrying capacity probably do not need blood unless the hematocrit is less than 25%.

BLOOD THERAPY

Determination of the blood types of the recipient and donor is the first step in selecting blood for transfusion therapy. Routine typing of blood is performed to identify the antigens (A, B, Rh) on the membrane of erythrocytes (Table 17-4). Naturally occurring antibodies (anti-B, anti-A) are formed whenever erythrocyte membranes lack A and/or B antigens. These antibodies are capable of causing rapid intravascular destruction of erythrocytes that contain the corresponding antigens.

Table 17-4. Blood Groups and Cross-match

			Incidence (%)	
Blood Group	Antigen on Erythrocyte	Plasma Antibodies	Whites	African-Americans
A	A	Anti-B	40	27
B	B	Anti-A	11	20
AB	AB	None	4	4
O	None	Anti-A Anti-B	45	49
Rh	Rh		42	17

Cross-match

The major cross-match occurs when the donor's erythrocytes are incubated with the recipient's plasma. Incubation of the donor's plasma with the recipient's erythrocytes is a minor cross-match. Agglutination occurs if either the major or minor cross-match is incompatible. The major cross-match also checks for immunoglobulin G antibodies (Kell, Kidd). Type-specific blood means that only the ABO-Rh type has been determined. The chance of a significant hemolytic reaction related to transfusion of type-specific blood is about 1 in 1000.

Type and Screen

Type and screen denotes blood that has been typed for A, B, and Rh antigens and screened for common antibodies. This approach is used when the scheduled surgical procedure is unlikely to require transfusion of blood (hysterectomy, cholecystectomy) but is one in which blood should be available. Use of type and screen permits more efficient use of stored blood because it is available to more than one patient. The chances of a significant hemolytic reaction related to use of type and screen blood is 1 in 10,000.

Blood Storage

Blood can be stored in a variety of solutions that contain phosphate, dextrose, and possibly adenine at temperatures of 1°C to 6°C. Storage time (70%

viability of transfused erythrocytes 24 hours after transfusion) is 21 to 35 days depending on the storage media. Adenine increases erythrocyte survival by allowing these cells to resynthesize adenosine triphosphate needed to fuel metabolic reactions. Changes that occur in blood during storage reflect the length of storage and the type of preservative used (Table 17-5). A unit of blood usually contains about 450 ml of blood and 65 ml of citrate-containing preservative.

Component Therapy

A unit of blood can be divided into several components that allow prolonged storage and specific treatment of underlying abnormalities without simultaneous infusion of unnecessary fractions such as plasma, which may contain antigens or antibodies.

Components Derived from Whole Blood

- Packed red blood cells
- Platelet concentrates
- Fresh frozen plasma
- Cryoprecipitate
- Albumin
- Plasma protein fraction
- Leukocyte poor blood
- Factor VIII
- Antibody concentrates

Packed Red Blood Cells

Packed red blood cells (volume 250 to 300 ml with a hematocrit of 70% to 80%) are used for treatment of anemia not associated with acute hemorrhage. The goal is to increase the oxygen carrying capacity of blood. A single unit of packed red blood cells will increase adult hemoglobin concentrations about 1 $g \cdot dl^{-1}$. Adequate oxygen carrying capacity can be maintained with a hemoglobin concentration of 7 $g \cdot dl^{-1}$ in most adult patients if intravascular fluid volume is maintained.[5]

Administration of packed red blood cells is facilitated by reconstituting them in crystalloid solutions such as 50 to 100 ml of saline.[6] Use of hypotonic glucose solutions may theoretically cause hemolysis, whereas calcium, as present in lactated Ringer's solution, may cause clotting if mixed with packed red blood cells.

Complications associated with packed red blood cells are similar to those of whole blood. An exception would be the chance of developing citrate intoxication, which would be smaller with packed red blood cells than whole blood because less citrate is infused. Infusion of less plasma reduces the likelihood of allergic reactions accompanying the administration of packed red blood cells. Conversely, removal of plasma also decreases the concentration of factors I (fibrinogen), V, and VIII.

Platelet Concentrates

Platelet concentrates allow specific treatment of thrombocytopenia without infusion of unnecessary blood components. During surgery, platelet transfu-

Table 17-5. Changes that Occur During Storage of Whole Blood in Citrate-Phosphate-Dextrose

	Days of Storage at 4°C			
	1	7	14	21
pH	7.1	7.0	7.0	6.9
PCO_2 (mmHg)	48	80	110	140
Potassium ($mEq \cdot L^{-1}$)	3.9	12	17	21
2,3-Diphosphoglycerate ($\mu M \cdot ml^{-1}$)	4.8	1.2	1	1
Viable platelets (%)	10	0	0	0
Factors V and VIII (%)	70	50	40	20

sions are probably not required unless the platelet count is less than 50,000 cells·mm^{-3} as determined by laboratory analysis. One unit of platelet concentrate will increase the platelet count 5000 to 10,000 cells·mm^{-3} as documented by platelet counts obtained 1 hour after infusion. Risks of platelet concentrate infusions are (1) sensitization reactions due to human leukocyte antigens (HLA) on cell membranes of platelets and (2) transmission of viral diseases, especially if pooled donor products are administered. The incidence of septic reactions can be decreased by the use of platelets with a shorter storage interval.[7]

Fresh Frozen Plasma

Fresh frozen plasma is the fluid portion obtained from a single unit of whole blood that is frozen within 6 hours of collection. All coagulation factors, except platelets, are present in fresh frozen plasma, explaining the use of this component for treatment of hemorrhage due to presumed coagulation factor deficiencies. Fresh frozen plasma transfusions during surgery are probably not necessary unless the prothrombin time and/or partial thromboplastin time are at least 1.5 times longer than normal. Risks of fresh frozen plasma include transmission of viral diseases and allergic reactions.

Cryoprecipitate

Cryoprecipitate is the fraction of plasma that precipitates when fresh frozen plasma is thawed. This component is useful for treating hemophilia A because it contains high concentrations of factor VIII in a small volume. Cryoprecipitate also can be used to treat hypofibrinogenemia (as induced by packed red blood cells) because it contains more fibrinogen than does fresh frozen plasma.

Colloids

There are several colloids that can be transfused that do not transmit disease. Albumin is available as 5% and 25% solutions. The 5% solution is isotonic with pooled plasma and is most often used when rapid expansion of the intravascular fluid volume is indicated. Hypoalbuminemia is the most frequent indication for administration of 25% albumin. It must be recognized that albumin solutions do not provide coagulation factors. Plasma protein fractions (Plasmanate) are 5% solutions of plasma proteins in saline. The risk of transmission of hepatitis with all these protein solutions is eliminated by heat treatment to 60°C for 10 hours. Hetastarch can cause decreases in circulating factor VIII concentrations if more than 1 to 1.5 L is infused. Colloids, including dextran, hold about 20 ml of water in the circulation for every gram of colloid given.

COMPLICATIONS OF BLOOD THERAPY

Complications of blood therapy, like an adverse effect of any therapy, must be considered when evaluating the risk-to-benefit ratio for treatment of individual patients with blood products. Anesthesiologists are among the most likely physicians to administer blood products to patients; therefore, it is imperative that complications of this therapy be fully appreciated.

Transfusion Reactions

Transfusion reactions are categorized as febrile, allergic, and hemolytic.

Complications of Blood Therapy

- Transfusion reactions
    - Febrile
    - Allergic
    - Hemolytic
- Metabolic abnormalities
    - Acidosis
    - Accumulation of potassium
    - Decreased 2,3-diphosphoglycerate
- Citrate intoxication
    - Alkalosis
    - Hypocalcemia
- Transmission of viral diseases
- Microaggregates
- Hypothermia
- Coagulation disorders
    - Dilutional thrombocytopenia
    - Dilution of factors V and VIII
    - Disseminated intravascular coagulation
- Immunosuppression

Febrile Reactions

Febrile reactions are the most common adverse nonhemolytic responses to transfusion of blood and accompany 0.5% to 1% of transfusions. The most likely explanation for febrile reactions is an interaction between recipient antibodies and antigens present on the leukocytes or platelets, or both, of the donor. The temperature rarely increases above 38°C, and the condition is treated by slowing the infusion and administering antipyretics. Severe febrile reactions accompanied by chills and shivering may require discontinuation of the blood infusion.

Allergic Reactions

Allergic reactions to properly typed and cross-matched blood manifest as body temperature increases, pruritus, and urticaria. Treatment often includes intravenous administration of antihistamines and, in severe cases, discontinuation of the blood infusion. Examination of the plasma and urine for free hemoglobin is useful to rule out hemolytic reactions.

Hemolytic Reactions

Hemolytic reactions occur when the wrong blood type is administered to a patient. The common factor in the production of intravascular hemolysis and development of spontaneous hemorrhage is activation of the complement system. With the exception of hypotension, the immediate signs (lumbar and substernal pain, fever, chills, dyspnea, skin flushing) of hemolytic reactions are masked by general anesthesia. Appearance of free hemoglobin in the plasma or urine is presumptive evidence of a hemolytic reaction. Acute renal failure reflects precipitation of stromal and lipid contents (not free hemoglobin) of hemolyzed erythrocytes in distal renal tubules. Disseminated intravascular coagulation is initiated by material released from hemolyzed erythrocytes (see the section *Disseminated Intravascular Coagulation*).

Treatment of acute hemolytic reactions is immediate discontinuation of the incompatible blood infusion and maintenance of urine output by infusion of crystalloid solutions and administration of mannitol or furosemide. The use of sodium bicarbonate to alkalinize the urine and improve the solubility of hemoglobin degradation products in the renal tubules is of unproven value, as is the administration of corticosteroids.

Metabolic Abnormalities

Metabolic abnormalities that accompany the storage of whole blood include accumulation of hydrogen ions and potassium, and decreased 2,3-diphosphoglycerate (2,3-DPG) concentrations (Table 17-5). Citrate present in the blood preservative may produce changes in the recipient.

Hydrogen Ions

Addition of most preservatives promptly increases the hydrogen ion content of stored whole blood. Continued metabolic function of erythrocytes results in additional production of hydrogen ions. Despite these changes, metabolic acidosis is not a consistent occurrence, even with rapid infusion of large volumes of stored blood. Therefore, intravenous administration of sodium bicarbonate to patients receiving transfusions of whole blood should be determined by measurement of pH and not based on arbitrary regimens.

Potassium

The potassium content of stored blood increases progressively with the duration of storage, but even massive transfusions rarely increase plasma potassium concentrations. Failure of plasma potassium concentrations to increase most likely reflects the small amount of potassium actually present in 1 unit of stored blood. For example, since 1 unit of whole blood contains only 300 ml of plasma, a measured potassium concentration of 21 $mEq \cdot L^{-1}$ would represent less than 7 mEq of potassium.

Decreased 2,3-Diphosphoglycerate

Storage of blood is associated with progressive decreases in concentrations of 2,3-DPG in erythrocytes, resulting in increased affinity of hemoglobin for oxygen (decreased P_{50} values). Conceivably, this change could jeopardize tissue oxygen delivery. Nevertheless, the clinical significance of 2,3-DPG changes remain unconfirmed.

Citrate

Citrate metabolism to bicarbonate may contribute to metabolic alkalosis, whereas binding of calcium by citrate could result in hypocalcemia. Indeed, metabolic alkalosis, rather than metabolic acidosis, is a common accompaniment of massive blood transfusions. Hypocalcemia due to citrate binding of calcium is rare, reflecting mobilization of calcium stores in bone and the ability of the liver to metabolize citrate to bicarbonate rapidly. Therefore, arbitrary administration of calcium in the absence of objective evidence of hypocalcemia (prolonged Q-T intervals on the ECG; measured decreases in plasma ionized calcium concentrations) is not indicated. Supplemental calcium may be needed when (1) the rate of blood infusion is higher than 50 ml·min^{-1} (as may be required during liver transplantation), (2) hypothermia or liver disease interferes with metabolism of citrate, or (3) the patient is a neonate (Fig. 17-3).[8]

Transmission of Viral Diseases

Transmission of viral diseases (acquired immunodeficiency syndrome [AIDS], hepatitis, cytomegalovirus, yersinia enterocolitica) is a risk of administration of blood or its components. The use of volunteer donors and routine screening for hepatitis B and C virus has significantly decreased the incidence of transfusion-transmitted hepatitis.[5,9] Transmission of the virus responsible for AIDS (human immunodeficiency virus [HIV]) by blood transfusion is unlikely since the introduction of routine screening for HIV antibody in March 1985. For example, the possibility that a screened donor will be positive for HIV is estimated to be 1 in 61,171 donors.[10] The current risk for post-transfusion hepatitis C is about 3 per 10,000 units of blood transfused.[9] Therefore, the risk of HIV and hepatitis C infection from blood transfusions, even in high-prevalence metropolitan areas, is extremely low. Nevertheless, possible transmission of diseases should assume a prominent place in the evaluation of the risk-to-benefit ratio associated with treatment of individual patients with blood. In some instances, nonblood solutions become the more acceptable treatment when the risk of transmission of disease is considered.

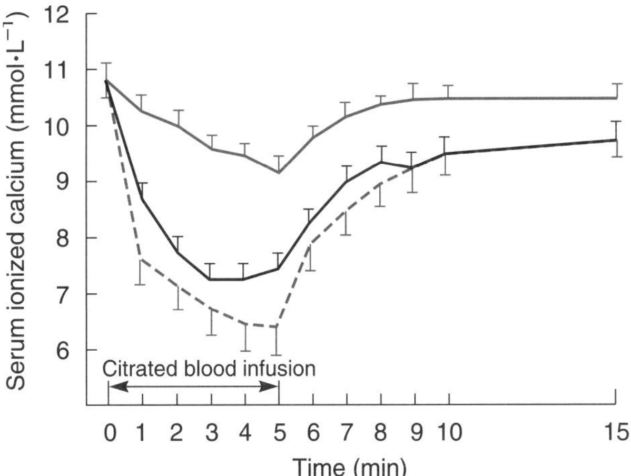

Figure 17-3. Serum ionized calcium concentrations were measured at three different rates of infusion over a 5-minute period. Solid red line, 50 ml·70 kg^{-1}·min^{-1}; solid black line, 100 ml·70 kg^{-1}·min^{-1}; dashed red line, 150 ml·70 kg^{-1}·min^{-1}. Mean ± SEM. (From Denlinger et al.,[8] with permission.)

Microaggregates

Microaggregates consisting of platelets and leukocytes form during storage of whole blood. Infusion of these microaggregates may be undesirable (pulmonary dysfunction), and micropore filters have been developed to remove particles with diameters in the 10- to 40–μm range. Use of micropore filters may decrease transfusion-induced splenic platelet sequestration and resulting thrombocytopenia and also reduce the incidence of febrile complications related to leukocytes. Nevertheless, use of micropore filters remains controversial.[11] It must be recognized, however, that stored blood should always be administered through 170-μm filters.

Hypothermia

Administration of blood stored at below 6°C can result in decreases in the patient's body temperature, with the possible development of cardiac irritability. Even a decrease of body temperature as small as 0.5°C to 1°C may induce shivering postoperatively, which in turn may increase oxygen consumption by as much as 400%. To meet the demands of an increased oxygen consumption, cardiac output must be increased. Passage of blood through specially designed warmers greatly decreases the likelihood of transfusion-related hypothermia. Occasionally, these warmers overheat the blood being transfused, causing hemolysis.[12]

Coagulation Disorders

Massive blood transfusions (10 units or more) can result in coagulation disorders due to dilutional thrombocytopenia and/or dilution of plasma concentrations of factors V and VIII. Disseminated intravascular coagulation due to hemolytic transfusion reactions must also be considered when intraoperative bleeding owing to unknown causes occurs.

Dilutional Thrombocytopenia

Dilutional thrombocytopenia reflects the virtual absence of viable platelets in blood stored at 4°C for longer than 24 hours (Table 17-5). It is likely that platelet counts will decline below 100,000 cells·mm^{-3} in adult patients receiving 10 to 15 units of whole blood or packed red blood cells. Bleeding may be associated with acute decreases in the platelet count to fewer than 100,000 cells·mm^{-3}. Dilutional thrombocytopenia is treated with infusion of platelet concentrates (see the section *Platelet Concentrates*).

Dilution of Factors V and VIII

Levels of factors V and VIII decrease in stored whole blood (all other clotting factors remain stable), but dilution of these factors in the patient's plasma from massive blood transfusions is rarely sufficient to cause bleeding (Table 17-5). Indeed, only 5% to 20% of the normal amount of factor V and 30% of factor VIII are necessary for hemostasis during surgery. Abnormalities due to dilution of clotting factors, including fibrinogen, are more likely to occur with infusion of erythrocytes that include minimal plasma volume. Fresh frozen plasma is the indicated treatment when specific measurements (prothrombin time or plasma thromboplastin time, or both, are at least 1.5 times longer than normal) confirm decreased plasma concentrations of clotting factors.

Disseminated Intravascular Coagulation

Disseminated intravascular coagulation is characterized by uncontrolled activation of the coagulation system, with consumption of platelets and clotting factors. Thrombocytopenia, prolongation of the prothrombin time and plasma thromboplastin time, and increased circulating concentrations of fibrin degradation products in the presence of diffuse hemorrhage (as around catheter placement sites) suggest the diagnosis. This condition is treated by removal of the underlying cause (hemolytic transfusion reactions, low cardiac output, hypovolemia, sepsis) and administration of platelet concentrates and fresh frozen plasma.

Immunosuppression

Blood transfusions exert a nonspecific immunosuppressive action that may be therapeutic for renal transplant recipients and detrimental for patients with cancer.[13] However, more recent evidence suggests that use of autologous blood, which does not depress the immune system, does not improve the prognosis in patients with colorectal cancer.[14] Perhaps patients who receive homologous blood have more extensive disease, which is the cause of this poorer prognosis rather than having received the blood. Packed red blood cells, which contain less plasma than whole blood, may produce less immunosuppression, suggesting that plasma contains an undefined immunosuppressive factor.

AUTOLOGOUS BLOOD

Many of the complications associated with homologous blood transfusions can be eliminated by the use of autologous blood, which can be obtained by several approaches.[15]

Predeposited Autologous Blood

Patients scheduled for elective surgery that may require transfusion of blood may elect to predonate (predeposit) blood for possible transfusion in the perioperative blood. This approach eliminates the chances of hemolytic reactions or transmission of blood-borne diseases. Most patients can donate 1 unit of blood about every 4 days (maximum about 3 units), with the last unit collected 72 hours or more before surgery to permit restoration of plasma volume. Oral iron supplementation is recommended when blood is withdrawn within a few days preceding surgery. Treatment with recombinant erythropoietin is very expensive but increases the amount of blood that patients can predeposit by as much as 40%. A hemoglobin concentration of about 8 g·dl^{-1} is now being accepted in the patient who predeposits blood for elective surgery.[15]

Intraoperative Salvage

By collection and reinfusion of blood lost during and immediately after surgery, the amount of homologous blood needed can be decreased. Typically, semiautomated systems are used that collect and wash the red blood cells and then deliver them to a reservoir for future administration either intraoperatively or postoperatively. Although controversial, blood containing disease-causing organisms or cancer cells probably should not be reinfused.

Complications of intraoperative salvage include dilutional coagulopathy, reinfusion of excessive anticoagulant (heparin), hemolysis, air embolism, and disseminated intravascular coagulation.

Hemodilution

Either immediately before or after induction of anesthesia, a portion of the patient's blood volume is removed through an arterial or venous catheter and stored in a sterile container with an anticoagulant. Most often, crystalloid solutions are infused to maintain normovolemia. Typically, the removed blood is reinfused when surgery is nearly completed. The volume of blood removed depends on the patient's body weight, preoperative hematocrit, and predicted blood loss. The proposed advantages of hemodilution include surgically induced loss of blood with a lower hematocrit and the subsequent availability of the patient's own fresh whole blood with its enhanced oxygen carrying capacity, platelets, and other coagulation factors as compared to stored homologous blood.

INDICATIONS FOR BLOOD TRANSFUSIONS

The increased concern relating to the possible infectivity of blood transfusions (AIDS, hepatitis) has resulted in anesthesiologists becoming especially conservative with respect to the indications for administration of homologous blood to patients. As a general rule, administration of homologous blood is usually not recommended unless the hemoglobin concentration is lower than 8 $g{\cdot}dl^{-1}$, or the patient has coronary artery disease or some other condition requiring additional oxygen carrying capacity. While it is reasonable to be less restrictive with autologous blood, complications such as bacterial contamination and hemolytic reactions due to clerical error can occur.[16] Neither homologous or autologous blood is recommended for transfusion to patients with hematocrits higher than 30%.

REFERENCES

1. Haynes GR, Conroy JM, Baker JD, Cooke, JE. Colloid oncotic pressures as a guide for the anesthesiologist in directing fluid therapy. Southern Med J 1989; 82:618–23.
2. Kharasch ED, Bowdle TA. Hypokalemia before induction of anesthesia and prevention by B2 adrenoceptor antagonism. Anesth Analg 1991;72:216–20.
3. Papademetrious V, Burris J, Kukich S, Freis ED. Effectiveness of potassium chloride or triamterene in thiazide hypokalemia. Arch Intern Med 1985;145: 1986–90.
4. Hirsch IA, Tomlinson DL, Slogoff S, Keats AS. The overstated risk of preoperative hypokalemia. Anesth Analg 1988;67:131–6.
5. Consensus Conference. Perioperative red blood cell transfusion. JAMA 1988;260:2700–3.
6. Cull DL, Lally KP, Murphy KD. Compatibility of packed erythrocytes and Ringer's lactate solution. Surg Gynecol Obstet 1991;173:9–12.
7. Morrow JF, Braine HG, Kickler TS, et al. Septic reactions to platelet transfusions. JAMA 1991;266:555–8.
8. Denlinger JK, Nahrwold ML, Gibbs PS, Lecky JH. Hypocalcemia during rapid blood transfusion in anaesthetized man. Br J Anaesth 1976;48:995–1000.
9. Donahue JG, Munoz A, Ness PM, et al. The declining risk of post-transfusion hepatitis C virus infection. N Engl J Med 1992;327:419–20.
10. Busch MP, Eble BE, Khayam-Bashi H, et al. Evaluation of screened blood donations of human immunodeficiency virus type 1 infection by culture and DNA amplification of pooled cells. N Engl J Med 1991; 325:1–5
11. Hassig A, Collins JA, Hogman C, et al. When is the microfiltration of whole blood and red cell concentrates essential? When is it superfluous? Vox Ang 1986;50:54–64.
12. Sazama K. Reports of 335 transfusions-associated deaths: 1976 through 1985. Transfusion 1990;30: 583–90.
13. Schriemer PA, Longnecker DE, Mintz PD. The possible immunosuppressive effects of perioperative blood transfusion in cancer patients. Anesthesiology 1988; 68:422–8.
14. Busch ORC, Hop WCJ, vanPapendrecht MAWH, et al. Blood transfusion and prognosis in colorectal cancer. N Engl J Med 1993;328:1372–6.
15. The use of autologous blood. The national blood resource education program expert panel. JAMA 1990; 263:414–7.
16. Miller AC, Scherba-Krugliak L, Toy PT, Drasner K. Hypotension during transfusion of autologous blood. Anesthesiology 1991;74:624–8.

Section IV

Special Anesthetic Considerations

18
Cardiovascular Disease

Management of anesthesia for patients with cardiovascular disease requires an understanding of the pathophysiology of the disease process and a careful selection of anesthetics, muscle relaxants, and monitors to match the unique needs of each individual patient.

CORONARY ARTERY DISEASE

Coronary artery disease (ischemic heart disease) is estimated to be present in 10 million adult Americans, and it is likely that 5% to 10% of patients who undergo anesthesia and surgery have associated coronary artery disease. The presence of coronary artery disease in patients who undergo anesthesia for noncardiac surgery may be associated with increased morbidity and mortality. History, physical examination, and evaluation of the patient's electrocardiogram (ECG) are important components of the routine preoperative cardiac evaluation.[1] More specialized procedures, such as ambulatory ECG monitoring (Holter monitoring), exercise ECG, echocardiography, radioisotope imaging, cardiac catheterization, and angiography, are performed on selected patients. Ultimately, data should determine whether patients are in the best medical condition possible before elective cardiac or noncardiac surgery.

Patient History

Important aspects of the history taken from patients with coronary artery disease before noncardiac surgery include cardiac reserve, characteristics of angina pectoris, and the presence of a prior myocardial infarction. Potential interactions of medications used in the treatment of coronary artery disease with drugs used to produce anesthesia must also be considered. Co-existing noncardiac diseases that often present in these patients include peripheral vascular disease, chronic obstructive pulmonary disease from cigarette smoking, renal dysfunction associated with chronic hypertension, and diabetes mellitus. A thorough evaluation is especially important because patients can remain asymptomatic despite 50% to 70% stenosis of a major coronary artery.

Cardiac Reserve

Limited exercise tolerance in the absence of significant pulmonary disease is the most striking evidence of decreased cardiac reserve. If a patient can climb two to three flights of stairs without symptoms, cardiac reserve is probably adequate.

Angina Pectoris

Angina pectoris is considered to be stable when no change has occurred for at least 60 days in precipitating factors, frequency, and duration. Chest pain produced with less than normal activity or lasting for increasingly longer periods is considered characteristic of unstable angina pectoris and may signal an impending myocardial infarction. Dyspnea following the onset of angina pectoris is indicative of acute left ventricular dysfunction due to myocardial ischemia. Angina pectoris due to spasm of the coronary arteries (variant or Prinzmetal's angina) differs from classic angina pectoris in that it may occur at rest but not during vigorous exertion. Silent myocardial ischemia does not evoke angina pectoris (asymptomatic) and usually occurs at a heart rate and blood pressure lower than those present during exercise-induced myocardial ischemia. It is estimated that about 70% of ischemic episodes are not associated with angina pectoris and as many as 15% of acute myocardial infarctions are silent.

The heart rate or systolic blood pressure, or both, at which angina pectoris or evidence of myocardial ischemia occurs on the ECG is useful preoperative information. An increased heart rate is more likely than hypertension to produce signs of myocardial ischemia. This is predictable because a rapid heart rate increases myocardial oxygen requirements and decreases the time during diastole for coronary blood flow and thus delivery of oxygen to occur. Conversely, increased myocardial oxygen requirements produced by increased systolic blood pressure may be offset by improved perfusion through pressure-dependent atherosclerotic coronary arteries.

Prior Myocardial Infarction

The incidence of myocardial reinfarction in the perioperative period is related to the time elapsed since the previous myocardial infarction (Table 18-1).[2-5] The incidence of perioperative myocardial reinfarction generally does not stabilize at 5% to 6% until 6 months after the prior myocardial infarction. Thus, a common recommendation is to delay elective surgery, especially thoracic and upper abdominal procedures, for about 6 months after a myocardial infarction. Even after 6 months, the 5% to 6% incidence of myocardial reinfarction is about 50 times greater than the 0.13% incidence of perioperative myocardial infarction in patients undergoing similar operations but in the absence of a prior myocardial infarction. Most perioperative myocardial reinfarctions occur in the first 48 to 72 hours postoperatively.

Several factors influence the incidence of myocardial infarction in the perioperative period. For example, the incidence of myocardial reinfarction is increased in patients undergoing intrathoracic or intra-abdominal operations lasting longer than 3 hours. Factors that have not been shown to predispose to a myocardial reinfarction include the (1) site of the previous myocardial infarction, (2) history of prior aortocoronary bypass graft surgery, (3) site of the operative procedure if the duration of the surgery is shorter than 3 hours, and (4) drugs or techniques, or both, used to produce anesthesia. Close hemodynamic monitoring using an intra-arterial and pulmonary artery catheter and prompt pharmacologic intervention or fluid infusion to treat hemodynamic alterations from a normal range may decrease the risk of perioperative myocardial reinfarctions in high-risk patients (Table 18-1).[4]

Table 18-1. Incidence of Perioperative Myocardial Reinfarction

Time Elapsed Since Prior Myocardial Infarction	Tarhan et al.[2] (%)	Steen et al.[3] (%)	Rao et al.[4] (%)	Shah et al.[5] (%)
0–3 mo	37	27	5.7	4.3
4–6 mo	16	11	2.3	0
>6 mo	5	6		5.7

Current Medications

Drugs most likely to be encountered in patients with coronary artery disease are beta antagonists, nitrates, and calcium channel blockers. In addition, patients with coronary artery disease may be receiving drugs classified as antihypertensives and diuretics. Knowledge of the pharmacology of these drugs and potential adverse interactions with anesthetics is an important preoperative consideration (see Chapters 3 and 21). Despite the potential for adverse drug interactions, cardiac medications being taken preoperatively probably should be continued without interruption through the perioperative period.

Electrocardiogram

The preoperative ECG should be examined for evidence of (1) myocardial ischemia, (2) prior myocardial infarction, (3) cardiac hypertrophy, (4) abnormal cardiac rhythm or conduction disturbances, or both, and (5) electrolyte abnormalities. The exercise ECG simulates sympathetic nervous system stimulation that may accompany perioperative events such as direct laryngoscopy and surgical stimulation. The resting ECG in the absence of angina pectoris may be normal despite extensive coronary artery disease. Nevertheless, an ECG demonstrating S-T seg-

Table 18-2. Area of Myocardial Ischemia as Reflected by the Electrocardiogram

Electrocardiogram Lead	Coronary Artery Responsible for Myocardial Ischemia	Area of Myocardium that May Be Involved
II, III, aVF	Right coronary artery	Right atrium Sinus node Atrioventricular node Right ventricle
V_3–V_5	Left anterior descending coronary artery	Anterolateral aspects of the left ventricle
I, aVL	Circumflex coronary artery	Lateral aspects of the left ventricle

ment depression greater than 1 mm, particularly during angina pectoris, confirms the presence of myocardial ischemia. Furthermore, the ECG lead demonstrating changes of myocardial ischemia can help determine the specific diseased coronary artery (Table 18-2). It should be remembered that a prior myocardial infarction, especially if subendocardial, may not be accompanied by persistent changes on the ECG. The preoperative presence of ventricular premature beats may signal their likely occurrence intraoperatively. A P-R interval on the ECG longer than 0.2 second is most often related to digitalis therapy. Conversely, the block of conduction of cardiac impulses below the atrioventricular node most likely reflects pathologic changes rather than drug effect.

Management of Anesthesia

Management of anesthesia in patients with coronary artery disease is based on a preoperative evaluation of left ventricular function and the maintenance of a favorable balance between myocardial oxygen requirements and myocardial oxygen delivery so as to prevent myocardial ischemia (Table 18-3). Any perioperative event associated with persistent tachycardia, systolic hypertension, arterial hypoxemia, or diastolic hypotension can adversely influence this delicate balance. The maintenance of this balance is more important than the specific technique or drugs selected to produce anesthesia and skeletal muscle paralysis. It is critical that persistent and excessive changes in heart rate and blood pressure be avoided (Fig. 18-1).[6] A common recommendation is to maintain heart rate and blood pressure within 20% of the awake values. Nevertheless, an estimated one-half of all new perioperative ischemic episodes are not preceded by or associated with significant changes in heart rate or blood pressure.[7] These episodes of silent myocardial ischemia are likely due to regional decreases in myocardial perfusion and oxygenation that are of questionable significance and identical to episodes that occur in these same patients during their daily activities in the absence of angina pectoris.

Induction of Anesthesia

Preoperative medication is intended to produce sedation so as to allay anxiety, which, if unopposed, could lead to secretion of catecholamines and an increase in myocardial oxygen requirements owing to an increase of blood pressure and heart rate. A frequent approach for preoperative medication in patients with coronary artery disease is intramuscular administration of morphine plus scopolamine with or without benzodiazepines. Scopolamine is valuable because of its profound sedative and amnesic effects without production of undesirable changes in heart rate. It may also be appropriate to apply a transdermal preparation of nitroglycerin at the time the preoperative medication is administered.

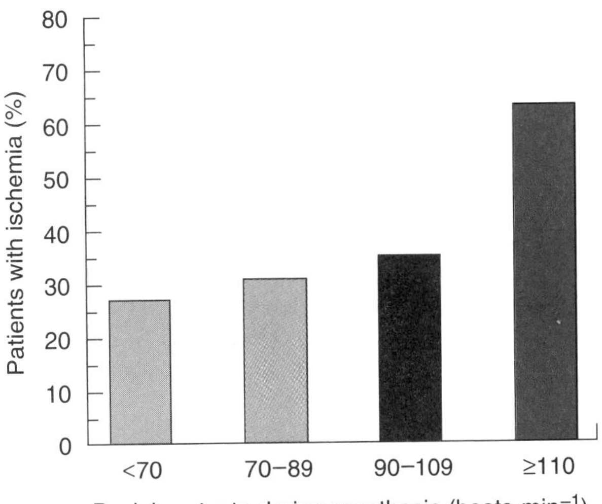

Figure 18-1. The incidence of myocardial ischemia is unrelated to heart rate until a value of about 110 beats·min^{-1} is reached or exceeded. (From Slogoff and Keats,[6] with permission.)

Table 18-3. Evaluation of Left Ventricular Function

	Good Function	Impaired Function
Prior myocardial infarction	No	Yes
Evidence of congestive heart failure	No	Yes
Ejection fraction	>0.55	<0.4
Left ventricular end-diastolic pressure	<12 mmHg	>18 mmHg
Cardiac index	>2.5 L·min^{-1}·m^{-2}	<2 L·min^{-1}·m^{-2}
Areas of ventricular dyskinesia	No	Yes

Induction of anesthesia is acceptably accomplished with the intravenous administration of rapidly acting drugs. Ketamine is not popular since an associated increase in heart rate and blood pressure might increase myocardial oxygen requirements. Intubation of the trachea is facilitated by the administration of succinylcholine or nondepolarizing muscle relaxants.

Myocardial ischemia may accompany the hypertension and tachycardia that result from the stimulation of direct laryngoscopy necessary for intubation of the trachea. A brief duration of direct laryngoscopy (preferably shorter than 15 seconds) is important in minimizing the magnitude of these circulatory changes. When the duration of direct laryngoscopy is not likely to be brief or when hypertension co-exists, the addition of other drugs to minimize the pressor response produced by intubation of the trachea should be considered. For example, laryngotracheal lidocaine (2 mg·kg^{-1}) administered just before inserting the tube into the trachea minimizes the magnitude and duration of the blood pressure increase. Likewise, lidocaine (1.5 mg·kg^{-1} IV), administered before direct laryngoscopy is begun, is efficacious. An alternative to lidocaine is nitroprusside (1 to 2 μg·kg^{-1} IV) administered about 15 seconds before direct laryngoscopy is begun or short-acting opioids such as fentanyl (1 to 3 μg·kg^{-1} IV) or sufentanil (0.1 to 0.3 μg·kg^{-1} IV) injected 2 to 4 minutes before direct laryngoscopy is begun. None of these pharmacologic interventions, however, reliably prevent heart rate increases produced by direct laryngoscopy. Continuous intravenous infusions of esmolol (200 μg·kg^{-1}·min^{-1} IV), a short-acting beta antagonist, are effective in attenuating heart rate increases associated with painful stimulation, including direct laryngoscopy.

Maintenance of Anesthesia

The choice of anesthesia is often based on the patient's left ventricular function (Table 18-3). For example, patients with coronary artery disease but normal left ventricular function are likely to develop tachycardia and hypertension in response to intense stimulation. Controlled myocardial depression produced by volatile anesthetics with or without nitrous oxide may be appropriate if the primary goal is to prevent increased myocardial oxygen requirements. Equally acceptable for the maintenance of anesthesia is the use of a nitrous oxide-opioid technique, with the addition of a volatile anesthetic as necessary to treat hypertension. When hypertension is treated with a volatile anesthetic, isoflurane and desflurane lower blood pressure by decreasing systemic vascular resistance, whereas halothane tends to lower blood pressure by decreasing cardiac output. The ability to rapidly increase the alveolar concentration of desflu-

Determinants of Myocardial Oxygen Requirements and Delivery

- Myocardial oxygen requirements
  - Heart rate
  - Systemic blood pressure
  - Myocardial contractility
  - Ventricular volume
- Myocardial oxygen delivery
  - Coronary blood flow
  - Oxygen content of arterial blood

rane (because of its low blood solubility) makes this volatile anesthetic uniquely efficacious for treating sudden increases in blood pressure. Use of volatile anesthetics to treat hypertension should consider the observation that abrupt increases in the concentrations of desflurane and isoflurane delivered to anesthetized but normotensive patients has been associated with transient increases in blood pressure and heart rate, presumably owing to activation of the sympathetic nervous system.[8,9]

Isoflurane is a more potent coronary arteriole vasodilator than halothane or desflurane. Conceivably, isoflurane-induced coronary arteriole vasodilation could result in diversion of blood flow from ischemic areas of myocardium (blood vessels already fully dilated) to nonischemic areas of myocardium supplied by vessels capable of vasodilation. Regional myocardial ischemia associated with drug-induced vasodilation is known as coronary artery steal. There are reports that the incidence of myocardial ischemia is either unchanged or increased in patients with coronary artery disease and anesthetized with isoflurane compared with those receiving a different volatile anesthetic or opioid.[10,11] All factors considered, volatile anesthetics may be (1) beneficial in patients with coronary artery disease because they decrease myocardial oxygen requirements or (2) detrimental because they lower blood pressure and coronary perfusion pressure or produce coronary artery steal (isoflurane).

Patients with impaired left ventricular function, as associated with a prior myocardial infarction, may not tolerate direct myocardial depression produced by volatile anesthetics. In these patients, the use of short-acting opioids with nitrous oxide may be more appropriate. It must be remembered that nitrous oxide, when administered to patients who have received opioids for anesthesia, may produce undesirable decreases in blood pressure and cardiac output. High-dose fentanyl (50 to 100 $\mu g \cdot kg^{-1}$ IV) or equivalent doses of sufentanil as the sole anesthetic have been advocated for patients who cannot tolerate even minimal anesthetic-induced myocardial depression.

A regional anesthetic is an acceptable technique in patients with coronary artery disease. It is important to realize, however, that flow through coronary arteries narrowed by atherosclerosis is pressure dependent. Therefore, decreases in blood pressure associated with a regional anesthetic that are more than 20% of the preblock value probably should be treated with an intravenous infusion of crystalloid solutions and/or sympathomimetics such as ephedrine.

Muscle Relaxant

The choice of nondepolarizing muscle relaxant during maintenance of anesthesia for patients with coronary artery disease is influenced by the circulatory effects of these drugs and the likely impact of these changes on myocardial oxygen requirements and myocardial oxygen delivery (see Chapter 7). Vecuronium, doxacurium, and pipecuronium are examples of muscle relaxants with benign circulatory effects. Likewise, the blood pressure lowering effects of atracurium and mivacurium are usually modest, especially if the drugs are injected over 30 to 45 seconds to minimize the likelihood of drug-induced histamine release. Muscle relaxants with benign circulatory effects are unlikely to alter myocardial oxygen requirements. Pancuronium increases heart rate and blood pressure, but these changes are usually less than 15% above predrug values, making this drug a possible choice for administration to patients with coronary artery disease. Furthermore, circulatory changes produced by pancuronium can be used to offset negative inotropic and/or chronotropic effects of drugs being used for anesthesia. In contrast to pancuronium, the other nondepolarizing muscle relaxants would not be expected to offset decreases in blood pressure or heart rate as associated with administration of high doses of opioids.

Nondepolarizing neuromuscular blockade can be safely reversed with anticholinesterase-anticholinergic drug combinations in patients with coronary artery disease. Glycopyrrolate apparently has less of a chronotropic effect than atropine. Nevertheless, marked increases in heart rate rarely occur with drug-enhanced reversal of nondepolarizing muscle relaxants and, therefore, atropine seems as acceptable as glycopyrrolate for combination with anticholinesterases.

Monitoring

The intensity of monitoring in the perioperative period is influenced by the complexity of the operative procedure and the severity of the coronary artery disease. The ECG is the only practical way to monitor the balance between myocardial oxygen requirements and myocardial oxygen delivery in unconscious patients (see Chapter 15). When this balance is unfavorably altered, myocardial ischemia occurs, as evidenced on the ECG by at least a 1-mm downsloping of the S-T segment from the baseline. A precordial V5 lead is a useful selection for detecting S-T segment changes characteristic of myocardial ischemia of the left ventricle during anesthesia. A pulmonary artery catheter is helpful for monitoring responses to intravenous fluid replacement and the therapeutic effects of drugs on left ventricular function. Right atrial pressure may not reliably reflect left heart filling pressure in the presence of left ventricular dysfunction due to coronary artery disease. Conversely, right atrial pressure is more likely to correlate with pulmonary artery occlusion pressure in patients with coronary artery disease when the ejection fraction is greater than 0.5 and there is no evidence of left ventricular dysfunction.[12]

The appearance of signs of myocardial ischemia on the ECG supports the aggressive treatment of adverse changes in heart rate and/or arterial blood pressure. Tachycardia is treated with the intravenous administration of propranolol or esmolol (0.2 to 0.5 $mg \cdot kg^{-1}$ IV), and excessive increases in blood pressure respond to nitroprusside. Nitroglycerin is a more appropriate choice than nitroprusside when myocardial ischemia is associated with normal blood pressure. Hypotension should be treated with sympathomimetics to rapidly restore pressure-dependent perfusion through atherosclerotic coronary arteries. In addition to drugs, the intravenous infusion of fluids to restore blood pressure is useful because myocardial oxygen requirements for volume work of the heart are lower than those for pressure work. A disadvantage of this approach is the time necessary for fluid treatment to be effective.

Decreases in body temperature that occur intraoperatively may predispose to shivering on awakening, leading to abrupt increases in myocardial oxygen requirements. Attempts to minimize decreases in body temperature and provision of supplemental oxygen are of obvious importance. Postoperative pain relief is important as pain-induced activation of the sympathetic nervous system can increase myocardial oxygen requirements.

VALVULAR HEART DISEASE

The most frequently encountered forms of valvular heart disease produce pressure overload (mitral stenosis, aortic stenosis) or volume overload (mitral regurgitation, aortic regurgitation) of the left ventricle. The net effect of valvular heart disease is interference with forward flow of blood from the heart into the systemic circulation. Echocardiography has revolutionized the noninvasive evaluation of valvular heart disease. Selection of anesthetic drugs and muscle relaxants for patients with valvular heart disease is often based on the likely effects of drug-induced changes in cardiac rhythm, heart rate, blood pressure, systemic vascular resistance, and pulmonary vascular resistance relative to maintenance of cardiac output in these patients. When cardiac reserve is minimal, high doses of short-acting opioids may be used as the sole anesthetic. Patients with valvular heart disease often receive antibiotics in the perioperative period for protection against infective endocarditis.

Doppler Echocardiography and Valvular Heart Disease

- Determine significance of cardiac murmurs (most often aortic stenosis)
- Identify hemodynamic abnormalities associated with physical findings (most often mitral regurgitation)
- Determine transvalvular pressure gradient
- Determine orifice area of cardiac valve
- Diagnose cardiac valve regurgitation
- Evaluate prosthetic valve function

Mitral Stenosis

Mitral stenosis is characterized by mechanical obstruction to left ventricular diastolic filling secondary to a progressive decrease in the orifice of the mitral valve. The obstruction produces an increase in left atrial and pulmonary venous pressure. Increased pulmonary vascular resistance is likely when the left atrial pressure is chronically higher than 25 mmHg. Distension of the left atrium predisposes to atrial fibrillation, whereas stasis of blood in this chamber favors the formation of thrombi, which can be displaced as systemic emboli. Mitral stenosis is almost always due to the fusion of the mitral valve leaflets during the healing process of acute rheumatic carditis. Symptoms of mitral stenosis do not usually develop until about 20 years after the initial episode of rheumatic fever. A sudden increase in the demand for cardiac output as produced by pregnancy or sepsis, however, may unmask previously asymptomatic mitral stenosis.

> **Anesthetic Considerations in the Patient with Mitral Stenosis**
>
> Avoid sinus tachycardia or rapid ventricular response rate during atrial fibrillation
> Avoid marked increases in central blood volume as associated with over-transfusion or head-down position
> Avoid drug-induced decreases in systemic vascular resistance
> Avoid events such as arterial hypoxemia or hypoventilation that may exacerbate pulmonary hypertension and evoke right ventricular failure

Patients taking digitalis preoperatively for the control of heart rate should continue to take this drug until surgery. Adequate digitalis effect for heart rate control is generally reflected by a ventricular rate less than 80 beats·min^{-1}. Because diuretic therapy is common, the serum potassium concentration is often measured preoperatively. Also, patients with mitral stenosis can be more susceptible than normal individuals to the ventilatory depressant effects of sedative drugs used for preoperative medication. When an anticholinergic drug is included in the preoperative medication, scopolamine or glycopyrrolate may have fewer chronotropic effects than atropine.

Management of Anesthesia

Induction of anesthesia in the presence of mitral stenosis can be achieved with intravenous drugs, with the possible exception of ketamine, which may be avoided because of its propensity to increase the heart rate. Intubation of the trachea is facilitated by the administration of a muscle relaxant. Drugs used for maintenance of anesthesia should cause minimal changes in heart rate and in systemic and pulmonary vascular resistance. Furthermore, these drugs should not greatly decrease myocardial contractility. These goals can be achieved with combinations of nitrous oxide and an opioid or low concentrations of a volatile anesthetic. Although nitrous oxide can increase pulmonary vascular resistance, this increase is not sufficiently great to justify avoiding this drug in all patients with mitral stenosis.[13] The effect of nitrous oxide on pulmonary vascular resistance, however, seems to be accentuated when co-existing pulmonary hypertension is severe.

Nondepolarizing muscle relaxants with minimal circulatory effects are useful in patients with mitral stenosis. Pancuronium is less appropriate because of its ability to increase the speed of transmission of cardiac impulses through the atrioventricular node, which could lead to excessive increases in heart rate. Such increases would seem particularly likely in the presence of atrial fibrillation because the ventricular response to atrial impulses is determined by the degree of atrioventricular conduction. There is no reason to avoid pharmacologic reversal of nondepolarizing muscle relaxants, but the adverse effects of possible drug-induced tachycardia should be anticipated. Intraoperative fluid therapy must be carefully titrated because these patients are susceptible to intravascular volume overload and to the development of left ventricular failure and pulmonary edema. Likewise, the head-down position is not well tolerated because the pulmonary blood volume is already increased.

Monitoring right atrial pressure is a helpful guide to the adequacy of intravascular fluid replacement. An increase in right atrial pressure could also reflect nitrous oxide-induced pulmonary vasoconstriction, suggesting the need to discontinue this drug.

Postoperatively, patients with mitral stenosis are at high risk of developing pulmonary edema and right heart failure. Mechanical support of ventilation of the lungs is often necessary, particularly after major thoracic or abdominal surgery.

Mitral Regurgitation

Mitral regurgitation is characterized by left atrial volume overload and decreased left ventricular for-

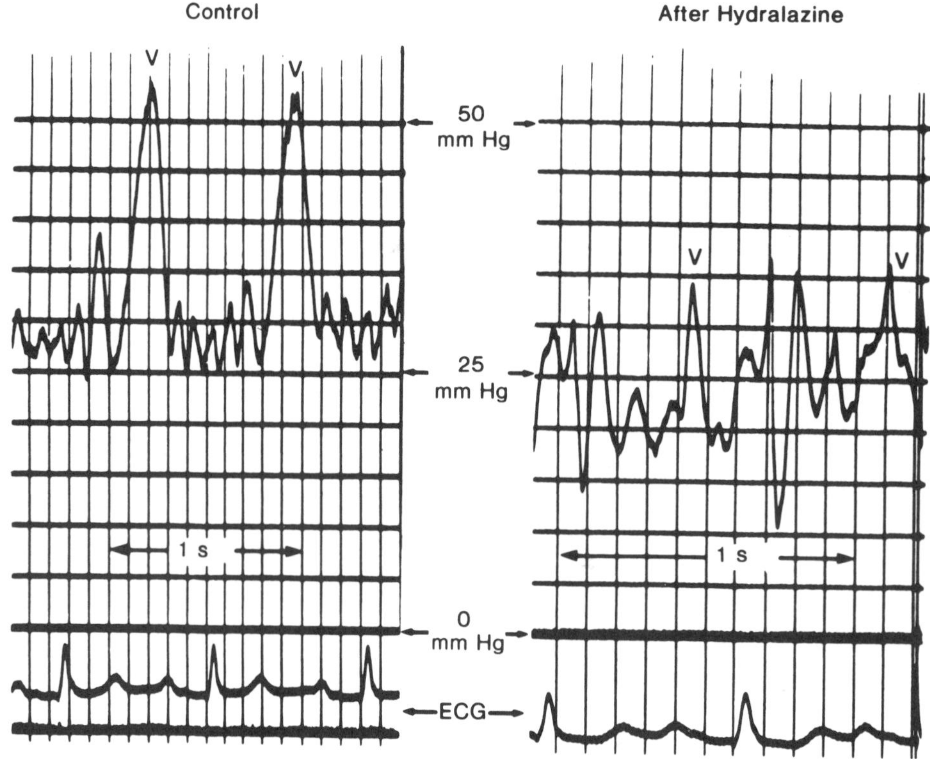

Figure 18-2. Regurgitant blood flow into the left atrium via an incompetent mitral valve produces a V wave on the trace of the pulmonary artery occlusion pressure. Vasodilation produced by hydralazine decreases impedance to forward ejection of blood from the left ventricle such that regurgitant flow into the left atrium is less and the size of the V wave is decreased. (From Greenberg and Rahmitoola,[14] with permission.)

ward stroke volume due to passage of part of each stroke volume through the incompetent mitral valve back into the left atrium. This regurgitant flow is responsible for the characteristic V waves seen on the recording of the pulmonary artery occlusion pressure (Fig. 18-2).[14] Mitral regurgitation is usually due to rheumatic fever and is almost always associated with mitral stenosis. Isolated mitral regurgitation is often acute, reflecting papillary muscle dysfunction after a myocardial infarction or rupture of chordae tendinae secondary to infective endocarditis.

Anesthetic Considerations in the Patient with Mitral or Aortic Regurgitation

- Avoid sudden decreases in heart rate
- Avoid sudden increases in systemic vascular resistance
- Minimize drug-induced myocardial depression
- Monitor the size of the V wave as a reflection of mitral regurgitant flow

Management of Anesthesia

Management of anesthesia in patients with mitral regurgitation should be designed to decrease the likelihood of decreases in the forward left ventricular stroke volume. Conversely, cardiac output can be improved by mild increases in heart rate and mild decreases in systemic vascular resistance.

A general anesthetic is the usual choice for patients with mitral regurgitation. Although decreases in systemic vascular resistance are theoretically beneficial, the uncontrolled nature of this response with a regional anesthetic detracts from the use of this technique except for surgery on peripheral sites. Maintenance of anesthesia can be provided with nitrous oxide plus a volatile anesthetic, the concentration of which can be adjusted to attenuate undesirable increases in blood pressure and systemic vascular resistance that can accompany surgical stimulation. Nondepolarizing muscle relaxants that lack significant circulatory effects are useful. Pancuronium is also acceptable as the increase in heart rate produced by this drug could increase forward left ventricular stroke volume. Intravascular fluid volume must be maintained by prompt replacement of blood loss to ensure adequate cardiac filling and ejection of an optimal forward left ventricular stroke volume.

Aortic Stenosis

Aortic stenosis is characterized by increased left ventricular systolic pressure to maintain the forward stroke volume through a narrowed aortic valve. The magnitude of the pressure gradient across the valve serves as an estimate of the severity of valvular stenosis. Hemodynamically significant aortic stenosis is associated with pressure gradients greater than 50 mmHg. Increased intraventricular pressures are accompanied by compensatory increases in the thickness of the left ventricular wall. Angina pectoris occurs often in these patients in the absence of coronary artery disease, reflecting an increased need for myocardial oxygen because of the increased amounts of ventricular muscle associated with myocardial hypertrophy. Furthermore, myocardial oxygen delivery is decreased as a result of compression of subendocardial coronary blood vessels by increased left ventricular systolic pressures.

Isolated nonrheumatic aortic stenosis usually results from progressive calcification and stenosis of a congenitally abnormal (usually bicuspid) valve. Aortic stenosis due to rheumatic fever almost always occurs in association with mitral valve disease. Likewise, aortic stenosis is usually accompanied by some degree of aortic regurgitation. Regardless of the etiology of aortic stenosis, the natural history of the disease includes a long latent period, often 30 years or more, before symptoms occur. Because many patients with aortic stenosis are asymptomatic, it is important to listen for this cardiac murmur (systolic murmur in the second right intercostal space) in patients scheduled for surgery. Indeed, the incidence of sudden death is increased in patients with aortic stenosis.

Anesthetic Considerations in the Patient with Aortic Stenosis

Maintain normal sinus rhythm
Avoid bradycardia
Avoid sudden decreases in systemic vascular resistance
Optimize intravascular fluid volume

Management of Anesthesia

Goals during management of anesthesia in patients with aortic stenosis are maintenance of normal sinus rhythm and avoidance of extreme and prolonged alterations in heart rate, systemic vascular resistance, and intravascular fluid volume. Preservation of normal sinus rhythm is critical because the left ventricle is dependent on properly timed atrial contractions to ensure an optimal left ventricular filling and stroke volume. Marked increases in heart rate (higher than 100 beats·min^{-1}) can decrease the time for left ventricular filling and ejection, whereas bradycardia (lower than 60 beats·min^{-1}) can lead to acute overdistension of the left ventricle. In view of the obstruction to left ventricular ejection, it must be appreciated that decreases in systemic vascular resistance may be associated with large decreases in blood pressure and coronary blood flow.

A general anesthetic is usually preferred to a regional anesthetic because sympathetic nervous system blockade can lead to undesirable decreases in systemic vascular resistance. Maintenance of anesthesia can be achieved with nitrous oxide plus an opioid or a low concentraion of volatile anesthetic. A potential disadvantage of volatile drugs (especially halothane) is depression of sinus node automaticity, which may lead to junctional rhythm and decreased left ventricular filling due to loss of properly timed atrial contractions.

Intravascular fluid volume must be maintained by prompt replacement of blood loss and liberal administration of intravenous fluids. If a pulmonary artery catheter is used, it should be remembered that the occlusion pressure may underestimate the left ventricular end-diastolic pressure because of the decreased compliance of the left ventricle that accompanies chronic aortic stenosis. A cardiac defibrillator should be promptly available when anesthesia is administered to patients with aortic stenosis since external cardiac compressions are unlikely to be effective in creating an adequate stroke volume across a stenosed valve.

Aortic Regurgitation

Aortic regurgitation is characterized by decreased forward left ventricular stroke volume due to regurgitation of part of the ejected stroke volume from the aorta back into the left ventricle through an incompetent aortic valve. A gradual onset of aortic regurgitation results in marked left ventricular hypertrophy. Increased myocardial oxygen requirements secondary to left ventricular hypertrophy, plus a characteristic decrease in aortic diastolic pressure that decreases coronary blood flow, can manifest as angina pectoris in the absence of coronary artery disease. Acute aortic regurgitation is most often due to infective endocarditis, trauma, or dissection of a thoracic aneurysm. Chronic aortic regurgitation is usually due to prior rheumatic fever. In contrast to aortic stenosis, the occurrence of sudden death with aortic regurgitation is rare. Management of anesthesia for noncardiac surgery in patients with aortic regurgitation is as described for patients with mitral regurgitation.

Mitral Valve Prolapse

Mitral valve prolapse (click-murmur syndrome, Barlow syndrome) is characterized by an abnormality of the mitral valve support structure that permits prolapse of the valve into the left atrium during contraction of the left ventricle. On the basis of the presence of a characteristic systolic murmur best heard at the apex, it is estimated that 5% to 10% of the adult population exhibits this valve abnormality. Echocardiography is helpful in confirming the diagnosis of mitral valve prolapse, particularly in the absence of the characteristic systolic murmur. There seems to be an increased incidence of mitral valve prolapse in patients with musculoskeletal abnormalities, including Marfan syndrome, pectus excavatum, and kyphoscoliosis.

Despite the prevalence of mitral valve prolapse, most patients are asymptomatic, emphasizing the usual benign course of this abnormality. Nevertheless, serious complications may accompany mitral valve prolapse. For example, mitral valve prolapse is probably the most common cause of pure mitral regurgitation, which may progress to the need for surgical intervention. Infective endocarditis is a potential complication, and transient ischemic attacks in patients younger than 45 years of age are often associated with mitral valve prolapse. Sudden death is an extremely rare complication that is presumed to be due to ventricular cardiac dysrhythmias.

Complications Associated with Mitral Valve Prolapse

Mitral regurgitation
Infective endocarditis
Transient ischemic events
Cardiac dysrhythmias
Sudden death (extremely rare)

Management of Anesthesia

The important principle in the management of anesthesia in patients with mitral valve prolapse is the avoidance of events that can increase cardiac emptying and accentuate prolapse of the mitral valve into the left atrium.[15] Perioperative events that can increase cardiac emptying include (1) sympathetic nervous system stimulation, (2) decreased systemic vascular resistance, and (3) performance of surgery with patients in the head-up or sitting position. With this in mind, it is important to optimize intravascular fluid volume in the preoperative period. Induction of anesthesia in the presence of mitral valve prolapse can be achieved with available intravenous induction drugs, keeping in mind the need to avoid sudden prolonged decreases in systemic vascular resistance. Ketamine and pancuronium are not recommended because of their ability to increase cardiac contractility and heart rate. Maintenance of anesthesia is most often achieved with nitrous oxide plus a volatile anesthetic to minimize sympathetic nervous system activation due to noxious intraoperative stimulation. The dose of volatile anesthetic is titrated to avoid excessive decreases in systemic vascular resistance. A regional anesthetic could also produce undesirable decreases in systemic vascular resistance. Prompt replacement of blood loss and generous administration of intravenous fluids will contribute to maintenance of an optimal intravascular fluid volume and decrease potential adverse effects of positive pressure ventilation of the lungs. Lidocaine and esmolol should be available to treat cardiac dysrhythmias. If sympathomimetics are needed to treat hypotension, an alpha agonist, such as phenylephrine, is useful.

CONGENITAL HEART DISEASE

Approximately 8 of every 1000 live births are associated with some form of congenital heart disease. Although more than 100 different congenital heart lesions are known, nearly 90% of all cardiac defects can be placed in 1 of 10 categories (Table 18-4). From the standpoint of management of anesthesia, it is helpful to categorize congenital heart defects as those that result in a left-to-right intracardiac shunt and those that result in a right-to-left intracardiac shunt. Patients with congenital heart disease often receive antibiotics in the perioperative period for protection against infective endocarditis.

Left-to-Right Intracardiac Shunt

A left-to-right intracardiac shunt may be due to an atrial septal defect or ventricular septal defect. Patent ductus arteriosus is an example of a left-to-right shunt at the level of the aorta. The result of these shunts is increased pulmonary blood flow with pulmonary hypertension, right ventricular hypertrophy, and eventually congestive heart failure.

Table 18-4. Common Congenital Heart Defects

Defect	Total Defects (%)
Ventricular septal defect	28
Secundum atrial septal defect	10
Patent ductus arteriosus	10
Tetralogy of Fallot	10
Pulmonary stenosis	10
Aortic stenosis	7
Coarctation of the aorta	5
Transposition of the great vessels	5
Other	15

Atrial Septal Defect

An atrial septal defect is often first suspected when there is a history of frequent pulmonary infections or when a systolic murmur is noted over the area of the pulmonary valve during a routine physical examination. Surgical closure of an atrial septal defect is indicated when the pulmonary blood flow is at least twice the systemic blood flow.

Management of Anesthesia. The presence of an atrial septal defect has only minor implications for the management of anesthesia. For example, as long as systemic blood flow remains normal, the pharmacokinetics of inhaled drugs will probably not be altered despite increased pulmonary blood flow. Increased pulmonary blood flow means that hemodynamic effects of positive intrathoracic pressure during controlled ventilation of the lungs are well tolerated. Drugs or events that increase arterial blood pressure and/or systemic vascular resistance may be avoided as this change could favor an increase in the magnitude of the left-to-right shunt at the atrial level. Conversely, decreases in these parameters as produced by volatile anesthetics or increases in pulmonary vascular resistance owing to positive pressure ventilation of the lungs will tend to decrease the magnitude of the shunt. It is imperative to avoid the entrance of air into the right atrium as can occur via the tubing used to deliver intravenous solutions. This air could bypass the lungs and cross directly into the systemic circulation to enter coronary and/or cerebral arteries.

Ventricular Septal Defect

Patients with small ventricular septal defects (ratio of pulmonary to systemic blood flow less than 1.5:1) are usually asymptomatic, with the only evidence of the cardiac abnormality being a pansystolic murmur that is of maximum intensity along the left sternal border. A large ventricular septal defect is characterized by a left-to-right intracardiac shunt that results in a pulmonary blood flow that exceeds systemic blood flow by three to five times. Recurrent pulmonary infections and, eventually, congestive heart failure are typical complications in patients with large ventricular septal defects. Management of anesthesia is as described for atrial septal defect.

Patent Ductus Arteriosus

Failure of the ductus arteriosus to close after birth results in passage of oxygenated blood from the aorta into the pulmonary artery. Most patients are asymptomatic, with the only manifestation being a continuous systolic and diastolic murmur. Management of anesthesia is as described for atrial septal defect.

Right-to-Left Intracardiac Shunt

A right-to-left intracardiac shunt is characterized by decreased pulmonary blood flow and arterial hypoxemia. Tetralogy of Fallot is the most common of the congenital cardiac defects that result in a right-to-left intracardiac shunt.

Tetralogy of Fallot

Tetralogy of Fallot is characterized by the presence of a ventricular septal defect, an aorta that overrides the pulmonary artery outflow tract, obstruction to blood flow through the pulmonary artery outflow tract, and right ventricular hypertrophy. Arterial blood gases and pH are likely to reveal a PaO_2 lower than 50 mmHg even when breathing oxygen. Squatting is a common feature of children with tetralogy of Fallot. Presumably, squatting increases systemic blood pressure and systemic vascular resistance by kinking the large arteries in the inguinal area. These circulatory changes decrease the magnitude of the right-to-left intracardiac shunt, leading to increased pulmonary blood flow and improved arterial oxygenation.

Hypercyanotic attacks ("tet spells") can occur without provocation but are often associated with crying or exercise. The most likely explanation for these attacks is a sudden decrease in pulmonary blood flow as a result of either a decrease in systemic vascular resistance or spasm of cardiac muscle in the region of the pulmonary artery outflow (infundibular) tract. A hypercyanotic attack that is due to a decrease in systemic vascular resistance is treated with intravenous administration of fluids or phenylephrine, or both. Sympathomimetics, such as ephedrine with beta agonist properties, are not recommended because sympathetic stimulation could accentuate spasm of the infundibular cardiac muscle. Propranolol or esmolol is effective when hypercyanotic attacks are due to cardiac muscle spasm in the region of the pulmonary artery outflow tract.

Management of Anesthesia. Management of anesthesia for patients with tetralogy of Fallot requires a thorough understanding of the events or drugs that can alter the magnitude of the right-to-left intracardiac shunt. For example, drug-induced responses that decrease systemic vascular resistance and blood pressure (volatile anesthetics, histamine release) may increase the magnitude of the right-to-left shunt and decrease the PaO_2. Pulmonary blood flow can also be decreased by increases in pulmonary vascular resistance that accompany positive pressure ventilation of the lungs or application of positive end-expiratory pressure. Nevertheless, the advantages of controlled ventilation of the lungs offset the potential hazards, as reflected by the fact that the PaO_2 usually improves.

Preoperatively, it is important to avoid dehydration by maintaining oral feedings in the very young or by providing intravenous fluids before arriving in the operating room. Crying associated with the intramuscular injection of medication can lead to hypercyanotic attacks. For this reason, it may be prudent to avoid intramuscular administration of drugs until the patient is in a highly supervised environment and an alpha agonist, such as phenylephrine, is promptly available for treatment of hypercyanotic attacks.

Induction of anesthesia in patients with tetralogy of Fallot is often accomplished with intramuscular (4 to 6 $mg{\cdot}kg^{-1}$) or intravenous (1 to 2 $mg{\cdot}kg^{-1}$) administration of ketamine. Indeed, the onset of anesthesia after the injection of ketamine is often associated with an improvement in the PaO_2, which presumably reflects increased pulmonary blood flow due to a ketamine-induced increase in systemic vascular resistance that leads to a decrease in the magnitude of the right-to-left intracardiac shunt.

Maintenance of anesthesia is often achieved with ketamine plus nitrous oxide. Disadvantages of nitrous oxide include possible increases in pulmonary vascular resistance evoked by this drug and decreases in inspired concentrations of oxygen that are necessitated by use of this anesthetic. Therefore, it would seem prudent to limit inspired concentrations of nitrous oxide to no more than 50%. Volatile anesthetics are not recommended for induction or maintenance of anesthesia because of the propensity of these drugs to increase the magnitude of the right-to-left intracardiac shunt by decreasing systemic vascular resistance and blood pressure.

Intraoperative skeletal muscle paralysis is often provided by pancuronium, since this drug maintains blood pressure and systemic vascular resistance. An increase in heart rate associated with administration of pancuronium may be helpful in maintaining cardiac output.

Ventilation of the lungs should be controlled, but it must be appreciated that excessive positive airway pressure may adversely increase resistance to blood flow through the lungs. Intravascular fluid volume must be maintained with intravenous fluid administration because acute hypovolemia will tend to increase the magnitude of the right-to-left intracardiac shunt. In view of co-existing polycythemia, it is probably not necessary to replace blood loss that is less than 20% of the estimated blood volume. It is crucial that care be taken to avoid infusion of air via the tubing used to deliver intravenous solutions, as this could lead to direct air embolization to coronary or cerebral arteries, or both. Phenylephrine should be available to treat undesirable decreases in systemic vascular resistance and blood pressure.

DISTURBANCES OF CARDIAC CONDUCTION AND RHYTHM

The ECG is a valuable tool for diagnosing disturbances of cardiac conduction and rhythm. Ambulatory ECG monitoring (Holter monitoring) is useful in documenting the occurrence of life-threatening cardiac dysrhythmias and assessing the efficacy of antidysrhythmic drug therapy. The following questions should be asked when interpreting the ECG:

1. What is the heart rate?
2. Are P waves present, and what is their relation ship to the QRS complex?
3. What is the duration of the P-R interval (normal 0.12 to 0.2 second)?
4. What is the duration of the QRS complex (normal 0.05 to 0.1 second)?
5. Is the ventricular rhythm regular?
6. Are there early cardiac beats or abnormal pauses after a preceding QRS complex?

Heart Block

Disturbances of conduction of cardiac impulses can be classified according to the site of the conduction block relative to the atrioventricular node. Heart block occurring above the atrioventricular node is usually benign and transient. Heart block occurring below the atrioventricular node tends to be progressive and permanent.

Classification of Heart Block

- First-degree atrioventricular heart block
- Second-degree atrioventricular heart block
    - Mobitz type I (Wenckebach)
    - Mobitz type II
- Unifasicular heart block
    - Left anterior hemiblock
    - Left posterior hemiblock
- Right bundle branch block
- Left bundle branch block
- Bifasicular heart block
    - Right bundle branch block plus left anterior hemiblock
    - Right bundle branch block plus left posterior hemiblock
- Third-degree (trifasicular, complete) atrioventricular heart block

A theoretical concern in patients with bifasicular heart block is that perioperative events, such as alterations in blood pressure, arterial oxygenation, or electrolyte concentrations, might compromise conduction in the one remaining intact fasicle, leading to the acute onset intraoperatively of third-degree atrioventricular heart block. There is no evidence, however, that surgery performed during a general or regional anesthetic predisposes to the development of third-degree atrioventricular heart block in patients with co-existing bifasicular block. Therefore, placement of a prophylactic artificial cardiac pacemaker is not recommended before anesthesia and surgery.

Third-degree atrioventricular heart block is treated by placement of an artificial cardiac pacemaker. An artificial cardiac pacemaker can be inserted intravenously (endocardial lead) or by the subcostal approach (epicardial or myocardial lead). An alternative to emergency transvenous artificial cardiac pacemaker placement is noninvasive transcutaneous cardiac pacing. A continuous intravenous infusion of isoproterenol acting as a pharmacologic cardiac pacemaker may be necessary to maintain an adequate heart rate until artificial electrical cardiac pacing can be established.

Sick Sinus Syndrome

Sick sinus syndrome is characterized by inappropriate sinus bradycardia associated with degenerative changes in the sinoatrial node. Frequently, bradycardia due to this syndrome is complicated by episodes of supraventricular tachycardia. Artificial cardiac pacemakers are indicated only when therapeutic plasma concentrations of drugs necessary to control tachycardia result in bradycardia. The high incidence of pulmonary embolism in these patients is the rationale for anticoagulation.

Ventricular Premature Beats

Ventricular premature beats are recognized on the ECG by (1) premature occurrence, (2) the absence of a P wave preceding the QRS complex, (3) a wide and often bizarre QRS complex, (4) an inverted T wave, and (5) a compensatory pause that follows the premature beat. Ventricular premature beats are often treated with lidocaine (1 to 2 $mg \cdot kg^{-1}$ IV) when they (1) are frequent (more than 6 $beats \cdot min^{-1}$), (2) are multifocal, (3) occur in salvos of three or more, or (4) take place during the ascending limb of the T wave (R on T phenomenon) that corresponds to the relative refractory period of the ventricle. At the same time, the underlying cause (myocardial ischemia, arterial hypoxemia, hypercarbia, hypertension, hypokalemia, mechanical irritation of the ventricles) should be eliminated.

Ventricular Tachycardia

Ventricular tachycardia is defined as the appearance of at least three consecutive wide QRS complexes (longer than 0.12 second) on the ECG occurring at an effective heart rate higher than 120 $beats \cdot min^{-1}$. Ventricular tachycardia not associated with hypotension is initially treated with the intravenous administration of lidocaine or procainamide. Symptomatic ventricular tachycardia is best treated with external electrical cardioversion (see Chapter 35).

Pre-excitation Syndromes

Pre-excitation syndromes are characterized by activation of a portion of the ventricles by cardiac impulses that travel from the atria via accessory (anomalous) conduction pathways.[16] These pathways bypass the atrioventricular node such that activation of the ventricles occurs earlier than it would if impulses reached the ventricles by normal pathways.

Wolff-Parkinson-White Syndrome

The Wolff-Parkinson-White syndrome is the most common of the pre-excitation syndromes, with an incidence that may approach 0.3% of the general population. The lack of a physiologic delay in transmission of cardiac impulses along the Kent fibers results in the characteristic short P-R interval (less than 0.12 second) on the ECG. The wide QRS complex and delta wave on the ECG reflect the composite of cardiac impulses conducted by normal and accessory pathways. Paroxysmal atrial tachycardia is the most frequent cardiac dysrhythmia associated with this syndrome. An increasing number of patients with Wolff-Parkinson-White syndrome are being treated by catheter ablation of accessory pathways as identified by electrophysiologic mapping.

Management of Anesthesia

The goal during management of anesthesia in the presence of a pre-excitation syndrome is to avoid events (anxiety) or drugs (anticholinergics, ketamine, pancuronium) that might increase sympathetic nervous system activity and predispose to tachydysrhythmias.[16] All antidysrhythmic drugs should be continued throughout the perioperative period. Induction of anesthesia can be achieved with intravenous drugs, with the possible exception of ketamine. Intubation of the trachea should be performed only after a sufficient depth of anesthesia has been achieved with nitrous oxide plus an opioid or a volatile anesthetic. Nondepolarizing muscle relaxants with minimal effects on heart rate or succinylcholine are useful to facilitate intubation of the trachea or to provide skeletal muscle paralysis during surgery.

The onset of paroxysmal atrial tachycardia or fibrillation in the perioperative period can be treated with the intravenous administration of drugs that abruptly prolong the refractory period of the atrioventricular node (adenosine) or lengthen the refractory period of accessory pathways (procainamide). Digitalis and verapamil may decrease the refractory period of accessory pathways responsible for atrial fibrillation, resulting in an increase in ventricular response during this dysrhythmia. Electrical cardioversion is indicated when tachydysrhythmias are life-threatening.

Prolonged Q-T Interval Syndrome

A prolonged Q-T interval (longer than 0.44 second on the ECG) syndrome is associated with ventricular dysrhythmias, syncope, and sudden death. Treatment of these patients is often empiric but may include beta antagonists or left stellate ganglion block. The effectiveness of a left stellate ganglion block supports the hypothesis that this syndrome results from a congenital imbalance of autonomic innervation to the heart produced by decreases in right cardiac sympathetic nerve activity. Management of anesthesia includes avoidance of events or drugs that are likely to activate the sympathetic nervous system and availability of beta antagonists (esmolol) and/or electrical cardioversion to treat life-threatening ventricular dysrhythmias.[17]

ARTIFICIAL CARDIAC PACEMAKERS

Preoperative evaluation of the patient with an artificial cardiac pacemaker in place includes determination of the reason for placing the pacemaker and an assessment of its present function. A preoperative history of vertigo or syncope may reflect dysfunction of the artificial cardiac pacemaker. The rate of discharge of an atrial or ventricular asynchronous cardiac pacemaker (usually 70 to 72 beats·min^{-1}) is a useful indicator of pulse generator function. A 10% decrease in heart rate from the initial fixed discharge rate may reflect battery failure. An irregular heart rate may reflect competition of the pulse generator with the patient's intrinsic heart rate or a pulse generator that is not sensing R waves. The ECG is evaluated to confirm one-to-one capture as evidenced by a pacemaker spike for every palpated peripheral pulse. The ECG is not helpful in the patient with an intrinsic heart rate greater than the preset pacemaker rate. In this patient, the proper function of a ventricular synchronous or sequential artificial cardiac pacemaker can be confirmed by demonstrating the appearance of captured beats on the ECG when the pacemaker is converted to the asynchronous mode by placement of an external converter magnet over the pulse generator.

Intraoperative monitoring of patients with artificial cardiac pacemakers includes the ECG so as to detect the appearance of asystole promptly. Atropine and isoproterenol are available should artificial cardiac pacemaker function cease. If electrocautery interferes with the ECG, monitoring a palpable peripheral pulse or auscultation through an esophageal stethoscope, or both, confirms continued cardiac activity. Inhibition of pulse generator activity by electromagnetic interference, which is interpreted as spontaneous cardiac activity by the artificial cardiac pacemaker, is most likely when the ground plate for electrocautery is placed too near the pulse generator. For this reason, the ground plate should be placed as far as possible from the pulse generator. Despite these concerns, it is alleged that improved shielding and circuit design of pulse generators results in conversion of artificial ventricular synchronous pacemakers to the asynchronous mode during continuous use of electrocautery, thus eliminating the hazard of electromagnetic inhibition or the need for an external converter magnet. Selection of drugs or techniques for anesthesia is not influenced by the presence of artificial cardiac pacemakers as there is no evidence that the threshold and subsequent response of these devices is altered by drugs administered in the perioperative period. Insertion of a pulmonary artery catheter will not disturb epicardial electrodes but might dislodge recently placed (less than 2 weeks duration) transvenous endocardial electrodes.[18]

ESSENTIAL HYPERTENSION

Essential hypertension is arbitrarily defined as sustained increases of arterial blood pressure (systolic blood pressure higher than 160 mmHg or a diastolic blood pressure higher than 90 mmHg, or both) independent of any known cause. Treatment of essential hypertension with appropriate drug therapy decreases the incidence of stroke and congestive heart failure, but there is no convincing evidence that adverse events associated with coronary artery disease are altered.

Management of Anesthesia

Management of anesthesia for patients with essential hypertension includes preoperative evaluation

Management of Anesthesia for the Patient with Essential Hypertension

Preoperative evaluation
- Determine adequacy of blood pressure control
- Review pharmacology of antihypertensive drugs
- Evaluate associated organ dysfunction (cardiac, central nervous system, renal)

Induction of anesthesia and intubation of the trachea
- Anticipate exaggerated blood pressure changes
- Minimize pressor response during intubation of the trachea by limiting duration of direct laryngoscopy to <15 seconds

Maintenance of anesthesia
- Use volatile anesthetic to control blood pressure
- Monitor electrocardiogram for evidence of myocardial ischemia

Postoperative management
- Anticipate excessive increases in blood pressure

of drug therapy and extent of the disease plus a consideration of the implications of exaggerated blood pressure increases intraoperatively in response to noxious stimulation.[19]

Preoperative Evaluation

Preoperative evaluation of patients with essential hypertension begins with a determination of the adequacy of blood pressure control and a review of the pharmacology of the antihypertensive drugs being used for therapy (see Chapter 3). It is important to maintain current therapy with antihypertensive drugs throughout the perioperative period. Evidence of major organ dysfunction (congestive heart failure, coronary artery disease, cerebral ischemia, renal dysfunction) must be sought. Patients with essential hypertension are assumed to have coronary artery disease until proven otherwise. Evidence of peripheral vascular disease should be recognized, particularly when placement of an intra-arterial catheter in the perioperative period is anticipated. It can be assumed that nearly one-half of patients with evidence of peripheral vascular disease will have 50% or greater stenosis of one or more coronary arteries even in the absence of angina pectoris and the presence of a normal resting ECG. Essential hypertension is associated with a shift to the right of the curve for the autoregulation of cerebral blood flow, emphasizing that these patients are more vulnerable to cerebral ischemia should perfusion pressures decrease. Detection of renal dysfunction due to chronic hypertension may influence the selection of drugs (it may be advisable to avoid enflurane and decrease the doses of nondepolarizing muscle relaxants) used during anesthesia.

The value of treating essential hypertension before an elective operation is suggested by the observation that the incidence of hypotension and evidence of myocardial ischemia on the ECG during the maintenance of anesthesia are increased in patients who remain hypertensive before induction of anesthesia.[19] Nevertheless, blood pressure increases during the intraoperative period are more likely to occur in patients with a history of essential hypertension regardless of the degree of blood pressure control established preoperatively. Furthermore, there is no evidence that the incidence of postoperative cardiac complications is increased when hypertensive patients undergo elective operations as long as the preoperative diastolic blood pressure is not higher than 110 mmHg. Pretreatment with an alpha-2 agonist, such as clonidine, may be useful in blunting exaggerated sympathetic nervous system responses in these patients.

Induction of Anesthesia

Induction of anesthesia with intravenous drugs is acceptable, remembering that an exaggerated decrease in blood pressure may occur, particularly if hypertension is preoperatively present. This response most likely reflects unmasking of decreased intravascular fluid volume due to chronic hypertension. Ketamine is rarely selected for induction of anesthesia since its circulatory effects could adversely increase blood pressure, especially in patients with co-existing hypertension.

Exaggerated blood pressure increases during direct laryngoscopy for intubation of the trachea are predictable in patients with the preoperative diagnosis of essential hypertension. Evidence of myocardial ischemia on the ECG may appear at this time. It would seem logical to ensure maximal attenuation of sympathetic nervous system responses evoked by direct laryngoscopy by administering volatile anesthetics or intravenous opioids before attempting intubation of the trachea. Regardless of the drugs administered before intubation of the trachea, however, it must be recognized that an excessive depth of anesthesia can produce decreases in blood pressure that are as undesirable as hypertension. An important concept for limiting pressor responses elicited by intubation of the trachea is to limit the duration of direct laryngoscopy to less than 15 seconds if possible. In addition, the administration of laryngotracheal lidocaine immediately before placement of the tube in the trachea will minimize any additional pressor response.

Maintenance of Anesthesia

The goal during maintenance of anesthesia is to adjust the depth of anesthesia in appropriate directions so as to minimize wide fluctuations in blood pressure. For this reason, a technique using nitrous oxide plus a volatile anesthetic is useful for permitting rapid adjustments in the depth of anesthesia in response to increases or decreases in blood pressure. Indeed, the management of intraoperative blood pressure lability by adjusting the concentrations of volatile anesthetics is probably more important than preoperative control of hypertension. The most likely intraoperative changes in blood pressure are hypertensive episodes produced by surgical stimulation. Volatile anesthetics are useful for attenuating activity of the sympathetic nervous system, which is responsible for these pressor responses. The ability to rapidly increase the alveolar concentration of desflurane (because of its low blood solubility) makes this volatile anesthetic uniquely efficacious for treating sudden increases in blood pressure (see the section *Coronary Artery Disease, Maintenance of Anesthesia*). A nitrous oxide-opioid technique is also acceptable for the maintenance of anesthesia, but the addition of a volatile anesthetic is often necessary to control undesirable increases in blood pressure, particularly during periods of maximal surgical stimulation. A continuous intravenous infusion of nitroprusside or the intermittent intravenous injection of drugs such as labetalol or esmolol are alternatives to the use of volatile anesthetics for maintaining normotension during the intraoperative period (see Chapter 3). Hypotension that occurs during maintenance of anesthesia is often treated by decreasing the concentrations of volatile anesthetics while infusing fluids intravenously to increase intravascular fluid volume. Sympathomimetics, such as ephedrine, may be necessary to restore perfusion pressures until the underlying cause of hypotension can be corrected.

The choice of intraoperative monitors for patients with co-existing essential hypertension is influenced by the complexity of the surgery. The ECG is monitored with the goal of recognizing changes suggestive of myocardial ischemia. Invasive monitoring using intra-arterial and pulmonary artery catheters may be indicated if major surgery is planned and there is evidence preoperatively of left ventricular dysfunction.

There is no evidence that a specific muscle relaxant is the best selection in patients with essential hypertension. Although pancuronium can increase the blood pressure, no data suggest that this mild pressor response is exaggerated by co-existing hypertension.

A regional anesthetic is a questionable choice when high levels of sympathetic nervous system blockade would be associated with the sensory level necessary for the planned surgery. This caution is based on the possibility of excessive decreases in blood pressure when vasodilation unmasks a decreased intravascular fluid volume associated with chronic hypertension.

Postoperative Management

Hypertension in the early postoperative period is a frequent occurrence in patients with a preoperative diagnosis of essential hypertension. If hypertension persists despite adequate analgesia, it may be necessary to administer a peripheral vasodilator such as hydralazine (5 to 10 mg IV every 10 to 20 minutes) or a continuous intravenous infusion of nitroprusside. Intermittent injections of labetalol (0.1 to 0.5 $mg \cdot kg^{-1}$ IV), a combined alpha and beta antagonist, may be a useful alternative to these drugs.

CONGESTIVE HEART FAILURE

Elective surgery should not be performed in patients who manifest evidence of congestive heart failure. Indeed, the presence of congestive heart failure has been reported to be the single most important factor for predicting postoperative morbidity. When surgery cannot be delayed, however, the drugs and techniques chosen to provide anesthesia must be selected with the goal of optimizing cardiac output. Ketamine may be useful for the induction of anesthesia in the presence of congestive heart failure. Use of volatile anesthetics for maintenance of anesthesia is not recommended because of the potential for cardiac depression. In the presence of severe congestive heart failure, the use of opioids in high doses as the sole anesthetic may be justified. Positive pressure ventilation of the lungs may be beneficial by decreasing pulmonary congestion and improving arterial oxygenation. Invasive monitoring of arterial pressure, as well as cardiac filling pressures, is justified when major surgery is necessary. Maintenance of myocardial contractility with continuous infusions of dopamine or dobutamine, or both, may be necessary in the perioperative period.

A regional anesthetic is a consideration for patients with congestive heart failure requiring peripheral surgery. The mild decrease in systemic vascular resistance secondary to peripheral sympathetic nervous system blockade could facilitate left ventricular stroke volume. Nevertheless, a regional anesthetic should probably not be selected in preference to a general anesthetic if the only reason is the belief that regional anesthesia will reliably improve cardiac output.

HYPERTROPHIC CARDIOMYOPATHY

Hypertrophic cardiomyopathy (idiopathic hypertrophic subaortic stenosis) is characterized by obstruction to left ventricular outflow produced by asymmetric hypertrophy of the intraventricular septal muscle. Associated left ventricular hypertrophy in an attempt to overcome the obstruction may be so massive that the volume of the left ventricular chamber is decreased. Despite these adverse changes, the stroke volume remains normal or increased owing to the hypercontractile state of the myocardium. This disease is often hereditary, and the genetic defect seems to be an increased density of calcium channels manifesting as myocardial hypertrophy.

Management of Anesthesia

The goal during management of anesthesia for patients with hypertrophic cardiomyopathy is to decrease the pressure gradient across the left ventricular outflow obstruction. Decreases in myocardial contractility and increases in preload (ventricular volume) and afterload will decrease the magnitude of left ventricular outflow obstruction. With this in mind, halothane is useful for maintenance of anesthesia, providing mild myocardial depression. Theoretically, enflurane, isoflurane, and desflurane would be less ideal choices than halothane since these drugs decrease systemic vascular resistance more than does halothane (see Chapter 4). Opioids are not likely choices, as they do not produce myocardial depression and can decrease systemic vascular resistance. Pancuronium is not a likely muscle relaxant selection because of its ability to increase heart rate and myocardial contractility.

Intraoperative hypotension is generally treated with intravenous fluids or an alpha agonist such as phenylephrine, or both. Drugs with beta agonist activity are not likely to be used to treat hypotension, because any increase in cardiac contractility or heart rate could increase left ventricular outflow obstruction. When hypertension occurs, an increased delivered concentration of halothane is a useful treatment. Vasodilators, such as nitroprusside

Events that Decrease Left Ventricular Outflow Obstruction in the Presence of Hypertrophic Cardiomyopathy

- Decreased myocardial contractility
  - Beta-adrenergic blockade (propranolol, esmolol)
  - Volatile anesthetics (halothane)
- Increased preload
  - Increased intravascular fluid volume
  - Bradycardia
- Increased afterload
  - Alpha-adrenergic stimulation (phenylephrine)
- Increased intravascular fluid volume

or nitroglycerin, are not likely choices for lowering blood pressure because decreases in systemic vascular resistance can increase left ventricular outflow obstruction.

COR PULMONALE

Cor pulmonale is the designation for right ventricular hypertrophy and eventual cardiac dysfunction that occurs secondary to chronic pulmonary hypertension. Elective operations in patients with cor pulmonale should not be performed until any reversible component of the co-existing pulmonary vascular disease has been treated.

Goals during management of anesthesia in patients with cor pulmonale are to avoid events or drugs that could increase pulmonary vascular resistance. Volatile anesthetics are useful for relaxing vascular smooth muscle and attenuating airway responsiveness to stimuli produced by a tracheal tube. Nitrous oxide may increase pulmonary vascular resistance.[13] Another disadvantage of nitrous oxide is the associated decrease in the inspired concentration of oxygen necessitated by the administration of this drug. Therefore, delivered concentrations of nitrous oxide are usually limited to 50%, and right atrial pressure is monitored to detect any adverse drug-induced effect on pulmonary vascular resistance.

CARDIAC TAMPONADE

Cardiac tamponade is characterized by (1) decreases in diastolic filling of the ventricles, (2) decreases in stroke volume, and (3) decreases in blood pressure due to increased intrapericardial pressure from accumulation of fluid in the pericardiac space. Decreased stroke volume results in activation of the sympathetic nervous system (tachycardia, vasoconstriction) in attempts to maintain the cardiac output. Cardiac output and blood pressure are maintained as long as the pressure in the central veins exceeds the right ventricular end-diastolic pressure. Institution of general anesthesia and positive pressure ventilation of the lungs in the presence of cardiac tamponade can lead to profound hypotension, reflecting anesthetic-induced peripheral vasodilation, direct myocardial depression, and decreased venous return. When percutaneous pericardiocentesis cannot be performed using local anesthesia, the induction and maintenance of general anesthesia are often achieved with ketamine. Potential adverse effects of increased intrathoracic pressure on venous return must be considered. Perhaps positive pressure ventilation of the lungs should be avoided until drainage of the pericardial space is imminent. With this in mind, it may be prudent to perform intubation of the trachea with topical anesthesia before the induction of anesthesia. Continuous intravenous infusions of catecholamines (isoproterenol, dopamine, dobutamine) may be necessary to maintain myocardial contractility.

Manifestations of Cardiac Tamponade

Hypotension
Tachycardia
Vasoconstriction
Equalization of diastolic filling pressures
Fixed stroke volume (cardiac output and blood pressure dependent on heart rate)

ANEURYSMS OF THE AORTA

Aneurysms of the aorta most often involve the abdominal aorta. Most patients are hypertensive, and many have associated atherosclerosis. A dissecting aneurysm denotes a tear in the intima of the aorta that allows blood to enter and penetrate between the walls of the vessel, producing a false lumen. Ultimately, the dissection may re-enter the lumen through another tear in the intima or rupture through the adventia.

Elective resection of an abdominal aneurysm is often recommended when the estimated diameter of the aneurysm is more than 5 cm. The incidence of spontaneous rupture increases dramatically when the size of the aneurysm exceeds this diameter. Extension of the abdominal aneurysm to include the renal arteries occurs in about 5% of patients.

Management of Anesthesia

Management of anesthesia for resection of an abdominal aortic aneurysm includes monitoring of arterial and left atrial filling pressures. Patients with co-existing coronary artery disease are likely to develop increases in the pulmonary artery occlusion pressure and evidence of myocardial ischemia during cross-clamping of the abdominal aorta. Intraoperative myocardial ischemia is treated by decreasing blood pressure and filling pressure to acceptable levels by pharmacologic interventions, which may include continuous intravenous infusions of nitroprusside or nitroglycerin. Preoperative hydration with a balanced salt solution and prompt intraoperative hydration and blood loss replacement as guided by data obtained from a pulmonary artery catheter are considered useful for maintaining intravascular fluid volume and thus renal function. Diuresis is often facilitated by intraoperative administration of a diuretic (mannitol or furosemide, or both) with or without dopamine. Nevertheless, animal data reveal that decreases in glomerular filtration rate and renal blood flow are not attenuated by these drugs.[20]

Hypotension can accompany unclamping of the abdominal aorta, presumably reflecting sudden increases in venous capacitance. Blood pressure decreases can be minimized by infusing intravenous fluids to maintain the pulmonary artery occlusion pressure between 10 to 20 mmHg before removal of the aortic cross-clamp. Gradual removal of the aortic cross-clamp minimizes decreases in blood pressure by allowing time for return of pooled venous blood to the circulation. The role of the washout of acid metabolites from the ischemic extremities when the clamp is released has been discredited as a cause of declamping hypotension.

CARDIOPULMONARY BYPASS

Cardiopulmonary bypass (extracorporeal circulation) is characterized by gravity drainage of blood from the venae cavae into an oxygenator followed by its return to the arterial system, usually the ascending aorta, by means of a roller pump (Fig. 18-3).[21] In the presence of a competent aortic valve, the heart is excluded from the patient's circulation by tightening occlusive ligatures that have been placed around the superior and inferior venae cavae so that all returning blood enters the large cannulae in these vessels. If the aortic valve is not competent, it is also necessary to cross-clamp the aorta distal to the aortic valve and proximal to the inflow cannula. Otherwise, retrograde blood flow through the incompetent aortic valve would prevent exclusion of the heart from the circulation. When the heart is isolated from the circulation, total cardiopulmonary bypass is present and ventilation of the lungs is no longer necessary to maintain oxygenation. Placing the operating table above the level of the cardiopulmonary bypass machine facilitates the gravity-dependent venous drainage.

The roller pump produces nonpulsatile flow (sine wave pattern) into the patient's aorta by compression of the fluid-containing tubing between the roller and curved metal back plate. The required cardiac index delivered by the roller pump depends on the patient's body temperature and oxygen consumption. For normothermia or mild hypothermia, a cardiac index of 2 to 2.4 $L \cdot min^{-1} \cdot m^{-2}$ is satisfactory, although flows of approximately half these levels have been used successfully. Low flows have the advantage of less blood trauma and less noncoronary collateral blood flow, which might result in better myocardial protection. An alternative to the roller pump is a centrifugal pump that produces pulsatile blood flow and less trauma to blood.

Blood is oxygenated in either a bubble or membrane oxygenator. The bubble oxygenator is most popular, and consists of an oxygenating column, a defoaming section to remove air bubbles, and an arterial reservoir. The PaO_2 is maintained between 100 and 150 mmHg by adjusting the flow of oxygen into the oxygenator. Addition of carbon dioxide to maintain $PaCO_2$ and pH at levels considered normal for 37°C may not be necessary during hypothermic cardiopulmonary bypass. Membrane oxygenators do not use a blood-gas interface and produce less trauma to the blood compared with the time-dependent trauma to blood caused by bubble oxygenators. Nevertheless, these more complex and expensive oxygenators have not proven to be more advantageous than bubble oxygenators, especially if the period of cardiopulmonary bypass is shorter than 2 hours.

Heat exchangers are incorporated into oxygenators to control the patient's body temperature by heating or cooling blood as it circulates. Hot or cold water entering the unit at one end with blood enter-

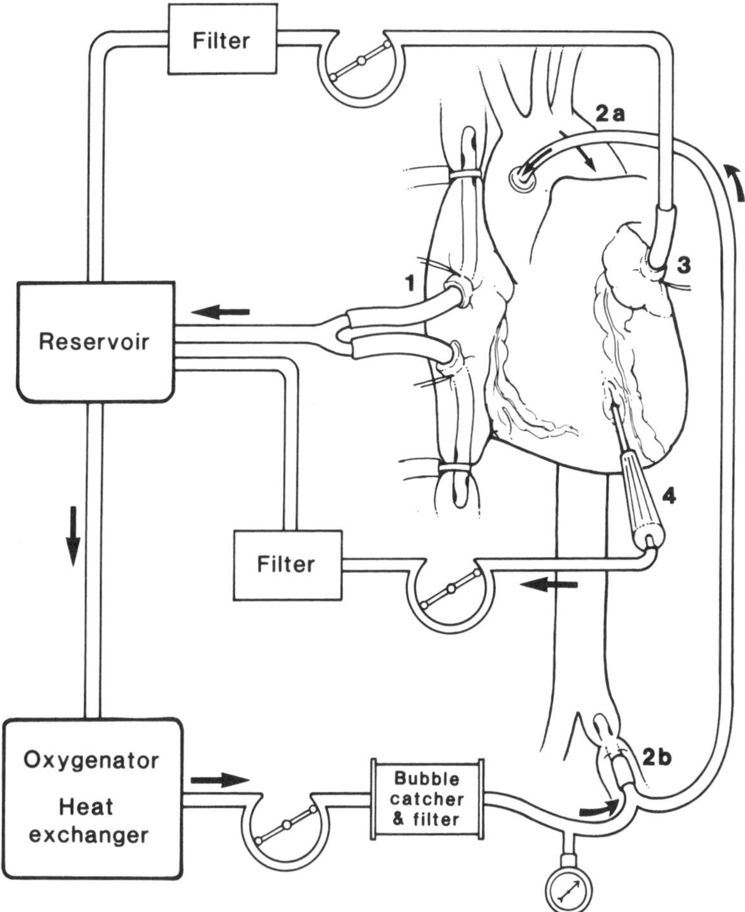

Figure 18-3. Schematic diagram of a cardiopulmonary bypass circuit. Blood from cannulae (1) placed in the superior and inferior vena cava drains by gravity into a reservoir and then to an oxygenator and heat exchanger. A roller pump returns oxygenated blood to the ascending aorta (2a) or, rarely, the femoral artery (2b). In addition, blood is returned to the reservoir from the left ventricular vent (3) and cardiotomy suction (4). (From Nosé,[21] with permission.)

ing at the other provides an efficient countercurrent flow system.

Blood from the pericardial cavity and the opened heart, as during a valve replacement, is returned to a cardiotomy reservoir, where it is filtered, defoamed, and returned to the oxygenator for recirculation. The cardiotomy suction is a major cause of hemolysis during cardiopulmonary bypass. When the heart is not opened, as during aortocoronary bypass graft operations, it may be necessary to insert a catheter (vent) into the left ventricle (most often via the right superior pulmonary vein) to prevent distension of the left ventricle with blood returning via thebesian veins or bronchial veins. Filters are incorporated in the oxygen delivery line and arterial delivery system to act as traps for cellular debris that could act as systemic emboli.

The tubing used for the cardiopulmonary bypass system is filled (primed) with blood and fluid in a predetermined ratio that is calculated to produce a specific hematocrit with institution of total cardiopulmonary bypass. Because whole body hypothermia (22°C to 28°C) is commonly used, the pump prime usually contains little or no blood, such that the hematocrit of blood during bypass is decreased. Hemodilution is important to lessen viscosity during hypothermia. It is mandatory that all air be cleared from the arterial side of the circuit before institution of cardiopulmonary bypass. Indeed, pumping of air into the patient by the cardiopulmonary bypass machine is an ever present hazard.

Heparin-induced anticoagulation of the patient is mandatory before placement of the venous and aortic cannulae used for cardiopulmonary bypass. The usual initial dose of heparin administered intravenously is 300 to 400 units·kg^{-1}. The adequacy of anticoagulation is subsequently confirmed by determination of the activated coagulation time, which is typically maintained for longer than 400 seconds (normal 90 to 120 seconds) during cardiopulmonary bypass.

Monitoring During Cardiopulmonary Bypass

Institution of cardiopulmonary bypass is often associated with decreases in mean arterial pressure, presumably reflecting the dramatic decreases in viscosity that result from infusion of prime solutions. In addition, peripheral vasodilation may accompany decreased oxygen delivery that occurs in the early period of hemodilution. Administration of an alpha agonist, such as phenylephrine, to increase perfusion pressures to higher than 50 mmHg in the early period after institution of cardiopulmonary bypass has been a common practice on the assumption that perfusion pressure is important for maintenance of cerebral blood flow. Supportive evidence for this practice, however, is not available, and many now believe that drug support of mean arterial pressure that remains above 30 mmHg is not necessary if hypothermia is being simultaneously produced.

After the initial decrease, blood pressure often begins to increase spontaneously, perhaps reflecting activation of the renin-angiotensin system or sympathetic nervous system. Mean arterial pressures higher than 100 mmHg can lead to impairment of tissue perfusion as well as the risk of intracranial hemorrhage. Furthermore, noncoronary collateral flow is likely to be increased as mean arterial pressure increases, resulting in perfusion of the heart with blood at higher temperatures than desired for optimal cellular protection. Hypertension is often treated by decreasing systemic vascular resistance with the continuous intravenous administration of nitroprusside or nitroglycerin. Alternatively, the vapors of volatile anesthetics can be introduced from vaporizers incorporated into the cardiopulmonary bypass circuit.

An increasing central venous pressure with or without facial edema (eyelids and sclera) may reflect improper placement of the vena cava cannulae, resulting in obstruction to venous drainage. For example, insertion of a cannula too far into the superior vena cava can obstruct the right innominate vein, leading to an increase of cerebral venous pressure with associated cerebral edema. Placement of a cannula too far into the inferior vena cava results in abdominal distension. Confirmatory evidence of misplacement of a vena cava cannula is inadequate venous return from the patient to the cardiopulmonary bypass machine. Prompt withdrawal of the vena cava cannula to a more proximal position should immediately improve venous drainage.

A pulmonary artery catheter detects increases in pulmonary artery pressures caused by malfunction of the left ventricular vent and the associated inadequate decompression of the left ventricle. Persistent left ventricular distension can result in damage to the contractile elements of the myocardium.

Blood gases and pH are monitored frequently during cardiopulmonary bypass. A mixed venous PO_2 lower than 30 mmHg associated with metabolic acidosis suggests inadequate tissue perfusion. Temperature correction of $PaCO_2$ and pH is probably not necessary (see Chapter 16). Urine output may serve as a guide to the adequacy of renal perfusion, with an output of 1 ml·kg^{-1}·h^{-1} being a reasonable expectation.

During total cardiopulmonary bypass the lungs are left quiescent with or without moderate continuous positive airway pressure. The best composition of gases in the lungs during this period is unsettled. Continued ventilation of the lungs with oxygen may be appropriate when there is some pulmonary blood flow, as evidenced by a pulsatile pulmonary artery trace (partial cardiopulmonary bypass).

Esophageal and rectal temperatures are monitored routinely. Drug-induced vasodilation as produced by a volatile anesthetic or nitroprusside may speed the rewarming process, as reflected by a more rapid approach of the rectal (core) to esophageal (blood) temperature. Measurement of urinary bladder temperature is an alternative to monitoring rectal temperature, although high urine flow rates during rewarming may cause the bladder temperature to more closely parallel blood than core temperature.

Myocardial Preservation

The goal of myocardial preservation is to decrease myocardial damage introduced by the period of ischemia associated with cardiopulmonary bypass.

This goal is achieved by decreasing myocardial oxygen consumption by infusing cold cardioplegia solutions containing potassium into the aortic root, which in the presence of a distally cross-clamped aorta and competent aortic valve ensures diversion of the solution into the coronary arteries. Potassium blocks the initial phase of myocardial depolarization, resulting in cessation of electrical and mechanical activity. The cold solution produces selective hypothermia of the cardiac muscle. At 30°C, the normally contracting heart muscle consumes oxygen at a rate of 8 to 10 ml·100 $g^{-1}·min^{-1}$. This consumption in the fibrillating heart at 22°C is 2 ml·100 $g^{-1}·min^{-1}$. The electromechanically quiet heart at 22°C consumes oxygen at a rate of 0.3 ml·100 $g^{-1}·min^{-1}$. The effectiveness of cold cardioplegia is monitored by measuring heart temperature with a temperature probe placed into the left ventricular muscle plus the absence of any visible electrical activity on the ECG. Cold cardioplegia infusions are supplemented by total body hypothermia and localized epicardial surface cooling using ice or cold irrigation solutions placed into the pericardial space. Adequate myocardial preservation is suggested by good myocardial contractility without the use of inotropic drugs at the conclusion of cardiopulmonary bypass.

A side effect of cardioplegia solutions is an increased incidence of atrioventricular heart block due to intramyocardial hyperkalemia. This heart block usually resolves in 1 to 2 hours and can be treated temporarily by use of an artificial cardiac pacemaker. Intramyocardial hyperkalemia also produces decreased myocardial contractility. Systemic hyperkalemia is likely to occur when coronary sinus blood containing cardioplegia solutions is returned to the oxygenator for subsequent circulation. Decreased renal function during cardiopulmonary bypass will also contribute to hyperkalemia. If hyperkalemia persists at the conclusion of cardiopulmonary bypass, it may be necessary to administer glucose (25 to 50 g IV) plus regular insulin (10 to 20 units IV) in attempts to shift potassium into the cells.

Maintenance of Anesthesia

Drugs selected for maintenance of anesthesia in patients undergoing cardiopulmonary bypass are determined by the patient's cardiac disease. Institution of cardiopulmonary bypass, however, produces a sudden dilution of circulating drug concentrations that can acutely decrease the depth of anesthesia. For this reason, supplemental anesthetics, such as benzodiazepines or opioids, may be administered intravenously at this time. Likewise, skeletal muscle paralysis may be supplemented with additional nondepolarizing muscle relaxants. Anesthetic depth can also be increased by volatile anesthetics from vaporizers incorporated into the cardiopulmonary bypass circuit. It must be appreciated that the impact of hemodilution on drug concentrations is likely to be offset by a decreased need for drugs during hypothermia. For reasons that are not clear, anesthetic requirements seem to be minimal following rewarming to a normal body temperature at the conclusion of cardiopulmonary bypass. Therefore, additional anesthesia is not routinely required during rewarming or the early period after the conclusion of cardiopulmonary bypass.

Discontinuation of Cardiopulmonary Bypass

Cardiopulmonary bypass is discontinued when the patient is hemodynamically stable and normothermia has been re-established. In the absence of adequate rewarming before discontinuation of cardiopulmonary bypass, body temperature is likely to decrease rapidly in the postcardiopulmonary bypass period, resulting in metabolic acidosis and poor myocardial contractility. When the left side of the heart has been opened, as during valve replacement surgery, it is mandatory to remove all air from the cardiac chambers and pulmonary veins before permitting the heart to eject blood into the aorta. Otherwise, systemic air emboli can occur, with disastrous cardiac and central nervous system effects. Unrecognized air in the coronary arteries may be a cause of poor myocardial contractility after discontinuation of cardiopulmonary bypass. Measurement of cardiac filling pressures, determination of thermodilution cardiac outputs, and calculation of systemic and pulmonary vascular resistance are helpful for guiding intravenous fluid replacement and the appropriate selection of drugs in the early postcardiopulmonary bypass period (Table 18-5). On occasion, a continuous intravenous infusion of a vasodilator, such as nitroprusside or nitroglycerin, or an inotrope, such as dopamine, dobutamine, or epinephrine, is necessary to maintain optimal cardiac output. Posterior papillary muscle dysfunction at the conclusion of cardiopulmonary bypass may result in

Table 18-5. Diagnosis and Therapy of Cardiovascular Dysfunction Following Cardiopulmonary Bypass

Blood Pressure	Atrial Pressure	Cardiac Output	Diagnosis	Therapy
Decreased	Increased	Decreased	Left ventricular dysfunction	Inotrope Vasodilator Mechanical assistance
Decreased	Decreased	Decreased	Hypovolemia	Administer volume
Decreased	Decreased	Increased	Vasodilation Low blood viscosity	Sympathomimetic Administer erythrocytes
Increased	Increased	Decreased	Vasoconstriction Left ventricular dysfunction	Vasodilator Inotrope
Increased	Decreased	Increased	Hyperdynamic	Volatile anesthetic Beta antagonist

mitral regurgitation as evidenced by the presence of prominent V waves on the pulmonary artery occlusion pressure tracing. This dysfunction may reflect less than optimal cardioplegic protection of the posterior myocardium, which is most vulnerable to warming effects from blood in the adjacent descending aorta, as well as perfusion with warm blood representing noncoronary collateral circulation.

A mechanical alternative to inotropic support of cardiac output is the intra-aortic balloon pump. The intra-aortic balloon pump (a 25-cm-long balloon mounted on a 90-cm stiff plastic catheter) is typically inserted percutaneously through the femoral artery and advanced so that the tip is just distal to the left subclavian artery. The balloon is timed to deflate immediately before systole, thus decreasing end-diastolic pressure (afterload reduction) so as to enhance forward left ventricular stroke volume and decrease myocardial oxygen requirements. Balloon inflation during diastole increases diastolic blood pressure (diastolic augmentation) and increases the gradient for coronary perfusion. Rapid heart rates and cardiac dysrhythmias interfere with proper balloon timing and optimal augmentation of cardiac output.

When an adequate blood pressure and cardiac output have been maintained for several minutes, the aortic and vena cava cannulae are removed and protamine is administered intravenously, usually over 3 to 5 minutes, to reverse heparin anticoagulation. Occasionally, infusion of protamine is accompanied by hypotension and pulmonary hypertension, possibly reflecting the release of histamine or prostaglandins, or both. Administration of nitrous oxide after cardiopulmonary bypass is questionable because this gas would unmask the presence of air in the heart or coronary arteries. For this reason, anesthesia is most often supplemented when necessary by the intravenous administration of opioids or low inhaled concentrations of volatile anesthetics. The blood and fluid that remains in the cardiopulmonary bypass circuit is washed and collected into plastic bags as packed cells for possible reinfusion to the patient. Low resistance to blood flow in the arm induced by rewarming may result in a falsely low blood pressure reading from the radial artery in the early period after cardiopulmonary bypass. The gradient between central aortic and radial artery blood pressure usually disappears within 60 minutes.

REFERENCES

1. Fleisher LA, Barash PG. Preoperative cardiac evaluation for noncardiac surgery: A functional approach. Anesth Analg 1992;74:586–98.
2. Tarhan S, Moffitt EA, Taylor WF, Guiliani ER. Myocardial infarction after general anesthesia. JAMA 1972;220:1451–4.
3. Steen PA, Tinker JH, Tarhan S. Myocardial reinfarction after anesthesia and surgery. An update: Incidence, mortality, and predisposing factors. JAMA 1978;239:2566–70.
4. Rao TLK, Jacobs KH, El-Etr AA. Reinfarction following anesthesia in patients with myocardial infarction. Anesthesiology 1983;59:449–505.

5. Shah KB, Kleinman BS, Sami H, Patel J, Rao TLK. Reevaluation of perioperative myocardial infarction in patients with prior myocardial infarction undergoing noncardiac operations. Anesth Analg 1991; 71:231–5.
6. Slogoff S, Keats AS. Does chronic treatment with calcium entry blocking drugs reduce perioperative myocardial ischemia? Anesthesiology 1988;68:676–80.
7. Slogoff S, Keats AS. Further observations on perioperative myocardial ischemia. Anesthesiology 1986; 65:539–42.
8. Ebert TJ, Muzi M. Sympathetic hyperactivity during desflurance anesthesia in healthy volunteers. A comparison with isoflurane. Anesthesiology 1993;79: 444–53.
9. Yli-Hankala A, Randell T, Seppala T, Lindgren L. Increases in hemodynamic variables and catecholamine levels after rapid increase in isoflurane concentration. Anesthesiology 1993;78:266–71.
10. Slogoff S, Keats AS, Dear WE, et al. Steal-prone coronary anatomy and myocardial ischemia associated with four primary anesthetic agents in humans. Anesth Analg 1991;72:22–7.
11. Diana P, Tullock WC, Gorcsan J, Ferson PF, Arvan S. Myocardial ischemia: A comparison between isoflurane and enflurane in coronary artery bypass patients. Anesth Analg 1993;77:221–6.
12. Practice guidelines for pulmonary artery catheterization. A report by the American Society of Anesthesiologists Task Force on pulmonary artery catheterization. Anesthesiology 1993;78:380–94.
13. Hilgenberg JC, McCammon RL, Stoelting RK. Pulmonary and systemic vascular responses to nitrous oxide in patients with mitral stenosis and pulmonary hypertension. Anesth Analg 1980;59:323–6.
14. Greenberg BH, Rahmitoola SH. Vasodilator therapy for valvular heart disease. JAMA 1981;246:269–72.
15. Kowalski SE. Mitral valve prolapse. Can Anaesth Soc J 1985;32:138–41.
16. Wellens HJJ, Brugada P, Penn OC. The management of preexcitation syndromes. JAMA 1987;257:2325–33.
17. Galloway PA, Glass PSA. Anesthetic implications of prolonged QT interval syndromes. Anesth Analg 1985;64:612–20.
18. Zaidan JR. Pacemakers. Anesthesiology 1984;60: 319–34.
19. Prys-Roberts C. Anaesthesia and hypertension. Br J Anaesth 1984;56:711–24.
20. Pass LJ, Eberhart RC, Brown JC, Rohn GN, Estrera AS. The effect of mannitol and dopamine on the renal response to thoracic aortic cross-clamping. J Thorac Cardiovas Surg 1988;95:608–12.
21. Nosé Y. Manual on Artificial Organs. Vol. 2. The Oxygenator. St. Louis, CV Mosby 1973.

19

Chronic Pulmonary Disease

Patients with chronic pulmonary disease present a challenge for management during the intraoperative and postoperative period regardless of the operative site. Nevertheless, thoracic and upper abdominal operations are a particular risk for patients with chronic pulmonary disease. Furthermore, patients with chronic pulmonary disease often manifest coexisting coronary artery disease or essential hypertension, or both (see Chapter 18).

OBSTRUCTIVE AIRWAY DISEASE

Obstructive airway disease is the most frequent cause of pulmonary dysfunction. The common pathophysiologic characteristic of all the obstructive airway disorders is an increased resistance to flow of gases in the airways (chronic obstructive pulmonary disease [COPD]). Regional differences in airway resistance lead to areas of ventilation-to-perfusion mismatching. As a result, arterial hypoxemia is likely to develop while the patient is breathing room air. Retention of carbon dioxide with the development of respiratory acidosis can also occur when regional hypoventilation is severe. Cough and sputum production are present. All obstructive airway diseases are characterized by dyspnea, reflecting the increased work of breathing introduced by the elevated airway resistance. COPD is estimated to affect at least 15 million Americans and is the fifth leading cause of death in the United States.[1]

Auscultation of the chest will probably reveal wheezing during exhalation, reflecting turbulent gas flow through narrowed airways. Radiographs of the chest show hyperinflated lungs with increased radiolucency due to decreased pulmonary blood flow. The diaphragm is likely to be flattened. Pulmonary function studies reveal decreases in expiratory flow rates owing to increased airway resistance. For example, the forced exhaled volume in 1 second (FEV_1) is typically less than 80% of the vital capacity in the presence of obstructive airway disease (Fig. 19-1).[2] Measurement of the FEV_1 alone can be misleading as the value may be low if the vital capacity is also decreased.

Bronchial asthma is the classic example of obstructive airway disease that is characterized by acute and reversible increases of airway resistance. Pulmonary emphysema and chronic bronchitis are examples of obstructive airway diseases characterized by progressive and persistent increases in airway resistance despite treatment.

Bronchial Asthma

Bronchial asthma is estimated to be present in 3% to 6% of the population of the United States.[3] Most individuals develop symptoms of asthma before 5 years of age, and male patients outnumber female patients by about two to one. Bronchial asthma is a disease that is defined by the (1) presence of increased responsiveness (hyperreactivity) of the airways to various stimuli, (2) reversible expiratory airflow obstruction, and (3) chronic inflammatory changes in the submucosa of the airways. Airway hyperreactivity accompanies this disease even in asymptomatic patients and is characterized by the

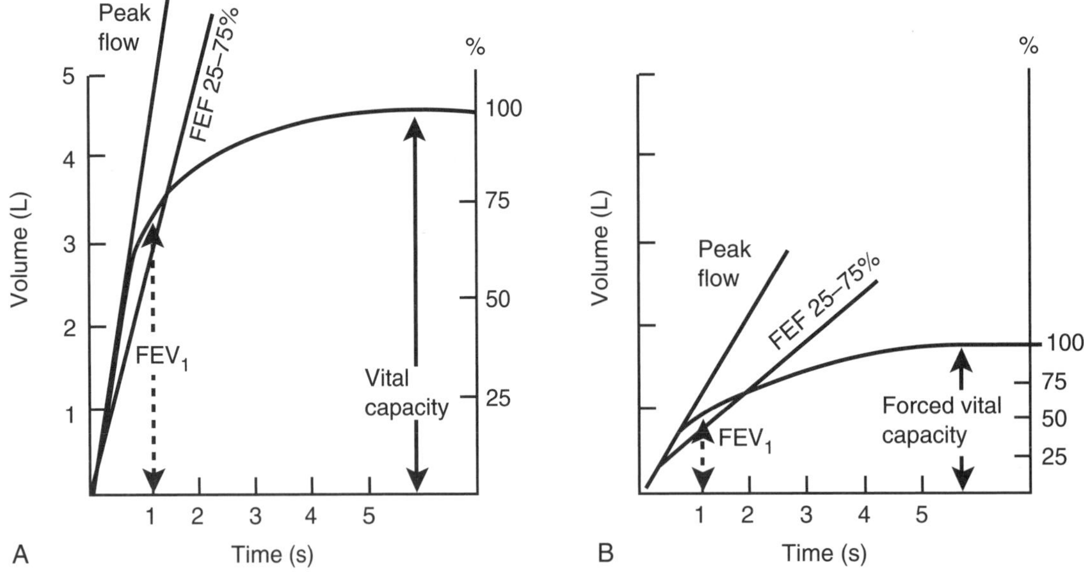

Figure 19-1. Spirogram changes of *(A)* a normal subject and *(B)* a patient in bronchospasm. The forced exhaled volume in 1 second (FEV_1) is typically less than 80% of the vital capacity in the presence of obstructive airway disease. Peak flow and maximum midexpiratory flow rate (FEF 25% to 75%) are also decreased in these patients (Fig. B). (From Kingston and Hirshman,[2] with permission.)

development of bronchoconstriction in response to stimuli (allergens, exercise, mechanical airway stimulation) that have little or no impact on normal airways. The degree of airway hyperreactivity probably parallels the extent of inflammation of the airways and the numbers of eosinophils in the peripheral blood. There is no pathognomonic feature or definitive diagnostic test for bronchial asthma, although more than a 15% increase in expiratory airflow in response to bronchodilator therapy is supportive evidence when bronchial asthma is suspected on clinical grounds.

Signs and Symptoms

During periods of normal to near normal pulmonary function, patients with bronchial asthma are likely to have no physical findings. As expiratory airflow obstruction increases a number of changes become detectable. Wheezing is the most common finding during an acute bronchial asthma attack. The characteristic cough of bronchial asthma ranges from nonproductive to production of copious amounts of tenacious sputum. Dyspnea tends to parallel the severity of expiratory airflow obstruction. The FEV_1 and forced expiratory flow between 25% and 75% of vital capacity are direct reflections of the severity of expiratory airflow obstruction (Fig. 19-1 and Table 19-1).[2] The flow-volume loop reveals a characteristic downward scooping of the expiratory limb of the loop (Fig. 19-2).[2] Mild bronchial asthma is usually accompanied by a normal PaO_2 and a normal to decreased $PaCO_2$ (Table 19-1).[2] Fatigue of the skeletal muscles necessary for breathing may contribute to the development of hypercarbia.

Treatment

Bronchial asthma is treated with anti-inflammatory drugs and bronchodilators. Recognition of the consistent presence of airway inflammation in the airways of patients with bronchial asthma is the basis for the use of inhaled corticosteroids or cromolyn as the first line of therapy for anything more than occasional mild asthma.[4] Bronchodilator therapy with a beta-2 agonist is added to the treatment regimen when anti-inflammatory therapy is insufficient. Albuterol delivered by metered dose inhaler is the inhaled beta-2 agonist most often administered for short-term relief of bronchoconstriction. Aminophylline is a less effective bronchodilator than beta-2 agonists and may be associated with cardiac dysrhythmias

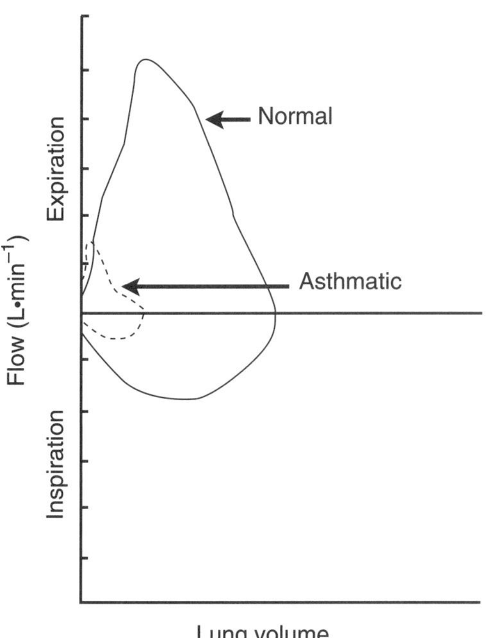

Figure 19-2. A flow-volume curve of a normal and asthmatic individual. (From Kingston and Hirshman,[2] with permission.)

and seizures, especially when its plasma concentration is higher than 20 mg·L^{-1}. Treatment of status asthmaticus includes repetitive administration of a beta-2 agonist by inhalation or subcutaneous injection, or both, plus intravenous administration of a corticosteroid. In rare circumstances where life-threatening status asthmaticus persists despite aggressive pharmacologic therapy, it may be acceptable to consider general anesthesia (isoflurane is as acceptable as halothane without the same risk of cardiac dysrhythmias) in an attempt to produce bronchodilation.

Table 19-1. Estimation of the Severity of Bronchial Asthma

Expiratory Airflow Obstruction	FEV_1 (% predicted)	PaO_2 (mmHg)	$PaCO_2$ (mmHg)
Mild (asymptomatic)	65–80	>60	<40
Moderate	50–64	>60	<45
Marked	35–49	<60	>50
Severe (status asthmaticus)	<35	<60	>50

Abbreviation: FEV_1, forced exhaled volume in 1 second.
(Data from Kingston and Hirshman.[2])

Management of Anesthesia

Preoperatively, the absence of (1) wheezing during auscultation of the chest or (2) complaints of dyspnea suggests that the patient is not experiencing an acute exacerbation of bronchial asthma. The observation that the blood eosinophil count may parallel the degree of airway inflammation and airway hyperreactivity provides an indirect assessment of the status of the disease preoperatively. Performance of pulmonary function studies (especially FEV_1) before and after bronchodilator therapy may be indicated in the patient who is scheduled for a thoracic or abdominal operation. Measurement of arterial blood gases before proceeding with elective surgery is a consideration if there are questions about the adequacy of ventilation or arterial oxygenation. Bronchodilator drugs should be continued until the induction of anesthesia. Supplementation with cortisol may be indicated before major surgery if adrenal cortex suppression from corticosteroids used to treat asthma is a possibility (see Chapter 22). The use of anticholinergics should be individualized, remembering that although these drugs can decrease airway resistance, they can also increase the viscosity of secretions, making it difficult to remove them from the airway. Administration of H_2 antagonists is questionable because antagonism of H_2-mediated bronchodilation could unmask H_1-mediated bronchoconstriction.

Regional anesthesia is an attractive choice when the surgery is superficial or on the extremities. Otherwise, the goal during induction and maintenance of general anesthesia in patients with bronchial asthma is to depress airway reflexes so as to avoid bronchoconstriction of hyperreactive airways in response to mechanical stimulation. Induction of anesthesia is with the intravenous administration of barbiturates, benzodiazepines, or propofol. These drugs, however, are unlikely to adequately depress airway reflexes, allowing the precipitation of bronchospasm should intubation of the trachea be attempted. Ketamine (1 to 2 mg·kg^{-1} IV) is an alternative selection for induction of anesthesia because of its sympathomimetic effects on bronchial smooth muscle. Increased secretions associated with administration of ketamine, however, may detract from use of this drug in patients with bronchial asthma. Before intubation of the trachea, a sufficient depth of anesthesia should be established to depress hyperreactive airway reflexes and minimize the likelihood of bronchoconstriction with stimulation of the upper airway. Halothane is a popular drug for administration to patients with bronchial asthma, although other volatile anesthetics such as isoflurane are equally acceptable bronchodilators and do not sensitize the heart to the cardiac dysrhythmic effects of sympathetic nervous system stimulation as produced by beta agonists and aminophylline. Administration of lidocaine (1 to 2 mg·kg^{-1} IV) before intubation of the trachea is also useful for preventing reflex bronchoconstriction provoked by instrumentation of the airway.[5] Muscle relaxants with limited ability to evoke the release of histamine are likely to be selected. For example, severe bronchospasm following the administration of atracurium has been reported in patients with asthma.[6] Nevertheless, in large comparative studies the incidence of bronchospasm following administration of atracurium compared with vecuronium is not different.[7] Although histamine release has been attributed to succinylcholine, there is no evidence that this drug is associated with the appearance of increased airway resistance when administered to patients with bronchial asthma.

Intraoperatively, the PaO_2 and $PaCO_2$ can be maintained at normal levels by mechanical ventilation of the lungs using a slow inspiratory flow rate to optimize distribution of inhaled gases. A slow breathing rate (6 to 10 breaths·min^{-1}) allows sufficient time for passive exhalation to occur in the presence of increased airway resistance. Positive end-expiratory pressure (PEEP) may not be ideal, because adequate exhalation may be impaired in the presence of narrowed airways. Liberal intravenous administration of crystalloid solutions during the perioperative period is useful for maintaining adequate hydration and ensuring the presence of less viscous secretions that can be more easily expelled from the airway. At the conclusion of elective surgery, the trachea may be extubated while the depth of anesthesia is still sufficient to suppress hyperreactive airway reflexes. Bronchospasm does not predictably follow administration of anticholinesterase drugs to reverse the effects of nondepolarizing muscle relaxants, which may reflect protective effects (decreased airway resistance) of simultaneously administered anticholinergics. When it is considered unsafe to extubate the trachea until the patient is awake because of the presumed presence of gastric contents, intravenous administration of lidocaine may minimize the likelihood of airway stimulation due to the continued presence of the tracheal tube.

Intraoperative Bronchospasm

Bronchospasm that occurs intraoperatively is usually due to factors other than an acute exacerbation of bronchial asthma. Indeed, it is important that treatment with drugs appropriate for the management of bronchospasm owing to bronchial asthma not be instituted until more likely causes of wheezing (mechanical obstruction, light anesthesia) have been considered. Fiberoptic bronchoscopy may be useful to rule out mechanical obstructive causes of bronchospasm. Bronchospasm due to bronchial asthma may respond to deepening of anesthesia with a volatile anesthetic but not skeletal muscle paralysis. Should bronchospasm due to bronchial asthma persist despite an increase in the depth of anesthesia, the delivery of albuterol into the patient's airway by attaching the metered dose inhaler to the anesthetic delivery system is indicated. When bronchospasm persists despite beta-2 therapy, it may be necessary to add corticosteroids and aminophylline to the treatment regimen.

Differential Diagnosis of Intraoperative Bronchospasm

Mechanical obstruction (anesthetic delivery system, tracheal tube)
Inadequate depth of anesthesia
Pulmonary aspiration
Endobronchial intubation
Pneumothorax
Pulmonary embolus
Acute bronchial asthma

Pulmonary Emphysema

Pulmonary emphysema is characterized by loss of elastic recoil of the lungs, which results in collapse of airways during exhalation, leading to increased airway resistance (Table 19-2). Severe dyspnea is typ-

Table 19-2. Comparative Features of Chronic Obstructive Pulmonary Disease

	Pulmonary Emphysema	Chronic Bronchitis
Forced exhaled volume in 1 second	Decreased	Decreased
Total lung capacity	Increased	Increased
Dyspnea	Severe	Moderate
Arterial hypoxemia	Late	Early
Hypercarbia	Late	Early
Hematocrit	Normal	Increased
Cor pulmonale	Late	Early
Prognosis	Good	Poor

ical of emphysema, reflecting increased work of breathing owing to loss of elastic recoil of the lungs. Preoperative evaluation of patients with emphysema should determine the severity of the disease and elucidate any reversible components such as infection or bronchospasm.

The presence of dyspnea, cough, sputum production, and decreased exercise tolerance suggests the need for preoperative pulmonary function studies. The risk of postoperative respiratory failure is increased if the preoperative ratio of FEV_1 to vital capacity is less than 50%. Arterial blood gases are usually normal ("pink puffers"), reflecting a high minute ventilation in an attempt to overcome increased airway resistance. The presence of a $PaCO_2$ higher than 50 mmHg cautions against performance of elective surgery as the risk of postoperative respiratory failure is increased. Preoperative detection and treatment of cor pulmonale with supplemental oxygen are important.

Management of Anesthesia

The presence of pulmonary emphysema does not dictate the use of specific drugs (inhaled or injected) or techniques (regional or general) for the management of anesthesia. More important than the drugs or techniques selected is the realization that these patients are susceptible to the development of acute respiratory failure in the postoperative period.

If general anesthesia is selected, a volatile anesthetic using humidification of the inhaled gases and mechanical ventilation of the lungs is useful. Nitrous oxide is frequently administered in combination with volatile anesthetics. Potential disadvantages of nitrous oxide include limitation of the inhaled concentrations of oxygen and passage of this gas into bullae that result from emphysema. Conceivably, nitrous oxide could lead to enlargement and rupture of bullae, resulting in the development of a tension pneumothorax. Opioids, although acceptable, are less ideal for maintenance of anesthesia owing to the frequent need for high inhaled concentrations of nitrous oxide (and associated decreases in inhaled concentrations of oxygen) to ensure amnesia. This disadvantage may be circumvented by substituting a low concentration of volatile anesthetic for nitrous oxide. Postoperative depression of ventilation may reflect residual effects of opioids as administered intraoperatively.

Humidification of inspired gases during anesthesia is important to prevent drying of secretions in the airways. It must be appreciated that systemic dehydration due to inadequate fluid administration during the perioperative period can result in excessive drying of secretions in the airways despite humidification of inhaled gases.

Controlled ventilation of the lungs using large tidal volumes (10 to 15 $ml \cdot kg^{-1}$) combined with a slow inspiratory flow rate is useful for optimizing arterial oxygenation. A slow breathing rate (6 to 10 $breaths \cdot min^{-1}$) allows sufficient time for venous return to the heart and is less likely to be associated with undesirable degrees of hyperventilation. Continued intubation of the trachea and mechanical ventilation of the lungs in the postoperative period are likely to be necessary following major surgery in patients with severe emphysema (see Chapter 33).

Chronic Bronchitis

Chronic bronchitis is characterized by chronic or recurrent secretion of excess mucus into the bronchi, resulting in increased resistance to gas flow through these airways. Patients with chronic bronchitis tend to develop arterial hypoxemia ("blue bloaters"), hypercarbia, and cor pulmonale early, in contrast to the delayed onset of these changes with emphysema (Table 19-2). Because the small airways account for only a minor proportion of total airway resistance, chronic bronchitis must be advanced before dyspnea becomes apparent. Cigarette smoking is the major predisposing factor to the development of chronic bronchitis. Preoperative evaluation and management of anesthesia are as described for patients with pulmonary emphysema.

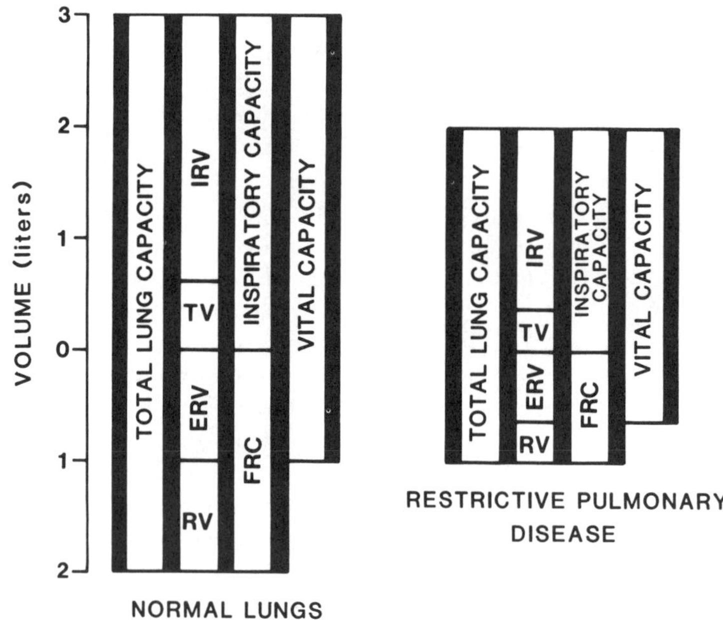

Figure 19-3. Compared with normal lungs, restrictive pulmonary disease is characterized by a decrease in total lung capacity and all the components that comprise this capacity, especially vital capacity. IRV, inspiratory reserve volume; TV, tidal volume; ERV, expiratory reserve volume; RV, residual volume; FRC, functional residual capacity.

RESTRICTIVE PULMONARY DISEASE

Restrictive pulmonary disease is characterized by decreases in lung compliance that result in decreased lung volumes (Fig. 19-3). A decrease in vital capacity (normal 50 to 70 ml·kg^{-1}) in the presence of a normal FEV_1 is the classic evidence of restrictive pulmonary disease.

Patients with restrictive pulmonary disease complain of dyspnea, reflecting the increased work of breathing necessary to expand poorly compliant lungs. A rapid and shallow pattern of breathing is characteristic because it minimizes the work of breathing in the presence of decreased lung compliance. A decrease in the $PaCO_2$ reflects hyperventilation produced by the rapid and shallow pattern of breathing. Indeed, the $PaCO_2$ is usually maintained at a decreased to normal value until restrictive pulmonary disease is far advanced.

Acute restrictive pulmonary disease is most often due to leakage of intravascular fluid into the interstitium of the lungs and into the alveoli, manifesting as pulmonary edema. Disorders associated with acute restrictive pulmonary disease include adult respiratory distress syndrome, aspiration pneumonitis, neurogenic pulmonary edema, opioid-induced pulmonary edema, and high-altitude pulmonary edema. Chronic restrictive pulmonary disease is characterized by the presence of pulmonary fibrosis (sarcoidosis) or processes that interfere with expansion of the lungs (effusions, kyphoscoliosis, obesity, ascites, pregnancy).

Management of Anesthesia

Regional anesthesia is appropriate for peripheral surgery, but it must be appreciated that sensory levels above T10 can be associated with impairment of respiratory muscle activity necessary for patients with restrictive pulmonary disease to maintain acceptable ventilation. Restrictive pulmonary disease does not influence the choice of drugs used for the induction or maintenance of general anesthesia. The need to minimize depression of ventilation that may persist into the postoperative period should be considered when selecting drugs such as opioids. Mechanical ventilation of the lungs is useful, but high inflation pressures may be necessary to inflate the poorly compliant lungs or thorax, or both. Continued ventilation of the lungs in the postoperative period is likely to be necessary when the vital capacity is lower than 15 ml·kg^{-1} or the $PaCO_2$ is higher than 50 mmHg preoperatively. It should be appreciated that restrictive pulmonary disease contributes to decreased lung volumes, making it difficult to generate an effective cough for removal of secretions from the airways in the postoperative period.

ANESTHESIA FOR THORACIC SURGERY

Anesthesia for thoracic surgery typically begins with the preoperative performance of pulmonary function tests and evaluation of the adequacy of medical management of chronic pulmonary disease. The choice of drugs to produce anesthesia, the selection of monitors, the impact of the lateral decubitus position on pulmonary physiology, and the indications and techniques for one-lung anesthesia are considerations in planning the management of anesthesia for thoracic surgery. Postoperatively, a high index of suspicion must be maintained for life-threatening complications (hemorrhage, bronchopleural fistula) associated with thoracic surgery. It may be necessary to continue mechanical ventilation of the lungs into the postoperative period. Methods to provide postoperative analgesia should receive high priority because pain is intense after thoracic surgery (see Chapter 32).

Preoperative Preparation

Patients undergoing thoracic surgery are at high risk of developing postoperative pulmonary complications, particularly if there is co-existing chronic pulmonary disease. Specific preoperative findings that make postoperative pulmonary complications likely include dyspnea, cough and sputum production, wheezing, history of cigarette smoking, obesity, and advanced age. In addition, a recent upper respiratory infection may be associated with increased airway resistance that persists for as long as 5 weeks. Respiratory defense mechanisms against bacteria may also be impaired after viral respiratory infections.

The main purpose of the preoperative evaluation is to identify patients at risk of complications and to institute appropriate perioperative therapy. Indeed, the incidence of postoperative pulmonary complications can be decreased by preoperative prophylactic measures (Table 19-3).

Discontinuation of Smoking

Smoking increases airway irritability and secretions, decreases mucociliary transport, and increases the incidence of postoperative pulmonary complications. Smoke free intervals of 12 to 18 hours result in substantial decreases in carboxyhemoglobin levels and normalization of the oxyhemoglobin dissociation curve, as evidenced by an increase in the P_{50} (partial pressure of oxygen at which 50% of the arterial hemoglobin is saturated with oxygen).[8] Carbon monoxide may also exert negative inotropic effects. In contrast to these favorable effects, improvement in ciliary and small airway function and decreases in sputum production require prolonged abstinence from smoking. For example, the incidence of postoperative pulmonary complications after coronary artery surgery decreases only when abstinence from cigarette smoking is longer than 8 weeks (Fig. 19-4).[9]

Pulmonary Function Tests

Pulmonary function tests are helpful in identifying patients at increased risk of developing pulmonary complications and in evaluating responses to preoperative pulmonary therapy. Patients with findings suggestive of the presence of chronic pulmonary disease on the history, physical examination, or chest radiograph who are scheduled for upper abdominal or thoracic surgery often undergo preoperative pulmonary function tests. In addition, elderly patients

Table 19-3. Preoperative Prophylactic Measures

Measures	Results
Consider discontinuation of smoking	Carboxyhemoglobin levels decrease in 12–18 hours so as to increase available hemoglobin
Treat pulmonary infection	Select antibiotics on basis of culture and sensitivity
Treat reversible component of increased airway resistance	Beta-2 agonist by metered dose inhaler
Thin and mobilize secretions	Hydration and chest percussion
Teach deep breathing and coughing exercises	

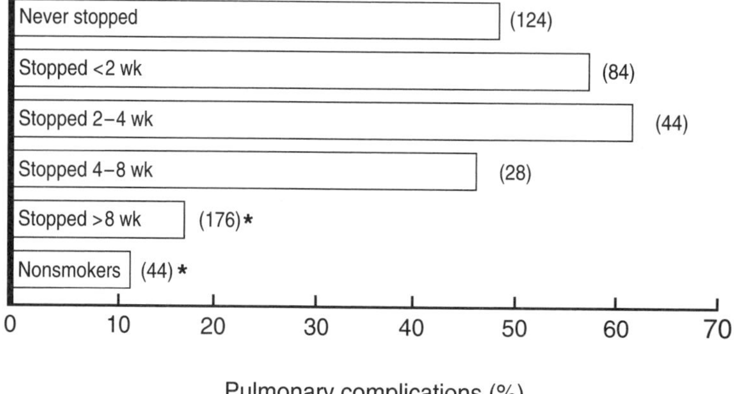

Figure 19-4. Preoperative duration of smoking cessation and pulmonary complication rates after cardiac surgery. The incidence of pulmonary complications begins to decrease only when abstinence from cigarette smoking is longer than 8 weeks. *P <0.001 compared with patients who never stopped smoking preoperatively. Number of patients studied are indicated in parentheses. (From Warner et al.,[9] with permission.)

and morbidly obese patients are candidates for preoperative pulmonary function tests. Arterial blood gases and pH may be measured in patients with complaints of severe dyspnea and decreased exercise tolerance.

Numerous pulmonary function tests can be used to quantitate pulmonary disease preoperatively. The simplest and often most informative tests are measurements of flow rates during exhalation (FEV_1) and vital capacity. The most detailed assessment of flow resistive properties of the airways during inhalation and exhalation is provided by analysis of flow-volume loops (Fig. 19-2).[2] The risk of postoperative pulmonary morbidity is predictably increased when preoperatively (1) the FEV_1 is lower than 2 L, (2) the ratio of the FEV_1 to forced vital capacity is lower than 0.5, (3) the vital capacity is lower than 15 $ml \cdot kg^{-1}$, or (4) maximum breathing capacity is lower than 50% of the predicted value. It is unusual for the $PaCO_2$ to increase before the ratio of FEV_1 to forced vital capacity is lower than 0.5. Pulmonary function studies and arterial blood gas measurements should be repeated after antibiotic and bronchodilator therapy to confirm a beneficial response to therapy.

Prophylactic Digitalis

Resection of pulmonary tissue decreases the available pulmonary vascular bed and can cause postoperative right atrial and ventricular enlargement with associated cardiac dysrhythmias, especially atrial fibrillation. For this reason, prophylactic use of digitalis (digoxin 0.75 mg PO in divided doses the day before surgery and 0.25 mg before the induction of anesthesia) has been recommended, particularly in elderly patients undergoing resection of large amounts of lung tissue.[10] A disadvantage of prophylactic digitalis is confusion with digitalis toxicity should cardiac dysrhythmias develop postoperatively. Indeed, events such as alterations in renal function, decreases in serum potassium concentrations owing to hyperventilation of the lungs, and increases in sympathetic nervous system activity are likely to occur intraoperatively and thus increase the likelihood of increased pharmacologic effects from circulating digitalis.[11]

Management of Anesthesia

General anesthesia with controlled ventilation of the lungs is appropriate for thoracic surgery. Use of volatile anesthetics with or without nitrous oxide is common, as these potent drugs decrease irritability of the airways and can be rapidly eliminated at the conclusion of surgery. In addition, volatile anesthetics do not seem to inhibit regional hypoxic pulmonary vasoconstriction, thus contributing to maintenance of arterial oxygenation during one-lung anesthesia (Fig. 19-5).[12] If nitrous oxide is administered, the inhaled concentrations are often limited to 50% until the adequacy of oxygenation can be

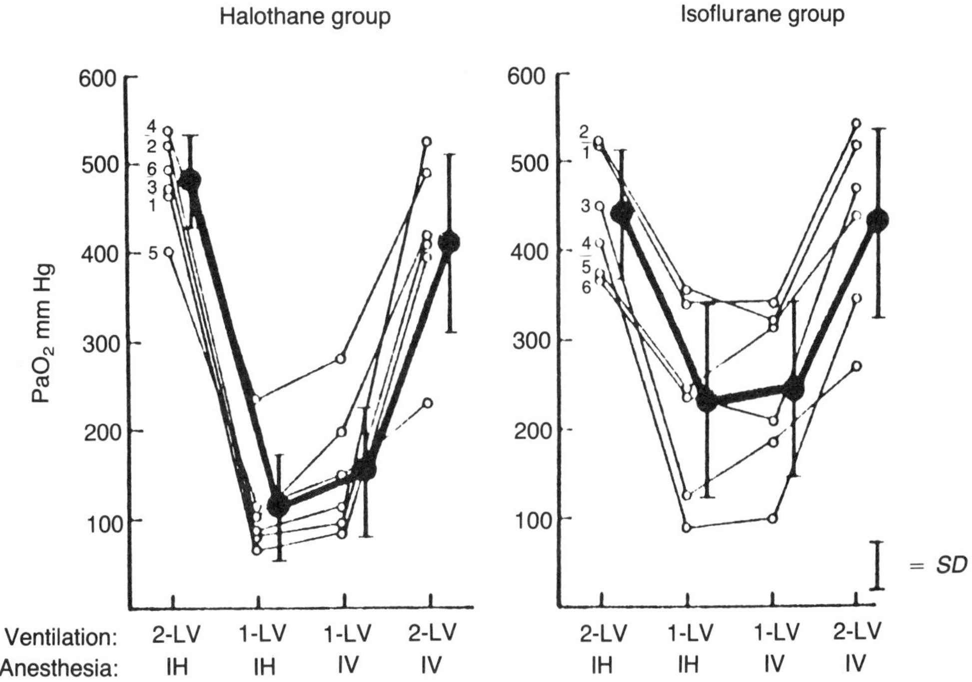

Figure 19-5. PaO_2 was measured during two-lung ventilation (2-LV) and then during one-lung ventilation (1-LV) during inhalation (IH) or intravenous (IV) anesthesia. Addition of halothane or isoflurane (about 1.0 MAC) did not greatly alter PaO_2, suggesting that these anesthetics do not significantly inhibit regional hypoxic pulmonary vasoconstriction. Open circles indicate individual patient data; solid circles indicate mean ± SD for each group. (From Benumof et al.,[12] with permission.)

confirmed by pulse oximetry or measurement of the PaO_2. Nondepolarizing muscle relaxants are usually administered to facilitate controlled ventilation of the lungs, to improve surgical exposure by maximizing mechanical separation of the ribs, and to decrease requirements for volatile anesthetics. Ketamine is useful for induction of anesthesia for emergency thoracotomy associated with hypovolemia (blunt trauma, gun shot, stab wound). Patients undergoing thoracotomy usually have an intra-arterial catheter in place to permit continuous monitoring of blood pressure and frequent measurement of arterial blood gases and pH. A central venous pressure catheter is helpful for guiding intravenous fluid replacement. Alternatively, a pulmonary artery catheter should be considered if co-existing coronary artery disease or cardiac valvular dysfunction is present. A catheter should be inserted into the bladder of patients who are expected to undergo long operations associated with alterations in blood volume, necessitating infusions of large amounts of intravenous fluids.

Lateral Decubitus Position

The lateral decubitus position necessary for thoracic surgery, as well as the need for mechanical ventilation of the lungs, results in an altered distribution of ventilation to perfusion (see Chapter 14).

One-Lung Anesthesia

One-lung anesthesia using a double-lumen endobronchial tube is indicated when one lung can contaminate the other lung with infected material or blood or when the distribution of ventilation between the two lungs must be separated as in the presence of a bronchopleural fistula. Relative indications for one-lung anesthesia are to provide a quiet lung and improved operating conditions as during lobectomy (especially upper lobectomy, which is technically the most difficult), pneumonectomy, resection of a thoracic aneurysm, or operations on the esophagus.

A clear plastic disposable Robertshaw tube with a low-pressure cuff is the most frequently used double-lumen endobronchial tube (Fig. 19-6). Inflation of

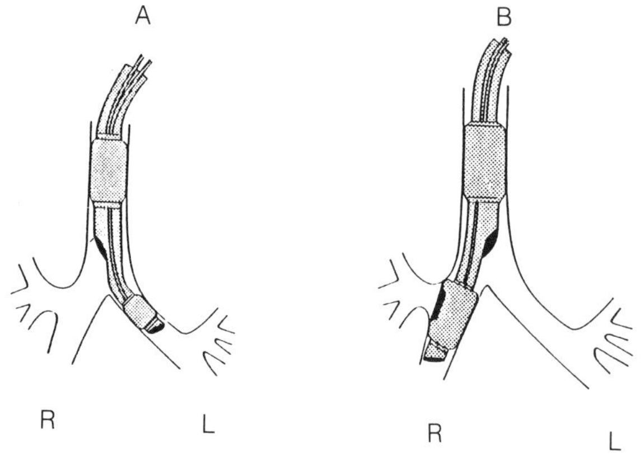

Figure 19-6. The Robertshaw double-lumen endobronchial tube is available as *(A)* a left or *(B)* a right design. Placed in the trachea, the distal end of the endobronchial tube is directed into the left (L) or right (R) mainstem bronchus. The distal end of the right Robertshaw endobronchial tube incorporates a slotted cuff to permit ventilation of the right upper lobe.

the proximal cuff on this tube provides a seal with the tracheal mucosa. Inflation of the cuff on the distal portion of the endobronchial tube that is present in the left or right mainstem bronchus provides a seal to isolate that lung from the contralateral lung. A left Robertshaw endobronchial tube is used for operations requiring isolation of the right lung and ventilation of the left lung. When isolation of the left lung is required, either a left or right Robertshaw endobronchial tube may be used. The nearness of the right upper lobe bronchus to the carina introduces the risk of inadequate ventilation of the right upper lobe when a right endobronchial tube is used. To avoid this complication, it is acceptable to use a left Robertshaw endobronchial tube for all one-lung anesthesia.[13] Should clamping of the left mainstem bronchus be necessary, the left Robertshaw endobronchial cuff is deflated and the tube is withdrawn into the trachea at the appropriate time, thus effectively converting this double-lumen endobronchial tube to a single-lumen tracheal tube for ventilation of the right lung.

Positioning of the endobronchial tube such that the 29-cm mark is present at the patient's lips will place the tube in the approximately correct position in most adult patients of average height.[14] It is recommended, however, to confirm proper placement of the endobronchial tube using fiberoptic bronchoscopy as auscultation of the lungs is not reliable.[15] Looking down the tracheal lumen of the endobronchial tube with a fiberoptic bronchoscope, the anesthesiologist should see a clear straight-ahead view of the carina and the upper surface of the blue left endobronchial cuff just below the tracheal carina. Left and right orientation is confirmed by observation of the tracheal rings, which are complete anteriorly and incomplete posteriorly.

An alternative to the conventional double-lumen endobronchial tube is a single-lumen tube that includes a bronchial blocker (Univent) that can be advanced into the right or left mainstem bronchus usually with the aid of fiberoptic bronchoscopy (Fig. 19-7). The need to switch tubes at the end of the surgical procedure is obviated since the tube functions as a single-lumen tracheal tube when the bronchial blocker is withdrawn into its channel.

The major disadvantage of one-lung anesthesia is the introduction of an iatrogenic right-to-left intrapulmonary shunt by virtue of continued perfusion to both lungs while only the dependent lung is ventilated. An unpredictable degree of variability in the magnitude of this shunt between patients reflects the multiple factors involved in determining the amount of perfusion to the nondependent and nonventilated lung. In addition to gravity, the amount of perfusion to the nonventilated lung is influenced by (1) hypoxic pulmonary vasoconstriction, (2) surgical compression, and (3) the method used to ventilate the dependent lung. Arterial hypoxemia may also be due to unrecognized blockade of the tracheal tube lumen with secretions. For all these reasons, use of high inspired concentrations of oxygen, continuous monitoring of peripheral arterial hemoglobin saturation with oxygen by pulse oximetry, and frequent measurements of the PaO_2 are indicated during one-lung anesthesia. If arterial hypoxemia persists despite inhalation of high concentrations of oxygen, the selective application of a low level of PEEP (2.5 to 10 cmH_2O) to the ventilated and dependent lung can be instituted in an attempt to divert more ventilation to this lung. Although selective dependent lung PEEP may improve arterial oxygenation, it may also increase pulmonary vascular resistance in the ventilated lung, resulting in further intrapulmonary shunt. In fact, selective continuous positive airway pressure ([CPAP] 2.5 to 10 cmH_2O) applied to the nondependent and nonventilated lung is the most efficacious maneuver for improving arterial

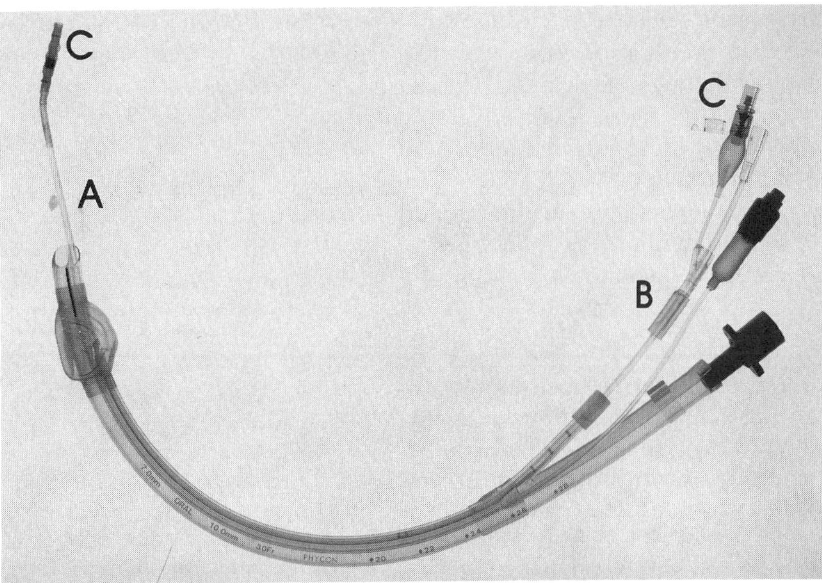

Figure 19-7. The Univent single-lumen cuffed tube includes a built-in bronchial blocker (A) that can be advanced manually (B) into the left or right mainstem bronchus to permit one-lung anesthesia when the bronchial blocker cuff is inflated (C).

oxygenation during one-lung anesthesia. Presumably, this selective CPAP causes some oxygenation of blood perfusing the nondependent lung while also increasing pulmonary vascular resistance in this lung, thus diverting more blood flow to the dependent and ventilated lung. Ligation of the pulmonary artery during one-lung anesthesia for a pneumonectomy improves oxygenation by removing perfusion to the nonventilated lung. Elimination of carbon dioxide is not usually a problem during one-lung anesthesia.

Conclusion of Surgery

Hyperinflation of the lungs is important to exclude air from the pleural space at the conclusion of thoracic surgery. Furthermore, alveoli incised during segmental resection of the lungs continue to leak air into the pleural space, necessitating the placement of drainage tubes (chest tubes) to ensure removal of this air and continued expansion of the lung. These drainage tubes are connected to a sterile disposable plastic unit, which incorporates a one-way valve that permits continuous suction. Chest tubes must not be allowed to kink, because sudden increases in intrathoracic pressure, as with coughing, may accentuate the leak and cause a tension pneumothorax if air cannot escape.

Placement of drainage tubes is not necessary after a pneumonectomy. Instead, intrapleural pressure on the operated side is adjusted by aspirating air to slightly below atmospheric pressure. Excessive negative pressure can cause hypotension by shifting the mediastinum and compromising cardiac output.

The trachea may be extubated when the adequacy of spontaneous ventilation is confirmed and protective upper airway reflexes have returned. In otherwise healthy patients, extubation of the trachea may be performed at the conclusion of surgery, especially if pain relief (intercostal nerve blocks, neuraxial opioids) has been instituted (see Chapter 32). If mechanical ventilation of the lungs must be continued into the postoperative period, it will be necessary to replace the double-lumen endobronchial tube with a single-lumen tracheal tube.

Postoperative Pulmonary Complications

Postoperative pulmonary complications after thoracic surgery (and other forms of surgery, especially upper abdominal operations) are most often characterized as atelectasis followed by pneumonia and arterial hypoxemia. The severity of these complications parallels the magnitude of decreases in vital capacity and functional residual capacity (see

Chapter 33). Presumably, decreases in these lung volumes interfere with generation of an effective cough, as well as contributing to atelectasis. The net effect is decreased clearance of secretions from the airways and atelectasis, leading to pneumonia and arterial hypoxemia. Adequate analgesia after thoracic surgery permits patients to breathe deeply and cough effectively so as to minimize the likelihood of postoperative atelectasis or pneumonia, or both.

MEDIASTINOSCOPY

Mediastinoscopy is often performed before thoracotomy to establish the diagnosis and/or resectability of carcinoma of the lung. Hemorrhage and pneumothorax are the most frequently encountered complications of this procedure. If a thoracotomy is not subsequently performed, it is important to maintain a high index of suspicion for pneumothorax in the immediate postoperative period. Radiographs of the chest in the recovery room are helpful in detecting the presence of a pneumothorax.

Positive pressure ventilation of the lungs during mediastinoscopy is recommended so as to minimize the risk of venous air embolism. The mediastinoscope can also exert pressure against the right subclavian artery, causing the loss of a pulse distal to the site of compression and an erroneous diagnosis of cardiac arrest. Likewise, unrecognized compression of the right carotid artery has been proposed as an explanation for postoperative neurologic deficits that may occur after this procedure. Bradycardia during mediastinoscopy may be due to stretching of the vagus nerve or trachea by the mediastinoscope. This is treated by repositioning the mediastinoscope followed by intravenous administration of atropine if bradycardia persists.

REFERENCES

1. Ferguson GT, Cherniack RM. Management of chronic obstructive pulmonary disease. N Engl J Med 1993;328:1017–22.
2. Kingston HGG, Hirshman CA. Perioperative management of the patient with asthma. Anesth Analg 1984; 63:844–55.
3. Weiss KB, Gergen PJ, Hodgson TA. An economic evaluation of asthma in the United States. N Engl J Med 1992;326:862–6.
4. Randall T. International consensus report urges sweeping reform in asthma treatment. JAMA 1992; 267:2153–4.
5. Downes H, Gerber N, Hirshman CA. I.V. lignocaine in reflex and allergic bronchoconstriction. Br J Anaesth 1980;52:873–8.
6. Oh TE, Horton JM. Adverse reactions to atracurium. Br J Anaesth 1989;62:467–70.
7. Lawson DH, Paice GM, Glavin RJ, et al. Atracurium—A post-marketing surveillance study: UK study and discussion. Br J Anaesth 1989;62:596–600.
8. Kambam JR, Chen LH, Hyman SA. Effect of short-term smoking halt on carboxyhemoglobin levels and P_{50} values. Anesth Analg 1986;65:1186–8.
9. Warner MA, Divertie MB, Tinker JH. Preoperative cessation of smoking and pulmonary complications in coronary artery bypass patients. Anesthesiology 1984 60:380–3.
10. Chee TP, Prakash NS, Desser KB, Benchimol A. Postoperative supraventricular arrhythmias and the role of prophylactic digoxin in cardiac surgery. Am Heart J 1982;104:974–7.
11. Chung DC. Anaesthetic problems associated with the treatment of cardiovascular disease: I. Digitalis toxicity. Can Anaesth Soc J 1981;28:6–16.
12. Benumof JL, Augustine SD, Gibbons JA. Halothane and isoflurane only slightly impair arterial oxygenation during one-lung ventilation in patients undergoing thoracotomy. Anesthesiology 1987;67:910–5.
13. Benumof JL, Partridge BL, Salvatierra C, Keating J. Margin of safety in positioning double-lumen endotracheal tubes. Anesthesiology 1987;67:729–38.
14. Brodsky JB, Benumof JL, Ehrenwerth J, Ozaki GT. Depth of placement of left double-lumen endobronchial tubes. Anesth Analg 1991;73:570–2.
15. Alliaume B, Coddens J, Deloof T. Reliability of auscultation in positioning of double-lumen endobronchial tubes. Can J Anaesth 1992;39:687–90.

20

Liver and Biliary Tract Disease

Management of anesthesia in the presence of liver disease requires an understanding of the physiologic functions of the liver. In addition, the impact of anesthesia and surgery on hepatic blood flow has important implications for the management of anesthesia. Liver function tests are useful for detecting unsuspected liver disease preoperatively and for establishing the diagnosis when postoperative liver dysfunction occurs. Liver transplantation represents one of the most demanding and intense anesthetic challenges with which anesthesiologists are confronted (see Chapter 28).

PHYSIOLOGIC FUNCTIONS OF THE LIVER

Physiologic functions of the liver that may be altered by co-existing liver disease include glucose homeostasis, protein synthesis, drug metabolism, and bilirubin formation and excretion. Hepatic sinuses are lined by Kupffer's cells that are capable of phagocytizing bacteria absorbed from the gastrointestinal tract into the portal vein. The response of patients during the perioperative period may be influenced by disease-induced alterations in these important functions of the liver.

Glucose Homeostasis

The liver is responsible for the storage and release of glucose. Glucose enters hepatocytes, where it is stored as glycogen. Breakdown of glycogen (glycogenolysis) releases glucose back into the systemic circulation to maintain normal blood glucose concentrations. The liver can store only about 75 g of glycogen, which can be depleted by 24 to 48 hours of starvation. Glucose homeostasis depends primarily on conversion of lactate, glycerol, and amino acids to glucose (gluconeogenesis) when liver glycogen stores are depleted. Exogenous sources of glucose during the fasting period associated with surgery become important when glycogen stores are depleted by poor preoperative nutrition and when gluconeogenesis is inhibited by anesthesia.[1] Indeed, patients with cirrhosis of the liver may be vulnerable to the development of hypoglycemia in the perioperative period.

Protein Synthesis

All proteins except gamma globulins and antihemophilic factor (factor VIII) are synthesized in the rough endoplasmic reticulum of hepatocytes. Approximately 10 to 15 g of albumin are produced daily to maintain plasma concentrations of this protein between 3.5 to 5.5 $g \cdot dl^{-1}$. Plasma albumin concentrations lower than 3.5 $g \cdot dl^{-1}$ may reflect significant liver disease. The half-time for albumin, however, is about 23 days, emphasizing that acute liver dysfunction will not be reflected by decreased plasma concentrations of this protein.

Protein synthesis in the liver is important for drug binding, coagulation, and production of enzymes necessary for hydrolysis of ester linkages.

Drug Binding

When liver disease results in decreased albumin production, fewer sites will be available for drug binding. As a result, the unbound, pharmacologically active fractions of drugs, such as thiopental, increase (Fig. 20-1).[2] Increased drug sensitivities due to decreased protein binding are most likely to manifest when plasma albumin concentrations are lower than 2.5 $g \cdot dl^{-1}$.

Coagulation

Clotting abnormalities must be suspected in patients with liver disease because hepatocytes are responsible for the synthesis of most procoagulants. The adequacy of clotting factor levels is evaluated by measuring the prothrombin time, partial thromboplastin time, and bleeding time. Liver function must be dramatically depressed before impaired coagulation manifests because many coagulation factors require only 20% to 30% of their normal levels to prevent bleeding. Nevertheless, the plasma half-time of hepatic-produced clotting factors, such as prothrombin and fibrinogen, is short and acute liver dysfunction is likely to be associated with clotting abnormalities.

Liver disease associated with splenomegaly can alter the normal coagulation mechanism independent of procoagulant synthesis by trapping platelets in the spleen. Another factor predisposing to a bleeding diathesis is the failure of a diseased liver to clear plasma activators of the fibrinolytic system.

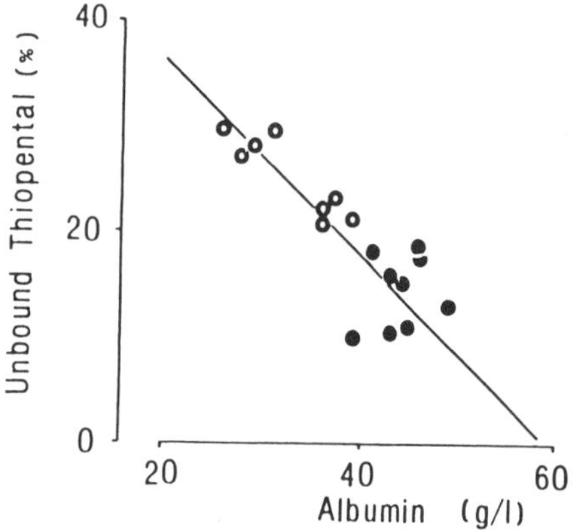

Figure 20-1. Unbound thiopental concentrations parallel serum concentrations of albumin in patients with cirrhosis of the liver (open circles) and normal patients (solid circles). Decreased serum albumin concentrations in patients with cirrhosis result in increased unbound (pharmacologically active) serum concentrations of thiopental. (From Pandele et al.,[2] with permission.)

Hydrolysis of Ester Linkages

Severe liver disease may decrease the production of cholinesterase (pseudocholinesterase) enzyme that is necessary for the hydrolysis of ester linkages in drugs such as succinylcholine, mivacurium, and ester local anesthetics. As a result, the duration of apnea after the administration of succinylcholine could be prolonged in the presence of liver disease. Prolonged effects of succinylcholine (longer than 30 minutes), however, are unlikely to be due to liver disease alone, and atypical plasma cholinesterase enzyme must be suspected. The plasma half-time for plasma cholinesterase is about 14 days, emphasizing that acute liver failure is unlikely to be associated with a decreased rate of succinylcholine hydrolysis. Presumably, this is also true for the hydrolysis of other drugs containing ester linkages.

Drug Metabolism

Drug metabolism, characterized by the conversion of lipid soluble drugs to more water soluble and pharmacologically less active substances, is under the control of microsomal enzymes, which are present in the smooth endoplasmic reticulum of hepatocytes. Chronic liver disease may interfere with metabolism of drugs by virtue of decreased numbers of enzyme-containing hepatocytes or decreased hepatic blood flow, or both, that typically accompanies cirrhosis of the liver. Indeed, prolonged elimination half-times for morphine, alfentanil, diazepam, lidocaine, pancuronium, and, to a lesser extent, vecuronium have been demonstrated in patients with cirrhosis of the liver (Fig. 20-2).[3] Repeated injections of these drugs would be likely to produce cumulative effects in patients with severe liver disease.

It is conceivable that accelerated drug metabolism could accompany cirrhosis of the liver. For example, in the presence of decreased numbers of hepatocytes, the amount of drug presented to each cell is increased. This may stimulate microsomal enzyme activity (enzyme induction). Enzyme induction may also be a response to chronic drug therapy or alcohol abuse. In this regard, it is a clinical impression that chronic alcohol abuse is associated with the development of cross-tolerance to other depressant drugs. Despite this impression, there is evidence that chronic alcohol abuse does not alter dose requirements for thiopental (Fig. 20-3).[4]

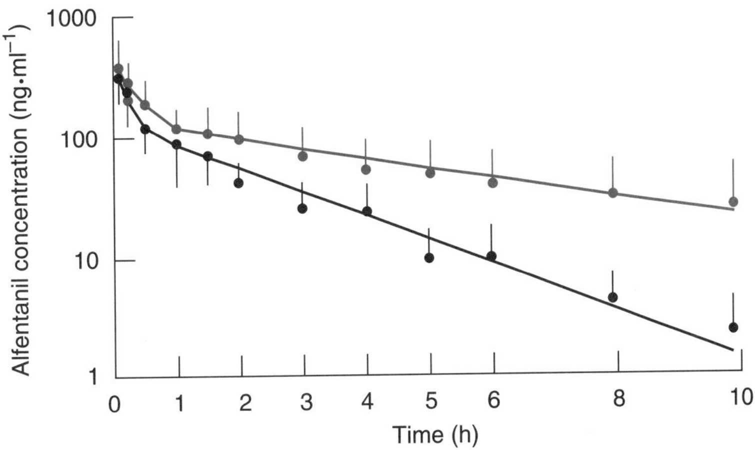

Figure 20-2. Clearance of alfentanil from the plasma is delayed in patients with cirrhosis of the liver (red line) compared with normal control patients (black line). Mean ± SD. (From Ferrier et al.,[3] with permission.)

Bilirubin Formation and Excretion

Bilirubin is produced in the reticuloendothelial system from the breakdown of hemoglobin. This bilirubin is bound to albumin for transport to the liver. Because protein-bound bilirubin (unconjugated) is not water soluble, urinary excretion is minimal. Conjugation of bilirubin with glucuronic acid in the liver renders bilirubin water soluble. This conjugation is under the control of the enzyme glucuronyl transferase, which is susceptible to enzyme induction. A small amount of conjugated bilirubin

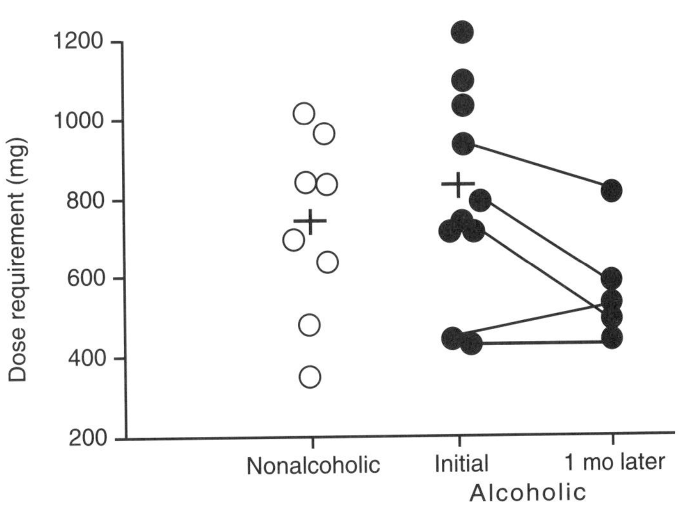

Figure 20-3. The average dose of thiopental (continuous infusion of 100 mg·min⁻¹ IV) needed to produce a brief period of isoelectric activity on the electroencephalogram is not different in nonalcoholic and alcoholic patients. (From Swerdlow et al.,[4] with permission.)

enters the circulation and undergoes renal excretion. The remainder is excreted into the biliary canaliculi and eventually into the small intestine.

HEPATIC BLOOD FLOW

The liver is unique in that it receives a dual afferent blood supply equivalent to about 25% of the cardiac output (Fig. 20-4). Most hepatic blood flow (70%) is via the portal vein, and the remainder is derived from the hepatic artery. Oxygen delivery to the liver may be marginal because most of the blood flow is with desaturated hemoglobin delivered via the portal vein.

Determinants of Hepatic Blood Flow

Hepatic blood flow is determined by perfusion pressure (mean arterial or portal vein pressure minus hepatic vein pressure) and splanchnic vascular resistance. The splanchnic vessels are innervated by vasoconstrictor nerve fibers from the sympathetic nervous system. Splanchnic nerve stimulation, as produced by arterial hypoxemia, hypercarbia, or increased circulating concentrations of catecholamines, results in increased splanchnic vascular resistance and decreased hepatic blood flow. The hepatic circulation is also supplied with beta receptors, and blockade of these receptors as produced by propranolol is associated with decreases in hepatic blood flow. Positive pressure ventilation of the lungs or congestive heart failure can decrease hepatic blood flow, presumably by increasing central venous pressure (hepatic vein pressure) and thus decreasing hepatic perfusion pressure. Cirrhosis of the liver associated with increased resistance to blood flow through the liver is predictably accompanied by decreases in hepatic blood flow (see the section *Cirrhosis of the Liver*). Portal vein blood flow parallels cardiac output emphasizing that drug-induced decreases in blood pressure or myocardial contractility, or both, as may occur during anesthesia, are likely to be associated with similar decreases in hepatic blood flow. Autoregulation of hepatic blood flow is limited, being characterized by increases in hepatic artery blood flow in an attempt to offset decreases in portal vein blood flow (Fig. 20-5).[5]

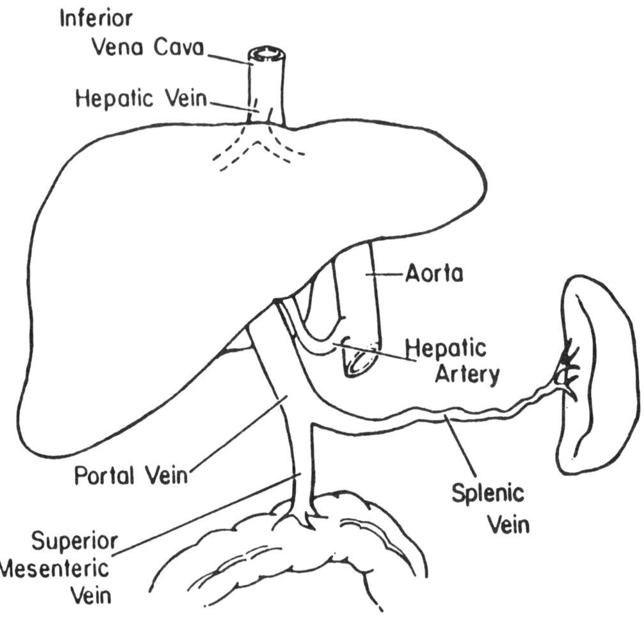

Figure 20-4. Schematic depiction of the dual afferent blood supply to the liver provided by the portal vein and hepatic artery. About 70% of hepatic blood flow is via the portal vein with the remainder via the hepatic artery. Total hepatic blood flow is directly proportional to perfusion pressure across the liver and inversely related to splanchnic vascular resistance. Cirrhosis of the liver increases resistance to blood flow through the portal vein and decreases hepatic blood flow.

Impact of Anesthetic Drugs on Hepatic Blood Flow

Inhaled anesthetics, as well as regional anesthesia, typically decrease hepatic blood flow 20% to 30% in the absence of surgical stimulation. These changes reflect drug- or technique-induced effects on perfusion pressure or splanchnic vascular resistance, or both. For example, decreases in hepatic blood flow associated with volatile anesthetics as well as regional anesthesia (T5 sensory level) are most likely due to decreased perfusion pressure. Isoflurane administered to animals is less likely to decrease hepatic blood flow than is halothane, thus better maintaining hepatocyte oxygen delivery (Fig. 20-5).[5] This reflects better maintenance of autoregulation of hepatic blood flow (increased hepatic artery blood flow offsets decreases in portal vein blood flow) during administration of isoflurane as compared with halothane (Fig. 20-5).[5] Selective hepatic artery constriction due to volatile anesthetics has been observed in occasional patients without liver disease. The mechanism and clinical significance of this selective hepatic artery constriction are not known.

Impact of Surgical Stimulation on Hepatic Blood Flow

Surgical stimulation and the nearness of the operative site to the liver are important determinants of the magnitude of decrease in hepatic blood flow during general anesthesia. For example, the greatest decreases in hepatic blood flow occur when the operative site is near the liver, as occurs during a cholecystectomy.

LIVER FUNCTION TESTS

Liver function tests are used to detect the presence of liver disease preoperatively and to establish the diagnosis when postoperative liver dysfunction occurs. It is important to remember that liver function tests are rarely specific. Furthermore, the large reserve of the liver means that considerable hepatic damage can be present before liver function tests are altered. Indeed, cirrhosis of the liver may produce little alteration in liver function, and only when some additional insult, such as anesthesia and surgery, produces further deterioration does the underlying liver disease become obvious. It is likely that inadequate hepatocyte oxygenation (oxygen supply relative to demand) during anesthesia and surgery is the principal mechanism responsible for postoperative liver dysfunction.

Postoperatively, the magnitude of liver dysfunction, as reflected by liver function tests, is exaggerated by operations near the liver (Fig. 20-6).[6] The specific anesthetic drug, however, does not influence

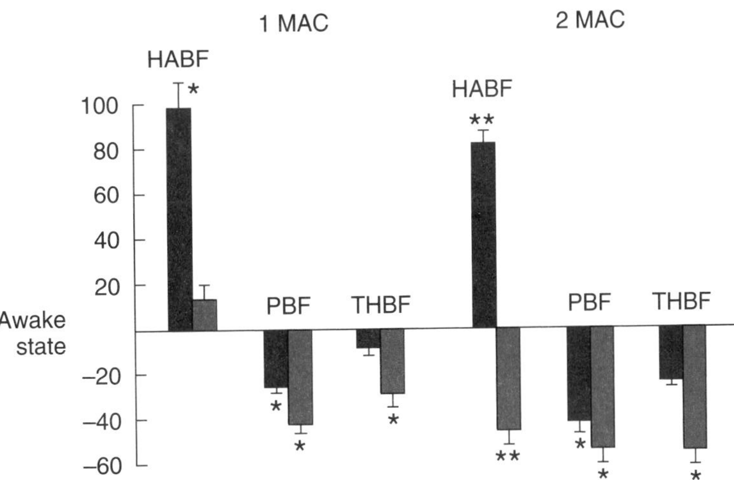

Figure 20-5. Hepatic artery blood flow (HABF), portal vein blood flow (PBF), and total hepatic blood flow (THBF) were measured in dogs (mean ± SE) as the percentage of change from awake values. HABF was increased during 1 MAC and 2 MAC isoflurane (black bars), and PBF was decreased by both drugs at each dose. THBF and, presumably hepatocyte oxygen delivery, was better maintained during administration of isoflurane (black bars) than halothane (red bars). **P* <0.05 vs. awake; ***P* <0.05 isoflurane vs. halothane. (From Gelman et al.,[5] with permission.)

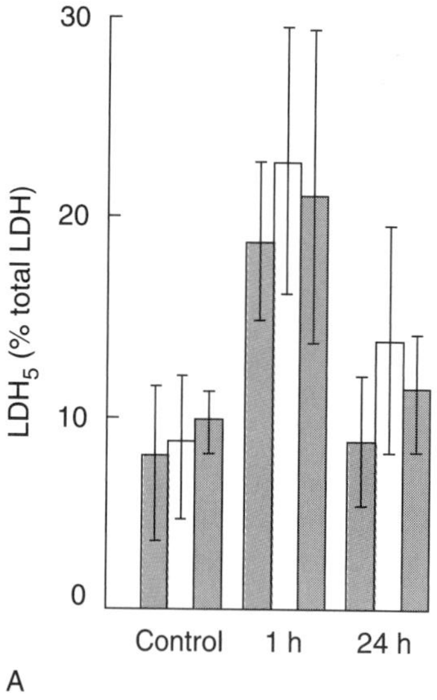

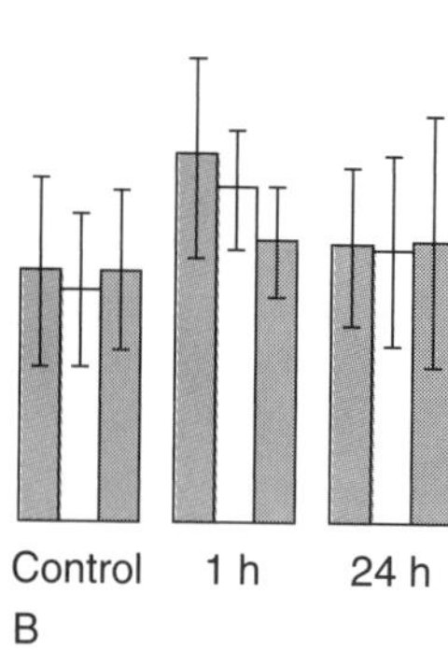

Figure 20-6. The magnitude of increase in the isoenzyme fraction of lactate dehydrogenase (LDH_5) is determined by the nearness of the operation to the liver and not the drugs used for maintenance of anesthesia. *(A)* Cholecystectomy. *(B)* Hysterectomy. Red bars, halothane-nitrous oxide; white bars, enflurane-nitrous oxide; gray bars, fentanyl-nitrous oxide. (From Viegas and Stoelting,[6] with permission.)

the magnitude of postoperative liver dysfunction as reflected by liver function tests. It is conceivable that cirrhosis of the liver could make hepatocytes more vulnerable to damage from decreases in blood flow owing to the effects of drugs or mechanical effects related to the site of surgery. Indeed, postoperative liver dysfunction, as reflected by changes in liver function tests, is greater in the presence of co-existing liver disease (Fig. 20-7).[7]

Commonly measured liver function tests include the serum concentrations of albumin, bilirubin, aminotransferase enzymes, and alkaline phosphatase and determination of the prothrombin time (Table 20-1). On the basis of these tests, postoperative liver dysfunction can be categorized as prehepatic, intrahepatic, and posthepatic (Table 20-2).

Prehepatic Dysfunction

Prehepatic dysfunction as a cause of postoperative jaundice most likely reflects delivery of bilirubin overloads to patients. Causes of hyperbilirubinemia include hemolysis, hematoma reabsorption, or whole blood administration. Hemolysis is often accompanied by decreases in the hematocrit or increases in the reticulocyte count. A 500-ml transfusion of fresh whole blood contains 250 mg of bilirubin. The bilirubin load increases as the age of transfused blood increases. Patients with normal hepatic function can receive large amounts of blood without any appreciable increase in serum bilirubin concentrations. This response can be different in patients with co-existing liver disease.

Overt jaundice is usually present when serum bilirubin concentrations are higher than 3 $mg \cdot dl^{-1}$. The unconjugated fraction of bilirubin is increased more than the conjugated fraction when prehepatic dysfunction is present.

Intrahepatic Dysfunction

Intrahepatic dysfunction reflects direct hepatocellular damage due to toxic effects of drugs, sepsis, arterial hypoxemia, congestive heart failure, or viruses. This form of postoperative dysfunction is recognized by hyperbilirubinemia and marked increases in serum aminotransferase concentrations. Although intrahepatic dysfunction occasionally causes accumulation of unconjugated bilirubin owing to impaired hepatic uptake or conjugation, accumulation of conjugated bilirubin is more common, reflecting impaired excretion of bilirubin conjugates into bile. Hepatocytes contain large amounts of aminotransferase enzymes that spill into the cir-

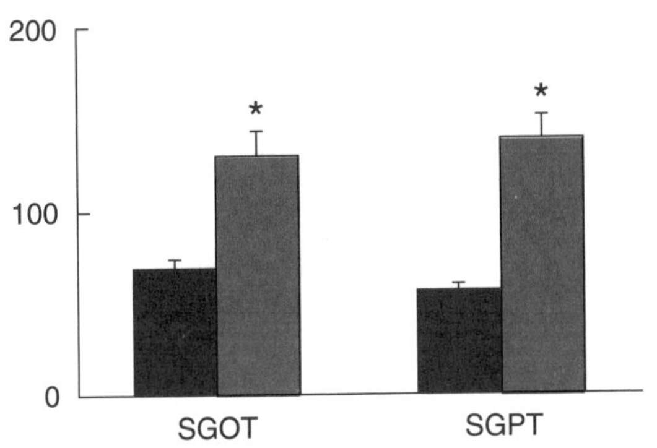

Figure 20-7. Liver aminotransferase enzymes (SGOT and SGPT) increase more in cirrhotic rats (red bars) than noncirrhotic rats (black bars) following exposure to 1.5% halothane in 50% oxygen for 3 hours. *P <0.05 compared with noncirrhotic rats. (From Baden et al.,[7] with permission.)

Table 20-1. Liver Function Tests

Test	Normal Values[a]
Albumin	3.5–5.5 g·dl^{-1}
Bilirubin	0.3–1.1 mg·dl^{-1}
Unconjugated bilirubin (indirect-reacting)	0.2–0.7 mg·dl^{-1}
Conjugated bilirubin (direct-reacting)	0.1–0.4 mg·dl^{-1}
Asparate aminotransferase (formerly serum glutamic oxaloacetic transaminase)	10–40 units·ml^{-1}
Alanine aminotransferase (formerly serum glutamic pyruvic transaminase)	5–35 units·ml^{-1}
Alkaline phosphatase	10–30 units·ml^{-1}
Prothrombin time	12–14 s

[a]Normal values for each individual laboratory should be considered when interpreting liver function tests.

culation when hepatocytes are acutely damaged. Other tissues, however, such as the heart, lungs, and skeletal muscles, also contain aminotransferase enzymes. Indeed, postoperative increases in the serum aminotransferase concentrations may reflect skeletal muscle damage from intramuscular injections given preoperatively or damage to skeletal muscles during surgery. Nevertheless, marked increases of the serum aminotransferase enzyme concentrations to three times normal or greater in the postoperative period should suggest acute hepatocellular damage. Nonspecific liver inflammatory diseases (hepatitis) are likely to be associated with increases in the serum alanine aminotransferase concentration, emphasizing the usefulness of this test in monitoring potential blood donors.

Table 20-2. Classification and Causes of Postoperative Liver Dysfunction

	Prehepatic	Intrahepatic	Posthepatic
Bilirubin	Increased (unconjugated fraction)	Increased (conjugated fraction)	Increased (conjugated fraction)
Aminotransferase enzymes	No change	Markedly increased	Normal to slightly increased
Alkaline phosphatase	No change	No change to slightly increased	Markedly increased
Prothrombin time	No change	Prolonged	No change to prolonged
Albumin	No change	Decreased	No change to decreased
Causes	Hemolysis Hematoma reabsorption Bilirubin overload from whole blood	Viruses Drugs Sepsis Arterial hypoxemia Congestive heart failure Cirrhosis	Stones Cancer Sepsis

Posthepatic Dysfunction

Posthepatic dysfunction reflects bile duct obstruction and is characterized by hyperbilirubinemia (predominately the conjugated fraction) and increased serum concentrations of alkaline phosphatase. Alkaline phosphatase is present in bile duct cells such that even slight degrees of biliary obstruction are manifested by threefold or greater increases of the serum concentrations of this enzyme. It must be remembered, however, that there are also extrahepatic stores of alkaline phosphatase, particularly in skeletal muscles.

Benign postoperative intrahepatic cholestasis may occur postoperatively, especially for surgery performed in elderly patients and complicated by hypotension, arterial hypoxemia, and massive blood transfusion. Jaundice associated with increased serum concentrations of conjugated bilirubin is typically present within 48 hours postoperatively and may persist for 14 to 28 days in these patients.

DRUG-INDUCED HEPATITIS

A variety of drugs (antibiotics, antihypertensives, anticonvulsants, analgesics, tranquilizers, anesthetics) are occasionally associated with hepatic dysfunction that may be indistinguishable histologically from viral hepatitis.

Halothane

Halothane is speculated to produce two types of hepatotoxicity. The first is a mild self-limited postoperative hepatotoxicity that is characterized by transient increases in the serum aminotransferase concentrations. It is likely that these changes are due to a nonspecific drug effect owing to drug-induced changes in hepatic blood flow that impair hepatocyte oxygenation. A less frequent and more severe form of hepatotoxicity (halothane hepatitis) occurs in 1 in 22,000 to 1 in 35,000 administrations of halothane and may lead to fulminant hepatic necrosis. This form of hepatic dysfunction is most likely an immune-mediated hepatotoxicity. Clinical manifestations that suggest an immune-mediated response include eosinophilia, fever, rash, arthralgia, and prior exposure to halothane. In susceptible patients, a reactive oxidative trifluoracetyl halide metabolite may acetylate liver proteins (self becomes nonself), resulting in the formation of neoantigens that stimulate the production of antibodies.[8] It is presumed that re-exposure to halothane results in an antigen-antibody interaction, leading to liver injury that is diagnosed clinically as halothane hepatitis. In the absence of documentation that specific antibodies exist in the patient's plasma, the diagnosis of halothane hepatitis is based on exclusion of other possible causes of hepatic dysfunction (Table 20-2). Halothane should not be administered to patients who have experienced postoperative hepatic dysfunction for unknown reasons after previous operations that included administration of halothane. Pediatric patients seem less likely than adults to develop halothane hepatitis, even with short intervals between exposures to halothane.

Other Volatile Anesthetics

Mild self-limited postoperative hepatic dysfunction that is associated with enflurane or isoflurane most likely reflects a nonspecific drug effect owing to drug-induced changes in hepatic blood flow that impair hepatocyte oxygenation. Nevertheless, like halothane, these fluorinated anesthetics may produce the same oxidative trifluoroacetyl halide metabolite that creates liver neoantigens in susceptible patients. Indeed, cross-sensitivity has been demonstrated to exist between enflurane and halothane in patients previously experiencing halothane hepatitis.[9] Considering the magnitude of metabolism of enflurane and isoflurane, it is predictable that the incidence of anesthetic-induced hepatitis owing to an immune-mediated mechanism would be greatest with halothane, intermediate with enflurane, and lowest with isoflurane. Desflurane undergoes less oxidative metabolism than isoflurane, and the likelihood of an immune-mediated hepatitis after administration of this drug seems remote.

CIRRHOSIS OF THE LIVER

Cirrhosis of the liver is a chronic disease process that destroys the hepatic parenchyma and subsequently replaces it with collagen. Excessive use of alcohol is the most frequent cause of cirrhosis. Cirrhosis is associated with decreases in the numbers of hepatocytes, leading to an impairment of all the physiologic functions of the liver (see the section *Physiologic Functions of the Liver*). Another important change associated with cirrhosis is a decrease in hepatic blood flow, owing to increased resistance to blood flow through the portal vein. As a result of this increased resistance, the proportion of hepatic blood flow delivered via the portal vein is decreased and the contribution to total hepatic blood flow from the hepatic artery is increased. Therefore, decreases in systemic perfusion pressure or arterial oxygenation during anesthesia and surgery are more likely to jeopardize the adequacy of hepatic blood flow and delivery of oxygen to the liver in patients with cirrhosis as compared with normal patients.

Portal Vein Hypertension

On physical examination, the most striking finding related to portal vein hypertension owing to cirrhosis of the liver is hepatomegaly with or without splenomegaly and ascites. Ascites reflects decreased plasma oncotic pressure secondary to low serum albumin concentrations, increased resistance to blood flow through the portal vein, and increased secretion of antidiuretic hormone. Despite the loss of skeletal muscle mass, body weight is often maintained owing to accumulation of ascitic fluid.

Gastroesophageal varices are predictable complications of portal vein hypertension. Varices are massively dilated submucosal veins that develop to allow splanchnic venous blood to bypass the liver and enter the azygous and hemiazygous thoracic veins. Chronic bleeding from these varices is reflected by moderate decreases in the hematocrit. Hemorrhage may be severe, requiring massive blood replacement, balloon tamponade, or sclerotherapy. Portasystemic shunts represent a surgical treatment for portal hypertension.

Extrahepatic Complications of Cirrhosis

A hyperdynamic circulation characterized by an increased cardiac output is often present in patients with cirrhosis. This increased cardiac output has been attributed to vasodilating substances such as glucagon, decreased viscosity of blood secondary to anemia, and arteriovenous communications, especially in the lungs. In contrast to developing a hyperdynamic circulation, patients with alcoholic cirrhosis may develop congestive heart failure due to cardiomyopathy. Megaloblastic anemia is frequent and is probably due to antagonism of folate by alcohol rather than to a dietary deficiency.

Arterial hypoxemia is a common finding in patients with cirrhosis of the liver. Indeed, many of these patients have chronic obstructive pulmonary disease associated with cigarette smoking. Furthermore, right-to-left intrapulmonary shunts may develop in the presence of portal vein hypertension, leading to arterial hypoxemia. Ascitic fluid may impair movement of the diaphragm, contributing to maldistribution of ventilation to perfusion. Arterial hypoxemia may be due to pneumonia, which is common in alcoholic patients. Alcohol ingestion suppresses immune defense mechanisms, rendering alcoholic patients vulnerable to bacterial and viral infections, tuberculosis, and development of cancer (especially hepatoma). In this regard, the individual using alcohol in excess should be viewed as being immunocompromised. The vulnerability to pneumonia may reflect the ability of alcohol to inhibit phagocytic activity normally present in the lungs. Indeed, most lung abscesses are found in chronic alcoholic patients. Spontaneous bacterial peritonitis develops in nearly 10% of patients with alcoholic liver disease and ascites, perhaps reflecting bacteria that enter the portal venous system via portasystemic collaterals and thus bypassing the major reticuloendothelial system in the liver.

Cirrhosis of the liver is associated with a decrease in renal blood flow and glomerular filtration rate. Hypoglycemia is a constant threat in alcoholic patients. The incidence of gallstones is increased, presumably reflecting an increased bilirubin load due to hemolysis of erythrocytes in the spleen. Peptic ulcer disease is twice as common in patients with cirrhosis of the liver. Hepatic encephalopathy, presumably due to the systemic accumulation of nitrogenous waste products, is evidenced by asterixis (flapping motion of the hands caused by intermittent loss of extensor muscle tone) and mental obtundation. The development of hepatic encephalopathy is associated with a high mortality rate.

Management of Anesthesia in the Sober Alcoholic Patient

It is estimated that 5% to 10% of patients with cirrhosis of the liver undergo surgery in the last 2 years of their lives. Postoperative morbidity is increased, especially with respect to bleeding, sepsis, and deterioration of hepatic function after surgery (Table 20-3).[10]

Table 20-3. Surgical Risk Based on Preoperative Evaluation of Liver Function

	Minimal	Modest	Marked
Bilirubin ($mg \cdot dl^{-1}$)	<2	2–3	>3
Albumin ($g \cdot dl^{-1}$)	>3.5	3–3.5	<3
Prothrombin time prolongation (s)	1–4	4–6	>6
Encephalopathy	None	Moderate	Severe
Nutrition	Excellent	Good	Poor
Ascites	None	Moderate	Marked

(Data from Strunin.[10])

Coagulation status should be evaluated preoperatively and parenteral vitamin K administered if the prothrombin time is prolonged. Failure of parenteral vitamin K to improve synthesis of prothrombin suggests the presence of severe hepatocellular disease. Conversely, impaired prothrombin production due to biliary obstruction and absence of bile salts to facilitate gastrointestinal absorption of vitamin K are promptly restored by parenteral vitamin K therapy. It is important to remember that hepatic blood flow is predictably decreased in patients with cirrhosis of the liver, and any further decrease due to anesthetic-induced depression of cardiac output or blood pressure could jeopardize hepatocyte oxygenation.

There is evidence that chronic alcohol abuse increases anesthetic requirements for volatile anesthetics (Fig. 20-8).[11] The most likely explanation for this increase is a cross-tolerance among depressant drugs. Accelerated metabolism of drugs in the presence of alcohol-induced microsomal enzyme stimulation might alter the amount of inhaled anesthetic needed to achieve a given brain partial pressure but would not alter the partial pressures required to produce anesthesia. Surprisingly, thiopental dose requirements have not been shown to be increased in the sober alcoholic patient (Fig. 20-3).[4] In contrast to resistance to depressant drugs, alcohol-induced cardiomyopathy could make these patients unusually sensitive to the cardiac depressant effects of volatile anesthetics. There may be decreased responsiveness to catecholamines, manifesting as an impaired tolerance to blood loss. Likewise, decreased protein binding of drugs in the presence of decreased serum albumin concentrations would increase the pharmacologically active fractions of injected drugs available to act at peripheral receptors (Fig. 20-1).[2] Severely jaundiced patients (total serum bilirubin concentrations higher than 8 $mg \cdot dl^{-1}$) are more likely to develop acute renal failure and sepsis postoperatively, emphasizing the possible value of establishing a diuresis with mannitol preoperatively and initiating antibiotic therapy.

The optimal anesthetic drug choice or technique in the presence of liver disease is not known. Among the volatile anesthetics, isoflurane may be associated with the best maintenance of hepatic blood flow and thus hepatocyte oxygenation (Fig. 20-5).[5] This may be more important in the chronic alcoholic patient, remembering that a constant feature of chronic liver disease is decreased hepatic blood flow owing to increased resistance to blood flow through the portal vein. As a result, hepatic blood flow and hepatocyte oxygenation are more dependent on hepatic artery blood flow than in normal patients. It is probably prudent to limit the dose of isoflurane (limit decrease in blood pressure to about 20% of awake values) by combining the volatile drug with nitrous oxide or an opioid. Injected anesthetics may serve as valuable adjuncts to nitrous oxide with or without volatile anesthetics, but it must be appreciated that cumulative drug effects are likely if liver disease is severe enough to slow metabolism. Regardless of the drugs selected for anesthesia, postoperative liver dysfunction is likely to be exaggerated in patients with chronic liver disease, presumably owing to detrimental nonspecific effects of anesthetic drugs on hepatic blood flow and subsequent hepatocyte oxygenation. Regional anesthesia is useful in patients with advanced liver disease assuming coagulation status is acceptable. Alcohol abuse may render peripheral nerves more vulnerable to ischemia should surgical positioning result in compression of these nerves despite padding of pressure points.

The role of the liver in the clearance of muscle relaxants must be considered when selecting these drugs for administration to patients with cirrhosis of the liver. Succinylcholine and mivacurium are acceptable muscle relaxants, but the dose should be adjusted if liver disease is sufficiently advanced to decrease cholinesterase activity. Hepatic dysfunction does not influence the clearance of atracurium, and the elimination half-time of vecuronium is unlikely to be prolonged unless doses higher than 0.1 $mg \cdot kg^{-1}$ are administered, making these drugs attractive selections for patients with cirrhosis. Resistance to the neuromuscular blocking effects of

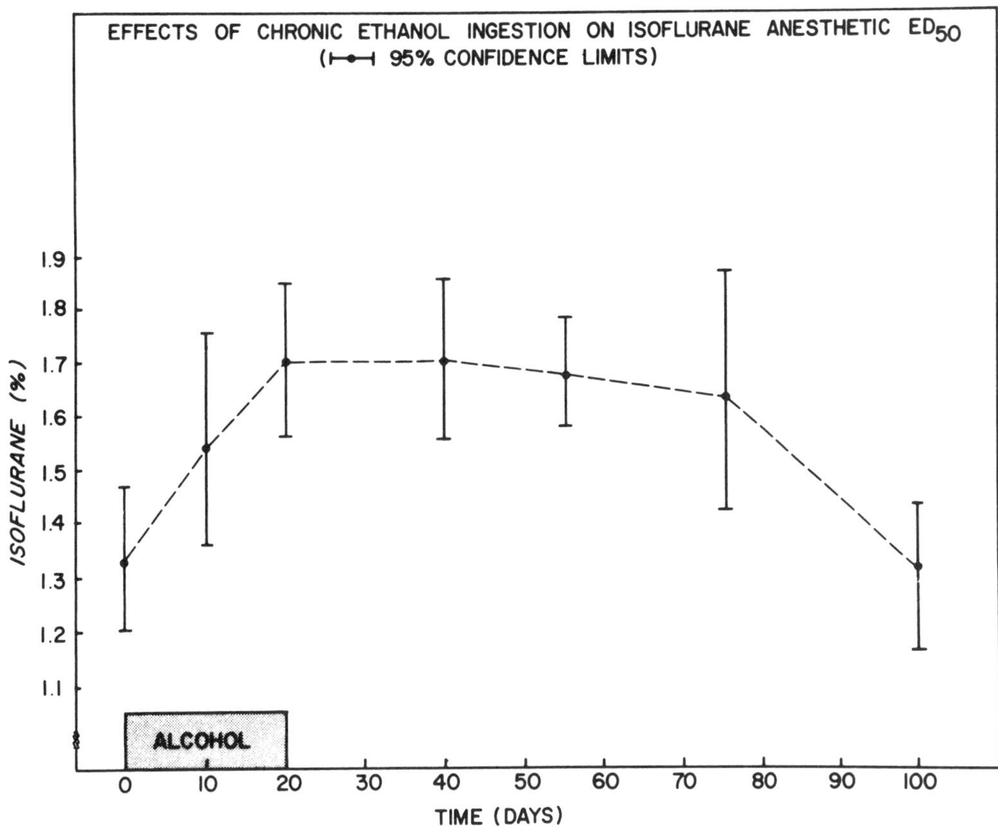

Figure 20-8. The effect of chronic alcohol ingestion on the anesthetic requirement for isoflurane in mice was determined during and after continuous exposure to alcohol. Isoflurane anesthetic requirements on days 20, 40, 55, and 75 were significantly ($P < 0.05$) increased above the control value. (From Johnstone et al.,[11] with permission.)

long-acting nondepolarizing muscle relaxants, such as pancuronium, may reflect alcohol-induced changes in the distribution volume of this drug. Indeed, the distribution volume of pancuronium is increased and the plasma clearance decreased in patients with alcoholic cirrhosis as compared with normal patients.[12] From these observations, the initial dose of pancuronium necessary to produce skeletal muscle relaxation in alcoholic patients might be increased, reflecting dilution of the drug in a larger distribution volume. Conversely, the duration of paralysis might be prolonged owing to slowed plasma clearance.

Monitoring of intraoperative blood gases, pH, and urine output and provision of exogenous glucose are important principles. Arterial hypoxemia may be exaggerated intraoperatively if drugs used for anesthesia produce vasodilation of co-existing portasystemic and intrapulmonary shunts. When blood replacement is necessary, it is logical to administer the stored blood as slowly as possible to compensate for decreased clearance of citrate by the diseased liver. A practical point is the avoidance of unnecessary esophageal instrumentation (stethoscope, gastric tube) in patients with known esophageal varices.

Alcohol Withdrawal Syndrome

Manifestations of a severe alcohol withdrawal syndrome (delerium tremens) usually appear 48 to 72 hours after cessation of drinking. This syndrome represents a medical emergency, as mortality may approach 15%. Postoperatively, patients will manifest tremulousness and hallucinations. There is increased activity of the sympathetic nervous system with catecholamine release, leading to diaphoresis, hyperpyrexia, tachycardia, and hypertension. In some patients grand mal seizures may be the first indication of the alcohol withdrawal syndrome. When seizures occur, hypoglycemia should be ruled out as a possible cause. Treatment of delirium tremens must be aggressive with administration of diazepam (5 to 10 mg IV every 5 minutes until the patient becomes sedated but remains awake) and a beta antagonist (propranolol or esmolol until the heart rate is lower than 100 beats·min^{-1}) to suppress manifestations of sympathetic nervous system hyperactivity. Protection of the upper airway with a cuffed tracheal tube may be necessary. Correction of fluid, electrolyte (magnesium, potassium), and metabolic (thiamin) derangements is important. Lidocaine is usually effective when cardiac dysrhythmias occur despite correction of electrolyte abnormalities. Despite aggressive treatment, mortality from delirium tremens is about 10%, principally because of hypotension, cardiac dysrhythmias, or seizures.

Management of Anesthesia in the Intoxicated Alcoholic Patient

In contrast to the chronic but sober alcoholic, acutely intoxicated patients require less anesthesia because there is an additive depressant effect between alcohol and anesthetics. Acutely intoxicated patients may withstand stress and blood loss poorly. Intoxicated patients are more vulnerable to regurgitation of gastric contents, since alcohol slows gastric emptying and decreases the tone of the lower esophageal sphincter. Surgical bleeding may reflect alcohol-induced interference with platelet aggregation.

DISEASE OF THE BILIARY TRACT

Gallstones are reported to be present in 10% of males and 20% of females between 55 and 65 years of age. Patients who experience repeated attacks of acute cholecystitis eventually develop a fibrotic gallbladder. Liver function tests are usually normal, but increased serum bilirubin or alkaline phosphatase concentrations suggest the presence of choledocholithiasis (common bile duct stone) or chronic cholangitis.

Management of Anesthesia

Management of anesthesia for cholecystectomy or common bile duct exploration, or both, is influenced by the effects of drugs used for anesthesia on intraluminal pressures in the biliary tract. Specifically, opioids (morphine, meperidine, fentanyl) can produce spasm of the choledochoduodenal sphincter, which increases common bile duct pressures (Fig. 20-9).[13] This spasm could impair passage of contrast media into the duodenum, erroneously suggesting the need for a sphincteroplasty or the presence of common bile duct stones. Nevertheless, opioids have been used in many instances without adverse effects, emphasizing that not all patients respond to opioids with choledochoduodenal sphincter spasm. Indeed, some believe that the incidence of opioid-induced sphincter spasm during cholecystectomy is so low (less than 3%) that the possibility of this response should not influence the use of opioids during anesthesia for this operation. The alternative to opioids for maintenance of anesthesia is the use of volatile anesthetics, although the possible presence of liver disease is often a concern when selecting volatile anesthetics for patients undergoing cholecystectomy. There is no evidence, however, that hepatic dysfunction after a cholecystectomy is

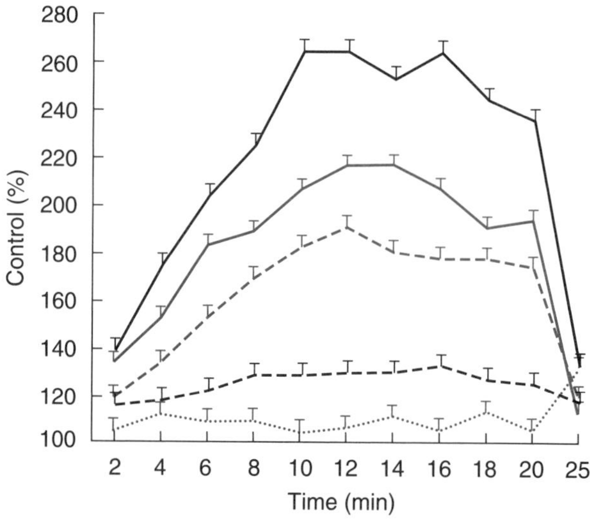

Figure 20-9. Administration of fentanyl (1.5 µg·kg^{-1} IV [solid black line]), morphine (0.15 mg·kg^{-1} IV [solid red line]), and meperidine (1 mg·kg^{-1} IV [dashed red line]) results in increased common bile duct pressures (percentage of control) in patients anesthetized with nitrous oxide-enflurane. Changes in common bile duct pressures after administration of butorphanol (0.03 mg·kg^{-1} IV [dashed black line]) are modest. Administration of naloxone (5 µg·kg^{-1} IV) 20 minutes after injection of the opioids results in prompt decreases in common bile duct pressures. Placebo, dotted red line. Mean ± SD. (From Radnay et al.,[13] with permission.)

different in patients anesthetized with nitrous oxide plus fentanyl, halothane, or enflurane (Fig. 20-6).[6]

Unique anesthetic considerations for laparoscopic cholecystectomy are similar to those for other laparoscopic procedures.[14] For example, insufflation of the abdominal cavity (pneumoperitoneum) with carbon dioxide introduced through a needle placed via a supraumbilical incision results in increased intra-abdominal pressure that may interfere with ventilation of the lungs and venous return. During laparoscopic cholecystectomy, the placement of the patient in the reverse Trendelenburg position favors movement of abdominal contents away from the operative site and may facilitate mechanical ventilation of the lungs. This position, however, may further interfere with venous return, emphasizing the need to maintain intravascular fluid volume. Monitoring of end-tidal carbon dioxide concentrations is useful in view of the unpredictable amounts of systemic absorption of carbon dioxide used to create the pneumoperitoneum. Intraoperative decompression of the stomach with a nasogastric or orogastric tube may decrease the risk of visceral puncture at the time of needle insertion for production of the pneumoperitoneum and subsequently improve laparoscopic visualization. Administration of nitrous oxide during laparoscopic cholecystectomy does not interfere with surgical working conditions by expanding the bowel gas volume.[15] Loss of hemostasis or injury to the hepatic artery or liver may require prompt intervention via a conventional laparotomy incision.

REFERENCES

1. Biebuyck JK. Effects of anesthetic agents on metabolic pathways: Fuel utilization and supply during anaesthesia. Br J Anaesth 1973;45:263–8.
2. Pandele G, Chaux F, Salvadori C, Farinott M, Duvaldestin P. Thiopental pharmacokinetics in patients with cirrhosis. Anesthesiology 1983;59:123–6.
3. Ferrier C, Marty J, Bouffard Y, Haberer JP, Levron JC, Duvaldestin P. Alfentanil pharmacokinetics in patients with cirrhosis. Anesthesiology 1985;62:480–4.
4. Swerdlow BN, Holley FO, Maitre PO, Stanski DR. Chronic alcohol intake does not change thiopental anesthetic requirement, pharmacokinetics, or pharmacodynamics. Anesthesiology 1990;72:455–61.
5. Gelman S, Fowler KC, Smith LR. Liver circulation and function during isoflurane and halothane anesthesia. Anesthesiology 1984;61:726–30.
6. Viegas OJ, Stoelting RK. LDH_5 changes after cholecystectomy or hysterectomy in patients receiving halothane, enflurane, or fentanyl. Anesthesiology 1979; 51:556–8.
7. Baden JM, Serra M, Fujinaga M, Mazze RI. Halothane metabolism in cirrhotic rats. Anesthesiology 1987; 67:600–4.
8. Hubbard AK, Roth TP, Gandolfi AJ, Brown BR, Webster NR, Nunn JF. Halothane hepatitis patients generate an antibody response toward a covalently bound metabolite of halothane. Anesthesiology 1988;68:791–6.
9. Christ DD, Kenna JG, Kammerer W, Satoh H, Pohl LR. Enflurane metabolism produces covalently bound liver adducts recognized by antibodies from patients with halothane hepatitis. Anesthesiology 1988;69:833–8.
10. Strunin L. Preoperative assessment of the patient with liver dysfunction. Br J Anaesth 1978;50:25–34.
11. Johnstone RE, Kulp RA, Smith TC. Effects of acute and chronic ethanol administration on isoflurane requirement in mice. Anesth Analg 1975;54:177–81.
12. Duvaldestin P, Agoston S, Henzel D, Kersten UW, Demonts JM. Pancuronium pharmacokinetics in patients with liver cirrhosis. Br J Anaesth 1978; 50:1131–6.
13. Radnay PA, Duncalf D, Novakovic M, Lesser ML. Common bile duct pressure changes after fentanyl, morphine, meperidine, butorphanol, and naloxone. Anesth Analg 1984;63:441–4.
14. Marco PA, Yeo CJ, Rock P. Anesthesia for the patient undergoing laparoscopic cholecystectomy. Anesthesiology 1990;73:1268–70.
15. Taylor E, Feinstein R, White PF, Soper N. Anesthesia for laparoscopic cholecystectomy. Is nitrous oxide contraindicated? Anesthesiology 1992;76:541–3.

21
Renal Disease

Essential physiologic functions of the kidneys include the (1) excretion of end products of metabolism (urea) with retention of nutrients (amino acids, glucose) and (2) control of electrolyte and hydrogen ion concentrations of body fluids. In addition to these physiologic functions, the kidneys secrete hormones (renin, erythropoietin) and metabolize hormones such as insulin. Therefore, impaired renal function is associated with characteristic changes (see the section *Changes Characteristic of Chronic Renal Disease*). It has been estimated that 5% of the adult American population have co-existing renal disease that could contribute to perioperative morbidity.[1] In addition to co-existing renal disease, the risk of acute renal failure is increased by certain events or patient characteristics independent of co-existing renal disease.

ANATOMY AND PHYSIOLOGY OF THE KIDNEY

The functional unit of the kidneys is the nephron (Fig. 21-1). Each kidney contains about 1.2 million nephrons, and this number does not change after birth. The two components of the nephron are the glomerulus and renal tubule. Physiologic function of the kidneys is dependent on renal blood flow, glomerular filtration rate (GFR), and responses evoked by nonrenal (parathormone and antidiuretic hormone [ADH]) and renal (renin and prostaglandins) humoral substances.

Renal Blood Flow

Renal blood flow is equivalent to about 20% of the cardiac output, even though the kidneys represent only 0.5% of total body weight. Approximately two-thirds of the renal blood flow is to the renal cortex. The impact, if any, of anesthetic drugs on distribution of blood flow between the renal cortex and medulla is not known. Renal blood flow and GFR remain constant at mean arterial pressures ranging from 60 to 150 mmHg. This ability to maintain renal blood flow constant despite changes in perfusion pressure is known as autoregulation. Autoregulation is achieved by adjustment of the afferent arteriolar tone and subsequent resistance imparted to blood flow. Autoregulation is important because it protects glomerular capillaries from large increases in arterial blood pressure during acute hypertensive episodes and maintains GFR and renal tubule function during modest decreases in blood pressure. Outside the range of mean arterial pressure associated with autoregulation, renal blood flow becomes pressure dependent.

Autoregulation does not preclude changes in renal blood flow due to other mechanisms. For example, renal blood flow is influenced by activity of the sympathetic nervous system and the release of renin. Indeed, the kidneys are richly innervated by the sympathetic nervous system (T4–L4). Sympathetic nervous system stimulation produces renal vascular vasoconstriction with marked decreases in renal

> **Increased Risk of Acute Renal Failure**
>
> Co-existing renal disease
> Prolonged renal hypoperfusion (hypovolemia, hypotension)
> High-risk surgery (abdominal aneurysm resection, cardiopulmonary bypass)
> Advanced age
> Congestive heart failure
> Extensive burns
> Sepsis and/or jaundice
> Treatment with prostaglandin inhibitors (?)

blood flow even if blood pressure is maintained in the range associated with autoregulation. Any decrease in renal blood flow will initiate release of renin, which can further decrease renal blood flow (see the section *Humoral Substances*).

Glomerular Filtration Rate

Hydrostatic pressure in the glomerular capillaries is about 50 mmHg. This pressure acts to force water and other low molecular weight substances such as electrolytes through the glomerular capillaries into Bowman's space (Fig. 21-1). The outward filtration force produced by hydrostatic pressure is opposed by the plasma oncotic pressure. Plasma oncotic pressure is about 25 mmHg at the afferent arteriole and with filtration increases to about 35 mmHg at the efferent arteriole. Despite the relatively low net fil-

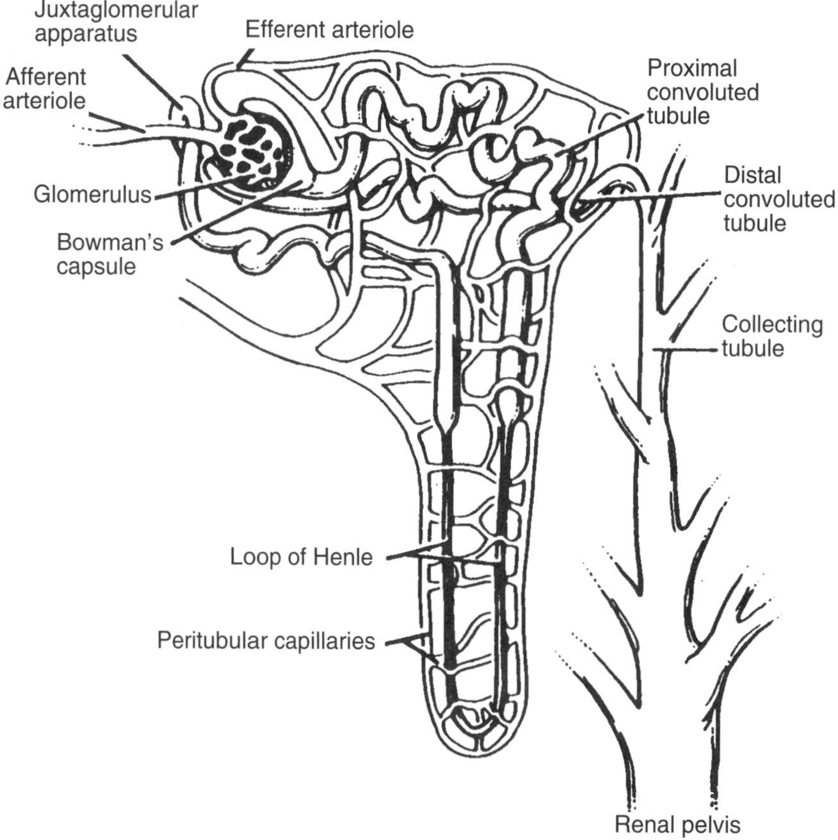

Figure 21-1. Anatomy of a nephron. The glomerulus is formed by the invagination of a tuft of capillaries into the dilated and blind end of the nephron known as Bowman's capsule. Hydrostatic pressure in these capillaries causes water and low molecular weight substances to filter through the glomerulus. Glomerular filtrate travels along the renal tubule (proximal convoluted tubule, loop of Henle, distal convoluted tubule), during which most of its water and various amounts of solutes are reabsorbed from the renal tubular lumen into peritubular capillaries. The remaining glomerular filtrate becomes urine.

tration pressure, the glomerular capillaries are able to filter plasma at a rate equivalent to about 125 ml·min^{-1}. GFR is reduced by decreased mean arterial pressure or decreased renal blood flow. Ultimately, about 90% of the fluid resulting from glomerular filtration is reabsorbed from renal tubules into peritubular capillaries and thus returned to the circulation (Fig. 21-1).

Humoral Substances

Renin is a proteolytic enzyme secreted by the juxtaglomerular apparatus of the kidneys in response to (1) sympathetic nervous system stimulation, (2) decreased renal perfusion pressure, and (3) decreases in the delivery of sodium to the distal convoluted tubules. Renin acts on an alpha-2 globulin in the plasma to form angiotensin I. Angiotensin I is then split by converting enzyme in the lungs to form angiotensin II. Angiotensin II is a potent vasoconstrictor and an important stimulus for the release of aldosterone from the adrenal cortex.

Prostaglandins are produced in the renal medulla and released in response to sympathetic nervous system stimulation and increased levels of angiotensin II. During periods of hemodynamic instability prostaglandins may modulate the vasoconstrictive actions of catecholamines. Drugs, such as aspirin, may attenuate this protective mechanism, thus allowing catecholamine-induced renal vascular vasoconstriction to persist and even increase.

TESTS USED FOR EVALUATION OF RENAL FUNCTION

Renal function can be evaluated preoperatively by laboratory tests that reflect GFR and renal tubular function. These tests are not sensitive measurements, and significant renal disease can exist (more than 50% of nephrons nonfunctional) despite normal laboratory values. Furthermore, trends are more useful than a single laboratory measurement for evaluating renal function.

Blood Urea Nitrogen

Blood urea nitrogen (BUN) concentrations (normal 10 to 20 mg·dl^{-1}) vary with the GFR. Nevertheless, the influence of dietary intake, co-existing illnesses, and intravascular fluid volume on BUN concentrations make this a potentially misleading test of renal function. For example, production of urea is increased by high-protein diets or gastrointestinal bleeding, resulting in increased BUN concentrations despite a normal GFR. Other causes of increased BUN concentrations despite a normal GFR include increased catabolism during febrile illnesses and dehydration. Increased BUN concentrations in the presence of dehydration most likely reflect increased urea absorption due to slow movement of fluid through the renal tubules. When slow movement of fluid through the renal tubules is responsible for increased BUN concentrations, the serum creatinine levels remain normal. BUN concentrations can remain normal in the presence of low-protein diets (hemodialysis patients) despite decreases in GFR. Despite these extraneous influences, BUN concentrations higher than 50 mg·dl^{-1} almost always reflect a decreased GFR.

Serum Creatinine

Serum creatinine concentrations are specific indicators of the GFR. In contrast to BUN concentrations, the serum creatinine levels are not influenced by protein metabolism or the rate of fluid flow through renal tubules. As a guide, a 50% increase in serum creatinine concentration reflects a similar decrease in the GFR. Creatinine is a product of skeletal muscle metabolism, and its release into the circulation is believed to be relatively constant. Serum creatinine concentrations are influenced by skeletal muscle mass in that normal levels (0.7 to 1.5 mg·dl^{-1}) tend to be higher in muscular males than less muscular females. Conversely, the maintenance of normal serum creatinine concentrations in elderly patients with known decreases in GFR reflects decreased cre-

Tests Used for Evaluation of Renal Function

- Glomerular filtration rate
  - Blood urea nitrogen
  - Serum creatinine
  - Creatinine clearance
  - Proteinuria
- Renal tubular function
  - Urine specific gravity
  - Urine osmolarity
  - Urine sodium

atinine production due to decreased skeletal muscle mass that accompanies aging. Indeed, mild increases in serum creatinine concentrations in elderly patients suggest significant renal disease. Likewise, in patients with chronic renal failure, serum creatinine concentrations may not accurately reflect the GFR because of decreased creatinine production in the presence of decreased skeletal muscle mass or nonrenal (gastrointestinal tract) excretion of creatinine. Serum creatinine concentrations may not be increased in the presence of acute renal failure, because at least 8 hours are required for serum creatinine concentrations to increase from normal levels to that suggestive of acute renal failure.

Creatinine Clearance

Creatinine clearance (normal 110 to 150 ml·min^{-1}) measures the ability of the glomeruli to excrete creatinine into the urine for a given serum creatinine concentration. This measurement does not depend on corrections for age or the presence of a steady state. As such, creatinine clearance is the most reliable measurement of the GFR. The major disadvantage of this test is the need for timed (2 hours is as acceptable as 24 hours) urine collections. Preoperatively, patients with creatinine clearances between 10 and 25 ml·min^{-1} must be considered at risk of developing prolonged or adverse responses to drugs, such as nondepolarizing muscle relaxants, that depend on renal excretion. In these patients, the doses of such drugs should be decreased and intravenous fluid and electrolyte replacement carefully monitored.

Proteinuria

Small amounts of protein are normally filtered through glomerular capillaries and then reabsorbed in the proximal convoluted tubules. Proteinuria (excretion of more than 150 mg·day^{-1} of protein) is most likely due to abnormally high filtration rather than impaired reabsorption by the renal tubules. Intermittent proteinuria occasionally occurs in healthy individuals when standing and disappears when supine. Other nonrenal causes of proteinuria include exercise, fever, and congestive heart failure. Severe proteinuria may result in hypoalbuminemia with associated decreases in plasma oncotic pressures and decreased protein binding of drugs.

Urine Concentrating Ability

The diagnosis of renal tubular dysfunction is established by demonstrating that the kidneys do not produce appropriately concentrated urine in the presence of a physiologic stimulus (vasopressin) for the release of ADH. In the absence of diuretic therapy or glycosuria, a urine specific gravity higher than 1.018 after an overnight fast, as precedes elective surgery, suggests that the ability of renal tubules to concentrate urine is adequate. Inability of the renal tubules to adequately concentrate urine may be due to (1) hypokalemia, (2) hypercalcemia, (3) excessive plasma inorganic fluoride concentrations (see the section *Effects of Anesthetics on Renal Function, Direct Nephrotoxicity*), (4) chronic pyelonephritis, or (5) treatment with diuretics or lithium.

Sodium Excretion

Urinary excretion of sodium that exceeds 40 mEq·L^{-1} reflects a decreased ability of the renal tubules to conserve sodium. Examples of sodium wasting by the renal tubules include (1) drug-induced diuresis (see the section *Pharmacology of Diuretics*), (2) adrenal insufficiency, and (3) hypoaldosteronism.

EFFECTS OF ANESTHETICS ON RENAL FUNCTION

Anesthetics can alter renal function by their effects on the systemic circulation and the sympathetic nervous system. In rare instances, drugs used for anesthesia may produce direct nephrotoxicity.

Systemic Circulation

Volatile anesthetics most likely depress renal function by producing dose-dependent decreases in blood pressure. The net effect is a decrease in renal blood flow, GFR, and urine output during anesthesia that is similar for all the volatile drugs (Fig. 21-2).[2] These changes are likely to be attenuated by preoperative hydration and administration of low concentrations of the anesthetic. Changes in renal function during barbiturate-opioid-nitrous oxide anesthesia are similar to those observed during administration of low concentrations of volatile anesthetics (Fig. 21-2).[2] Epidural or spinal anesthesia results in minimal changes in renal blood flow and GFR, assuming renal perfusion pressure is maintained. Anesthetic-induced depression of renal blood flow, GFR, and urine output is transient and usually clinically insignificant.

Decreased urine output during anesthesia suggests the release of ADH. However, serum concen-

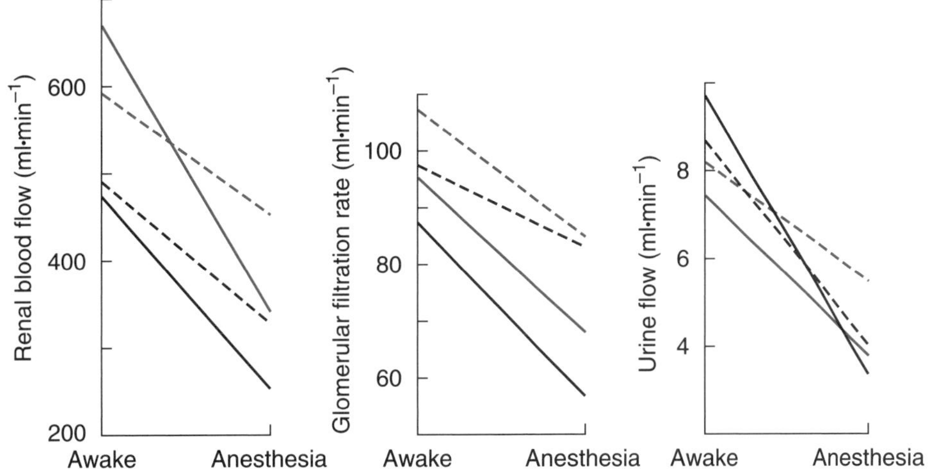

Figure 21-2. Anesthetics produce similar decreases in renal blood flow, glomerular filtration rate, and urine flow. Isoflurane, 1 MAC (solid black line); enflurane, 0.8 MAC (dashed red line); halothane, 1 MAC (solid red line); nitrous oxide-opioid (dashed black line). (From Eger,[2] with permission.)

trations of ADH are not increased during halothane or morphine anesthesia (Fig. 21-3).[3] Instead, painful stimulation associated with the onset of surgery produces significant increases in circulating levels of ADH. Hydration before the induction of anesthesia attenuates the increase in serum ADH concentrations produced by surgical stimulation. Atrial natriuretic factor antagonizes the release of ADH and renin and produces an increased urine output. Positive end-expiratory pressure alters atrial filling pressure and results in inhibition of the release of atrial natriuretic factor, which is consistent with the recognized antidiuretic effects that accompany this method of mechanical ventilation.[4] There is no evidence that anesthetics in the absence of surgical stimulation evoke the release of renin. Autoregulation of renal blood flow does not seem to be altered by inhaled anesthetics (Fig. 21-4).[5]

Sympathetic Nervous System

The renal vasculature is richly innervated by the sympathetic nervous system such that drug-induced changes in systemic vascular resistance can lead to alterations in renal blood flow and GFR. For example, ketamine is associated with decreased renal blood flow and GFR despite increases in cardiac output and mean arterial pressure. Presumably, these changes reflect constriction of renal vasculature by ketamine-induced increases in sympathetic nervous system activity. Conversely, volatile anesthetics that decrease sympathetic nervous system activity might decrease renal vascular resistance.

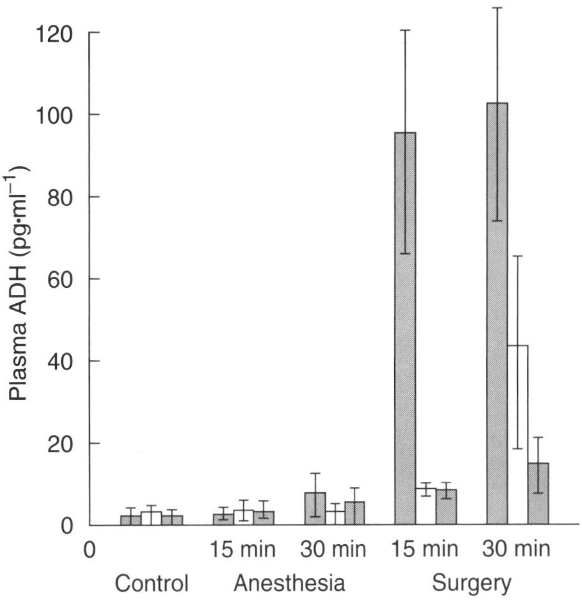

Figure 21-3. Plasma antidiuretic hormone (ADH) levels (mean ± SE) in adult patients are not altered from control measurements during anesthesia. Surgical stimulation increases ADH concentrations, particularly in patients receiving halothane. Red bars, halothane (0.5%); white bars, morphine (1 mg·kg^{-1}); gray bars, morphine (2 mg·kg^{-1}). (From Philbin and Coggins,[3] with permission.)

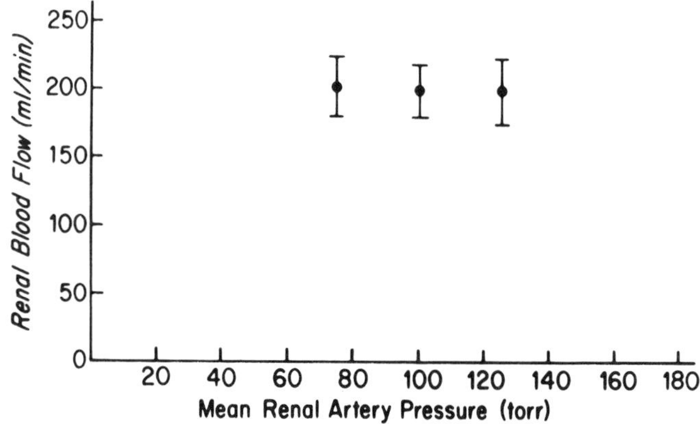

Figure 21-4. Halothane administered to dogs does not alter autoregulation, as evidenced by an unchanging renal blood flow despite changes in mean renal artery pressure. (From Bastron et al.,[5] with permission.)

Direct (Fluoride-Induced) Nephrotoxicity

High output renal failure (dehydration, hypernatremia) following prolonged exposures (longer than 2.5 MAC hours) to methoxyflurane reflects the extensive metabolism of this anesthetic to inorganic fluoride. Plasma inorganic fluoride concentrations that exceed 50 $\mu m \cdot L^{-1}$ may interfere with the ability of renal tubules to concentrate urine. The nephrotoxic potential of methoxyflurane has led to the almost total abandonment of the use of this drug to produce general anesthesia.

Enflurane and sevoflurane are less extensively metabolized to inorganic fluoride, and high output renal failure manifesting as an inability to concentrate urine is unlikely following general anesthesia with these drugs (Fig. 21-5).[2] Nevertheless, the administration of enflurane or sevoflurane to patients with known renal disease or undergoing operations likely to be associated with renal dysfunction is controversial. This controversy is based on the realization that elimination of inorganic fluoride depends on GFR. Therefore, it is likely that patients with decreased GFR will maintain increased circulating levels of inorganic fluoride for longer periods than normal patients. Fluoride-induced nephrotoxicity depends on the duration of exposure of the renal tubules to fluoride (area under the curve), as well as on the absolute increase in the plasma fluoride concentration. As a result, it is possible that patients with decreased GFR are at an increased risk in the presence of fluoride concentrations usually considered to be nontoxic (lower than 50 $\mu m \cdot L^{-1}$). Nevertheless, patients with co-existing renal disease do not manifest evidence of postoperative renal dysfunction following anesthesia that includes enflurane despite the presence of modest

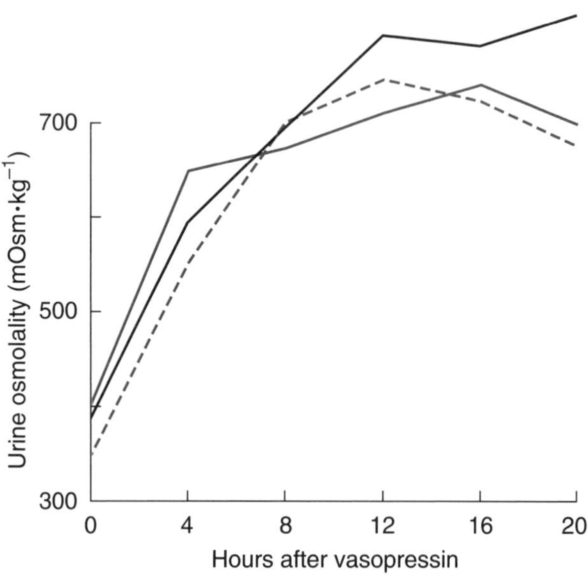

Figure 21-5. The ability to concentrate urine in response to subcutaneous vasopressin (2.5 units) is not altered following anesthesia with a volatile drug. Solid red line, halothane; solid black line, isoflurane; dashed red line, enflurane. (From Eger,[2] with permission.)

increases in the plasma inorganic fluoride concentration (Fig. 21-6).[6] Plasma inorganic fluoride concentrations do not change significantly following the administration of isoflurane, halothane, or desflurane.

CHRONIC RENAL DISEASE

Changes Characteristic of Chronic Renal Disease

Chronic renal disease is characterized by progressive decreases in the number of functioning nephrons leading to irreversible decreases in GFR (Table 21-1). Renal reserve is decreased, but patients remain asymptomatic when more than 40% of the nephrons continue to function. Renal insufficiency is present when only 10% to 40% of the nephrons are functioning. These patients are compensated, but there is no renal reserve, such that catabolic loads or toxic substances (antibiotics, potassium from hemolysis) can exacerbate renal insufficiency. Loss of more than 90% of functioning nephrons results in uremia (urine in the blood) and the need for dialysis.

Rational management of anesthesia in patients with chronic renal disease requires an understanding of the pathologic changes that accompany renal disease. Furthermore, the management of anesthesia is influenced by whether the renal disease is sufficient to require hemodialysis.

Changes Characteristic of Chronic Renal Disease

- Anemia
- Increased cardiac output
- Decreased platelet adhesiveness
- Hyperkalemia
- Unpredictable intravascular fluid volume
- Metabolic acidosis
- Systemic hypertension
- Pericardial effusion
- Decreased sympathetic nervous system activity

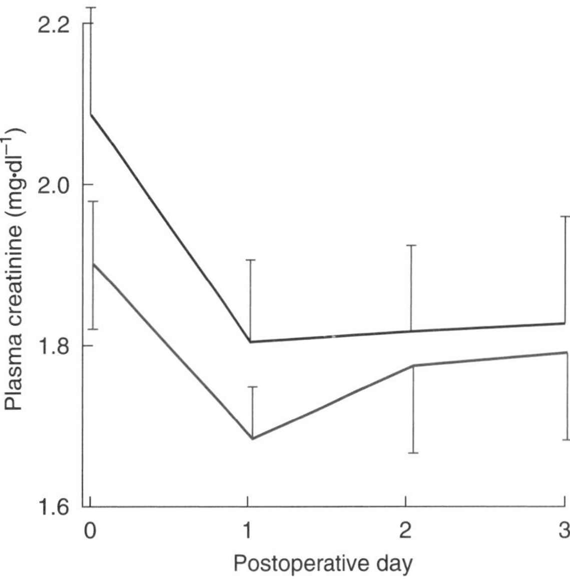

Figure 21-6. Plasma creatinine concentrations in patients with chronic renal disease decreased by similar amounts following anesthesia that included enflurane (black line) or halothane (red line). (Data from Mazze et al.[6])

Anemia

A hemoglobin concentration in the range of 5 to 8 g·dl^{-1} (hematocrit 15% to 25%) is a well-recognized complication of chronic renal failure. Decreased renal production of erythropoietin is responsible for the decreased production of erythrocytes. Administration of recombinant human erythropoietin can correct the anemia of end-stage chronic renal failure, thus improving the patient's ability to function and virtually eliminating the need for blood transfusions designed to increase the oxygen carrying capacity of the patient's blood. Erythropoietin is administered until a hematocrit of 30% to 33% is achieved. Correction of anemia results in striking improvement in the general well-being of these patients. A side effect of erythropoietin treatment is development of hypertension or exacerbation of coexisting hypertension. Erythropoietin treatment lowers the plasma concentration of histamine and may decrease the intensity of pruritus that is so often present in these patients.

Table 21-1. Stages of Chronic Renal Failure

	Glomerular Filtration Rate (ml·min^{-1})	Signs	Laboratory Abnormalities
Normal	125	None	None
Deceased renal reserve	50–80	None	None
Renal insufficiency	12–50	Nocturia	Increased BUN and serum creatinine
Renal failure	<12	Uremia	Increased BUN and serum creatinine Anemia Hyperkalemia Increased bleeding time

Coagulopathies

Patients with chronic renal failure exhibit a bleeding tendency despite a normal prothrombin time, plasma thromboplastin time, and platelet count. The most likely coagulation defect is decreased platelet adhesiveness as reflected by a prolonged bleeding time. Treatment may include administration of desmopressin or cryoprecipitate, especially when surgery is planned. Correction of anemia with erythropoietin also shortens bleeding time in these patients. Hemodialysis has not consistently improved coagulation in these patients.

Electrolyte and Hydration Status

Hyperkalemia is the most serious electrolyte abnormality associated with chronic renal disease (see Chapter 17). Even when hemodialysis has been performed in the previous 6 to 8 hours, it is helpful to measure the serum potassium concentration before induction of anesthesia since unexpected hyperkalemia can occur rapidly. If surgery cannot be delayed, the serum potassium concentration can be lowered by hyperventilation of the lungs (a 10-mmHg decrease in $PaCO_2$ or 0.1-unit increase in pH decreases serum potassium about 0.5 mEq·L^{-1}) or administration of a glucose-insulin mixture (25 to 50 g glucose plus 10 to 20 units of regular insulin IV), or both. Intravenous administration of calcium is effective in restoring normal cardiac conduction in the presence of hyperkalemia. Sodium bicarbonate is indicated if metabolic acidosis accompanies hyperkalemia.

Regardless of hydration status, patients with chronic renal disease often respond to induction of anesthesia as if they were hypovolemic. The likelihood of hypotension during induction of anesthesia may be increased if sympathetic nervous system function is attenuated by antihypertensive drug therapy. Attenuated sympathetic nervous system activity produced by these drugs impairs compensatory peripheral vasoconstriction, such that a small decrease in blood volume, positive pressure ventilation of the lungs, or sudden changes in body position can result in exaggerated decreases in blood pressure.

Metabolic Acidosis

Chronic renal disease interferes with the normal renal excretion of hydrogen ions, leading to the appearance of metabolic acidosis. Hemodialysis is effective in restoring the pH to nearly normal values. Acidosis in patients with chronic renal disease is particularly undesirable because a low pH favors an extracellular rather than intracellular distribution of potassium.

Systemic Hypertension

Hypertension is a frequent complication of chronic renal disease. Preoperative hypertension is often due to fluid overload and is best treated by hemodialysis. Refractory hypertension occurs in 10% to 15% of patients with chronic renal disease despite hemodialysis and requires treatment with antihypertensive drugs. Management of hypertension in the perioperative period is with vasodilators such as hydralazine, labetalol, or nitroprusside. Cyanide toxicity from nitroprusside is unlikely because excretion of thiosulfate (necessary for conversion of cyanide to thiocyanate) is decreased in the presence of renal dysfunction.

Sepsis

The most common cause of death in patients with chronic renal disease is sepsis, often originating from pulmonary infections A high incidence of viral hepatitis most likely reflects the frequent use of blood products, as well as the effects of immunosuppression. Strict attention to asepsis is important when placing vascular cannulae and tracheal tubes in these patients.

Management of Anesthesia

Patients on hemodialysis scheduled for elective surgery usually undergo hemodialysis before surgery. Knowledge of the serum potassium concentration before induction of anesthesia is important because cardiac dysfunction may accompany hyperkalemia. Antihypertensive drug therapy is often continued. Signs of digitalis toxicity should be sought in treated patients, emphasizing the role of renal clearance of this drug.

Induction of anesthesia and intubation of the trachea can be safely accomplished with any of the commoly used intravenous drugs (see Chapter 5). An alternative to succinylcholine would be intermediate- or short-acting muscle relaxants, such as atracurium, vecuronium, or mivacurium. None of these induction drugs or muscle relaxants depend significantly on renal excretion for clearance from the plasma. Potassium release after administration of succinylcholine is not exaggerated in normokalemic patients with chronic renal disease.[7] Caution is necessary, however, because preoperative serum potassium concentrations in a high range (near 5.5 mEq·L^{-1}) combined with a high normal increase of serum potassium concentrations (0.5 to 1 mEq·L^{-1}) after administration of succinylcholine could theoretically result in dangerous hyperkalemia. A possible but undocumented concern is the potential for exaggerated potassium release after administration of succinylcholine to patients with neuropathies associated with chronic uremia. Exaggerated pharmacologic effects produced by drugs used for induction of anesthesia could reflect decreased protein binding, resulting in more unbound drug to act at receptors. Furthermore, the blood-brain barrier may not be intact in the presence of uremia. Exaggerated decreases in blood pressure after induction of anesthesia may also reflect autonomic nervous system dysfunction and impaired baroreceptor-mediated reflex responses.

Maintenance of anesthesia is often achieved with nitrous oxide combined with a volatile anesthetic or short-acting opioid. Some avoid nitrous oxide so as to permit administration of higher inspired concentrations of oxygen. Potent volatile anesthetics are useful in controlling intraoperative hypertension and decreasing the dose of muscle relaxants needed for adequate surgical relaxation. The use of halothane is sometimes questioned in patients requiring hemodialysis, in view of the high incidence of co-existing liver disease due to viral hepatitis in these patients. Likewise, enflurane, because of its modest metabolism to inorganic fluoride, may be avoided in patients with chronic renal disease. Nevertheless, excessive plasma inorganic fluoride concentrations do not occur in anephric patients after administration of enflurane because storage of fluoride in bone is able to offset the lack of renal excretion. Anemia decreases the blood solubility of volatile anesthetics, which could speed the rate at which the alveolar concentration can be increased or decreased. Excessive depression of cardiac output is a potential hazard of volatile anesthetics. Opioids decrease the likelihood of cardiovascular depression and avoid the concern of hepatotoxicity, but have the disadvantage of being unreliable for controlling intraoperative hypertension. Furthermore, occasional prolonged central nervous system and ventilatory depression from even small doses of opioids may reflect accumulation of pharmacologically active metabolites of opioids when renal function is absent.

Meticulous attention must be given to management of ventilation and intravenous fluid replacement. Normocapnia is desirable, since hyperventilation of the lungs with associated respiratory alkalosis adversely affects the position of the oxyhemoglobin dissociation curve, whereas respiratory acidosis from hypoventilation could result in acute increases in serum potassium concentrations. Patients dependent on hemodialysis have a narrow margin of safety between insufficient and excessive fluid administration. Replacement of insensible water losses with 5% glucose in water is appropriate, whereas any urine output is generally replaced with 0.45% sodium chloride. Lactated Ringer's solution (4 mEq of potassium in each liter) or other potassium-containing fluids probably should not be administered to anuric patients. Measurement of central venous pressure is useful in guiding fluid replacement. Monitoring of the electrocardiogram is important for recognizing signs of hyperkalemia. Arteriovenous shunts must be carefully protected to ensure continued patency during the perioperative period.

Blockade of the brachial plexus with local anesthetic is useful for the placement of vascular shunts in the arm as are necessary for hemodialysis. In addition to providing analgesia, this form of regional anesthesia abolishes vasospasm and provides optimal surgical conditions by producing maximal vascular vasodilation. A suggestion that the duration of brachial plexus anesthesia is shortened in patients with chronic renal failure has not been confirmed in controlled studies.[8] Adequacy of coagulation should be confirmed and the presence of uremic neuropathies ascertained before regional anesthesia is selected for these patients. Whether regional anesthesia should be selected in patients with uremic neuropathy is controversial. Some anesthesiologists fear that the regional anesthetic may be blamed for any subsequent progression of the co-existing neuropathy. Co-existing metabolic acidosis may also decrease the seizure threshold for local anesthetics.

A perplexing problem regarding altered drug responses in patients with chronic renal disease relates to the use of nondepolarizing muscle relaxants, since many of these drugs undergo extensive renal excretion (see Chapter 7). In this regard, intermediate- and short-acting muscle relaxants are often selected since the durations of action of atracurium and mivacurium are not prolonged and that of vecuronium is only slightly prolonged. Excretion of laudanosine, which is the major metabolite of atracurium, however, is delayed in the presence of renal failure. Laudanosine lacks effects at the neuromuscular junction but at high plasma concentrations may produce stimulation of the central nervous system. Regardless of the muscle relaxant selected, it would seem prudent to decrease the initial dose of drug and to administer subsequent doses on the basis of the response observed using a peripheral nerve stimulator.

A diagnosis of residual neuromuscular blockade after apparent reversal of nondepolarizing neuromuscular blockade with an anticholinesterase drug should be considered in anephric patients who manifest signs of skeletal muscle weakness in the early postoperative period. In normal patients whose blockade is adequately reversed with an anticholinesterase drug, reappearance of neuromuscular blockade does not occur because continued renal elimination of the muscle relaxant offsets waning effects of the anticholinesterase drug. Even in anephric patients, there is some protection because renal elimination of the anticholinesterase drug is delayed as long as, if not longer than, that of the nondepolarizing muscle relaxant. Indeed, other explanations (antibiotics, acidosis, electrolyte imbalance, diuretics) should be considered when neuromuscular blockade persists or reappears in patients with renal dysfunction.

Caution must be exercised in the use of opioids for postoperative analgesia in these patients in view of the possibility of exaggerated central nervous system and ventilatory depression after even small doses of opioids. Hypertension is a frequent problem in the postoperative period, and hemodialysis is the best treatment if fluid excess is the cause.

DIFFERENTIAL DIAGNOSIS OF PERIOPERATIVE OLIGURIA

Perioperative oliguria (less than 0.5 $ml \cdot kg^{-1} \cdot h^{-1}$) is classified as prerenal oliguria or acute tubular necrosis (Table 21-2).[1]

Prerenal Oliguria

Prerenal oliguria is characterized by excretion of concentrated urine containing minimal amounts of sodium. Excretion of a highly concentrated and sodium-poor urine confirms that renal tubular function is intact and reflects an attempt by the kidneys to conserve sodium and restore intravascular fluid volume in response to decreased renal blood flow. Decreased renal blood flow most likely reflects an acute decrease in intravascular fluid volume or a decreased cardiac output.

Table 21-2. Differential Diagnosis and Causes of Preoperative Oliguria

	Prerenal Oliguria	Acute Tubular Necrosis
Urinary sodium ($mEq \cdot L^{-1}$)	<40	>40
Urine osmolarity ($mOsm \cdot L^{-1}$)	>400	<400
Causes	Decreased renal blood flow (hypovolemia, hypotension, decreased cardiac output)	Renal ischemia Nephrotoxins Free hemoglobin or myoglobin

Treatment

The key strategy in decreasing the likelihood of oliguria progressing to acute renal failure is limiting the duration and magnitude of decreases in renal blood flow.[1] A brisk diuresis in response to rapid infusion of 3 to 6 $ml \cdot kg^{-1}$ of crystalloid, such as lactated Ringer's solution (fluid challenge), suggests that an acute decrease in intravascular fluid volume is the cause of prerenal oliguria. When fluid replacement does not result in an increased urine output, the possibility of decreased renal blood flow due to a low cardiac output should be considered. Dopamine (3 to 5 $\mu g \cdot kg^{-1} \cdot min^{-1}$ IV) is a useful drug to administer when oliguria is caused by a decreased cardiac output. A small dose of furosemide (0.1 $mg \cdot kg^{-1}$ IV) may re-establish urine output in the presence of oliguria due to pain-induced release of ADH. Conversely, this small dose of diuretic is unlikely to reverse oliguria due to decreased renal blood flow. If a urinary catheter is in place, it is important to confirm its patency.

Use of diuretics to maintain or stimulate urine flow in the perioperative period is controversial. Some believe that prevention of renal tubule urine stasis with diuretics, such as furosemide, can prevent prerenal oliguria from progressing to acute tubular necrosis. Nevertheless, urine output that is enhanced by administration of a diuretic does not necessarily predict postoperative renal function (Fig. 21-7).[9] Preoperative and intraoperative administration of mannitol has been advocated as a beneficial prophylaxis for prevention of acute tubular necrosis in jaundiced patients or patients undergoing resection of abdominal aortic aneurysms. Despite the clinical impression that mannitol may protect against renal failure, there is no evidence that mannitol is prefer-

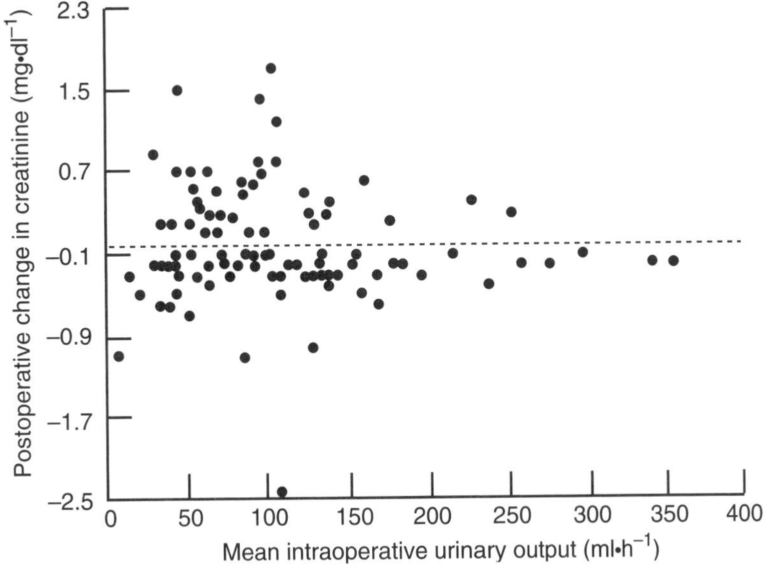

Figure 21-7. Changes in the postoperative plasma creatinine concentration do not correlate with intraoperative urinary output. (From Alpert et al.,[9] with permission.)

able to extracellular fluid volume expansion with saline alone in prevention of changes in renal function (decreased GFR) associated with elective infrarenal aortic cross-clamping.[10] Under any circumstance, it is crucial to restore intravascular fluid volume before administration of diuretics, because drug-induced diuresis could exaggerate hypovolemia and further decrease cardiac output and renal blood flow. Another disadvantage of diuretics is the impairment of sodium reabsorption for at least 6 to 12 hours, making the urine of prerenal oliguria indistinguishable from the urine excreted in the presence of acute tubular necrosis. Measurement of central venous or pulmonary artery occlusion pressure is helpful in evaluating the adequacy of volume replacement before administration of diuretics.

Acute Tubular Necrosis

Acute tubular necrosis is another cause of perioperative oliguria. In contrast to oliguria due to hypovolemia, the urine of patients developing acute tubular necrosis contains excessive amounts of sodium and is poorly concentrated. Hyperkalemia can accompany acute tubular necrosis. In the absence of renal function, the serum potassium concentration increases at a daily rate of 0.3 to 0.5 $mEq \cdot L^{-1}$. After surgery, however, the daily increase may be 1 to 2 $mEq \cdot L^{-1}$, reflecting the release of potassium from surgically damaged tissues. For this reason, the serum concentrations of potassium should be monitored frequently when acute tubular necrosis is suspected.

PHARMACOLOGY OF DIURETICS

Frequent administration of diuretics to patients undergoing anesthesia and operation emphasizes the need to appreciate the pharmacology of these drugs (Table 21-3).

Thiazide Diuretics

Thiazide diuretics are administered orally for treatment of essential hypertension and mobilization of edema fluid associated with renal, hepatic, or cardiac dysfunction. Diuresis occurs as a result of inhibition of reabsorption of sodium and chloride from the renal tubules. Hypochloremic, hypokalemic metabolic alkalosis is a consequence of prolonged administration of thiazide diuretics. Side effects associated with hypokalemia may include (1) skeletal muscle weakness, (2) increased likelihood of developing digitalis toxicity, and (3) potentiation of nondepolarizing muscle relaxants (see Chapter 7). Preoperative detection of orthostatic hypotension should arouse suspicion of diuretic-induced decreases in intravascular fluid volume.

Loop Diuretics

Loop diuretics (ethacrynic acid, furosemide) inhibit reabsorption of sodium and chloride and augment secretion of potassium primarily in the loop of Henle (hence the designation as loop diuretics). Intravenous administration of these drugs produces a diuretic response in 2 to 10 minutes. Contraction of the intravascular fluid volume (manifesting as orthostatic hypotension) may occur. Chronic administration of loop diuretics may result in hypochloremic, hypokalemic metabolic alkalosis, and in rare instances deafness occurs. Furosemide is used to (1) treat acute pulmonary edema, (2) decrease intracranial pressure, and (3) aid in the differential diagnosis of acute renal failure.

Osmotic Diuretics

The most frequently administered osmotic diuretic is the six-carbon sugar mannitol. Mannitol produces diuresis because it is filtered by the glomeruli and not reabsorbed from the renal tubules, leading to increased osmolarity of renal tubule fluid and associated excretion of water. In addition, mannitol increases plasma osmolarity, which will then draw fluid from intracellular spaces into extracellular spaces and thus acutely increase the intravascular fluid volume. This redistribution of fluid from intracellular to extracellular compartments decreases brain size and intracranial pressure. In patients who are oliguric secondary to congestive heart failure, mannitol-induced increases in intravascular fluid volume may precipitate pulmonary edema.

Aldosterone Antagonists

Spironolactone blocks the renal tubular effects of aldosterone, thus tending to offset the loss of potassium that is associated with the administration of thiazide diuretics. Fluid overload due to cirrhosis of the liver is often treated with spironolactone on the assumption that decreased hepatic function and

Table 21-3. Side Effects of Diuretics

	Hypokalemic Hypochloremic, Metabolic Alkalosis	Hyperkalemia	Hyperglycemia
Thiazide diuretics	Yes	No	Yes
Loop diuretics	Yes	No	Minimal
Osmotic diuretics	No	No	No
Aldosterone antagonists	No	Yes	No

metabolism leads to increased plasma concentrations of aldosterone.

TRANSURETHRAL SURGERY

Transurethral resection of the prostate (TURP) or of bladder tumors entails the excision of tissue and coagulation of bleeding vessels through a modified cystoscope. Benign prostatic hypertrophy affects an estimated 15 million American males, and TURP is the most common surgical procedure performed in males older than 50 years of age. During TURP, the use of continuous irrigation with fluid is necessary to improve visibility through the cystoscope, distend the prostatic urethra or bladder, and maintain the operative field free of blood and dissected tissue. Complications of transurethral surgery include (1) intravascular absorption of irrigating fluid, (2) hemorrhage, and (3) perforation of the bladder or urethra.[11]

Intravascular Absorption of Irrigating Fluid

The opening of venous sinuses in association with transurethral surgery leads to intravascular absorption of irrigating fluid. The amount of irrigating fluid absorbed depends on the (1) hydrostatic pressure of the fluid (determined by the height of the fluid container above the patient), (2) number and size of the venous sinuses opened, and (3) duration of the resection.

Fluids suitable for irrigation must be nonelectrolytic to prevent the dispersion of high-frequency electrical current from the operative area. These fluids should also be transparent and nontoxic to tissues. In the past, distilled water was a popular irrigating fluid because of superior visibility. Nevertheless, distilled water cannot be recommended, as intravascular absorption of this hypotonic fluid produces hemolysis. Commonly used electrolyte-free irrigating fluids that are nonhemolytic and nearly isotonic include glycine and Cytal. Glycine is an amino acid that normally occurs in the body. A metabolite of glycine is ammonia, but complications from this substance are rarely observed clinically. Nevertheless, prolonged central nervous system depression after use of glycine as the irrigating fluid should suggest the possibility of ammonia toxicity.[11] Glycine may also act as an inhibitory neurotransmitter in the retina and transient blindness after TURP has been attributed to intravascular absorption of this irrigating fluid.[11] Cytal is the trade name for the irrigating solution that consists of two sugars, man-

Manifestations of the TURP Syndrome

- Hypervolemia
  - Hypertension
  - Bradycardia
  - Increased central venous pressure
  - Pulmonary edema
  - Congestive heart failure
- Hyponatremia
- Hypoosmolarity
  - Cerebral edema
  - Headache
  - Restlessness
  - Confusion
  - Obtundation
  - Seizures

nitol and sorbitol. The major problem associated with Cytal is the possibility of bacterial contamination, since the sugars provide an excellent culture medium. Absorption of large volumes of isotonic irrigating fluids produces symptoms characterized as the TURP syndrome.[11] Prompt detection of excessive intravascular fluid absorption of irrigating fluid can be facilitated by use of an ethanol-tagged irrigating solution and measurement of the ethanol concentration in the patient's exhaled breath.[12]

Management of Anesthesia

Management of anesthesia for transurethral surgery is accomplished with a regional or general anesthetic. Because patients are often elderly, they are likely to have co-existing medical diseases, especially cardiopulmonary disorders. General anesthesia may mask signs of excessive intravascular absorption of irrigating fluid, but, nevertheless, may be a more desirable approach in a patient who cannot cooperate. A T10 sensory level is necessary when a regional anesthetic is selected for transurethral surgery that includes distension of the bladder. Cited advantages of regional anesthesia include the ability of awake patients to voice symptoms suggestive of bladder perforation and/or excessive intravascular absorption of irrigating fluid. For example, bladder perforation is often accompanied by complaints of shoulder discomfort that reflects referred pain due to subdiaphragmatic irritation by extravasated irrigating fluid. Inclusion of 0.1 to 0.2 mg of morphine in the local anesthetic solution injected into the subarachnoid space provides prolonged postoperative analgesia.[13] Despite the alleged advantages of regional anesthesia, there is no evidence of differences in morbidity or mortality when general anesthesia is selected.

Regardless of the technique of anesthesia selected, it is important to monitor these patients carefully for signs and symptoms of excessive intravascular absorption of irrigating fluid.[11] In addition to monitoring blood pressure, heart rate, and the electrocardiogram, it may be prudent to measure central venous pressure and to obtain periodic blood samples for determination of serum osmolarity and sodium concentration. When hyponatremia is suggestive of excessive hemodilution (plasma sodium concentration lower than 120 $mEq \cdot L^{-1}$), the administration of mannitol or furosemide may be indicated. Resection time should be as brief as possible. On the basis of an estimated intravascular absorption of irrigating fluid equal to 20 $ml \cdot min^{-1}$, the usual recommended resection time is 1 hour. It must be appreciated, however, that resection times as short as 15 minutes have resulted in symptoms of excessive intravascular absorption of irrigating fluid.[11]

REFERENCES

1. Byrick RJ, Rose DK. Pathophysiology and prevention of acute renal failure: The role of the anaesthetist. Can J Anaesth 1990;37:457–67.
2. Eger EI. Isoflurane (Forane). A Compendium and Reference. Madison, WI, Anaquest, a division of BOC, Inc. 1986:1–160.
3. Philbin DM, Coggins CH. Plasma antidiuretic hormone levels in cardiac surgical patients during morphine and halothane anesthesia. Anesthesiology 1974;40:95–8.
4. Kharash ED, Yeo K-T, Kenny MA, Buffington CW. Atrial natriuretic factor may mediate the renal effects of PEEP ventilation. Anesthesiology 1988;69:862–9.
5. Bastron RD, Perkins FM, Pyne JL. Autoregulation of renal blood flow during halothane anesthesia. Anesthesiology 1977;46:142–4.
6. Mazze RI, Sievenpiper TS, Stevenson J. Renal effects of enflurane and halothane in patients with abnormal renal function. Anesthesiology 1984;60:161–3.
7. Powell DR, Miller RD. The effect of repeated doses of succinylcholine on serum potassium in patients with renal failure. Anesth Analg 1975;54:746–8.
8. McEllistrem RF, Schell J, O'Malley KO, O'Toole DO, Cunningham AJ. Interscalene brachial plexus blockade with lidocaine in chronic renal failure—A pharmacokinetic study. Can J Anaesth 1989;36:59–63.
9. Alpert RA, Roizen MF, Hamilton WK, et al. Intraoperative urinary output does not predict postoperative renal function in patients undergoing abdominal aortic revascularization. Surgery 1984; 95:701–11.
10. Paul MD, Mazer D, Byrick RJ, Rose DK, Goldstein MB. Influence of mannitol and dopamine on renal function during elective infrarenal aortic clamping in man. Am J Nephrol 1986;6:427–34.
11. Jensen V. The TURP syndrome. Can J Anaesth 1991; 38:90–7.
12. Hulten J, Samra VJ, Hyertberg H, Palmquist B. Monitoring of irrigating fluid absorption during transurethral prostatectomy. A study in anaesthetized patients using a 1% ethanol tag solution. Anaesthesia 1991;46:349–53.
13. Kirson LE, Goldman JM, Slover RB. Low-dose intrathecal morphine for postoperative pain control in patients undergoing transurethral resection of the prostate. Anesthesiology 1989;71:192–5.

22

Endocrine and Nutritional Disease

Disorders of endocrine gland function or the presence of nutritional disease may be the primary reason for surgery or may co-exist in patients requiring operations unrelated to these disorders. The presence or absence of endocrine disease is suggested by specific observations during the preoperative evaluation of patients.

DIABETES MELLITUS

Diabetes mellitus (diabetes) is a chronic systemic disease that is characterized by an array of abnormalities, the most notable of which is disturbed glucose metabolism resulting in inappropriate hyperglycemia. It is estimated that 2.4% of the United States population are diabetic and that 50% of these patients undergo at least one surgical procedure. Diabetes is classified as insulin-dependent diabetes mellitus (IDDM) and non-insulin-dependent diabetes mellitus (NIDDM) (Table 22-1). Patients with NIDDM are almost always overweight and constitute over 90% of all diabetics. Treatment of diabetes includes diet (avoidance of obesity), oral hypoglycemic drugs (appropriate only in patients with NIDDM), and exogenous insulin.

Complications

The most serious acute metabolic complication of diabetes is ketoacidosis, whereas chronic complications manifest as macroangiopathy, microangiopathy, and disorders of the nervous system. Diabetic retinopathy occurs in 80% to 90% of those who have had IDDM for at least 20 years. In young and middle-aged adults in the United States, diabetes is the leading cause of kidney failure requiring hemodialysis.

Ketoacidosis

Hyperglycemia in the presence of metabolic acidosis and a history of diabetes are sufficient to establish the diagnosis of ketoacidosis. Causes of ketoacidosis include poor patient compliance with insulin regimens, infection, silent myocardial infarction, and inhibition of premature labor with a beta-2 agonist. Initial treatment of ketoacidosis includes repletion of the intravascular fluid volume, regular insulin (0.2 units·kg^{-1} IV followed by a low-dose continuous infusion), potassium, and sodium bicarbonate if the arterial pH is lower than 7.2. Even in the presence of hypovolemia, there is usually some urine output because of the osmotic effect of glucose.

Autonomic Neuropathy

Autonomic neuropathy reflects dysfunction of the autonomic nervous system as a result of diabetes.[1] Once autonomic neuropathy develops, the prognosis is poor, with mortality (often sudden death) exceeding 50% during a 5-year period. It is important to seek evidence of autonomic neuropathy (impotence, orthostatic hypotension, resting tachycardia, gastroparesis) in the preoperative evaluation as these patients may be at increased risk of the development of unexpected hemodynamic instability (hypotension requiring vasopressor therapy, bradycardia that is unresponsive to atropine) in the intraoperative period.[2,3] The presence of autonomic

Preoperative Evaluation of Endocrine Function

Absence of glucose in the urine
Blood pressure and heart rate normal
Body weight unchanged
Sexual function normal
No history of relevant drug therapy

neuropathy may prevent the development of angina pectoris (painless myocardial infarction) and thus obscure the presence of coronary artery disease.

Management of Anesthesia

The principal goal in the management of anesthesia for the diabetic patient undergoing elective surgery is to mimic normal metabolism as closely as possible by avoiding hypoglycemia, excessive hyperglycemia, ketoacidosis, dehydration, and electrolyte disturbances.[4] Hypoglycemia is prevented by ensuring an adequate supply of exogenous glucose. Hyperglycemia and associated ketoacidosis, dehydration, and electrolyte abnormalities are prevented by the exogenous administration of insulin. Perioperative monitoring of blood glucose concentrations (every 1 to 2 hours intraoperatively) is useful in maintaining good glycemic control. Nevertheless, despite the technical ability to normalize blood glucose concentrations in the perioperative period, prospective data showing a benefit to surgical outcomes are not available.

Complications of Diabetes Mellitus

Hyperglycemia
Hypoglycemia
Ketoacidosis
Autonomic neuropathy
Coronary artery disease
Cerebral vascular disease
Peripheral vascular disease
Nephropathy
Retinopathy
Sensory neuropathy
Stiff joint syndrome

Preoperative Evaluation

It is a frequent recommendation that the diabetic patient should be scheduled for surgery early in the day when possible. The well-controlled, diet-treated patient with NIDDM does not require prior hospitalization or any special treatment (including exogenous insulin) before and during surgery. Even the patient with well-controlled IDDM undergoing a brief outpatient surgical procedure may not require any adjustment in the usual subcutaneous insulin regimen. If an oral hypoglycemic drug is being administered, it may be continued until the evening before surgery, remembering that these drugs may produce delayed hypoglycemia in the absence of any caloric intake. Preadmission to the hospital is probably indicated only for the patient with poorly controlled IDDM.

Table 22-1. Classification of Diabetes Mellitus

	Insulin-Dependent Diabetes Mellitus	Non-insulin-Dependent Diabetes Mellitus
Alternative designations	Juvenile onset Type I	Maturity onset Type II
Age at onset	Before 16	After 35
Appearance	Abrupt	Gradual
Require exogenous insulin	Always	Occasionally
Ketoacidosis prone	Yes	No
Blood glucose concentration	Wide fluctuations	Relatively stable
Nutrition	Thin	Obese

Signs and Symptoms of Autonomic Nervous System Neuropathy

Impotence
Orthostatic hypotension
Resting tachycardia
Absent variation in heart rate with deep breathing
Gastroparesis (vomiting, diarrhea, abdominal distension)
Asymptomatic hypoglycemia
Sudden death syndrome

Preoperative evaluation and treatment of hyperglycemia, ketoacidosis, and electrolyte disturbances are important before elective surgery is performed. Measurement of the glycohemoglobin concentration provides information about the average blood glucose concentration in the previous 1 to 3 weeks. Manifestations of coronary artery disease (electrocardiogram), cerebral vascular disease, and renal dysfunction are sought in the preoperative evaluation. The most common cause of perioperative morbidity in the diabetic patient is coronary artery disease. Signs of peripheral neuropathy (which may influence selection of regional anesthesia) and autonomic neuropathy are noted. The diabetic patient with preoperative evidence of autonomic neuropathy may be at increased risk of aspiration on induction of anesthesia and intraoperative cardiovascular lability (hypotension requiring vasopressor therapy, bradycardia that is resistant to atropine).[2,3] Evaluation of the patient with IDDM for evidence of limited joint mobility is important in predicting possible difficulty in performing direct laryngoscopy for intubation of the trachea. The common presence of obesity in this patient population may influence the ease of tracheal intubation or performance of regional anesthetic techniques.

Exogenous Insulin. There is a consensus that the patient with IDDM undergoing major surgery should be treated with insulin, but the accepted route of administration (subcutaneous, intravenous) remains unsettled (Table 22-2).[4] The traditional and most common approach to preoperative management is subcutaneous injection of insulin. Regardless of the regimen selected, it is important to adjust subsequent administration of insulin or changes in intravenous glucose infusion rates, or both, on the basis of intraoperative measurements (every 1 to 2 hours) of the blood glucose concentrations. Estimation of urine glucose concentrations and the use of a sliding scale to manage intraoperative insulin needs are not ideal since the sliding scale regimen is based on retrospective hyperglycemia. Furthermore, this approach may require the placement of a bladder catheter in an anesthetized patient, with the associated potential for infection.

Table 22-2. **Regimens for Exogenous Insulin Replacement**

Subcutaneous insulin administration
- Administer one-fourth to one-half the usual daily intermediate-acting dose of insulin on the morning of surgery
- Initiate infusion of glucose (5–10 g·h^{-1}) with administration of insulin

Continuous intravenous infusion of insulin[a]
- Regular insulin (50 units in 500 ml normal saline) at 0.5–1 unit·h^{-1}
- Initiate infusion of glucose (5–10 g·h^{-1}) with initiation of insulin infusion
- Measure blood glucose concentration as necessary (usually every 1 to 2 hours) and adjust insulin infusion accordingly

<80 mg·dl^{-1}	Discontinue insulin infusion Administer 25 ml of 50% glucose Remeasure blood glucose concentration in 30 min
80–120 mg·dl^{-1}	Decrease insulin infusion rate by 0.3 unit·h^{-1}
120–180 mg·dl^{-1}	No change in insulin infusion rate
180–120 mg·dl^{-1}	Increase insulin infusion rate by 0.3 unit·h^{-1}
>220 mg·dl^{-1}	Increase insulin infusion rate by 0.5 unit·h^{-1}

[a]Data for intravenous infusion from Hirsch et al.[4]

Induction and Maintenance of Anesthesia

The choice of drugs or techniques for induction and maintenance of anesthesia is less important than monitoring the blood glucose concentrations and treatment of potential physiologic derangements associated with diabetes. When general anesthesia is chosen, intubation of the trachea with a cuffed tube seems prudent, especially if there is preoperative evidence of gastroparesis. Although volatile anesthetics impair the release of insulin in response to administration of glucose, there is no evidence that maintenance of anesthesia with a specific volatile drug in a diabetic patient is advantageous. Epidural and spinal anesthesia preserve glucose tolerance, but the high incidence of peripheral neuropathy may influence selection of a regional anesthetic technique for fear that a diabetic sensory neuropathy could be erroneously attributed to the regional technique. Episodes of bradycardia and hypotension that develop suddenly and are unresponsive to atropine have been described during regional or general anesthesia in diabetic patients with preoperative evidence of cardiac autonomic neuropathy.[2,3] Prompt intervention with intravenous administration of epinephrine may be the most effective therapy in these patients.

HYPEROSMOLAR HYPERGLYCEMIC NONKETOTIC COMA

Hyperosmolar hyperglycemic nonketotic coma occurs most often in elderly patients with an impaired thirst mechanism. Two-thirds of patients who develop this syndrome do not have a history of diabetes, ketoacidosis does not occur, and exogenous insulin is not needed after recovery. Hyperglycemia and insulin resistance present during cardiopulmonary bypass in patients with NIDDM makes this patient population vulnerable to the development of hyperosmolar hyperglycemic nonketotic coma. This syndrome is treated with intravenous administration of insulin and restoration of intravascular fluid volume with sodium-containing solutions.

Signs and Symptoms of Hyperosmolar Hyperglycemic Nonketotic Coma

Plasma hyperosmolarity (>330 $mOsm \cdot L^{-1}$)
Hyperglycemia (>600 $mg \cdot dl^{-1}$)
Normal arterial pH
Osmotic diuresis (hypokalemia)
Hypovolemia
Seizures and coma (decreased intracellular brain water due to hyperosmolarity)

HYPERTHYROIDISM

Hyperthyroidism is a generic term for all conditions in which tissues are exposed to increased circulating concentrations (5 to 15 times) of triiodothyronine (T_3) or thyroxine (T_4), or both. Graves disease (diffuse toxic goiter) is the most common form of hyperthyroidism, manifesting most often in females between 20 and 40 years of age. Hyperthyroidism occurs in about 0.2% of parturients. An autoimmune pathogenesis for Graves disease is suggested by the presence of circulating antibodies that mimic the effects of thyroid stimulating hormone (TSH). Diagnosis of hyperthyroidism is based on clinical signs and symptoms plus confirmation of excessive thyroid gland function as demonstrated by appropriate tests (Table 22-3).

Signs and Symptoms of Hyperthyroidism

Anxiety
Fatigue
Skeletal muscle weakness
Tachycardia
Tachydysrhythmias
Exophthalmos

Management of Anesthesia

Elective surgery should probably be deferred until patients have been rendered euthyroid with drug therapy and the hyperdynamic circulation controlled with a beta antagonist as evidenced by a resting heart rate lower than 85 $beats \cdot min^{-1}$. When surgery cannot be delayed, the continuous infusion of esmolol (100 to 300 $\mu g \cdot kg^{-1} \cdot min^{-1}$ IV) is useful for control of cardiovascular responses evoked by sympathetic nervous system stimulation.[5] Preoperative sedation is often produced by the oral administration of a benzodiazepine. Anticholinergic drugs are not recommended, as they could interfere with heat

Table 22-3. Tests for the Diagnosis of Thyroid Gland Dysfunction

	Thyroxine	Triiodothyronine	Thyroid Stimulating Hormone
Hyperthyroidism	Increased	Increased	Normal
Primary hypothyroidism	Decreased	Decreased	Increased
Secondary hypothyroidism	Decreased	Decreased	Decreased

regulation and contribute to increases in heart rate. Evaluation of the upper airway for evidence of obstruction is an important part of the preoperative evaluation. In this regard, computed tomography may be helpful in evaluating airway anatomy.

Induction of Anesthesia

Induction of anesthesia is acceptably achieved with a number of intravenous induction drugs. Thiopental is an attractive selection because its thiourea structure lends antithyroid activity to the drug. Nevertheless, it is unlikely that a significant antithyroid effect is produced by an induction dose of this drug. Ketamine is not a likely selection because it can stimulate the sympathetic nervous system. Assuming the absence of airway obstruction from an enlarged goiter, the administration of succinylcholine or a nondepolarizing muscle relaxant that lacks effects on the cardiovascular system is useful to facilitate intubation of the trachea.

Maintenance of Anesthesia

Goals during maintenance of anesthesia are to avoid administration of drugs that stimulate the sympathetic nervous system and to provide sufficient anesthetic depression of the sympathetic nervous system to prevent an exaggerated response to surgical stimulation. The possibility of organ toxicity owing to altered or accelerated drug metabolism in the presence of hyperthyroidism is a consideration when selecting drugs for maintenance of anesthesia. In an animal model rendered hyperthyroid, the administration of halothane, enflurane, and isoflurane was followed by evidence of hepatic centrilobular necrosis in some animals, with the greatest incidence (92%) being in animals exposed to halothane.[6] Nevertheless, liver function tests are not altered postoperatively in previously hyperthyroid patients who are rendered euthyroid before surgery and given anesthesia that includes administration of halothane or enflurane.[7]

Despite animal evidence of hepatic necrosis after exposure to volatile anesthetics, the ability of isoflurane to offset exaggerated sympathetic nervous system responses to surgical stimulation and not sensitize the heart to catecholamines makes this drug an attractive selection to combine with nitrous oxide for maintenance of anesthesia in a hyperthyroid patient. Nitrous oxide combined with a short-acting opioid is an alternative to administration of a volatile anesthetic but has the disadvantage of not reliably suppressing sympathetic nervous system activity.

Controlled studies in animals do not support the clinical impression that anesthetic requirements for inhaled drugs (MAC) are increased in the presence of hyperthyroidism.[8] The discrepancy between clinical impression and objective data is presumed to reflect the increased cardiac output characteristic of hyperthyroidism. For example, increased cardiac output accelerates uptake of inhaled anesthetics, resulting in the need to increase the inspired concentration of the drug so as to achieve a brain partial pressure similar to that achieved with a lower inspired concentration in the euthyroid patient. It should be appreciated that accelerated metabolism of the anesthetic does not alter the partial pressure of the drug necessary in the brain to produce the desired pharmacologic effect. Another factor to be considered in evaluating anesthetic requirements in the presence of altered thyroid gland function is body temperature. For example, an increase in body temperature, as could accompany thyroid storm, would be expected to increase MAC about 5% for each degree the temperature increases above 37°C.

Selection of a muscle relaxant for production of intraoperative surgical muscle relaxation should consider the theoretical advantage of drugs that lack cardiovascular effects. Conceivably, a prolonged response could occur when a traditional dose of muscle relaxant is administered to a patient with co-existing skeletal muscle weakness. For this reason, it may be prudent to decrease the initial dose of muscle relaxant and closely monitor the effect produced at the neuromuscular junction using a peripheral nerve stimulator. Antagonism of neuromuscular blockade with an anticholinesterase drug combined with an anticholinergic drug introduces the concern for drug-induced tachycardia. Although experience is too limited to make a recommendation, it would seem unwarranted to avoid pharmacologic reversal of nondepolarizing muscle relaxants in hyperthyroid patients. Perhaps glycopyrrolate, which has less chronotropic effect than atropine, would be a more appropriate anticholinergic drug selection.

Monitoring during maintenance of anesthesia in hyperthyroid patients is directed at early recognition of increased activity of the thyroid gland suggesting the onset of thyroid storm. Constant monitoring of body temperature is particularly useful, and methods to lower body temperature, including a cooling mattress and cold crystalloid solutions for intravenous infusion are recommended. The electrocardiogram may reveal tachycardia or cardiac dysrhythmias, or both, indicating the need for the intraoperative administration of a beta antagonist (continuous intravenous infusion of esmolol) or lidocaine. Patients with exophthalmos are susceptible to corneal ulceration and drying, emphasizing the need to protect the eyes during the perioperative period.

Treatment of hypotension with a sympathomimetic drug must consider the possibility of the exaggerated responsiveness of hyperthyroid patients to endogenous or exogenous catecholamines. For this reason, a decreased dose of a direct-acting vasopressor, such as phenylephrine, may be a more logical selection than ephedrine, which acts in part by providing the release of catecholamines.

Regional Anesthesia

Regional anesthesia with its associated blockade of the sympathetic nervous system is a potentially useful selection for hyperthyroid patients, assuming there is no evidence of high output congestive heart failure. A continuous lumbar epidural anesthetic may be preferable to a spinal anesthetic because of the slower onset of sympathetic nervous system blockade, making severe hypotension less likely. If hypotension occurs, a decreased dose of phenylephrine is recommended, keeping in mind the possible hypersensitivity of these patients to sympathomimetic drugs. Epinephrine should not be added to the local anesthetic solution since systemic absorption of this catecholamine could produce exaggerated circulatory responses. Increased anxiety and associated activation of the sympathetic nervous system can be treated in awake patients with the intravenous administration of a benzodiazepine such as midazolam.

Thyroid Storm

Thyroid storm (thyrotoxicosis) is an abrupt exacerbation of hyperthyroidism owing to the sudden excessive release of thyroid gland hormones into the circulation. Hyperthermia, tachycardia, congestive heart failure, dehydration, and shock are likely. Thyroid storm associated with surgery can occur intraoperatively but is more likely to manifest 6 to 18 hours after surgery. When thyroid storm occurs during the perioperative period, it may mimic malignant hyperthermia. Thyroid storm is treated with infusion of cooled crystalloid solutions and continuous infusion of esmolol to maintain the heart rate at an acceptable level.[5] When hypotension is persistent, the administration of cortisol (100 to 200 mg IV) may be considered. Dexamethasone may inhibit the conversion of T_4 to T_3, an effect that is additive to that of propylthiouracil. Aspirin may displace T_4 from its carrier protein and is not recommended for lowering body temperature. It is important to also treat any suspected infection. Ultimately, drugs such as propylthiouracil and sodium iodide are administered to prevent thyroid gland hormone synthesis and release.

Complications after Total or Subtotal Thyroidectomy

Damage to the laryngeal nerves, tracheal compression, and accidental removal of the parathyroid glands are early complications that can follow thyroid surgery.

Laryngeal Nerves

The entire sensory and motor supply to the larynx is from the two superior and two recurrent laryngeal nerves. The superior laryngeal nerves provide the motor supply to the cricothyroid muscles and sensation above the level of the vocal cords. The recurrent laryngeal nerves supply motor innervation to all the muscles of the larynx except the cricothyroid muscles plus sensation below the level of the vocal cords. Function of the vocal cords after thyroid surgery can be evaluated by asking patients to say "e." The most common nerve injury after thyroid surgery is unilateral damage to the recurrent laryngeal nerve, manifesting as hoarseness and a paralyzed vocal cord, which assumes an intermediate position. Bilateral recurrent laryngeal nerve injury results in aphonia and paralyzed vocal cords that can flap together during inspiration to produce airway obstruction. Superior laryngeal nerve paralysis manifests as hoarseness and loss of sensation above the vocal cords, making patients vulnerable to inhalation of any material present in the pharynx.

Compression of the Trachea

Compression of the trachea leading to airway obstruction may reflect a hematoma at the operative site or tracheomalacia due to weakening of the tracheal rings by chronic pressure from a goiter. Airway obstruction after extubation of the trachea and in the presence of normal vocal cord function should suggest the diagnosis of tracheomalacia.

Accidental Removal of the Parathyroid Glands

Hypoparathyroidism due to accidental removal of the parathyroid glands occurs in about 1% of patients who undergo total thyroidectomy. In these patients, signs of hypocalcemia can manifest as early as 1 to 3 hours after surgery but typically do not appear until 24 to 72 hours postoperatively. Laryngeal muscles are very sensitive to hypocalcemia, and inspiratory stridor progressing to laryngospasm may be the first suggestion that surgically induced hypoparathyroidism is present.

HYPOTHYROIDISM

Hypothyroidism is a generic term for all conditions in which tissues are exposed to decreased circulating concentrations of T_3 and T_4. Chronic thyroiditis (Hashimoto's thyroiditis) is the most common cause of hypothyroidism, manifesting as an autoimmune disease characterized by progressive destruction of the thyroid gland. Medical or surgical treatment of hyperthyroidism may also become a cause of iatrogenic hypothyroidism. Diagnosis of hypothyroidism is based on clinical signs and symptoms plus confirmation of decreased thyroid gland function as demonstrated by appropriate tests (Table 22-3). The development of hypothyroidism in adulthood is often insidious and gradual and may go unrecognized in part because of the associated apathy that minimizes the patient's complaints. Subclinical hypothyroidism manifesting only as an increased plasma TSH concentration is present in about 5% of the United States population, with a prevalence of 13.2% in otherwise healthy elderly patients, especially females.[9] There is no evidence that these asymptomatic patients are at increased anesthetic or surgical risk.

Signs and Symptoms of Hypothyroidism

Lethargy
Intolerance to cold
Bradycardia
Decreased cardiac output
Peripheral vasoconstriction
Hyponatremia
Atrophy of the adrenal cortex

Management of Anesthesia

Elective surgery should probably be deferred in patients with symptomatic hypothyroidism. Nevertheless, controlled clinical studies do not confirm an increased risk when patients with mild to moderate hypothyroidism undergo elective surgery.[10] There are no controlled data to support the position that hypothyroid patients are unusually sensitive to inhaled anesthetic drugs and opioids. Nevertheless, a high index of suspicion for possible adverse effects, including exaggerated effects of depressant drugs, adrenal insufficiency, hypovolemia, and prolonged gastric emptying time, would still seem warranted.[11] Furthermore, a severe nonthyroid illness may precipitate acute hypothyroidism in a vulnerable patient.[12]

Preoperative medication for the hypothyroid patient should emphasize the value of the preoperative visit and resultant psychological support. Opioid premedication has been administered safely, but there is a historical concern that the depressant effects of these drugs may be exaggerated in hypothyroid patients. Supplemental cortisol may be considered if there is concern that surgical stress could unmask decreased adrenal function that may accompany hypothyroidism. In some patients, it may be better to administer sedative and anticholinergic drugs intravenously after the arrival in the operating room so that any unexpected effect can be promptly recognized and treated.

Induction of Anesthesia

Induction of anesthesia is often accomplished by the intravenous administration of ketamine with the presumption that this drug's inherent support of the cardiovascular system will be beneficial. Intubation of the trachea is facilitated by administration of succinylcholine or a nondepolarizing muscle relaxant, keeping in mind that co-existing skeletal muscle weakness could be associated with an exaggerated muscle relaxant effect.

Maintenance of Anesthesia

Maintenance of anesthesia is often achieved by inhalation of nitrous oxide plus supplementation if necessary with minimal doses of ketamine, opioids, or benzodiazepines. Volatile anesthetics are not recommended because of the exquisite sensitivity of hypothyroid patients to drug-induced myocardial depression. The failure of decreases in thyroid activity to decrease anesthetic requirements (MAC) may reflect the maintenance of cerebral metabolic requirements for oxygen that are independent of thyroid activity.[8] Decreased production of carbon dioxide associated with the decreased metabolic rate makes hypothyroid patients vulnerable to excessive decreases in the $PaCO_2$ during controlled ventilation of the lungs. Pancuronium, because of its mild sympathomimetic effects, would seem a useful selection for production of skeletal muscle paralysis. Antagonism of nondepolarizing neuromuscular blockade with an anticholinesterase drug combined with an anticholinergic drug does not pose a risk in these patients. Regional anesthesia is also an acceptable technique for management of anesthesia in selected hypothyroid patients.

Monitoring of hypothyroid patients is directed toward early recognition of congestive heart failure and detection of the onset of hypothermia. Continuous recording of arterial blood pressure and cardiac filling pressures are indicated for invasive operations. In addition to glucose, intravenous solutions should contain sodium so as to prevent the development of hyponatremia. The possibility of acute primary adrenal insufficiency should be remembered when hypotension persists despite intravenous infusion of fluids or administration of sympathomimetic drugs, or both. Maintenance of body temperature is facilitated by increasing the temperature of the operating room and passing intravenous fluid solutions through warming devices.

Postoperative Complications

Recovery from the sedative effects of anesthetics may be delayed in hypothyroid patients, necessitating continued mechanical ventilation of the lungs. Removal of the tracheal tube is logically deferred until the patient is responding appropriately and body temperature is near 37°C. The concern about possible increased sensitivity to the effects of opioids is a consideration in the management of postoperative pain, perhaps with emphasis on utilization of nonopioid analgesics such as ketorolac.

CORTICOSTEROID THERAPY BEFORE SURGERY

Corticosteroid supplementation should be increased whenever patients being treated for chronic hypoadrenocorticism undergo surgical procedures. This recommendation is based on the concern that these patients are susceptible to cardiovascular collapse because they cannot release additional endogenous cortisol in response to the stress of surgery. More controversial is the management of patients who may manifest suppression of the pituitary-adrenal axis owing to current or previous administration of corticosteroids for treatment of diseases unrelated to abnormalities in the anterior pituitary or adrenal cortex. The dose of corticosteroids or duration of therapy with corticosteroids that produces suppression of the pituitary-adrenal axis is not known. Suppression, however, may persist for as long as 12 months after discontinuation of therapy. Therefore, it is common practice to empirically administer supplemental corticosteroids in the perioperative period when surgery is planned in patients who are being treated with corticosteroids or who have been treated for longer than 1 month in the past 6 to 12 months.[13] Nevertheless, it should be appreciated that cause and effect relationships between intraoperative hypotension and acute hypoadrenocorticism in patients previously treated with corticosteroids is very difficult to document. Furthermore, there is no objective evidence to support the practice of increasing the maintenance doses of corticosteroids preoperatively and then gradually decreasing the dose back to maintenance levels during the first few days postoperatively.

Empiric Regimen for Perioperative Corticosteroid Supplementation

- Administer daily corticosteroid maintenance dose with preoperative medication
- Administer cortisol (25 mg IV) with induction of anesthesia
- Initiate a continuous infusion of cortisol (100 mg IV delivered over the next 24 hours)
- Resume usual daily corticosteroid maintenance dose postoperatively

(Data from Symreng et al.[13])

PHEOCHROMOCYTOMA

Pheochromocytoma is a catecholamine-secreting tumor that originates in the adrenal medulla or aberrant tissue along the paravertebral sympathetic chain. Although fewer than 0.1% of patients with hypertension have a pheochromocytoma, nearly 50% of deaths in patients with unsuspected pheochromocytoma occur during anesthesia and surgery or parturition. Pheochromocytoma can occur as part of an autosomal dominant multiglandular neoplastic syndrome (medullary thyroid carcinoma is most often present) designated multiple endocrine neoplasia. Hypertension and hypermetabolism associated with pheochromocytoma may mimic other diseases, including thyroid storm and malignant hyperthermia.

The hallmark of pheochromocytoma is paroxysmal or sustained hypertension. The triad of diaphoresis, tachycardia, and headache in a hypertensive patient is highly suggestive of pheochromocytoma. Definitive diagnosis of pheochromocytoma requires chemical confirmation of excessive catecholamine release. Oral clonidine suppresses the plasma concentration of catecholamines in hypertensive patients but not in patients with a pheochromocytoma.

Signs and Symptoms of Pheochromocytoma

- Paroxysmal hypertension
- Triad of diaphoresis, tachycardia, and headache
- Tremulousness
- Weight loss
- Decreased intravascular fluid volume
    - Orthostatic hypotension
    - Hematocrit >45%
- Cardiomyopathy
- Intracerebral hemorrhage

Treatment of pheochromocytoma is surgical excision of the catecholamine-secreting tumor. Before surgery is scheduled, however, it is important to establish alpha blockade (phenoxybenzamine, prazosin, labetalol), restore blood volume (disappearance of orthostatic hypotension, decrease in the hematocrit), and treat cardiac dysrhythmias (beta antagonists). Preoperative normalization of intravascular fluid volume and blood pressure also decreases the risk of intraoperative hypertension during manipulation of the tumor. The recommendation that beta blockade should not be instituted in the absence of alpha blockade is based on the theoretical concern that a heart depressed by beta blockade might not be able to maintain an adequate cardiac output should unopposed alpha-mediated vasoconstriction from the release of catecholamines result in an abrupt increase in systemic vascular resistance. Alpha blockade will facilitate the release of insulin and decrease the likelihood of hyperglycemia. Echocardiography may be useful in patients with suspected cardiomyopathy.

Management of Anesthesia

Management of anesthesia for patients requiring excision of pheochromocytoma is based on avoidance of drugs or events that might activate the sympathetic nervous system and on the use of invasive monitoring techniques (arterial and pulmonary artery catheters) that permit early and appropriate interventions when catecholamine-induced changes in cardiovascular function occur.[14] Continuation of alpha and beta antagonists until the induction of anesthesia is recommended. If bilateral adrenalectomy is anticipated, supplemental cortisol treatment may be instituted at the time of preoperative medication. The times of significant intraoperative risk for these patients are (1) during intubation of the trachea, (2) during manipulation of the tumor, and (3) following ligation of the tumor's venous drainage.

Induction of Anesthesia

Placement of a catheter in a peripheral artery to provide continuous monitoring of blood pressure is useful before proceeding with the induction of anesthesia. Unconsciousness is produced with administration of any intravenous anesthetic (except ketamine) followed by ventilation of the lungs with nitrous oxide plus a volatile anesthetic. Selection of isoflurane, enflurane, or desflurane is based on the ability of these drugs to decrease sympathetic nervous system activity and on their low likelihood of sensitizing the heart to the cardiac dysrhythmic effects of catecholamines. Halothane is no longer recommended because of its propensity to produce cardiac dysrhythmias in the presence of increased plasma concentrations of catecholamines. Mechanical ventilation of the lungs is facilitated by the production of skeletal muscle paralysis with a nondepolarizing muscle relaxant deemed to be devoid of vagolytic or histamine releasing effects (vecuronium, doxacurium, pipecuronium).

Direct laryngoscopy for intubation of the trachea is initiated only after establishment of a surgical depth of anesthesia with a volatile anesthetic (about 1.3 MAC). An adequate depth of anesthesia is necessary to minimize increases in blood pressure associated with intubation of the trachea. It may be helpful to administer lidocaine (1 to 2 $mg \cdot kg^{-1}$ IV) about 1 minute before initiating laryngoscopy, as this drug may attenuate the hypertensive response to intubation of the trachea and decrease the likelihood of cardiac dysrhythmias. In addition, the administration of a short-acting opioid (fentanyl 100 to 200 μg IV, sufentanil 10 to 20 μg IV) just before starting direct laryngoscopy may attenuate the pressor response. Nitroprusside (50 to 100 μg IV) or phentolamine (1 to 5 mg IV) should be readily available for injection should persistent hypertension accompany intubation of the trachea.

Maintenance of Anesthesia

Maintenance of anesthesia is most often accomplished with nitrous oxide plus a volatile anesthetic. An opioid combined with nitrous oxide is a less likely selection, since this combination does not suppress hypertensive responses owing to catecholamine release. In addition, it is not easy to decrease the depth of anesthesia should persistent hypotension occur when injected drugs are used for maintenance of anesthesia. A continuous intravenous infusion of nitroprusside will be necessary should hypertension persist despite delivery of maximum concentrations of the volatile anesthetic (about 1.5 to 2.0 MAC). Reflex tachycardia that may accompany nitroprusside-induced peripheral vasodilation is treated with a continuous infusion of esmolol. Cardiac dysrhythmias are initially treated with lidocaine. A decrease in blood pressure that accompanies ligation of the tumor's venous drainage (reflects sudden decreases in circulating catecholamine concentrations) is treated by decreasing the delivered concentration of volatile anesthetic and rapid infusion of intravenous fluids. Rarely, a continuous intravenous infusion of phenylephrine or norepinephrine may be required until the peripheral vasculature can adapt to a decreased level of endogenous alpha stimulation. A pulmonary artery catheter is helpful in evaluating the response to therapeutic interventions. Monitoring of blood glucose concentrations is useful as hyperglycemia is common before excision of the pheochromocytoma whereas hypoglycemia may occur within minutes of tumor removal as alpha-induced suppression of insulin release wanes.

Regional anesthesia for excision of a pheochromocytoma has the attractive features of blocking the sympathetic nervous system without sensitizing the heart to catecholamines. Nevertheless, postsynaptic alpha receptors can still respond to the direct effects of circulating catecholamines. Furthermore, hypotension that may accompany ligation of the veins draining the pheochromocytoma cannot be offset by sympathetic nervous system activation in the presence of epidural or spinal anesthesia. Selection of a regional anesthetic is practical only if the surgical procedure is performed with the patient supine.

Postoperative Care

Invasive monitoring is continued in the postoperative period as abrupt increases or decreases in blood pressure remain a possibility. An estimated 50% of patients will remain hypertensive during the early postoperative period despite removal of the pheochromocytoma. A high index of suspicion for hypoglycemia is maintained. Relief of postoperative pain as with neuraxial opioids may contribute to early tracheal extubation in these often young and otherwise healthy patients.

MORBID OBESITY

Obesity is the most common nutritional disorder in the United States, affecting about 25% of the population as reflected by a body weight more than 20% above the ideal weight. Morbid obesity is present when body weight is twice the ideal weight.

Adverse Effects

Adverse effects of obesity are associated with increased morbidity and mortality, often reflecting the concomitant presence of hypertension, lipid abnormalities, and diabetes mellitus.

Cardiovascular

There is a positive correlation between increases in systemic blood pressure, cardiomegaly, and weight gain. Increased cardiac output and blood volume is the presumed cause of hypertension. It is estimated that cardiac output increases 0.1 $L{\cdot}min^{-1}$ for every 1 kg of weight gain related to adipose tissue (1 kg of fat contains about 3000 m of blood vessels). When measuring blood pressure in an obese patient, care should be taken to use a blood pressure cuff of the correct size. As a general rule, the width of the blood pressure cuff should be greater than one-third the circumference of the arm. When the cuff is too narrow, more pressure will be required to compress the extra tissues and a false-high systemic blood pressure will be recorded. Pulmonary hypertension is common and most likely reflects the effects of chronic arterial hypoxemia or increased pulmonary blood volume, or both.

Adverse Effects of Obesity

- Cardiovascular
  - Systemic hypertension
  - Cardiomegaly
  - Congestive heart failure
  - Coronary artery disease
  - Pulmonary hypertension
- Ventilation
  - Decreased lung volumes and capacities
  - Arterial hypoxemia
  - Obesity-hypoventilation syndrome
- Liver
  - Abnormal liver function tests
  - Fatty liver infiltration
- Metabolic
  - Insulin resistance (diabetes mellitus)
  - Hypercholesterolemia (coronary artery disease, cholelithiasis)

Ventilation

Obesity imposes a restrictive ventilation defect (decreased expiratory reserve volume, vital capacity, and functional residual capacity) due to the compressive effects on the chest and abdomen produced by the excess adipose tissue. This added weight impedes motion of the diaphragm, especially with the assumption of the supine position. Fatty infiltration of the muscles of breathing further diminishes ventilation and limits exercise tolerance.

There is a predictable decrease in the PaO_2 of obese patients, presumably reflecting ventilation-to-perfusion mismatching, which is accentuated by decreases in lung volumes and capacities. Conversely, the $PaCO_2$ and the ventilatory response to carbon dioxide remain normal, reflecting the high diffusing capacity and favorable characteristics of the dissociation curve for carbon dioxide. The margin of reserve, however, is small, and administration of ventilatory depressant drugs or assumption of the head-down position can result in hypoventilation.

Obesity-Hypoventilation Syndrome. Obesity-hypoventilation syndrome (pickwickian syndrome) occurs in about 8% of obese patients. The presence of episodic daytime somnolence and hypoventilation in a morbidly obese patient suggests the presence of this syndrome. Ultimately, hypoventilation leads to sustained pulmonary hypertension and right ventricular failure. Obstructive sleep apnea may be associated with this syndrome. The etiology of the obesity-hypoventilation syndrome is unknown but may represent a disorder of the central nervous system regulation of breathing or inability of the muscles of breathing to respond to neural impulses, or both.

Management of Anesthesia

Management of anesthesia is influenced by the presence of adverse effects due to underlying obesity.

Induction of Anesthesia

Obese patients are likely to be at increased risk of pulmonary aspiration considering the increased incidence of gastroesophageal reflux and hiatal hernia in this patient population. Furthermore, gastric acidity, gastric fluid volume, and intragastric pressure are likely to be increased. The massive amount of soft tissue about the head and upper trunk can impair mandibular and cervical mobility, making maintenance of a patent upper airway and intubation of the trachea difficult. For these reasons, the preoperative administration of an H_2-receptor antagonist or metoclopramide, or both, may be considered in the hope of increasing gastric fluid pH and decreasing gastric fluid volume. In addition, rapid induction of anesthesia followed by prompt intubation of the trachea with a cuffed tube is often selected to minimize the risk of pulmonary aspiration. In prospectively selected patients, awake intubation of the trachea, most often with a fiberoptic laryngoscope, may be indicated. The decreased functional residual capacity predisposes the obese patient to a rapid decrease in PaO_2 during any period of apnea such as may accompany direct laryngoscopy for intubation of the trachea (Fig. 22-1).[15] This risk of rapid decreases in PaO_2 emphasizes the importance of maximizing the oxygen content of

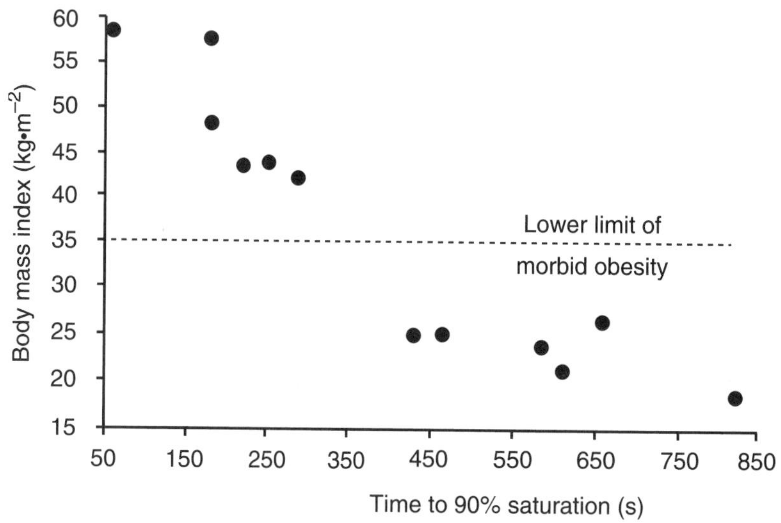

Figure 22-1. Arterial oxygen saturation decreases to 90% more rapidly in morbidly obese patients as quantitated by the body mass index. (From Berthoud et al.,[15] with permission.)

the lung before initiating direct laryngoscopy and of monitoring peripheral arterial hemoglobin oxygen saturation continuously with a pulse oximeter. A decrease in the functional residual capacity also decreases the mixing time for any inhaled drug, thus accelerating the rate of increase in the alveolar concentration of that drug.

The impact of obesity on the necessary dose of injected drugs is difficult to assess. Blood volume is often increased in obese patients, which would tend to decrease the plasma concentrations achieved with single rapid intravenous injections of drugs such as thiopental. Conversely, adipose tissue has a low blood flow such that increased doses calculated on an absolute weight basis in obese patients could result in exposure of well-perfused tissues to excessive concentrations of drugs. Perhaps the most logical approach is to calculate the initial doses on an ideal rather than actual body weight. Subsequent doses would be based on the patient's observed responses. Repeated injections of drugs, however, could result in cumulative effects and prolonged responses reflecting storage of lipid soluble drugs in adipose tissue for subsequent release into the circulation as the plasma concentrations of drugs decline.

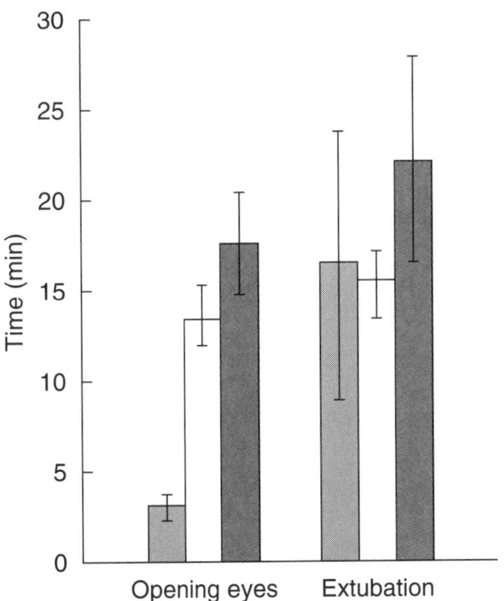

Figure 22-2. Awakening times (mean ± SE) were measured in obese patients anesthetized with nitrous oxide plus fentanyl (gray bars), enflurane (white bars), or halothane (red bars) for gastric stapling operations. The time to opening eyes on request was shortest in patients receiving fentanyl, whereas the time to extubation of the trachea was similar in all three anesthesia study groups. (From Cork et al.,[16] with permission.)

Maintenance of Anesthesia

The preferred choice of drugs or techniques for maintenance of anesthesia in obese patients is not clear. An increased incidence of fatty liver infiltration suggests caution in selection of drugs associated with postoperative liver dysfunction. Increased defluorination of volatile anesthetics in obese patients, however, has not been shown to result in hepatic or renal dysfunction. The possibility of prolonged responses to drugs stored in fat (volatile anesthetics, opioids, barbiturates) is not supported by delayed awakening from anesthesia in obese patients (Fig. 22-2).[16] Controlled ventilation of the lungs using a large tidal volume acts to offset the decreases in functional residual capacity and PaO_2 that accompany obesity and may be accentuated by anesthesia.

The selection of spinal or epidural anesthesia is limited in obese patients because bony landmarks are obscured and the level of anesthesia that will be produced by a given dose of drug is difficult to predict.

Postoperative Care

The semisitting position is often used in the postoperative care of obese patients to optimize the mechanics of breathing and to minimize the development of arterial hypoxemia. Arterial oxygenation should be closely monitored as with pulse oximetry and supplemental oxygen administered, remembering that the maximum decrease in PaO_2 typically occurs 2 to 3 days postoperatively. The likelihood of deep vein thrombosis and the risk of pulmonary embolism are increased, emphasizing the possible importance of early postoperative ambulation.

MALNUTRITION

Caloric support, in the presence of increased energy requirements, is commonly provided by enteral or total parenteral nutrition (hyperalimentation). It is often recommended that patients who have lost more than 20% of their body weight should be treated nutritionally before elective surgery.[17] Patients who are unable to eat or absorb food 1 week postoperatively may require parenteral nutrition.

Enteral Nutrition

The gastrointestinal tract is the site used for nutritional supplementation whenever possible. Enteral nutrition is delivered as a continuous infusion (100 to 120 $ml \cdot h^{-1}$) via a nasogastric or orogastric tube. Complications of enteral feedings are infrequent but may include hyperglycemia leading to osmotic diuresis and hypovolemia. Therefore, blood glucose concentrations should be monitored and exogenous insulin administration considered when hyperglycemia (higher than 250 $mg \cdot dl^{-1}$) occurs. The high osmolarity (550 to 850 $mOsm \cdot L^{-1}$) of elemental diets is often a cause of diarrhea.

Total Parenteral Nutrition

Total parenteral nutrition is indicated when the gastrointestinal tract is not functioning. Total parenteral nutrition with an isotonic solution delivered through a large peripheral vein is acceptable when the patient requires less than 2000 calories per day and the anticipated need for nutritional support is shorter than 2 weeks. When caloric requirements are higher than 2000 calories per day or prolonged nutritional support is required, a venous catheter is placed in the subclavian vein to permit infusion of a hypertonic parenteral solution (about 1900 $mOsm \cdot L^{-1}$) in a daily volume of about 40 $ml \cdot kg^{-1}$.

Adverse Effects

Potential adverse effects of total parenteral nutrition are numerous. Blood glucose concentrations are monitored; hyperglycemia (higher than 250 $mg \cdot dl^{-1}$) may require treatment with exogenous insulin, whereas hypoglycemia may occur if the parenteral nutrition solution infusion is abruptly discontinued (mechanical obstruction in delivery tubing) but increased circulating endogenous concentrations of insulin persist. A reason for considering a decrease in the infusion rate prior to induction of anesthesia is to avoid the possibility of plasma hyperosmolarity developing intraoperatively. Likewise, it may be appropriate to decrease the infusion rate of maintenance fluids so as to minimize the risk of fluid overload. Indeed, parenteral feeding of patients with compromised cardiac function is associated with the risk of congestive heart failure owing to fluid overload. Hyperchloremic metabolic acidosis may occur because of the liberation of hydrochloric acid during the metabolism of amino acids present in most parenteral nutrition solutions. Increased production of carbon dioxide resulting from metabolism of large amounts of glucose may result in the need to initiate mechanical ventilation of the lungs or failure to wean a patient from long-term ventilatory support.[18] Parenteral nutrition solution can support growth of bacteria and fungi, and catheter-related sepsis is a constant threat. In view of the risk of contamination, use of a hyperalimentation catheter for administration of medications, withdrawal of blood samples, or monitoring of central venous pressure as during the perioperative period is not recommended. Electrolyte abnormalities owing to total parenteral nutrition are detected by preoperative measurement of plasma electrolyte concentrations.

Adverse Effects of Total Parenteral Nutrition

Hyperglycemia
Hypoglycemia
Fluid overload
Increased carbon dioxide production
Catheter-related sepsis
Electrolyte abnormalities, (hypokalemia, hypocalcemia, hypophosphatemia, hypomagenesemia)
Hepatic dysfunction
Renal dysfunction
Thrombosis of central veins

ENDOCRINE AND METABOLIC CHANGES IN THE PERIOPERATIVE PERIOD

Surgical stimulation produces profound endocrine and metabolic responses that parallel the magnitude of the operative trauma.[19] Conversely, inhaled or injected drugs used to produce anesthesia result in minimal effects on hormone secretion in the absence of surgical stimulation. An exception to this statement is etomidate, which interferes with the synthesis of cortisol in the adrenal cortex.

The initial endocrine response to surgical stimulation is an increase in the circulating concentrations of cortisol and catecholamines and a decrease in the plasma concentrations of insulin despite hyperglycemia. In view of the latter, excessive infusion of glucose via intravenous solutions could result in intraoperative hyperglycemia.

Surgical trauma evokes protein degradation as reflected by loss of lean body weight and increased urinary excretion of nitrogen postoperatively. Sodium and water retention and excretion of potassium in the postoperative period presumably reflect release of antidiuretic hormone and activation of the renin-angiotensin-aldosterone system.

Although it is difficult to quantitate adverse effects produced by endocrine and metabolic responses to surgical stimulation, it would seem prudent to minimize the magnitude and duration of these changes whenever possible. Attenuation or prevention of the endocrine responses to surgery can be produced by afferent neuronal blockade, as with regional anesthesia (T4 sensory level) or by inhibition of hypothalamic function with large doses of opioids. It is likely, however, that regional anesthesia merely postpones endocrine responses to surgery until the postoperative period. Furthermore, the concept that the administration of the lowest dose of anesthetic is best may not be valid during periods of acute surgical stimulation.[20]

REFERENCES

1. Watkins PJ. Diabetic autonomic neuropathy. N Engl J Med 1990;322:1078–9.
2. Burgos LG, Ebert TJ, Asiddao C, et al. Increased intraoperative morbidity in diabetics with autonomic neuropathy. Anesthesiology 1989;70:591–7.
3. Lucas LF, Tsueda K. Cardiovascular depression after brachial plexus block in two diabetic patients with renal failure. Anesthesiology 1990;73:1032–5.
4. Hirsch IB, Magill JB, Cryer PE, White PF. Perioperative management of surgical patients with diabetes mellitus. Anesthesiology 1991;74:346–59.
5. Thorne AC, Bedord RF. Esmolol for perioperative management of thyrotoxic goiter. Anesthesiology 1989;71:291–4.
6. Berman ML, Khunert L, Phythyon JM, Holaday DA. Isoflurane and enflurane-induced hepatic necrosis in triiodothyronine-pretreated rats. Anesthesiology 1983;58:1–5.
7. Seino H, Dohi S, Aiyoshi Y, et al. Postoperative hepatic dysfunction after halothane or enflurane anesthesia in patients with hyperthyroidism. Anesthesiology 1986;64:122–5.
8. Babab AA, Eger EI II. The effects of hyperthyroidism and hypothyroidism on halothane and oxygen requirements in dogs. Anesthesiology 1968;29:1087–93.
9. Cooper DS. Subclinical hypothyroidism. JAMA 1987; 258:246–7.
10. Weinberg AB, Berman MD, Gorman CA, Marsch HM, O'Fallon WM. Outcome of anesthesia and surgery in hypothyroid patients. Arch Intern Med 1983;143: 893–7.
11. Murkin JM. Anesthesia and hypothyroidism: A review of thyroxine physiology, pharmacology, and anesthetic implications. Anesth Analg 1982;61:371–83.
12. Mogensen T, Hjortso NC. Acute hypothyroidism in a severely ill surgical patient. Can J Anaesth 1988;35: 74–5.
13. Symreng T, Karlberg BE, Kagedal B, Schildt B. Physiological cortisol substitution of long-term steroid-treated patients undergoing major surgery. Br J Anaesth 1981;53:949–53.
14. Pullerits J, Ein S, Balfe JW. Anaesthesia for phaeochromocytoma. Can J Anaesth 1988;35:526–34.
15. Berthoud MC, Peacock JE, Reilly CS. Effectiveness of preoxygenation in morbidly obese patients. Br J Anaesth 1991;67:464–6.
16. Cork RC, Vaughn RW, Bentley JB. General anesthesia for morbidly obese patients—An examination of postoperative outcomes. Anesthesiology 1981;54:310–3.
17. Powell-Tuck J, Goode AW. Principles of enteral and parenteral nutrition. Br J Anaesth 1981;53:169–80.
18. Askanzi J, Nordenstrom J, Rosenbaum SH, et al. Nutrition for the patient with respiratory failure: Glucose vs. fat. Anesthesiology 1981;54:373–7.
19. Traymor C, Hall GM. Endocrine and metabolic changes during surgery: Anaesthetic implications. Br J Anaesth 1981;53:153–60.
20. Roizen MF, Horrigan RW, Frazer BM. Anesthetic doses blocking adrenergic (stress) and cardiovascular responses to incision-MAC BAR. Anesthesiology 1981;54:390–8.

23

Central Nervous System Disease

Anesthesia for surgical treatment of central nervous system disease requires an understanding of relationships between cerebral blood flow (CBF), cerebral metabolic rate for oxygen ($CMRO_2$), and intracranial pressure (ICP). Physiologic and pharmacologic influences, which are often under the control of the anesthesiologist, may alter the fragile relationship between CBF, $CMRO_2$, and ICP. Indeed, the selection of drugs, the technique of ventilation of the lungs, and the choice of monitors have uniquely important implications in the care of patients with disease involving the central nervous system.

INTRACRANIAL TUMORS

Intracranial tumors occur most often in patients 40 to 60 years old, with initial signs and symptoms reflecting increases in ICP. Seizures that appear in adult years suggest the presence of an intracranial tumor. Eventually, the presence of an intracranial tumor is confirmed by specific diagnostic tests, most often computed tomography or magnetic resonance imaging.

Management of Anesthesia

Management of anesthesia for removal of an intracranial tumor is designed to prevent undesirable changes in CBF or ICP.

Cerebral Blood Flow

Determinants of CBF include (1) PaO_2, (2) $PaCO_2$, (3) cerebral perfusion pressure and autoregulation, and (4) anesthetic drugs (Fig. 23-1). Cerebral blood vessels receive innervation from the autonomic nervous system, but the impact on CBF seems to be minimal. The role of $CMRO_2$ is emphasized by decreases in CBF of about 7% for every 1°C decrease in body temperature below 37°C.

$PaCO_2$. Changes in $PaCO_2$ produce corresponding directional changes in CBF. As a guide, CBF (normal 50 $ml \cdot 100\ g^{-1} \cdot min^{-1}$) increases or decreases 1 $ml \cdot 100\ g^{-1} \cdot min^{-1}$ for every 1-mmHg increase or decrease of $PaCO_2$ from 40 mmHg. These changes in CBF reflect the impact of carbon dioxide mediated alterations in pH, leading to dilation or constriction of cerebral arterioles. The ability of decreases in $PaCO_2$ to lower CBF and ICP is the basis of neuroanesthesia.

The influence of $PaCO_2$ on local CBF may be altered by the acidosis that often surrounds intracranial tumors. For example, acid metabolites from tumors cause vasomotor paralysis in surrounding vessels, leading to maximal vasodilation and increased local blood flow (luxury perfusion). If $PaCO_2$ increases, normal vessels but not vessels surrounding tumors will dilate, and blood flow could be diverted to normal areas (intracranial steal syndrome). Conversely, hyperventilation of the lungs to lower the $PaCO_2$ might constrict normal vessels, thus diverting blood flow to diseased or ischemic areas of the brain (reverse steal syndrome). The relative importance of these steal syndromes is not established.

PaO_2. Decreases in PaO_2 do not produce significant increases in CBF until a threshold value of about 50 mmHg is present.

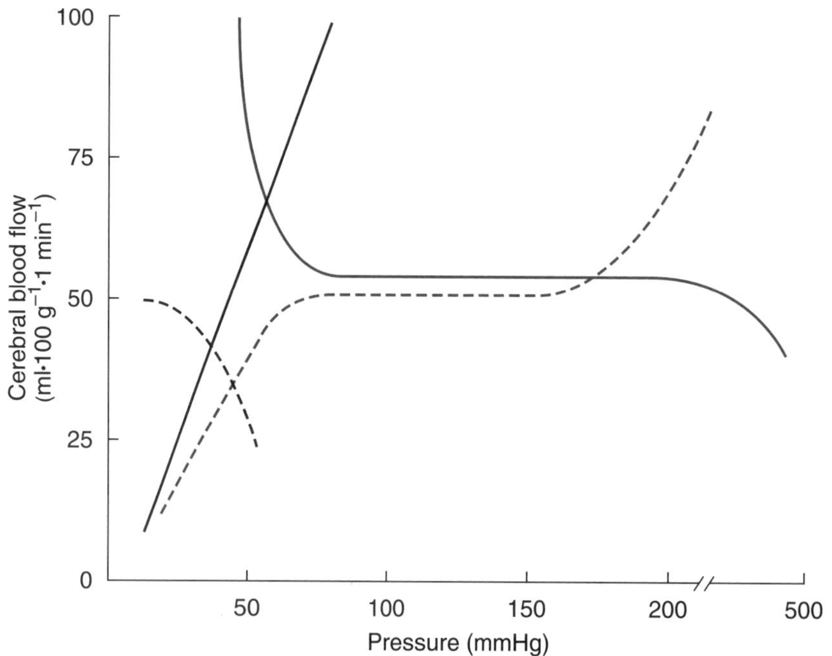

Figure 23-1. Schematic depiction of the impact of intracranial pressure (dashed black line), PaO_2 (solid red line), $PaCO_2$ (solid black line), and mean arterial pressure (dashed red line) on cerebral blood flow.

Cerebral Perfusion Pressure and Autoregulation. Cerebral perfusion pressure is the difference between mean arterial pressure and right atrial pressure or ICP, whichever is greater. Nevertheless, CBF remains relatively constant between mean arterial pressures of 60 and 150 mmHg, reflecting autoregulation. Below or above this range of autoregulation, CBF is directly related to mean arterial pressure. Chronic hypertension shifts the autoregulation curve to the right such that higher mean arterial pressures are tolerated before CBF becomes pressure dependent. Autoregulation of CBF is impaired in the presence of intracranial tumors or volatile anesthetics.

Anesthetic Drugs. Volatile anesthetics administered during normocapnia in concentrations higher than 0.6 MAC are potent cerebral vasodilators (halothane > enflurane and desflurane > isoflurane) and produce dose-dependent increases in CBF (Fig. 23-2).[1] These increases in CBF occur despite concomitant decreases in $CMRO_2$ (greater with isoflurane than halothane).[2] Nitrous oxide is a cerebral vasodilator, but limitation of its dose usually to lower than 0.7 MAC seems to minimize associated increases in CBF. Ketamine is a potent cerebral vasodilator, increasing CBF more than 60% despite normocap-

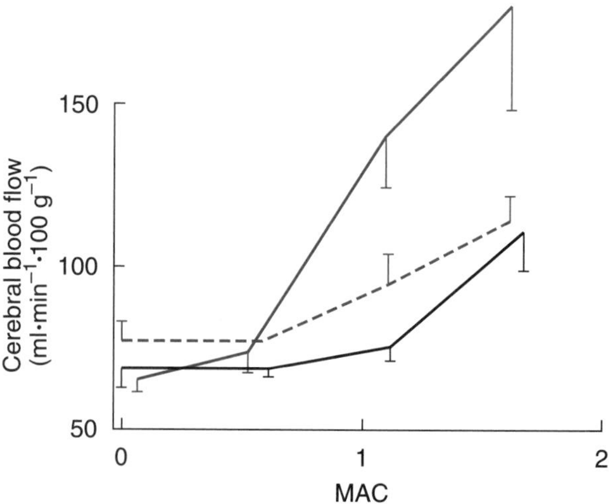

Figure 23-2. Volatile anesthetics administered during normocapnia in doses higher than 0.6 MAC are potent cerebral vasodilators and produce dose-dependent increases in CBF. These drug-induced increases in CBF are greatest with halothane (solid red line), intermediate with enflurane (dashed red line), and least with isoflurane (black line). (From Eger,[1] with permission.)

nia. Drug-induced cerebral vasodilation and associated increases in CBF predictably increases ICP in patients with intracranial tumors. In normal patients, compensatory mechanisms, including displacement of cerebrospinal fluid from the cranium, prevent increases in ICP. Thiopental decreases both $CMRO_2$ and CBF (cerebral vasoconstriction), which accounts for its ability to decrease ICP. Propofol apparently has similar properties when compared with thiopental. Etomidate decreases $CMRO_2$ and to a lesser degree CBF but produces myoclonus and occasionally seizure activity. Benzodiazepines do not significantly increase ICP. Opioids usually do not significantly increase ICP, although they may modestly and transiently increase ICP in head trauma patients (Fig. 23-3).[3]

Pressure-Volume Compliance Curves

Pressure-volume compliance curves reflect changes produced by expanding intracranial tumors (Fig. 23-4). Eventually, a point on the curve is reached where even small increases in intracranial volume, as produced by drug-induced cerebral vasodilation and increased CBF, result in marked increases in ICP.

Intracranial Pressure

Marked increases in ICP can so decrease cerebral perfusion pressure that CBF is dangerously decreased. A normal ICP is lower than 15 mmHg. In patients with intracranial tumors, ICP is commonly monitored so as to recognize sudden and often unexpected increases in ICP and thus facilitate prompt and aggressive interventions to lower ICP. Methods to decrease ICP include (1) elevation of the head to encourage venous drainage; (2) hyperventilation of the lungs; (3) cerebrospinal fluid drainage; and (4) administration of drugs, including osmotic diuretics, renal tubular diuretics, corticosteroids, and barbiturates (see Chapter 33). The duration of the efficacy of hyperventilation of the

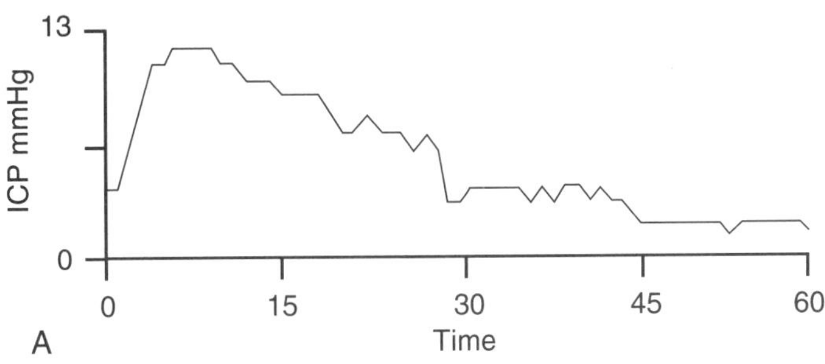

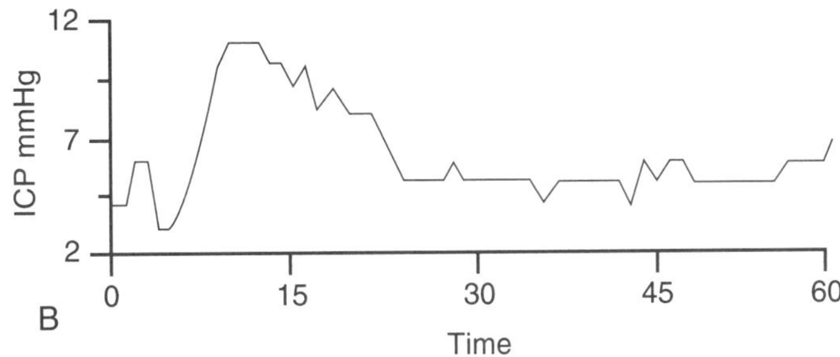

Figure 23-3. The time course (minutes) of the intracranial pressure (ICP) in a single-head-injury patient following the administration (0 minute) of *(A)* fentanyl (3 $\mu g \cdot kg^{-1}$ IV) or *(B)* sufentanil (0.6 $\mu g \cdot kg^{-1}$ IV). (From Sperry et al.,[3] with permission.)

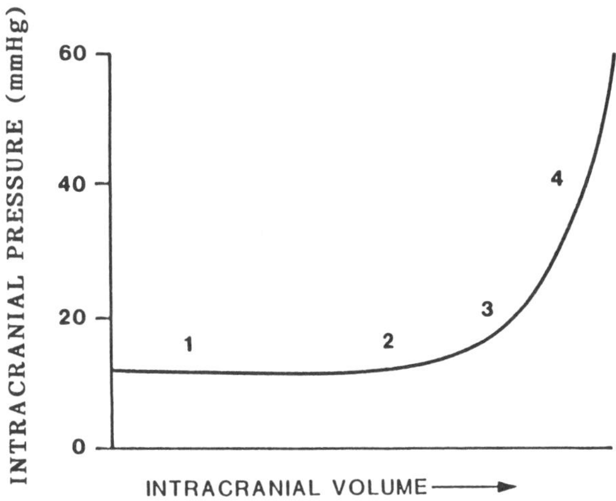

Figure 23-4. The pressure-volume compliance curve depicts the impact of increasing intracranial volume on intracranial pressure (ICP). As volume increases from point 1 to point 2 on the curve, the ICP does not increase because cerebrospinal fluid is shifted from the cranium into the spinal subarachnoid space. Patients with intracranial tumors but between point 1 and point 2 on the compliance curve are unlikely to manifest clinical symptoms of increased ICP. Patients who are on the rising portion of the pressure-volume curve (point 3) can no longer compensate for increases in intracranial volume, and ICP begins to increase. Clinical symptoms due to increased ICP are likely. Additional increases in volume at this point, as produced by increased CBF during anesthesia, can precipitate abrupt increases in ICP (point 4).

lungs for decreasing ICP is unknown. In volunteers, however, the effect of hyperventilation wanes with time and CBF returns to normal after about 6 hours.

Preoperative Preparation

Evidence of increased ICP is sought during the preoperative visit. Preoperative medication that produces sedation or depression of ventilation is usually avoided. For example, drug-induced depression of ventilation can lead to increased $PaCO_2$ and subsequent increases in CBF and ICP. Nevertheless, in otherwise alert patients, small doses of benzodiazepines may provide useful anxiety relief.

Induction of Anesthesia

Induction of anesthesia is generally achieved with intravenous administration of drugs (thiopental 4 to 6 $mg{\cdot}kg^{-1}$, or equivalent doses of etomidate, propofol, or midazolam) that produce reliable onset of anesthesia and are unlikely to increase ICP. These drugs are followed by intravenous administration of nondepolarizing muscle relaxants or succinylcholine (may produce transient increases in ICP) to facilitate mechanical ventilation of the lungs and to produce skeletal muscle relaxation for intubation of the trachea. The trachea is intubated when intense skeletal muscle paralysis is confirmed by a peripheral nerve stimulator. If paralysis is not intense, reaction to the tracheal tube (attempted coughing) may result in marked increases in ICP. Administration of additional intravenous doses of thiopental, opioids, or lidocaine just before beginning direct laryngoscopy may be effective in attenuating the increases in arterial blood pressure and ICP that may accompany intubation of the trachea (Fig. 23-5).[4] After intubation of the trachea, the patient's lungs are mechanically ventilated at a rate and tidal volume sufficient to maintain the $PaCO_2$ between 25 and 30 mmHg. There is no evidence of additional therapeutic benefit when the $PaCO_2$ is decreased below this recommended range. Positive end-expiratory pressure is not encouraged as this could impair cerebral venous drainage and increase ICP.

Preoperative Evidence of Increased Intracranial Pressure

Nausea and vomiting
Hypertension
Bradycardia
Personality change
Altered levels of consciousness
Altered patterns of breathing
Papilledema
Seizures

Maintenance of Anesthesia

Maintenance of anesthesia is often achieved with nitrous oxide plus opioids, benzodiazepines, and/or barbiturates. Volatile anesthetics may be avoided because of their ability to increase CBF and to interfere with autoregulation of CBF. Nevertheless, low concentrations of volatile anesthetics (less than 0.6 MAC) may be useful for preventing or treating increases in blood pressure evoked by surgical stimulation. The minimal effects of isoflurane

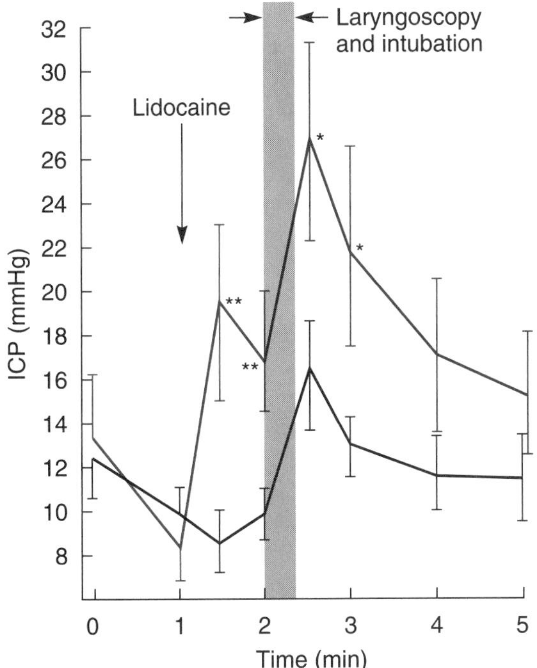

Figure 23-5. Increases in intracranial pressure (ICP) in response to laryngoscopy and intubation of the trachea are attenuated by administration of intravenous (black line) but not laryngotracheal (red line) lidocaine. $^{**}P < 0.05$ versus intravenous group; $^{*}P < 0.05$ versus control. Mean ± SE. (From Hamill et al.,[4] with permission.)

on CBF plus the acceptability of initiating hyperventilation of the lungs simultaneously with introduction of this drug (halothane should be preceded by hyperventilation of the lungs) make isoflurane a useful volatile anesthetic in patients undergoing intracranial operations. Peripheral vasodilating drugs (nitroprusside, nitroglycerin, trimethaphan) increase CBF and ICP despite causing simultaneous decreases in blood pressure. Therefore, use of these drugs before opening the dura is not encouraged in patients with increased ICP.

Skeletal muscle movement is hazardous during intracranial procedures as it can lead to increases in ICP, bleeding in the operative site, and a brain that bulges into the operative site, making surgical exposure difficult. Therefore, in addition to an adequate depth of anesthesia, it is common to maintain skeletal muscle paralysis during intracranial surgery.

Cerebral Swelling. If cerebral swelling occurs despite hyperventilation of the lungs, it may be useful to administer drugs designed to decrease brain water content. Mannitol (0.25 to 1 $g \cdot kg^{-1}$ IV) or furosemide (0.5 to 1 $mg \cdot kg^{-1}$ IV) is effective in decreasing cerebral swelling and improving surgical exposure (see Chapter 33). Intermittent intravenous injections of thiopental may also be useful in decreasing ICP. If surgically possible, placing the patient in a head-up position may be beneficial in decreasing ICP.

Fluid Therapy. Fluid infusions should be minimal (1 to 3 $ml \cdot kg^{-1} \cdot h^{-1}$) so as to avoid increases in brain water content and increased ICP. Glucose-in-water solutions are not recommended since they are rapidly distributed throughout body water. If blood glucose concentrations decrease more rapidly than brain glucose concentrations, brain water becomes hyperosmolar such that water enters and cerebral edema results. Furthermore, increased blood glucose concentrations may be associated with increased neuronal cell injury should cerebral ischemia occur. Therefore, isotonic or even hypertonic crystalloid solutions are recommended. Colloids such as 5% albumin or hetastarch are also acceptable replacement fluids.

Monitors

Continuous monitoring of blood pressure via a catheter in a peripheral artery is recommended, as is measurement of exhaled carbon dioxide concentrations. A continuous monitor of ICP is helpful but cannot be considered a routine monitor in every patient undergoing intracranial surgery. The electrocardiogram allows prompt detection of cardiac dysrhythmias due to surgical stimulation of vital medullary centers. Neuromuscular blockade is monitored with a peripheral nerve stimulator. A bladder catheter is necessary if drug-induced diuresis is planned during the operation. A central venous pressure catheter is useful for guiding fluid administration and aspiration of air from the heart should venous air embolism occur during surgery (see the section *Venous Air Embolism*).

Awakening

On awakening from anesthesia, coughing or straining by the patient must be avoided as these responses will increase ICP. For this reason, it may be advisable to extubate the trachea with the patient still anesthetized. Also, prior intravenous administration of thiopental or lidocaine, or both, may further decrease the likelihood of coughing during extubation of the trachea. Delayed return of consciousness postoperatively or neurologic deterioration in the postoperative period is often evaluated by computed tomography or magnetic resonance imaging. Tension pneumocephalus as a cause of neurologic deterioration is a consideration if nitrous oxide was administered during anesthesia.

Venous Air Embolism

Patients undergoing surgery for resection of intracranial tumors are at increased risk of venous air embolism, not only because the operative site is often above the level of the heart, but also because veins in the cut edge of bone constituting the skull may not collapse when transected. Presumably, air enters the right ventricle, leading to interference with blood flow into the pulmonary artery. Pulmonary edema and reflex bronchoconstriction may result from movement of air into the pulmonary circulation. Death is usually due to cardiovascular collapse and arterial hypoxemia. Air may reach the coronary and cerebral circulations (paradoxical air embolism) by crossing a patent foramen ovale (probe patent foramen ovale is present in up to 25% of adults) or by traversing the pulmonary circulation.

Detection. A Doppler transducer placed over the right heart (over the second or third intercostal space to the right of the sternum) is the most sensitive indicator of the presence of intracardiac air.[5] Sudden decreases in end-exhaled concentrations of carbon dioxide reflect increased deadspace due to continued ventilation of alveoli no longer being perfused because of obstruction of their vascular supply by air. An increase in end-tidal nitrogen concentrations may reflect nitrogen from venous air embolism. During controlled ventilation of the lungs, sudden attempts (gasps) by patients to initiate spontaneous breaths may be the first indication of the occurrence of venous air embolism. Hypotension, tachycardia, cardiac dysrhythmias, cyanosis, and "mill-wheel" murmur are late signs of venous air embolism.

Treatment. Venous air embolism is treated by (1) aspiration of air through a right atrial catheter and (2) irrigation of the operative site with fluid, as well as by applying occlusive material to all bone edges so as to occlude sites of venous air entry. A right atrial catheter with the tip positioned at the junction of the superior vena cava with the right atrium seems to provide the most rapid aspiration of air.[6] A pulmonary artery catheter, because of its small lumen size and slow blood return, is not uniquely useful for aspirating air but may provide additional evidence that venous air embolism has occurred because of increases in pulmonary artery pressure. Nitrous oxide is promptly discontinued to avoid the risk of increasing the size of venous air bubbles due to the diffusion of this gas into the air bubbles. Despite the logic of positive end-expiratory pressure to decrease entrainment of air, the efficacy of this maneuver has not been confirmed. Furthermore, positive end-expiratory pressure could reverse the pressure gradient between the left and right atria and predispose to passage of air across a patent foramen ovale. Cardiovascular collapse may require treatment with positive inotropic drugs (see Chapter 3).

CAROTID ENDARTERECTOMY

Carotid endarterectomy is the most commonly performed surgical procedure for treatment of patients with histories of transient ischemic attacks or an occlusive lesion of greater than 70% in the carotid artery.[7] Special attention should be given preoperatively to these patients' cardiovascular (coronary artery disease, hypertension) and neurologic (transient ischemic attacks) status. These observations will allow proper interpretation of postoperative complications that may be related to co-existing conditions rather than perioperative events. The goal during management of anesthesia for carotid endarterectomy surgery is to maintain cerebral perfusion pressure and CBF. The critical period during surgery is cross-clamping of the diseased carotid artery, when the patient is dependent on collateral circulation for perfusion of the ipsilateral brain. Rather than relying on collateral circulation, some surgeons routinely place an intraluminal shunt across the surgically clamped carotid artery. Alternatively, a shunt may be placed only when monitors (electroencephalogram, somatosensory evoked potentials, stump pressure, transcranial Doppler) suggest the likelihood of cerebral ischemia (see Chapter 15). Stump pressure is the pressure in the carotid artery distal to the surgical clamp. Therefore, stump pressure reflects transmitted pressure via the circle of Willis and implies adequate (higher than 60 mmHg) or inadequate collateral circulation (Fig. 23-6).[8] It must be appreciated that variations in cerebral vascular resistance (increased by barbiturates and decreased by volatile drugs) influence interpretation of stump pressure.

Choice of Anesthesia

Anesthesia for carotid endarterectomy surgery can be performed with local or general anesthesia. The choice of local or general anesthesia has not been confirmed to alter morbidity or mortality after this operation.

Local Anesthesia

Local anesthesia includes a cervical plexus block combined with regional infiltration of local anesthetic (see Chapter 13). This approach provides the advantage of being able to monitor cerebral function of the awake patient by voice contact when the carotid artery is occluded. Nevertheless, strokes still can occur postoperatively despite the apparent maintenance of normal cerebral function intraoperatively.

General Anesthesia

General anesthesia is acceptably produced by intravenous injection of barbiturates, benzodiazepines, etomidate, or propofol followed by administration of nitrous oxide plus volatile drugs or opioids for maintenance of anesthesia. Skeletal muscle paralysis is often produced to allow decreases in the depth of anesthesia in response to hypotension without introducing the possibility of unwanted patient movement. Although differences among volatile anesthetics as regards neurologic outcome after carotid endarterectomy surgery are not detectable, it is possible that isoflurane offers some brain protection if volatile anesthetics are selected for maintenance of anesthesia (Fig. 23-7).[9] Nevertheless, thiopental remains the appropriate drug to select in specific circumstances where pharmacologic brain protection is indicated. In this regard, it may be reasonable to administer thiopental (3 to 6 $mg \cdot kg^{-1}$ IV) immediately before clamping the carotid artery. Despite this practice, no data show that barbiturates used in this manner reduce morbidity after carotid endarterectomy.

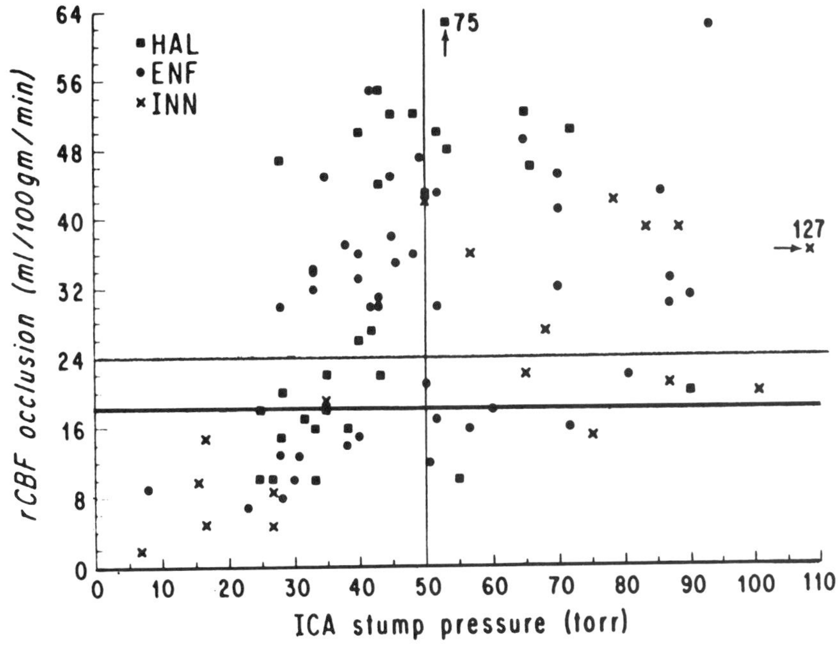

Figure 23-6. Stump pressures in the internal carotid artery (ICA) higher than 60 mmHg (torr) are associated with regional cerebral blood flows (rCBF) higher than 18 $ml \cdot 100\ g^{-1} \cdot min^{-1}$ in most patients anesthetized with nitrous oxide plus halothane (HAL), enflurane (ENF), or Innovar (INN). (From McKay et al.,[8] with permission.)

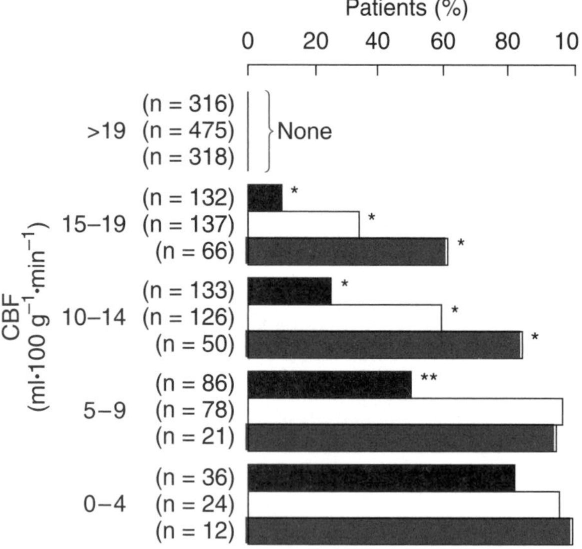

Figure 23-7. Percentage of patients developing evidence of cerebral ischemia on the electroencephalogram (EEG) at different cerebral blood flows (CBF) during inhalation of three different anesthetics. Critical CBF (the CBF below which most patients develop EEG signs of ischemia within 3 minutes of carotid occlusion) is lowest with isoflurane (black bars) (implies brain protection), intermediate with enflurane (white bars), and highest during inhalation of halothane (red bars). *Significantly different from each other; **significantly different from the other two. (From Michenfelder et al.,[9] with permission.)

Regardless of the drugs selected for anesthesia, the goal must be to maintain arterial blood pressure in a normal range for that patient. When decreases in blood pressure below the normal range do not respond to decreases in concentrations of anesthetic drugs, it may be necessary to return blood pressure to a normal level by the continuous intravenous infusion of a sympathomimetic drug such as phenylephrine. Sustained increases of blood pressure above normal levels are undesirable since hypertension may contribute to cerebral edema, particularly in diseased areas of the brain with altered ability to autoregulate CBF. Furthermore, hypertension increases myocardial oxygen requirements and may contribute to myocardial ischemia in patients with coronary artery disease.

Ventilation of the lungs during carotid endarterectomy surgery is performed with a tidal volume and breathing rate that maintain $PaCO_2$ near 35 mmHg. Manipulation of $PaCO_2$ in attempts to alter CBF by vasodilation of vasoconstriction is not recommended (see the section *Cerebral Blood Flow*).

Postoperative Problems

Postoperative problems after carotid endarterectomy surgery include (1) lability of blood pressure, (2) airway compression due to hematoma formation at the operative site, (3) loss of carotid body function, (4) myocardial infarction, and (5) stroke. Hypertension is common, especially in previously hypertensive patients, and may require treatment with peripheral vasodilators such as nitroprusside. The mechanism for hypertension is not known but may reflect altered activity of the carotid sinus or loss of carotid sinus function due to denervation at the time of surgery. Likewise, hypotension may be due to increased nerve activity perceived by a carotid sinus previously shielded by an atheromatous plaque. Unilateral loss of carotid body function is not likely to alter the patient's ventilatory response to hypoxemia.

INTRACRANIAL ANEURYSMS

Intracranial aneurysms that rupture are the most common cause of intracranial hemorrhage. These aneurysms usually present as headache, nausea, vomiting, focal neurologic signs, and/or depressed consciousness. Electrocardiographic changes may include sinus bradycardia or T wave changes that mimic myocardial ischemia.[10] Vasospasm of the cerebral arteries generally occurs 5 to 7 days after bleeding and is a major cause of morbidity. Treatment of vasospasm includes increasing cerebral perfusion pressure by increasing cardiac output (intravenous administration of fluids or inotropic drugs, or both) and possibly by the administration of a calcium entry blocker (nimodipine, nicardipine).[11]

Management of Anesthesia

Management of anesthesia for resection of an intracranial aneurysm is designed to (1) prevent increases in arterial blood pressure and (2) facilitate surgical exposure and control of the aneurysm. Preoperative medication is desirable to decrease anxiety but must be titrated to prevent hypoventilation and associated increases in CBF. Induction of anesthesia and maintenance of anesthesia must be designed to minimize arterial blood pressure increases evoked by noxious stimulation, especially during direct laryngoscopy for intubation of the trachea.

Controlled Hypotension

Surgical exposure and control of an intracranial aneurysm are facilitated by production of controlled hypotension. The duration of controlled hypotension may be brief, corresponding to isolation and clamping of the aneurysm. In the presence of adequate anesthesia, as provided by volatile anesthetics, the addition of a continuous infusion of nitroprusside (seldom more than 3 $\mu g \cdot kg^{-1} \cdot min^{-1}$ IV) is usually adequate to decrease arterial blood pressure to the desired hypotensive level. The hypotensive effect of nitroprusside is easily reversed by slowing or discontinuing the drug infusion. Nitroprusside is degraded to cyanide, and arterial pH should be monitored to detect metabolic acidosis due to cyanide toxicity when high doses of nitroprusside (higher than 8 $\mu g \cdot kg^{-1} \cdot min^{-1}$ IV) are required for longer than 1 to 3 hours. Alternative drugs to nitroprusside are nitroglycerin, trimethaphan, and labetalol. Compensatory tachycardia may offset the blood pressure-lowering effects of peripheral vasodilators used to produce controlled hypotension. Beta antagonists, such as propranolol or esmolol, are useful for slowing this reflex-mediated tachycardia. Oxygenation as reflected by pulse oximetry may decrease during controlled hypotension as peripheral vasodilators may accentuate ventilation-to-perfusion mismatching. A significant disadvantage of controlled hypotension may be the associated loss of cerebral autoregulation and a possible accentuation of focal cerebral ischemia. An alternative to deliberate hypotension may be temporary occlusion of the aneurysm's afferent blood supply so as to decompress the vascular defect.

A useful guideline during controlled hypotension is that mean arterial pressure can be decreased to about 50 mmHg in previously normotensive patients. It should also be appreciated that patients will safely tolerate even lower mean arterial pressures for short periods as may be needed to place a clip on an intracranial aneurysm. The need to monitor arterial blood pressure accurately requires attention to calibration of the transducer used to measure blood pressure and recognition that proper positioning of the height of the transducer relative to heart level is crucial. For example, cerebral perfusion pressure decreases about 0.7 mmHg for every 1 cm that the head is above heart level. Therefore, if the head is elevated 20 cm above heart level, cerebral perfusion pressure will be about 14 mmHg lower than mean arterial pressure at heart level. In this regard, a useful approach is to place the transducer at brain level (external auditory canal reflects the level of the circle of Willis) when controlled hypotension is planned and the head is elevated.

SPINAL CORD TRANSECTION

Spinal cord transection is the damage to the spinal cord that manifests as paralysis of the lower extremities (paraplegia) or all the extremities (quadraplegia). Anatomically, the spinal cord is not divided, but the effect physiologically is the same as if it were transected. The most common cause of spinal cord transection is trauma.

Acute Paralysis

Patients with acute spinal cord transection who require surgery present unique problems during the management of anesthesia. For example, further damage to the spinal cord could result from extension of the head in the presence of a cervical spine fracture. Topical anesthesia and placement of a tube into the trachea of an awake patient using a fiberoptic laryngoscope is an alternative to rapid sequence induction of anesthesia. Nevertheless, there is no evidence of increased neurologic morbidity following elective or emergency orotracheal intubation in the anesthetized or awake patient with an unstable cervical spine.[12] Succinylcholine is unlikely to provoke an excessive release of potassium in the first 24 hours after acute spinal cord transection. Nevertheless, it is common practice to avoid use of this drug except when the rapid onset of short-duration skeletal muscle paralysis is considered to be necessary for protection of the patient's lungs from aspiration. The support of blood pressure and heart rate provided by pancuronium makes this drug an attractive choice if intraoperative skeletal muscle relaxation is required. Minimal concentrations of anesthetics are required, as these patients are often anesthetic in the operative area. The absence of sympathetic nervous system activity below the level of spinal cord transection makes these patients vulnerable to hypotension, particularly in response to acute changes in body posture, blood loss, or institution of positive airway pressure. Hypothermia is a hazard, as these patients tend to become poikilothermic below the spinal cord transection. Breathing is best managed by mechanical ventilation of the lungs because abdominal and intercostal muscle paralysis, combined with general anesthesia, makes maintenance of adequate spontaneous ventilation unlikely. In the early hours following spinal cord transection, these patients may be receiving high doses of corticosteroids in hopes of improving sensory and motor function.

Chronic Paralysis

The most important goal during management of anesthesia for patients with chronic transection of the spinal cord is prevention of autonomic hyperreflexia. Autonomic hyperreflexia manifests as abrupt arterial hypertension with an associated compensatory bradycardia due to activation of the carotid sinuses (Fig. 23-8). Spinal cord transection above T6 is most likely to be associated with autonomic hyperreflexia, with as many as 85% of patients manifesting this response. Autonomic hyperreflexia is initiated by cutaneous or visceral stimulation below the level of the spinal cord transection. Distension of a hollow viscus, such as the bladder, during cystoscopy is a common initiating event. Stimulation elicits reflex sympathetic nervous system activity and vasoconstriction below the level of the spinal cord transection, resulting in hypertension. Vasoconstriction and hypertension persist because vasodilatory impulses from the central nervous system cannot traverse the spinal cord to reach the area below the level of the cord transection. Spinal anesthesia is particularly effective in preventing autonomic hyperreflexia. General anesthesia with volatile anesthetics or epidural anesthesia is also effective but less so than spinal anesthesia. Treatment of hypertension with nitroprusside is necessary if autonomic hyperreflexia occurs despite preventive steps.

SLEEP APNEA SYNDROME

Sleep apnea syndrome (cessation of air flow at the mouth for longer than 10 seconds) can reflect loss of central nervous system drive to maintain ventilation (Ondine's curse) or mechanical upper airway obstruction, or both. Manifestations of sleep apnea syndrome reflect the chronic effects of intermittent

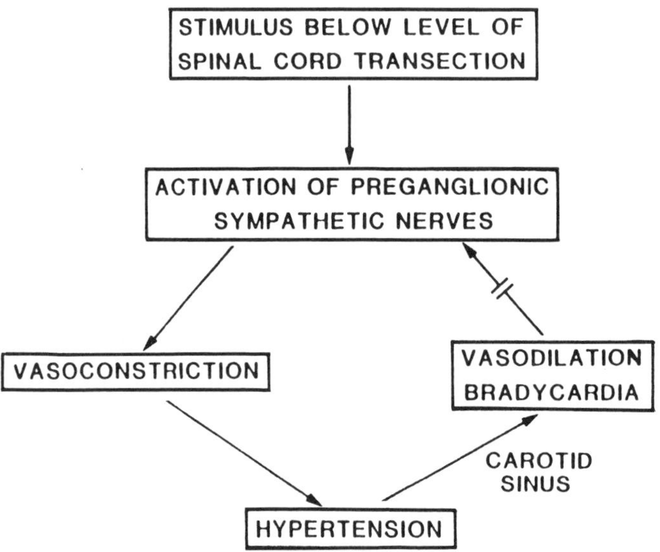

Figure 23-8. Sequence of events associated with clinical manifestations of autonomic hyperreflexia. Impulses that produce vasodilation cannot reach the neurologically isolated distal portion of the spinal cord so that vasoconstriction and hypertension persist.

apnea in these patients. Treatment of obstructive sleep apnea may include uvulopalatopharyngoplasty. Management of anesthesia in the patient with a history of sleep apnea syndrome must consider the likely exquisite sensitivity to drugs that depress ventilation and the possibility of upper airway obstruction with the induction of anesthesia.[13] Tracheal extubation in these patients is delayed until there is a full return of consciousness. Neuraxial opioids are a consideration for postoperative pain relief in an effort to minimize systemic effects of opioids on ventilation.

Manifestations of Sleep Apnea Syndrome

Hypertension
Arterial hypoxemia
Hypercarbia
Polycythemia
Cor pulmonale
Obesity
Intense snoring

REFERENCES

1. Eger EI. Isoflurane (Forane). A Compendium and Reference. Madison, WI, Anaquest, a division of BOC, Inc. 1986;1–160.
2. Muzzi DA, LoSasso TJ, Dietz NM, et al. The effect of desflurane and isoflurane on cerebrospinal fluid pressure in humans with supratentorial mass lesions. Anesthesiology 1992;76:720–4.
3. Sperry RJ, Bailey PL, Reichman MV, Peterson JC, Petersen PB, Pace NL. Fentanyl and sufentanil increase intracranial pressure in head trauma patients. Anesthesiology 1992;77:416–20.
4. Hamill JF, Bedford RF, Weave DC, Colohan AR. Lidocaine before endotracheal intubation: Intravenous or laryngotracheal? Anesthesiology 1981;55:578–81.
5. English JB, Westenskow D, Hodges MR, Stanley TH. Comparison of venous air embolism monitoring methods in supine dogs. Anesthesiology 1978; 48:425–9.
6. Bunegin L, Albin MS, Helsel PE, Hoffman A, Hung T-K. Positioning the right atrial catheter: A model for reappraisal. Anesthesiology 1981;55:343–8.
7. North American Symptomatic Carotid Endarterectomy Trial Collaborators. Beneficial effect of carotid endarterectomy in symptomatic patients with high-grade carotid stenosis. N Engl J Med 1991;325: 445–53.
8. McKay RD, Sundt TM, Michenfelder JD, et al. Internal carotid artery stump pressure and cerebral blood flow during carotid endarterectomy: Modification by halothane, enflurane and Innovar. Anesthesiology 1976;45:390–9.
9. Michenfelder JD, Sundt TM, Fode N, Sharbrough FW. Isoflurane when compared to enflurane and halothane decreases the frequency of cerebral ischemia during carotid endarterectomy. Anesthesiology 1987;67:336–40.
10. Davies KR, Gelb AW, Manninen PH, et al. Cardiac function in aneurysmal subarachnoid haemorrhage: A study of electrocardiographic and echocardiographic abnormalities. Br J Anaesth 1991;67:58–63.
11. Mohr JP. Clinical trial of nimodipine in acute ischemic stroke. Stroke 1992;23:3–8.
12. Meschino A, Devitt JH, Kock JP, Schwartz ML. The safety of awake tracheal intubation in cervical spine injury. Can J Anaesth 1992;39:114–7.
13. Hoffstein V, Zamel N. Sleep apnea and the upper airway. Br J Anaesth 1990;65:139–50.

24

Ophthalmology and Otolaryngology

Anesthesia for surgery related to ophthalmology or otolaryngology requires an appreciation of the anatomy and physiology of structures present in the operative area, as well as the unique requirements of specific operative procedures. Most of the operative procedures are elective, and often the patients represent extremes of age, being very young or elderly.

OPHTHALMOLOGY

Management of anesthesia for patients undergoing ophthalmic surgery requires an understanding of factors that influence intraocular pressure (IOP), a consideration of adverse drug interactions between ophthalmic drugs and drugs administered perioperatively, and an appreciation of the oculocardiac reflex.

Intraocular Pressure

Normal IOP is between 10 and 22 mmHg, reflecting the balance between aqueous humor formation by the ciliary body and its elimination via the canal of Schlemm. The greatest increase in IOP (as much as 35 to 50 mmHg) occurs when venous pressure is acutely increased, as during vomiting or coughing. Direct laryngoscopy for intubation of the trachea can increase IOP even in the absence of coughing or hypertension.[1] Nevertheless, an increase in IOP is most likely when coughing accompanies intubation of the trachea. Overhydration leading to increased venous pressure may increase IOP. Succinylcholine produces an average peak IOP increase of about 8 mmHg within 1 to 4 minutes following its intravenous administration; this is followed by a return to baseline within 7 minutes.[2] This ocular hypertensive response occurs whether succinylcholine is given as a single intravenous injection, as a continuous intravenous infusion, or intramuscularly. In contrast to intravenous administration of succinylcholine, it appears that intramuscular injection of succinylcholine results in a longer duration of increased IOP, necessitating about a 15-minute wait before the globe is opened. Prolonged tonic contraction of the extraocular muscles produced by succinylcholine is the most likely mechanism for the increase in IOP. Administration of nonparalyzing doses of nondepolarizing muscle relaxants (pretreatment) before the injection of succinylcholine probably attenuates but does not reliably prevent this drug-induced increase in IOP.[3] Conversely, paralyzing doses of nondepolarizing muscle relaxants in the absence of succinylcholine decrease IOP, presumably via their relaxant effects on the extraocular muscles. Inhaled anesthetics and most injected anesthetics (barbiturates, benzodiazepines, etomidate, propofol, opioids) tend to lower IOP. The effect of ketamine on IOP is controversial, but even if this drug lowers IOP its use for ophthalmic anesthesia may be considered objectionable for other reasons such as blepharospasm and nystagmus. Changes in arterial blood pressure or the $PaCO_2$ within a normal physiologic range have minimal effect on IOP.

Carbonic anhydrase inhibitors (acetazolamide) and osmotic diuretics (mannitol, urea, glycerin) are used in the perioperative period to acutely decrease IOP. Acetazolamide lowers IOP by interfering with the secretion of aqueous humor. Glycerin is effective orally but introduces the hazard of an increased gastric fluid volume in the perioperative period.

Adverse Drug Interactions

Ophthalmic medications applied topically to the cornea may undergo sufficient absorption to produce systemic effects. Unexpected drug interactions during and after surgery may reflect systemic effects of these drugs. For example, topical application of a beta antagonist, timolol, to treat glaucoma has been associated with bradycardia and bronchospasm.[4] Timolol has been implicated in the exacerbation of myasthenia gravis and the production of postoperative apnea in neonates.[5] Rarely, a long-acting anticholinesterase, echothiophate, is used to treat glaucoma. Systemic absorption of this drug decreases cholinesterase activity, resulting in marked prolongation of the duration of action of succinylcholine and mivacurium should the usual doses of these muscle relaxants be administered. At least 3 weeks is required after cessation of echothiophate therapy for cholinesterase activity to return to 50% of predrug levels. Topical application of phenylephrine to produce capillary decongestion and mydriasis can result in hypertension if systemic absorption is sufficient. A 2.5% phenylephrine solution minimizes the likelihood of hypertension owing to systemic absorption. Cyclopentolate is a popular mydriatic that may produce central nervous system toxicity, manifesting as dysarthria, disorientation, and psychotic reactions. Epinephrine applied topically to the cornea to produce mydriasis introduces the possibility of systemic absorption and potential sensitization of the heart in the presence of halothane. Nevertheless, systemic absorption of epinephrine seems to be minimal. Chronic treatment with acetazolamide can be associated with renal loss of bicarbonate ions and potassium, leading to metabolic acidosis with hypokalemia.

Oculocardiac Reflex

The oculocardiac reflex consists of a trigeminal vagal reflex arc that is characterized by a 10% to 50% decrease in heart rate. Pressure on the globe and surgical traction (stretch) of extraocular muscles, particularly the medial rectus muscle, are the most likely stimuli to elicit this reflex. Hypercarbia or arterial hypoxemia may also increase the incidence and severity of this reflex. In addition to bradycardia, other manifestations of this reflex include junctional rhythm and ventricular premature contractions. Cardiac arrest has been attributed to the oculocardiac reflex, but the evidence to support this is not convincing. Indeed, the importance of this reflex is controversial, with the most important principle being continuous monitoring of the electrocardiogram so as to detect the appearance of bradycardia or cardiac dysrhythmias. Removal of the surgical stimulus is usually sufficient treatment. Furthermore, this reflex tends to fatigue, such that the subsequent stimulation is less likely to elicit the same response. Premedication with intramuscular injection of atropine is of little or no value in preventing this reflex. Prophylactic use of atropine administered intravenously, however, may be justified in pediatric patients having strabismus correction because of the more active vagal reflexes in children. Should bradycardia persist after removal of the surgical stimulus, the appropriate treatment is the administration of atropine (3 to 5 $\mu g \cdot kg^{-1}$ IV).

Management of Anesthesia

Management of anesthesia for ophthalmic surgery includes recognition of unique requirements for successful treatment of ocular disorders. Inclusion of opioids in the preoperative medication may be avoided in view of the association of these drugs with nausea and vomiting. Intubation of the trachea to ensure control of the airway is necessary because of the proximity of the surgical field and draping. Co-existing diseases may influence the management of anesthesia independent of the ophthalmic surgery. For example, elderly patients requiring

Goals in Management of Anesthesia for Ophthalmic Surgery

- Control of intraocular pressure
- Intense analgesia
- Motionless eye (akinesia)
- Avoidance of the oculocardiac reflex
- Awareness of drug interactions
- Awakening without coughing, nausea, or vomiting

ophthalmic surgery often have associated illnesses such as diabetes mellitus, coronary artery disease, essential hypertension, or chronic obstructive pulmonary disease. Selection of drugs used for anesthesia must consider potential adverse interactions with medications being used to treat ocular disease, particularly glaucoma.

During operations in which the globe is not opened, there can be more flexibility in surgical conditions, but for intraocular procedures, perfection is required. For example, when the globe is open any uncontrolled increase in IOP can lead to an extrusion of ocular contents and permanent damage. Avoidence of the intraoperative use of succinylcholine is recommended while the eye is open or in patients who have undergone recent eye surgery. Otherwise, increases in IOP produced by succinylcholine are transient, allowing this drug to be safely administered to most patients undergoing ophthalmic surgery.

Available data have not demonstrated a significant difference in ocular morbidity between local and general anesthesia. Nevertheless, an impressive record of safety is associated with local anesthesia for ophthalmic surgery in patients with heart disease. Retrobulbar block provides local anesthesia and akinesia of the globe. Akinesia of the eyelids, if needed, is obtained by blocking the branches of the facial nerve supplying the orbicularis muscle. Complications associated with retrobulbar block include elicitation of the oculocardiac reflex, hemorrhage, and local anesthetic toxicity due to accidental intravascular injection of the drug. Accidental brain stem anesthesia after retrobulbar block manifests as unconsciousness and apnea.[6] Intravenous administration of a drug to produce transient central nervous system depression (methohexital, propofol) may be recommended just before performance of the retrobulbar block so as to optimize patient comfort. When local anesthesia is selected, the ophthalmologist is responsible for the management of the patient, although the anesthesiologist may be asked to monitor the patient's vital signs (monitored anesthesia care).

When general anesthesia is selected, it is mandatory that the patient not cough during intubation of the trachea, as any increase in venous pressure will increase IOP. Short duration laryngoscopy in the presence of adequate anesthesia and skeletal muscle relaxation plus the use of topical tracheal lidocaine or intravenous lidocaine may be helpful for ensuring minimal changes in IOP in response to intubation of the trachea. Likewise, emergence from anesthesia should not be associated with any reaction to the tracheal tube. The administration of intravenous lidocaine prior to extubation of the trachea may be helpful in attenuating coughing. Maintenance of anesthesia with volatile drugs with or without nitrous oxide is useful to provide an adequate depth of anesthesia plus rapid awakening and a low incidence of postoperative nausea and vomiting. Opioids may be avoided in an attempt to decrease factors that may contribute to postoperative nausea and vomiting. Nitrous oxide must be used with caution if an intravitreal injection of sulfa hexafluoride is planned (see the section *Retinal Detachment Surgery*). The eye is a highly innervated, pain-sensitive organ, and ophthalmic surgery requires surgical levels of anesthesia. Monitoring the electrocardiogram is essential for early recognition of the oculocardiac reflex. Administration of nondepolarizing muscle relaxants to maintain nearly complete suppression of the twitch response elicited by a peripheral nerve stimulator may be used to prevent unexpected patient movement. Large doses of atropine used in conjunction with anticholinesterase drugs to reverse neuromuscular blockade do not alter IOP. The increased incidence of nausea and vomiting following ophthalmic surgery, especially eye muscle surgery, suggests the existence of an oculogastric reflex. Indeed, a surgical repair may be jeopardized by sudden increases in IOP produced by vomiting. For these reasons, intravenous administration of antiemetics, such as droperidol or ondansetron, near the end of general anesthesia in an attempt to minimize the incidence of postoperative nausea and vomiting may be indicated. Propofol, as used for induction of anesthesia, may have an antiemetic effect that is useful for management of these patients. Passage of an orogastric tube to decompress the stomach before awakening from anesthesia may also be helpful in decreasing the incidence of postoperative vomiting. A catheter placed in the bladder may be indicated if an osmotic diuretic is administered to lower IOP.

Strabismus Surgery

Strabismus surgery is the most common pediatric ocular operation performed. Special considerations in the management of anesthesia for strabismus surgery include the (1) questionable use of succinylcholine, (2) increased incidence of the oculocardiac reflex, (3) increased incidence of postoperative nausea and vomiting, and (4) possible susceptibility to malignant hyperthermia. For example, succinylcholine may produce sustained contractions of the extraocular muscles, making interpretation of the forced duction test unreliable for 20 to 30 minutes.[7] Furthermore, routine use of succinylcholine in children is not recommended because of the remote risk of adverse responses evoked by this drug in the presence of unrecognized skeletal muscle disease. Indeed, malignant hyperthermia has been reported in patients undergoing strabismus surgery, suggesting a possible generalized skeletal muscle disturbance in some of these patients. Administration of atropine (3 to 5 $\mu g \cdot kg^{-1}$) or local infiltration of the extraocular muscle with lidocaine may be useful in preventing or treating the oculocardiac reflex. Prophylactic intravenous administration of droperidol decreases but does not eliminate the incidence of postoperative vomiting after strabismus surgery.[8]

Glaucoma

Special considerations in the management of anesthesia for the patient with glaucoma include (1) maintenance of drug-induced miosis throughout the perioperative period, (2) avoidance of venous congestion, and (3) awareness of potential adverse interactions between drugs used to treat glaucoma and those administered during anesthesia (see the section *Adverse Drug Interactions*). Continuation of the application of topical miotic eye drops on the morning of surgery is appropriate. Inclusion of an anticholinergic drug in the preoperative medication is acceptable because the amount of drug reaching the eye is too small to dilate the pupil. For example, an estimated 0.0001 mg of atropine is absorbed by the eye after parenteral administration of 0.4 mg as preoperative medication. Nevertheless, scopolamine has a greater mydriatic effect than atropine, suggesting the need for caution in consideration of its administration to patients with glaucoma.[9] Likewise, the use of anticholinergic drugs in combination with anticholinesterase drugs to reverse nondepolarizing muscle relaxants is safe because only small amounts of drug reach the eye. The implications of transient increases in IOP produced when succinylcholine is administered to patients with glaucoma are not known. Presumably, patients with adequate medical control of glaucoma are not jeopardized by this transient drug-induced increase in IOP. Prolonged hypotension may predispose to retinal artery thrombosis in these patients.

Cataract Extraction

Special considerations in the management of anesthesia for cataract extraction include the (1) likely presence of co-existing diseases in elderly patients, (2) need for absolute immobility during the operative procedure, and (3) steps to minimize the occurrence of postoperative nausea and vomiting. Sudden movement or attempts to cough when the globe is open can result in extrusion of ocular contents and permanent damage. For these reasons, when general anesthesia is selected for cataract surgery, it is essential to maintain an adequate depth of anesthesia. In addition, skeletal muscle paralysis is often included to minimize the chance of sudden unexpected patient movement. Succinylcholine, to facilitate intubation of the trachea, is acceptable because IOP has returned to normal by the time surgery begins. A short-acting nondepolarizing muscle relaxant may be an alternative to succinylcholine in these patients. Modest hyperventilation of the lungs to produce hypocarbia and a 10- to 15-degree head-up tilt to promote venous drainage will likely decrease IOP during intraocular surgery. Steps to decrease the likelihood of postoperative nausea and vomiting may include avoidance of opioids in the preoperative medication or intravenous administration of an antiemetic near the end of surgery, or both.

Retinal Detachment Surgery

Retinal detachment surgery requires a decrease in IOP as is often provided by intravenous administration of acetazolamide or mannitol. Rotation of the globe with traction on the extraocular muscles may elicit the oculocardiac reflex. Nitrous oxide must be used with caution when an intravitreal injection of air and sulfur hexafluoride is performed to compensate for loss of vitreous volume during surgery. Sulfur hexafluoride is included with air because the low water solubility of this gas ensures persistence of the intraocular bubble for several days postoperatively. Nitrous oxide, which is 34 times more soluble than nitrogen, can diffuse into the intraocular bubble more rapidly than nitrogen can leave, resulting in an enlargement of the bubble and increased IOP.[10] This increased IOP may be sufficient to compromise retinal blood flow, particularly if systemic blood pressure is decreased. When nitrous oxide is discontinued, IOP decreases to below awake levels, which presumably reflects loss of aqueous humor while the IOP was increased. This rapid decrease in IOP may jeopardize the retinal detachment surgical repair. For these reasons, it may be prudent to discontinue the inhalation of nitrous oxide about 15 minutes before the creation of an intraocular bubble. Furthermore, nitrous oxide should be avoided for up to 10 days after intravitreal injection of sulfur hexafluoride.[10]

Special anesthetic considerations are introduced when the laser is used for repair of retinal detachment and treatment of diabetic retinopathy (see the section *Laser Surgery*).

Open Eye Injury

Special considerations in the management of anesthesia for open eye injury include the (1) possibility of recent ingestion of food and (2) need to avoid even minimal increases in IOP if the injured eye is considered salvageable. Therefore, rapid intubation of the trachea facilitated by succinylcholine must be balanced against the possible hazards of increases in IOP. Nevertheless, rapid sequence induction of anesthesia that includes a barbiturate and pretreatment with a nondepolarizing muscle relaxant prior to the administration of succinylcholine to patients with open eye injuries has not been reported to be associated with vitreous loss.[11] Despite this evidence, many anesthesiologists would not use succinylcholine for induction of anesthesia in patients with open eye injuries. An awake intubation of the trachea, although attractive from the standpoint of airway protection, would be unacceptable because potential patient reaction to placement of the tube in the trachea would increase IOP. An alternative to the administration of succinylcholine is the injection of an intubating dose of a nondepolarizing muscle relaxant. The disadvantage of this approach is a prolonged duration of skeletal muscle paralysis (less likely following administration of mivacurium compared with atracurium, vecuronium, or pancuronium) for what may be a short operation. Regardless of the muscle relaxant selection, it is helpful to confirm the presence of skeletal muscle paralysis by the use of a peripheral nerve stimulator before initiating direct laryngoscopy for intubation of the trachea. Premature placement of the tube in the trachea will provoke a cough response and defeat all the prior attempts to minimize the occurrence of vomiting or increases in IOP during direct laryngoscopy.

Corneal Abrasion

Corneal abrasion is the most common ocular complication associated with general anesthesia. Abrasions typically occur in the inferior one-third of the cornea corresponding to the area exposed when the eyes are not mechanically closed. Reduction in tear production by general anesthetics plus the loss of protective eyelid closure renders patients susceptible to corneal abrasions during anesthesia. For these reasons, placement of protective goggles and instillation of ophthalmic ointment (artificial tears) is commonly performed. Disadvantages of ophthalmic ointments include occasional allergic reactions, potential flammability (which may make their use undesirable during surgery that utilizes electrocautery around the face), and blurred vision in the early postoperative period.[12] The blurring and foreign body sensation associated with ophthalmic ointments could increase the likelihood of corneal abrasions should excessive rubbing of the eyes occur as the patient emerges from anesthesia. Alternatively, mechanical closure of the eyelids by gentle application of adhesive strips protects the cornea and avoids the disadvantages of ophthalmic ointment.

The patient who sustains a corneal abrasion will complain of the sensation of a foreign body, tearing, photophobia, and pain. When a corneal abrasion is suspected, it is desirable to obtain an ophthalmology consultation while the patient is still in the postanesthesia care unit. After gross examination, a local anesthetic should be instilled and the eye examined with fluorescein to demonstrate the injured area. Corneal abrasions are usually treated by patching the injured eye and applying a prophylactic antibiotic ointment such as erythromycin. Repeated instillation of local anesthetics to control pain is not recommended, since these drugs inhibit corneal healing. Healing normally occurs within 48 hours.

Retinal Ischemia

Postoperative visual loss may reflect perioperative retinal ischemia as associated with external pressure on the eye, especially when the patient is prone. An episode of hypotension in this situation could further decrease retinal blood flow. The importance of carefully positioning patients to avoid excessive external pressure on the eyes is obvious. Retinal ischemia may also result from ocular trauma secondary to prolonged pressure from an improperly fitting anesthetic face mask, embolism during cardiac surgery, or the combination of sulfur hexafluoride and nitrous oxide resulting in excessive increases in IOP.

OTOLARYNGOLOGY

Optimal management of anesthesia for otolaryngologic surgery is based on reliable control of the upper airway. These patients may present with compromised airways before surgery because of edema, infection, or tumor invasion of the upper airway. After intubation of the trachea, monitoring to ensure continued patency of the airway and intactness of the anesthetic delivery system (precordial or esophageal stethoscope, capnography, pulse oximetry) is especially important. Monitoring the electrocardiogram is necessary to detect cardiac dysrhythmias that frequently accompany surgical manipulation in the larynx, pharynx, and neck. Blood loss during major otolaryngologic surgery can be substantial and is often underestimated because of hidden losses onto drapes or into the patient's stomach. Extubation of the trachea may be hazardous after otolaryngologic surgery, especially when the airway is compromised as a result of edema or bleeding after endoscopy or upper airway surgery.

Ear Surgery

Special considerations in the management of anesthesia for ear surgery include (1) facial nerve preservation, (2) the use of epinephrine by the surgeon, and (3) the effect of nitrous oxide on middle ear pressure.

Facial Nerve Preservation

Surgical identification and preservation of the facial nerve is essential during ear surgery and many other otolaryngologic operations. This requirement necessitates maintenance of some skeletal muscle activity if muscle relaxants are administered. Ideally, the twitch response produced by stimulation of the ulnar nerve using a peripheral nerve stimulator should remain at 10% to 20% of control levels when muscle relaxants are administered. A volatile anesthetic is useful because muscle relaxants to prevent unexpected patient movement are not routinely required, thus preserving the ability to easily identify the facial nerve by virtue of skeletal muscle responses to electrical stimulation of tissue presumed to be nerve. Furthermore, if nitrous oxide must be discontinued, the patient remains adequately anesthetized by increasing the inhaled concentration of the volatile anesthetic. Another advantage of volatile anesthetics is the ability to maintain systolic blood pressure between 80 and 85 mmHg so as to minimize intraoperative blood loss if this is deemed important for the success of the surgery.

Use of Epinephrine

Epinephrine is often infiltrated in the operative area by the surgeon to produce vasoconstriction and thus decrease blood loss. Halothane is more likely than other volatile anesthetics to evoke cardiac dysrhythmias in the presence of exogenous epinephrine.

Nitrous Oxide and Middle Ear Pressure

Nitrous oxide, which is 34 times more soluble than nitrogen, enters air-filled cavities such as the middle ear more rapidly than air can leave, resulting in an increase in middle ear pressure (Fig. 24-1).[13] Under normal conditions, any pressure increase in the middle ear is passively vented via the eustachian tube into the nasopharynx. Narrowing of the eustachian tube by acute inflammation or the presence of scar tissue, as is possible after an adenoidectomy, impairs the ability of the middle ear to vent passively any pressure increases produced by nitrous oxide. Tympanic membrane rupture, manifesting as bright red blood in the external auditory canal, has been attributed to pressure increases produced by nitrous oxide.[14] Disruption of previous middle ear reconstructive surgery has been alleged when nitrous oxide is administered at a later date for operative procedures not involving the ear.[15] Nevertheless, it is undeniable that many patients with a history of middle ear surgery have received nitrous oxide on subsequent occasions without detectable effects on hearing. During tympanoplasty surgery, the effect of nitrous oxide on middle ear pressures may cause displacement of the tympanic membrane graft. Therefore, inhaled nitrous oxide concentrations are often limited to 50%, with dis-

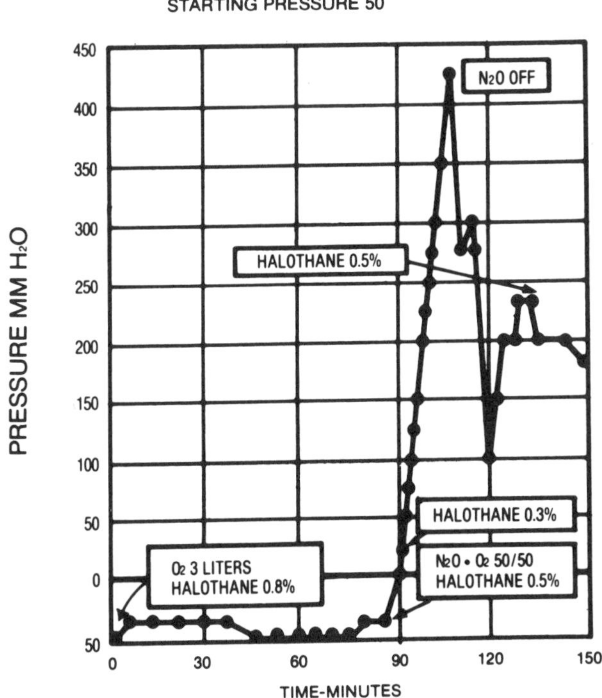

Figure 24-1. Measurements in a single patient demonstrate an abrupt increase in middle ear pressure (mmH_2O) when nitrous oxide is added to the inhaled gases. (From Patterson and Bartlett,[13] with permission.)

continuance about 15 minutes before placement of the graft. The speculation that postoperative nausea and vomiting could be due to increased middle ear pressure that persists after the administration of nitrous oxide remains unproven.

Rapid absorption of nitrous oxide when administration of this gas is discontinued can produce negative pressure in the middle ear, manifesting as serous otitis or transient postoperative hearing loss (Fig. 24-2).[13]

Nasal and Sinus Surgery

Special considerations in the management of anesthesia for nasal and sinus surgery include the (1) intraoperative application of topical cocaine to produce maximal vasoconstriction in the operative area, (2) use of a posterior pharyngeal pack, (3) possibility of large intraoperative blood loss, and (4) need for extubation of the trachea only when protective upper airway reflexes have returned. Systemic absorption of cocaine may manifest as tachycardia, hypertension, and myocardial ischemia. The use of a combination of topical cocaine and epinephrine does not increase the vasoconstrictive effectiveness of cocaine. Furthermore, topically applied epinephrine does not retard the systemic absorption nor prolong the anesthetic action of cocaine. Maintenance of anesthesia is acceptably provided by using volatile anesthetics, which offer the advantage of providing better control of the blood pressure than opioid techniques. Alternatively, a nitrous oxide-opioid technique may be selected with intermittent administration of a volatile anesthetic to control blood pressure. Although nasal sinuses represent air-filled cavities, there is no evidence that nitrous oxide produces adverse increases in pressures in these structures (see the section *Nitrous Oxide and Middle Ear Pressure*). Before extubation of the trachea, the pharynx should be suctioned, the posterior pharyngeal pack removed, and the return of protective upper airway reflexes confirmed.

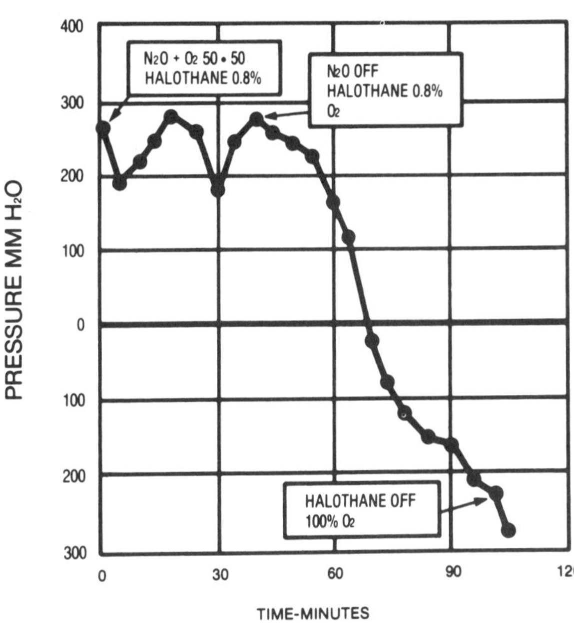

Figure 24-2. Measurements in a single patient demonstrate an abrupt decrease in middle ear pressure (mmH_2O) to below normal when inhalation of nitrous oxide is discontinued. (From Patterson and Bartlett,[13] with permission.)

Endoscopy

Special considerations in the management of anesthesia for endoscopy (laryngoscopy, laser surgery, bronchoscopy, esophagoscopy) include the (1) possibility of a co-existing airway abnormality, (2) management of an upper airway that is shared with the surgeon, (3) need to minimize oral secretions, (4) need for suppression of cough and laryngeal reflexes, (5) need for a relaxed mandible, (6) protection of teeth with a dental guard, and (7) need for rapid awakening with return of protective upper airway reflexes. Cardiac dysrhythmias are frequently associated with the stimulus of endoscopy. In some patients, endoscopy is best performed with the patient awake using local anesthesia. Oral secretions can usually be effectively minimized by inclusion of an anticholinergic drug in the preoperative medication. Pulse oximetry is particularly useful in monitoring the maintenance of acceptable arterial oxygenation during anesthesia for endoscopy.

Laryngoscopy

General anesthesia for laryngoscopy may be performed with a small (5- to 6-mm internal diameter) tracheal tube. This approach permits the use of muscle relaxants to ensure optimal surgical working conditions and facilitates ventilation of the patient's lungs. It is usually preferable to tape the tracheal tube to the left side of the mouth as the surgeon will insert the laryngoscope down the right side of the mouth. The disadvantage of using a tracheal tube is interference with the surgeon's view of the larynx, especially the posterior commissure. Intermittent injections or a continuous intravenous infusion of succinylcholine (mivacurium may be an alternative drug selection) is an effective method of producing skeletal muscle relaxation for these short procedures. The only significant difference between laryngoscopy and microlaryngoscopy is the use of an operating microscope in microlaryngoscopy.

Laser Surgery

A laser (light amplification by stimulated emission of radiation) is a device capable of producing an intense beam of light that can be focused to produce precisely controlled coagulation, incision, or vaporization of tissues. Edema is minimal and healing is rapid because damage to surrounding tissues is minimal. Patients must remain absolutely immobile, since the laser is critically focused on specific target tissues and any amount of patient movement may divert the beam to adjacent normal tissues. Bronchospasm or laryngospasm, or both, are common during and after laser surgery in the larynx and trachea.

Hazards

Hazards associated with the use of the laser require special precautions in the operating room.[16] Vaporization of tissue by the laser produces a plume of smoke and fine particulates (mean size 0.31 μm) that may be deposited in the alveoli if inhaled. An efficient smoke evacuator at the surgical site and wearing of high-efficiency masks by operating room personnel (conventional surgical masks efficiently filter particles down to about 3 μm) are the most effective means of preventing dissemination of the plume. Misdirected laser energy may perforate a viscus or a large blood vessel (uncoagulable by laser). Venous gas embolism is a risk of laparoscopic laser surgery. Energy transfer to an inappropriate location may manifest as ocular injury or endotracheal tube fire during airway surgery. In this regard, eye protection (safety goggles) should be used by all operating room personnel and the patient's (nonoperated) eyes should be taped so the lids are closed and then covered with a protective shield.

Hazards Associated with Laser Surgery

- Atmospheric contamination from vaporization of tissues (smoke and fine particulates)
- Misdirected laser energy (viscus perforation, transection of uncoagulable blood vessels)
- Venous gas embolism
- Ocular injury (cornea, retina)
- Endotracheal tube fire during airway surgery

The risk of endotracheal tube fire during airway surgery is decreased by decreasing the potential flammability of the endotracheal tube (metallic foil wrap tube [Merocel]; laser-resistant coating of aluminum powder in silicone incorporated into the tube [Xomed tube]). Polyvinylchloride endotracheal tubes are highly flammable and are not recommended during laser surgery. The mixture of airway gases is an important consideration when any type of potentially flammable endotracheal tube is used during airway surgery. For this reason, the delivered concentration of oxygen is decreased to the minimum concentration (ideally lower than 40%) consistent with acceptable oxygenation (as reflected by pulse oximetry). Nitrous oxide, which supports combustion, is avoided. Use of an air-oxygen mixture is acceptable. Alternatively, helium may be substituted for air since the higher thermal conductivity of this gas could delay ignition of the endotracheal tube.[17] Helium also has a lower viscosity than nitrogen and will permit the use of a smaller endotracheal tube without turbulence and high resistance to flow. Regardless of the tracheal tube selected, the cuff is vulnerable to puncture by the laser beam. When the cuff is inflated with saline instead of air to act as a heat sink for laser energy, it can still be perforated by the laser beam but ignition will not occur. The fine spray of saline released by a perforation may serve to quench any possible fire in the airway. Should an airway fire occur, the surgeon and anesthesiologist must act promptly and in a coordinated fashion, remembering that the tube becomes a blowtorch because of the high gas flows that occur in it during ventilation of the lungs.[16]

The administration of a volatile anesthetic during airway laser surgery has been questioned since these drugs may pyrolyze to potentially toxic compounds during an airway fire. In cases in which Venturi ventilation is used, administration of volatile anesthetics is usually not mechanically possible.

Airway Fire Protocol During Laser Surgery

Remove the ignition source
Discontinue ventilation of the lungs (removes enriched oxygen source)
Extubate the trachea and extinguish the removed flaming material in water
Ventilate the lungs by mask with oxygen
Perform rigid bronchoscopy to survey damage and remove debris (reintubate if any airway damage present)
Assess oropharynx and face
Obtain chest radiograph

Bronchoscopy

Methods of general anesthesia and management of ventilation of the lungs for bronchoscopy do not differ from those for laryngoscopy. Volatile anesthetics are useful to provide adequate suppression of upper airway reflexes and also permit use of high inhaled concentrations of oxygen. Spontaneous ventilation is preferred in cases of foreign body removal, because it is theoretically possible that positive airway pressure would push the foreign body deeper into the bronchial tree. Bronchoscopes in current use include the (1) flexible fiberoptic, (2) rigid-ventilating, and (3) rigid-Venturi (Sanders injector) type. The flexible fiberoptic bronchoscope offers the advantage of being placed via a large (8.5-mm internal diameter or larger) tracheal tube, permitting reliable ventilation of both lungs during endoscopy. Patient movement or excessive airway pressures during bronchoscopy performed with a rigid bronchoscope may result in a tracheal tear or pneumothorax, or both. Trauma associated with bronchoscopy can manifest as airway edema, which may warrant administration of dexamethasone (0.1 $mg \cdot kg^{-1}$ IV).

Head and Neck Surgery

Head and neck surgery, such as laryngectomy or radical neck dissection, may last 6 to 8 hours and involve substantial blood loss. Patients with carcinoma of the larynx often smoke cigarettes excessively and develop associated chronic obstructive pulmonary disease. Patency of the upper airway may be compromised by tumor, necessitating placement of a tracheal tube or performance of a tracheostomy before the induction of anesthesia. Surgery near the carotid sinus can elicit vagal responses, manifesting as bradycardia and hypotension. During head and neck surgery, open neck veins create the possibility of venous air embolism. Positive pressure ventilation of the lungs decreases the likelihood of venous air embolism by maintaining an increased pressure in the veins. Maintenance of blood pressure in a low-normal range by varying the inhaled concentrations of volatile anesthetics plus a 10- to 15-degree head-up tilt is helpful in minimizing intraoperative blood loss. Blood and intravenous fluids can be warmed to help maintain body temperature during prolonged operations. A catheter placed in the bladder is indicated if large volumes of fluid replacement will be necessary. Cardiac dysrhythmias associated with prolonged Q-T intervals may follow right but not left radical neck dissection, presumably reflecting damage to the cervical autonomic nervous system during surgical dissection (Fig. 24-3).18

Adenotonsillectomy

Special considerations in the management of anesthesia for adenotonsillectomy include (1) preoperative evaluation of coagulation, (2) determination of the presence of loose teeth, (3) provision of mandibular and pharyngeal muscle relaxation, (4) suppression of laryngeal reflexes, and (5) rapid awakening with return of protective upper airway reflexes. Because it is an intraoral procedure, inclusion of an antisialagogue in the preoperative medication is useful. In addition to recurrent tonsillitis, an emerging indication for a similar procedure (uvulopalatopharyngoplasty) is obstructive sleep apnea (see Chapter 23). Adults with obstructive sleep apnea are often obese and have short necks and large tongues, potentially making maintenance of a patent upper airway and subsequent direct laryngoscopy for tracheal intubation technically difficult. Elective adenotonsillectomy should probably be delayed if there is preoperative evidence of an upper respiratory tract infection.

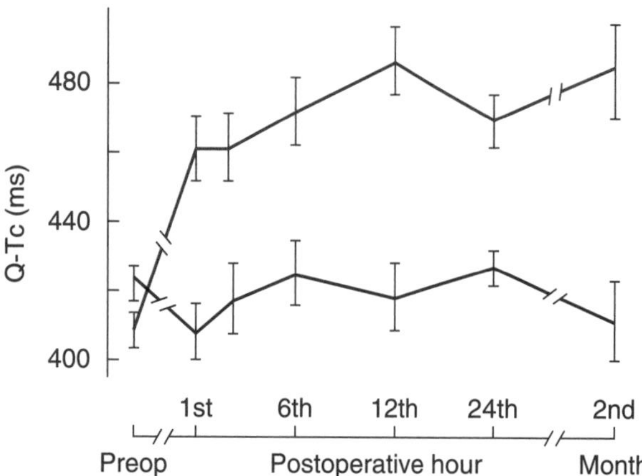

Figure 24-3. Right radical neck dissection (red line), but not left radical neck dissection (black line), is associated with prolongation of Q-Tc intervals on the electrocardiogram. (From Otteni et al.,[18] with permission.)

Blood loss during adenotonsillectomy averages 4 $ml \cdot kg^{-1}$ but is usually underestimated because of drainage of an undetermined amount of blood into the stomach. Maintenance of anesthesia for these short surgical procedures is acceptably achieved with nitrous oxide plus a volatile anesthetic delivered via a tracheal tube. Postoperatively, patients are often placed in the lateral position with the head lower than the hips ("tonsil position") so that blood drains out the mouth. As a result, blood loss is less likely to irritate the vocal cords or to be masked by unrecognized accumulation in the stomach.

Reoperation for continued bleeding from the tonsil bed is a major anesthetic challenge. Nearly 90% of significant postoperative bleeding, when it does occur, manifests in the first 9 hours postoperatively.[19] These patients are often hypovolemic, as reflected by tachycardia and orthostatic hypotension. Rehydration with lactated Ringer's solution (15 to 20 $ml \cdot kg^{-1}$) is important before the induction of anesthesia. Since large volumes of blood may have been swallowed, it is common to treat these patients as if they have a full stomach. A rapid sequence induction of anesthesia using thiopental and succinylcholine plus cricoid pressure is acceptable. Ketamine may be selected rather than thiopental, especially if the possibility of hypovolemia exists despite attempts at rehydration. Alternatively, awake intubation of the trachea may be performed. The stomach should be emptied via an orogastric tube after placement of the tracheal tube. After the completion of surgery, protective airway reflexes are allowed to return before the trachea is extubated.

Tracheostomy

Tracheostomy must be regarded as a procedure that is best performed electively in the operating room. Ideally, a translaryngeal tracheal tube should be in place to facilitate ventilation of lungs and permit an unhurried surgical procedure. Cricothyrotomy can be performed rapidly as a life-saving procedure when acute upper airway obstruction occurs and translaryngeal intubation of the trachea is not possible (see Fig. 11-13). Early complications of tracheostomy include tube displacement, hemorrhage, and pneumothorax.

REFERENCES

1. Myers EF, Krupin T, Johnson M, Zink H. Failure of nondepolarizing neuromuscular blockers to inhibit succinylcholine-induced increased intraocular pressure—A controlled study. Anesthesiology 1978; 48:149–51.
2. Pandey K, Badola RP, Kumar S. Time course of intraocular hypertension produced by suxamethonium. Br J Anaesth 1972;44:191–5.
3. Miller RD, Way WL, Hickey RF. Inhibition of succinylcholine-induced increased intraocular pressure by nondepolarizing muscle relaxants. Anesthesiology 1968;29:123–6.
4. Kim JW, Smith PH. Timolol-induced bradycardia. Anesth Analg 1980;59:301–3.
5. Bailey PL. Timolol and postoperative apnea in neonates and young infants. Anesthesiology 1984; 61:622.
6. Chang J-L, Gonzalez-Abola E, Larson CE. Brain stem anesthesia following retrobulbar block. Anesthesiology 1984;61:789–90.
7. France NK, France TD, Woodburn JD, et al. Succinylcholine alteration of the forced duction test. Ophthalmology 1980;87:1282–5.
8. Abramowitz MD, Oh TH, Epstein BS. Antiemetic effect of droperidol following outpatient strabismus surgery in children. Anesthesiology 1983;59:579–83.
9. Garde JF, Aston R, Endler GC, Sison OS. Racial mydriatic response to belladonna preparations. Anesth Analg 1978;57:572–5.
10. Wolf GL, Capuano C, Hartung J. Nitrous oxide increases intraocular pressure after intravitreal sulfur hexafluoride injection. Anesthesiology 1983;59:547–8.
11. Libonati M, Leahy JJ, Ellison N. The use of succinylcholine in open eye surgery. Anesthesiology 1985; 62:637–40.
12. Siffring PA, Poulton TJ. Prevention of ophthalmic complications during general anesthesia. Anesthesiology 1987;66:569–70.
13. Patterson ME, Bartlett PC. Hearing impairment caused by intratympanic pressure changes during general anesthesia. Laryngoscope 1976;86:399–404.
14. Owens WD, Gustave F, Schlaroff A. Tympanic membrane rupture with nitrous oxide anesthesia. Anesth Analg 1978;57:283–6.
15. Man A, Segal S, Ezra S. Ear injury caused by elevated intratympanic pressure during general anaesthesia. Acta Anaesth Scand 1980;24:224–6.
16. Rampil IJ. Anesthetic considerations for laser surgery. Anesth Analg 1992;74:424–35.
17. Pashayan AG, Gravenstein JS. Helium retards endotracheal tube fires from carbon dioxide lasers. Anesthesiology 1985;62:272–7.
18. Otteni JC, Pottecher T, Bronner G, Flesch H, Diebolt JR. Prolongation of the Q-T interval and sudden cardiac arrest following right radical neck dissection. Anesthesiology 1983;59:358–61.
19. Crysdale WS. Complications of tonsillectomy and adenoidectomy in 949 children observed overnight. Can Med Assoc J 1986;135:1129–42.

25

Obstetrics

Optimal analgesia or anesthesia, or both, for labor, vaginal delivery, and cesarean section requires an understanding of the physiologic changes in the parturient during pregnancy and labor, the effects of anesthetics on the fetus and neonate, the benefits and risks of various techniques of anesthesia, and the significance of obstetric complications on the management of anesthesia. Unlike the patient scheduled for elective surgery, the parturient is rarely in optimal condition at the time anesthetic care becomes necessary. For example, the parturient must always be considered to have a full stomach and to be at increased risk of inhalation (pulmonary aspiration) of gastric contents. During labor, emergencies such as fetal distress, maternal hemorrhage, and prolapsed cord demand immediate anesthesia.

PHYSIOLOGIC CHANGES IN THE PARTURIENT

Pregnancy and subsequent labor and delivery are accompanied by predictable physiologic changes.

Cardiovascular System

Changes in the cardiovascular system during pregnancy provide for the needs of the developing fetus and prepare the mother for events that will occur during labor and delivery. These changes include alterations in the (1) intravascular fluid volume and its constituents, (2) cardiac output, and (3) peripheral circulation (Table 25-1).[1] The supine hypotension syndrome reflects circulatory changes due to the impact of the enlarging gravid uterus.

Intravascular Fluid Volume

The increase in maternal intravascular fluid volume begins in the first trimester and results in an average expansion of about 1000 ml at term. The plasma volume increases 45% and the erythrocyte volume increases 20%. This disproportionate increase in plasma volume accounts for the relative anemia of pregnancy. The increased intravascular fluid volume offsets the 400 to 600 ml blood loss that accompanies vaginal delivery and the average 1000 ml blood loss that accompanies cesarean section. The total plasma protein concentration is decreased, reflecting the dilutional effect of the increased intravascular fluid volume.

Cardiac Output

Cardiac output is increased about 40% above nonpregnant levels by the 10th week of gestation and is maintained at this level throughout the second and third trimesters. This augmentation of cardiac output is primarily due to an increased stroke volume, as heart rate is not greatly increased. It is likely that placental and ovarian steroids are important in producing and sustaining this increase. Earlier studies suggesting return of cardiac output toward nonpregnant levels during the third trimester were in error. Instead, this decrease reflected decreased venous return due to compression of the inferior vena cava by the gravid uterus when the supine position was assumed.

The onset of labor is associated with further increases in cardiac output, which may reach 45% above the prelabor value. The largest increase in

Table 25-1. Changes in the Cardiovascular System During Pregnancy

	Value Near Term Compared with Nonpregnant value
Intravascular fluid volume	Increased 35%
Plasma volume	Increased 45%
Erythrocyte volume	Increased 20%
Cardiac output	Increased 40%
Stroke volume	Increased 30%
Heart rate	Increased 15%
Peripheral circulation	
Systolic blood pressure	No change
Systemic vascular resistance	Decreased 20%
Pulmonary vascular resistance	Decreased 35%
Central venous pressure	No change
Femoral venous pressure	Increased 15%

cardiac output occurs immediately after delivery, when output is increased as much as 60% above prelabor values. A regional anesthetic is capable of attenuating increases in cardiac output during labor and may therefore be a useful way of protecting a compromised cardiovascular system during the peripartum period. Typically, cardiac output returns to nonpregnant values by 2 weeks postpartum.

Peripheral Circulation

Systolic blood pressure does not increase above nonpregnant levels during an uncomplicated pregnancy. Because cardiac output is increased, systemic vascular resistance must decrease for arterial blood pressure to remain normal. There is no change in the central venous pressure during pregnancy, but femoral venous pressure is increased about 15%, presumably reflecting compression of the inferior vena cava by the gravid uterus. The failure of central venous pressure to increase in response to an increased blood volume probably reflects the presence of dilated systemic and pulmonary circulations.

Supine Hypotension Syndrome

Decreases in maternal blood pressure associated with the supine position occur in about 10% of parturients near term. Diaphoresis, nausea, vomiting, and changes in cerebration may accompany this hypotension. These symptoms are termed the supine hypotension syndrome.

The mechanism for the supine hypotension syndrome is decreased venous return due to compression of the inferior vena cava by the gravid uterus when the parturient assumes the supine position (Fig. 25-1). The resulting decrease in venous return leads to a decrease in cardiac output and a decline in blood pressure. Fortunately, most parturients (about 90%) are able to initiate compensatory responses on assuming the supine position. These compensatory responses prevent the appearance of the supine hypotension syndrome. For example, increased venous pressure below the level of compression of the inferior vena cava serves to divert venous blood from the lower one-half of the body via the paravertebral venous plexuses to the azygos vein. Flow from the azygos vein enters the superior vena cava and venous return is maintained. This compensatory response means that inadvertent intravascular injection of local anesthetics during an attempted lumbar epidural anesthetic can result in bolus delivery of the drug to the heart, with resulting profound myocardial depression. An additional compensatory response that offsets inferior vena cava compression by the gravid uterus is an increase in peripheral sympathetic nervous system activity. This increased activity results in increased systemic vascular resistance, which permits blood pressure to be maintained despite a decreased cardiac output. It is important to recognize that compensatory increases in systemic vascular resistance are impaired by regional anesthetic techniques. Indeed, arterial hypotension is more common and profound during regional anesthesia administered to parturients compared with nonpregnant patients.

In addition to compression of the inferior vena cava, the gravid uterus may compress the lower abdominal aorta (Fig. 25-1). This compression leads to arterial hypotension in the lower extremities, but maternal symptoms or decreases in blood pressure as measured in the arm do not occur.

The significance of aortocaval compression is the associated decrease in uterine and placental blood flow. Even in the presence of a healthy uteroplacental unit, decreases in maternal systolic blood pressure to lower than 100 mmHg for longer than 10 to 15 minutes may be associated with progressive fetal acidosis and bradycardia.

The incidence of the supine hypotension syndrome can be minimized by nursing the parturient in the lateral position. Alternatively, left uterine dis-

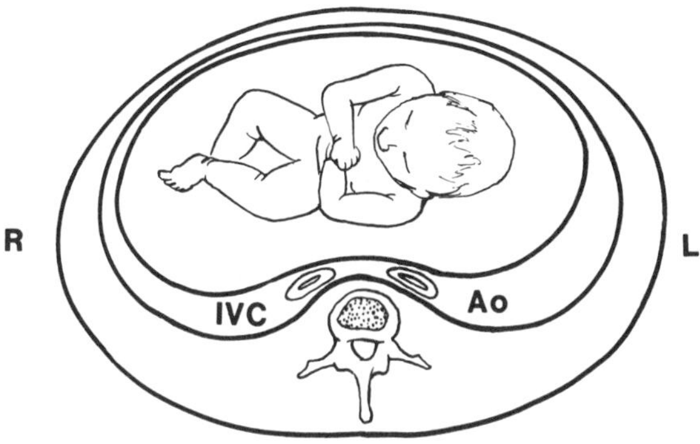

Figure 25-1. Schematic diagram showing compression of the inferior vena cava (IVC) and abdominal aorta (Ao) by the gravid uterus when the parturient assumes the supine position.

placement is effective by moving the gravid uterus off the inferior vena cava or aorta. Displacement of the uterus to the left can be accomplished manually or by elevation of the right hip 10 to 15 cm with a blanket or foam-rubber wedge (Fig. 25-2).

Pulmonary System

Changes in the pulmonary system during pregnancy are manifested as alterations in the (1) upper airway, (2) minute ventilation, (3) lung volumes, and (4) arterial oxygenation (Table 25-2).

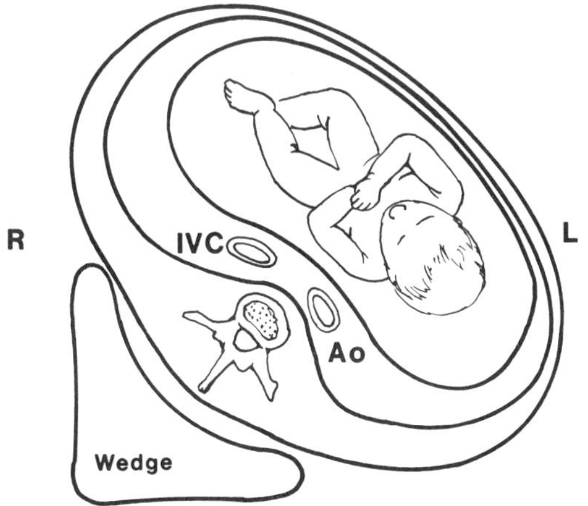

Figure 25-2. Schematic diagram depicting left uterine displacement by elevation of the parturient's right hip with a foam-rubber wedge. This position moves the gravid uterus off the inferior vena cava (IVC) and aorta (Ao).

Table 25-2. Changes in the Pulmonary System

	Value Near Term Compared with Nonpregnant Value
Minute ventilation	Increased 50%
Tidal volume	Increased 40%
Breathing frequency	Increased 10%
Lung volumes	
Expiratory reserve volume	Decreased 20%
Residual volume	Decreased 20%
Functional residual capacity	Decreased 20%
Vital capacity	No change
Total lung capacity	No change
Arterial blood gases and pH	
PaO_2	Normal or slightly decreased
$PaCO_2$	Decreased 10 mmHg
pH	No change
Oxygen consumption	Increased 20%

Upper Airway

Capillary engorgement of the mucosal lining of the upper respiratory tract accompanies pregnancy and emphasizes the need for gentleness during instrumentation (suctioning, placement of nasal or oral airways, direct laryngoscopy) of the upper airway. It may be prudent to select a smaller cuffed tracheal tube (6.5 to 7.0 mm internal diameter) because vocal cords and arytenoids are often edematous. Weight gain associated with pregnancy in short, obese parturients can result in difficulty in inserting the laryngoscope because of a short neck and large breasts.

Minute Ventilation

Minute ventilation is increased about 50% above nonpregnant levels during the first trimester and maintained at this elevated level for the remainder of the pregnancy. This increased minute ventilation is achieved by an increased tidal volume, since breathing frequency is not greatly altered (Table 25-2). Increased circulating levels of progesterone are presumed to be the stimulus for increased minute ventilation.

The resting maternal $PaCO_2$ decreases from 40 mmHg to about 30 mmHg during the first trimester as a reflection of increased minute ventilation. Arterial pH, however, remains near normal because of increased renal excretion of bicarbonate ions. Pain associated with labor and delivery results in further hyperventilation, which can be attenuated by lumbar epidural anesthesia.

Lung Volumes

Lung volumes, in contrast to the early appearance of increased minute ventilation, do not begin to change until about the fifth month of pregnancy (Table 25-2). With increasing enlargement of the uterus, the diaphragm is forced cephalad. This change is largely responsible for the 20% decrease in functional residual capacity present at term. Vital capacity is not significantly changed.

The combination of increased minute ventilation and decreased functional residual capacity increases the rate at which changes in alveolar concentrations of inhaled anesthetics can be achieved. Indeed, induction of anesthesia, emergence from anesthesia, and changes in depth of anesthesia are notably faster in parturients.

Arterial Oxygenation

Early in gestation, maternal PaO_2 while breathing room air is normally higher than 100 mmHg, reflecting the presence of hyperventilation. Later, PaO_2 is normal or even slightly decreased, most likely reflecting airway closure. Induction of general anesthesia in the parturient may be associated with marked decreases in the PaO_2 if apnea, as during intubation of the trachea, is prolonged. This tendency for a rapid decrease in PaO_2 reflects a decreased oxygen reserve secondary to the decrease in functional residual capacity. A decrease in cardiac output owing to aortocaval compression and increased oxygen consumption may also contribute to rapid decreases in PaO_2 during apnea. For these reasons, the administration of supplemental oxygen during a regional anesthetic or before any anticipated period of apnea (preoxygenation for 3 minutes or four deep breaths during 30 seconds) is often recommended.[2]

Nervous System Changes

Central nervous system changes during pregnancy are reflected by decreased anesthetic requirements (MAC) for volatile anesthetics as demonstrated in animals.[3] It is presumed, but not documented, that similar changes occur in humans. Sedative effects produced by progesterone may be partially responsible for this decrease in MAC. The important clinical implication of decreased MAC is that alveolar concentrations of inhaled drugs that would not produce unconsciousness in nonpregnant patients may approximate anesthetizing concentrations in parturients. This degree of central nervous system depression may also impair protective upper airway reflexes and subject parturients to the hazards of pulmonary aspiration. Furthermore, the decreased functional residual capacity increases the rate at which potential excessive alveolar concentrations of anesthetics can be achieved.

Engorgement of epidural veins as intra-abdominal pressure increases with progressive enlargement of the uterus decreases the size of the epidural space and decreases the volume of cerebrospinal fluid in the subarachnoid space. The decreased volume of these spaces facilitates the spread of local anesthetics and is consistent with the 30% to 50% decrease in dose requirements of local anesthetics necessary for epidural or spinal anesthesia in parturients at term. The observation of exaggerated spread of local anesthetics placed in the epidural space as early as the first trimester suggests a role for biochemical as well as mechanical changes.[4] Indeed, experimental evidence confirms increased sensitivity to local anesthetics in pregnant versus nonpregnant animals. There are also data that do not demonstrate a difference in the level of sensory anesthesia achieved when equal volumes of local anesthetics are injected into the epidural space of pregnant and nonpregnant patients if care is exercised to prevent aortocaval compression in parturients.[5]

Renal Changes

Renal blood flow and glomerular filtration rate are increased about 50% by the fourth month of pregnancy. Therefore, the normal upper limits of the blood urea nitrogen and serum creatinine concentrations are decreased about 50% in parturients.

Hepatic Changes

Plasma cholinesterase (pseudocholinesterase) activity is decreased about 25% from the 10th week of gestation to as long as 6 weeks postpartum. This decreased activity is unlikely to be associated with significant prolongation of the neuromuscular blocking effects of succinylcholine or mivacurium.

Gastrointestinal Changes

Gastrointestinal changes during pregnancy make parturients vulnerable to regurgitation of gastric contents and to the development of acid pneumonitis should pulmonary aspiration occur. For example, the enlarged uterus displaces the pylorus upward and backward, which retards gastric emptying. In addition, progesterone decreases gastrointestinal motility. As a result, gastric fluid volume tends to be increased even in the fasting state. In addition, gastrin, which is secreted by the placenta, stimulates gastric hydrogen ion secretion such that the pH of gastric fluid is predictably low in parturients. The enlarging uterus changes the angle of the gastroesophageal junction, leading to relative incompetence of the physiologic sphincter mechanism. For this reason, gastric fluid reflux into the esophagus and subsequent esophagitis (heartburn) are common in parturients.

Regardless of the time interval since ingestion of food, the parturient in labor must be treated as having a full stomach. Pain, anxiety, and drugs (especially opioids) administered during labor can all retard gastric emptying beyond an already prolonged transit time.

The increased risk of pulmonary aspiration of gastric contents is the reason for recommending the placement of a cuffed tube in the trachea of every parturient who is rendered unconscious by anesthesia. The recognition that the pH of inhaled gastric fluid is important in the production and severity of acid pneumonitis is the basis for the administration of antacids to parturients before the induction of anesthesia. Considering the potential accumulation of antacids in the stomach, particularly if gastric emptying is slowed by opioids, there seems little reason to recommend repeated use of antacids at regular intervals during labor.[6] Furthermore, repeated use of antacids has not been conclusively proven to decrease morbidity or mortality despite the accepted ability of these drugs to increase the pH of gastric fluid. It must be appreciated that inhalation of antacids containing particulate matter can produce adverse pulmonary changes. In an attempt to obviate the hazards of inhalation of particulate antacids, the use of the nonparticulate antacid sodium citrate has been recommended. Alternatively, H_2-receptor antagonists usually increase gastric fluid pH in parturients without producing adverse effects. It must be remembered that H_2-receptor antagonists, unlike antacids, do not alter the pH of gastric fluid already present in the stomach. The combination of an H_2-receptor antagonist and sodium citrate may be more useful than an antacid alone for producing a persistent increase in gastric fluid pH.[7]

Metoclopramide may be useful for decreasing the gastric fluid volume of parturients in active labor requiring general anesthesia and considered at high risk of increased gastric fluid volumes (apprehension, opioid analgesia, recent food ingestion). Gastric hypomotility due to opioids, however, may be resistant to treatment with metoclopramide.

PHYSIOLOGY OF UTEROPLACENTAL CIRCULATION

The placenta provides for the union of maternal and fetal circulations for the purpose of physiologic exchange. Maternal blood is delivered to the placenta by the uterine arteries, and fetal blood arrives via two umbilical arteries. Nutrient-rich and waste-free blood is delivered to the fetus via a single umbilical vein. The most important determinants of placental function are uterine blood flow and the characteristics of substances available for exchange across the placenta.

Uterine Blood Flow

Maintenance of uterine blood flow at term (500 to 700 $ml \cdot min^{-1}$) is critical, since this flow determines the adequacy of placental circulation and fetal well-being. It is estimated that in the presence of a normal placenta, uterine blood flow can decrease about 50% before fetal distress, as reflected by acidosis, is detectable.

Uterine blood flow is not autoregulated and is therefore directly proportional to the mean perfusion pressure across the uterus and inversely proportional to the uterine vascular resistance. Therefore, uterine blood flow is decreased by drugs or events that decrease perfusion pressure (decreased systemic blood pressure or increased venous pressure) or increase uterine vascular resistance.

Hypotension

Hypotension due to aortocaval compression or peripheral sympathetic nervous system blockade decreases uterine blood flow by virtue of decreases in perfusion pressure. Drugs administered to parturients to produce analgesia and anesthesia during labor and delivery could decrease uterine blood flow via drug-induced changes in blood pressure. Epidural or spinal anesthesia does not alter uterine blood flow as long as maternal hypotension is avoided.

Uterine Vascular Resistance

Alpha-adrenergic stimulation produced by methoxamine and metaraminol can increase uterine vascular resistance and decrease uterine blood flow (Fig. 25-3).[8] Conversely, ephedrine is considered a useful sympathomimetic for increasing blood pressure in parturients because uterine blood flow is maintained in the presence of this vasopressor (Fig. 25-3).[8] Increased uterine vascular resistance with decreases in uterine blood flow can result from maternal stress or pain that stimulates the endogenous release of catecholamines (Fig. 25-4).[9] This response suggests that a regional or general anesthetic may be protective to the fetus. Uterine contractions also decrease uterine blood flow secondary to increased uterine venous pressure.

Placental Exchange

Placental exchange of substances occurs principally by diffusion from the maternal circulation to the fetus and vice versa. Diffusion of a substance across the placenta to the fetus depends on maternal-to-fetal concentration gradients, maternal protein binding, molecular weight, lipid solubility, and

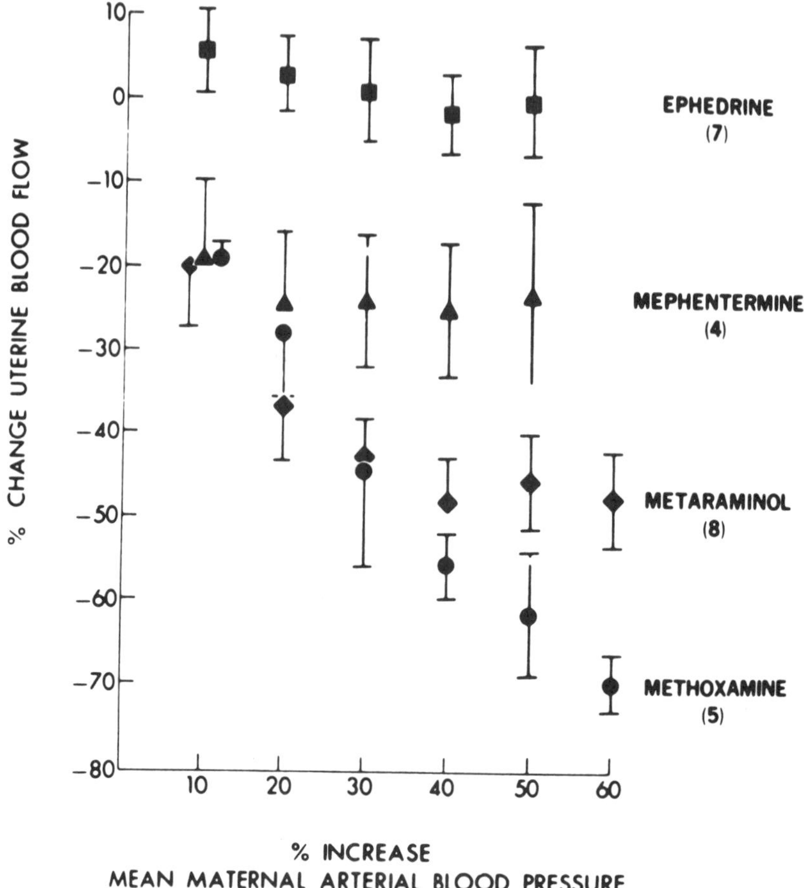

Figure 25-3. Uterine blood flow (mean ± SE) was measured in pregnant ewes (number of animals studied in parentheses) before and after increases in maternal blood pressure produced by the intravenous administration of sympathomimetics. With the exception of ephedrine, these drugs decreased uterine blood flow despite increasing mean arterial pressure. (From Ralston et al.,[8] with permission.)

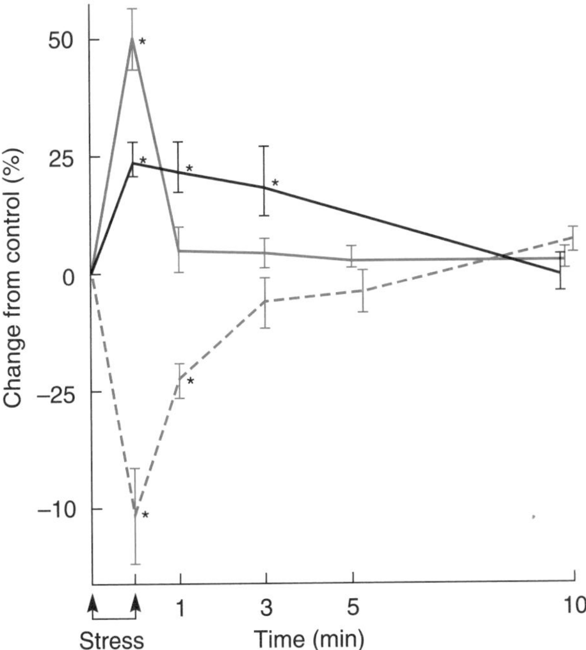

Figure 25-4. Electrically induced stress lasting 30 to 60 seconds in pregnant ewes results in increased maternal blood pressure (solid red line) and serum norepinephrine concentrations (solid black line) (mean ± SE). Uterine blood flow (dashed red line) is decreased about 50% at the time of maximum blood pressure and catecholamine increase. *Significantly different from control (*P* <0.05). (From Shnider et al.,[9] with permission.)

degree of ionization of that substance (Table 25-3). Minimizing the maternal blood concentration of a drug is the most important method of limiting the amount that ultimately reaches the fetus. Furthermore, transfer to the fetus can be decreased by intravenous injection of a drug during a uterine contraction because maternal blood flow to the placenta is markedly decreased at this time.

Maternal Protein Binding

Maternal protein binding of local anesthetics is important because only the portion of the drug not bound to protein is available for diffusion across the placenta. At typical clinical concentrations, 50% to 70% of lidocaine is bound to protein as compared with 95% of bupivacaine. The greater degree of protein binding for bupivacaine could impair placental transfer by decreasing the amount of free drug available for diffusion. This is consistent with the observation that the umbilical vein-to-uterine artery concentration ratio of bupivacaine is lower than the ratio measured for lidocaine. Nevertheless, dissociation of local anesthetics from protein is rapid, and it is questionable whether protein binding of drugs significantly impairs diffusion across the placenta.

Table 25-3. Determinants of Diffusion Across the Placenta

	Rapid Diffusion	Slow Diffusion
Maternal protein binding	Low	High
Molecular weight	<500	>1000
Lipid solubility	High	Low
Ionization	Minimal	Maximum

Molecular Weight and Lipid Solubility

The high molecular weight and poor lipid solubility of nondepolarizing muscle relaxants are consistent with their limited ability to cross the placenta. Succinylcholine has a low molecular weight but is highly ionized and therefore does not readily cross the placenta. Conversely, placental transfer of barbiturates, local anesthetics, and opioids is facilitated by the relatively low molecular weights of these substances.

FETAL UPTAKE AND DISTRIBUTION OF DRUGS

Fetal uptake of a substance that crosses the placenta is facilitated by the lower pH (0.1 unit) of fetal compared with maternal blood. The lower fetal pH means that weakly basic drugs (local anesthetics, opioids) that cross the placenta in the nonionized form will become ionized in the fetal circulation. Since an ionized drug cannot readily cross the placenta back to the maternal circulation, this drug will accumulate in the fetal blood against a concentration gradient. This phenomenon is known as ion trapping and may explain the higher concentrations of lidocaine found in the fetus when acidosis due to fetal distress is present (Fig. 25-5).[10] Furthermore, conversion of lidocaine to the ionized fraction maintains the concentration gradient from mother to fetus for the continued passage of nonionized lidocaine to the fetus. Despite decreased enzyme activity

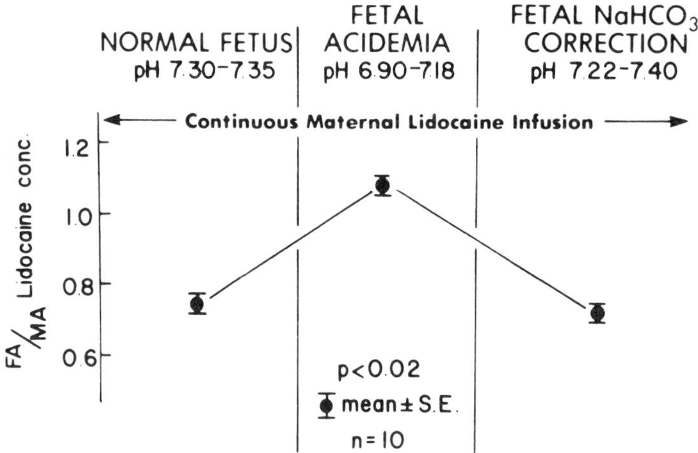

Figure 25-5. Fetal-to-maternal arterial (FA/MA) lidocaine ratios are higher during fetal acidemia than during control (normal fetus) or during pH correction with sodium bicarbonate. This reflects ion trapping of the ionized fraction of lidocaine in the fetus in the presence of acidosis. (From Biehl et al., with permission.)

compared with that in adults, the neonatal enzyme systems are adequately developed to metabolize most drugs, with the possible exception of mepivacaine.

The unique characteristics of the fetal circulation influence the distribution of drugs in the fetus and protect the vital organs of the fetus from exposure to high concentrations of drugs initially present in the umbilical venous blood. For example, about 75% of umbilical venous blood passes through the liver, such that significant portions of drugs can be metabolized before reaching the fetal arterial circulation for delivery to the heart and brain. Furthermore, drugs in the portion of the umbilical venous blood that enters the inferior vena cava via the ductus venosus will be diluted by drug-free blood returning from the lower extremities and pelvic viscera of the fetus.

MATERNAL MEDICATION DURING LABOR

Despite the increasing use of epidural analgesia to provide pain relief during labor and vaginal delivery, there is still an occasional role for systemic medications to decrease pain and anxiety. There is no ideal drug, since all systemic medications cross the placenta to some extent and produce depressant effects on the fetus. The amount of fetal depression depends primarily on the dose of drug and route and time of administration before delivery. Drugs likely to be administered as systemic medications are benzodiazepines, opioids, and ketamine. For example, a low dose of midazolam (0.5 to 1 mg IV) may be useful for decreasing anxiety, as during cesarean section performed with regional anesthesia. Meperidine is a popular opioid for administration to the parturient, particularly since the respiratory center of the newborn seems to be less sensitive to this opioid than to morphine. In an occasional parturient, intermittent doses of ketamine (10 to 15 mg IV) can be titrated to produce intense analgesia for 10 to 15 minutes without associated loss of consciousness or neonatal depression. Adverse maternal psychological effects, however, may accompany even these low doses of ketamine.

PROGRESS OF LABOR

Progress of labor refers to increasing cervical dilation, effacement, and descent of the fetal presenting part through the vagina with time (Fig. 25-6).[11] The onset of regular contractions signals the beginning of the first stage of labor. This stage is subdivided into the latent and active phases, lasting 7 to 13 hours in the primigravida and 4 to 5 hours in the multigravida. The second stage of labor begins with complete dilation of the cervix. The third stage extends from delivery of the baby until the placenta is expelled.

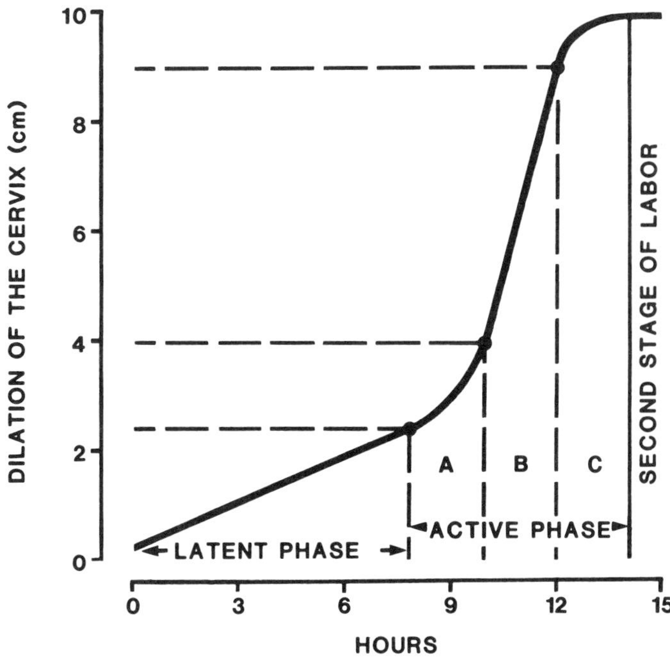

Figure 25-6. The progress of labor is divided into the first and second stages of labor, depending on the dilation of the cervix. The first stage of labor is further subdivided into a latent and an active phase. The active phase consists of the accelerated phase (A), the phase of maximum slope (B), and the deceleration phase (C). (Adapted from Friedman,[11] with permission.)

The progress of labor is unpredictable, being influenced by many variables, including maternal pain, parity, size and presentation of the fetus, and drugs and techniques used to provide analgesia or anesthesia. Excessive sedation or the premature initiation of a regional anesthetic is the most common cause for prolongation of the latent phase. Nevertheless, labor can slow spontaneously during the latent phase in the absence of anesthesia. Furthermore, catecholamine release in response to pain can inhibit uterine contractions such that analgesia provided by appropriate regional anesthetic techniques might even enhance the early progress of labor. During the active phase the most likely causes of delayed progress of labor are cephalopelvic disproportion, fetal malposition, and fetal malpresentation.

The impact of anesthesia on the progress of labor is more predictable after labor has become active. For example, during the active phase a T10 sensory level produced by spinal or epidural anesthesia has no significant effect on progress of labor provided fetal malpresentation is absent and hypotension is avoided. However, a regional anesthetic, by removing the reflex urge to bear down, may prolong the second stage of labor. Nevertheless, even if labor is prolonged by a regional anesthetic, there is no evidence that this is harmful to the fetus.

Volatile anesthetics produce dose-dependent decreases in uterine activity. Analgesia provided by low inhaled concentrations of halothane (0.5%) or enflurane (1%) during vaginal delivery does not decrease uterine activity, prolong labor, increase postpartum blood loss, or interfere with the uterine response to oxytocin. Higher inhaled concentrations of volatile anesthetics are the most reliable way of rapidly producing uterine relaxation when necessary.

REGIONAL ANESTHESIA FOR LABOR AND VAGINAL DELIVERY

Compared with analgesia produced by inhaled or parenteral drugs, the use of regional anesthetic techniques for labor and vaginal delivery decreases the likelihood of fetal drug depression and maternal pulmonary aspiration. Standards for regional anesthesia in obstetrics have been endorsed by the American Society of Anesthesiologists (see Appendix 2).

Regional anesthetic techniques effective during the first stage of labor include paracervical block, lumbar epidural analgesia, and caudal analgesia (Table 25-4). Pain during the second stage of labor is relieved by lumbar epidural analgesia, caudal analgesia, spinal anesthesia, and pudendal nerve block (Table 25-4).

Pain During Labor and Delivery

Parturition is associated with two distinct kinds of pain. The first type of pain, visceral in origin, is caused by uterine contractions plus dilation of the cervix. The other type of pain is somatic and is due to stretching of the vagina and perineum by descent of the fetus. The parturient has an uncontrollable urge to bear down as the presenting fetal part begins its descent through the vagina. It is customary to consider visceral pain to be part of the first stage and somatic pain to be part of the second stage of labor.

Rational use of regional anesthetic techniques requires an understanding of the pathways responsible for the transmission of visceral and somatic pain during labor and vaginal delivery (Fig. 25-7). During the first stage of labor, afferent visceral pain impulses from the uterus and cervix travel in nerves that accompany sympathetic nervous system fibers and enter the spinal cord at T10–L1. In the late first stage and the second stage of labor, somatic pain impulses originate primarily from receptors in the vagina and perineum and travel via the pudendal nerves to the spinal cord at S2–S4.

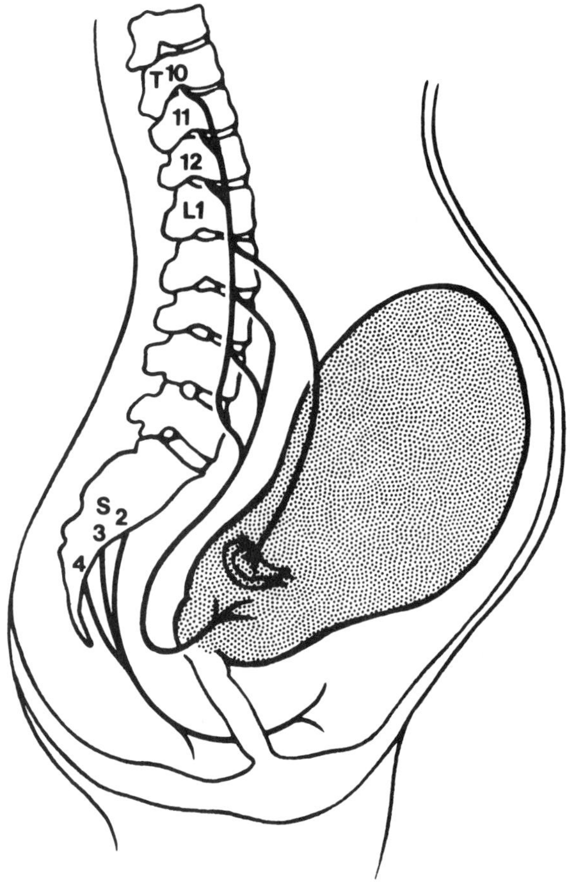

Figure 25-7. Schematic diagram of pain pathways during parturition. Visceral pain during the first stage of labor is due to uterine contraction and dilation of the cervix. Afferent pain impulses from the uterus and cervix are transmitted by nerves that accompany sympathetic nervous system fibers and enter the spinal cord at T10–L1. Somatic pain during the second stage of labor is vaginal and perineal in origin, and impulses travel via the pudendal nerves to S2–S4.

Table 25-4. Types of Regional Anesthesia for Labor and Vaginal Delivery

	Area of Anesthesia	Type of Pain Blocked
Paracervical block	T10–L1	Visceral
Lumbar epidural		
Segmental	T10–L1	Visceral
Standard	T10–S5	Visceral and somatic
Caudal	T10–S5	Visceral and somatic
Spinal		
Saddle	S1–S5	Somatic
Modified	T10–S5	Visceral and somatic
Pudendal nerve block	S2–S4	Somatic

Paracervical Block

Injection of local anesthetic solution into the fornix of the vagina lateral to the cervix (3 and 9 position) eliminates visceral pain by anesthetizing the sensory fibers from the uterus, cervix, and upper vagina. Somatic pain and the urge to bear down are not obtunded. Maternal hypotension does not result because sympathetic nervous system blockade does not occur. Paracervical block is not effective during the second stage of labor because sensory fibers from the perineum are not blocked. The major disadvantage of a paracervical block is the 8% to 40% incidence of fetal bradycardia that develops 2 to 10 minutes after injection of the local anesthetic solution. The cause of the bradycardia is not known but is probably related to decreased uterine blood flow secondary to uterine vasoconstriction from local anesthetic solutions applied in close proximity to the artery plus direct cardiac toxicity due to high fetal blood levels of the local anesthetics. Bradycardia produced by paracervical block is often associated with fetal acidosis. It would seem prudent to avoid this block in parturients with uteroplacental insufficiency or when there is co-existing fetal distress.

Lumbar Epidural Analgesia

Advantages of continuous lumbar epidural analgesia via an appropriately placed epidural catheter include the (1) ability to achieve segmental bands of analgesia (T10–L1) during the first stage of labor when total anesthesia is not required, (2) minimal local anesthetic requirements, and (3) maintenance of pelvic muscle tone so that rotation of the fetal head is more easily accomplished. Institution of continuous lumbar epidural analgesia is appropriate when the first stage of labor is well established as evidenced by dilation of the cervix (6 to 8 cm in a primipara or 4 to 6 cm in a multipara) and uterine contractions are strong and regular.

The visceral pain of the first stage of labor can be relieved by injection of 6 to 8 ml of 0.25% bupivacaine solution into the lumbar epidural space. Initially, a 2-ml test dose is injected and 3 minutes is allowed to elapse before the remaining drug is injected. This small test dose is used to improve the likelihood that an accidental subarachnoid injection will be recognized clinically. Assuming the absence of signs of spinal anesthesia after the test dose, the remaining 4 to 6 ml of local anesthetic solution is injected. The low dose of local anesthetic produces a sensory band of analgesia that is unlikely to cause sufficient peripheral sympathetic nervous system blockade to result in maternal hypotension. Nevertheless, parturients should be encouraged to remain in the lateral position. Addition of small doses of opioids (50 to 150 μg of fentanyl) to low concentrations of bupivacaine (0.125%) may accelerate the onset of analgesia.

The addition of fentanyl (50 μg) to the low concentration of bupivacaine provides more rapid and complete analgesia than the local anesthetic alone. A continuous epidural infusion of bupivacaine solution (0.0625% or 0.125%) plus a low dose of opioid (fentanyl 1 to 2 $\mu g \cdot ml^{-1}$) when delivered at a rate of about 10 $ml \cdot h^{-1}$ has the advantage of providing analgesia with the preservation of skeletal muscle tone.[12]

During the first 20 minutes after the initial dose of local anesthetic and after any additional doses, the parturient should be under continuous surveillance. If hypotension occurs (systolic blood pressure lower than 100 mmHg or more than a 30% decrease in a previously hypertensive parturient), left uterine displacement must be confirmed, intravenous fluids infused rapidly, the parturient placed in a 10- to 20-degree head-down position, and oxygen administered via a face mask. If blood pressure is not restored in 1 to 2 minutes, ephedrine (5 to 10 mg IV) should be administered every 1 to 2 minutes until an appropriate blood pressure response occurs. Often, the fetal heart rate is continuously monitored electronically before and after epidural analgesia is instituted.

Caudal Analgesia

Caudal analgesia is produced by injection of local anesthetic solution (0.25% bupivacaine 10 to 12 ml) into the sacral epidural space. Compared with continuous lumbar epidural analgesia, there is a lower incidence of inadvertent dural puncture and perineal analgesia is more profound. Disadvantages of caudal analgesia include difficulty in keeping the sacral area clean, technical difficulties in identifying the sacral hiatus, and accidental injection of local anesthetic solution into the fetal head. It may not be possible to produce a sufficient level of anesthesia with caudal analgesia should cesarean section become necessary.

Spinal (Saddle) Anesthesia

Spinal anesthesia is administered immediately before vaginal delivery by injecting small doses of a hyperbaric tetracaine solution (3 to 5 mg) or lidocaine (20 to 30 mg) into the lumbar subarachnoid space with the parturient in the sitting position. The sitting position is maintained for 1 to 2 minutes to ensure that only perineal analgesia (the area of the body that would be in contact with a saddle) occurs. True saddle anesthesia does not produce complete pain relief as afferent fibers from the uterus are not blocked.

Modified saddle anesthesia is achieved by the subarachnoid injection of 4 to 6 mg of tetracaine or 30 to 50 mg of lidocaine with the sitting position maintained for 30 seconds. With this approach, sensory blockade typically extends to T10, which prevents pain from contractions of the uterus. Addition of a small dose of opioid (fentanyl 6 to 10 μg, sufentanil 3 to 10 μg) to the local anesthetic solution can greatly prolong the period of analgesia into the postpartum period.

The major disadvantage of spinal anesthesia for vaginal delivery is the subsequent appearance of a headache, which is presumably due to loss of fluid through the hole in the dura produced by the needle used to gain entry into the subarachnoid space (see Chapter 12).

Pudendal Nerve Block

Pudendal nerve block is typically administered transvaginally by the obstetrician to provide perineal analgesia for delivery. Overlapping innervation of the perineum means that the urge to bear down is not completely abolished. Alone, this block provides complete analgesia for episiotomy and its repair and is usually sufficient for low forceps delivery. Supplementation with inhalation analgesia is required for mid-forceps delivery. A pudendal nerve block is not associated with peripheral sympathetic nervous system blockade and labor is not prolonged.

INHALATION ANALGESIA FOR VAGINAL DELIVERY

The goal of inhalation analgesia is to maintain the parturient in an awake but comfortable state with intact laryngeal reflexes during the first and second stages of labor. The major risk of inhalation analgesia is loss of protective airway reflexes, made more likely by excessive sedation associated with the decreased functional residual capacity and decreased MAC characteristic of pregnancy. Because all inhaled anesthetics readily cross the placenta, the possibility of neonatal effects must also be considered. However, analgesic concentrations of inhaled anesthetics (about 0.3 to 0.4 MAC) are free from excessive depressant effects on the fetus even if administered for prolonged periods.

An effective form of inhalation analgesia is the continuous administration of 30% to 40% nitrous oxide. Less satisfactory analgesia results when nitrous oxide is administered only during uterine contractions because about 50 seconds are necessary to achieve an effective analgesic concentration of this drug. Intermittent delivery of methoxyflurane (0.1% to 0.3% inspired) by self-administration or passively from an anesthetic machine is an alternative to the continuous administration of nitrous oxide. It must be appreciated that maternal and neonatal serum inorganic fluoride concentrations are increased after the administration of methoxyflurane. Enflurane (0.5% inspired) provides analgesia during the second stage of labor similar to that achieved with nitrous oxide.

ANESTHESIA FOR CESAREAN SECTION

Cesarean section is one of the most frequent of all surgical procedures. Indications for cesarean section include fetal distress, cephalopelvic disproportion, and failure of labor to progress. The notion that a previous cesarean section mandates the same route of delivery for all subsequent deliveries has been modified, and for selected patients (prior low segment transverse uterine incision and cephalic presentation) it is acceptable to allow vaginal delivery.

The decision to select a general or regional anesthetic to provide analgesia for cesarean section depends on the desire of the parturient and the presence or absence of fetal distress. When fetal distress is present, a general anesthetic may be preferable because anesthesia can be established quickly and maternal hypotension is less likely. A regional anesthetic is more often chosen for elective cesarean section, particularly when maternal awareness is desirable. Furthermore, a regional anesthetic minimizes the likelihood of maternal pulmonary aspiration and fetal depression. Independent of the choice of anesthesia, venous air emboli occur in 20% to 50% of patients undergoing cesarean section, although the magnitude of this occurrence is rarely sufficient to cause symptoms.[13] The incidence of venous air embolism can be decreased by maintaining the parturient in a 5-degree head-up position during the operation.

General Anesthetic

Preoperative medication often includes pharmacologic attempts to increase the gastric fluid pH. A nonparticulate antacid is widely used for this purpose. H_2-receptor antagonists are also effective for increasing the gastric fluid pH, but the time required for these drugs to act, unlike an antacid, precludes their use when induction of anesthesia is imminent. Metoclopramide could be administered to facilitate gastric emptying, although its usefulness in the parturient undergoing elective cesarean section is not established. If an anticholinergic drug is judged to be necessary, glycopyrrolate may be preferred because its quaternary ammonium structure prevents significant transfer across lipid barriers such as the placenta. If the cesarean section is elective, a benzodiazepine may be administered if the parturient is particularly apprehensive.

After preoxygenation, induction of anesthesia is typically accomplished with thiopental (3 to 5 $mg \cdot kg^{-1}$ IV) plus succinylcholine (1 to 1.5 $mg \cdot kg^{-1}$ IV) to facilitate intubation of the trachea with a cuffed tube. Cricoid pressure may be applied until the trachea is protected with the cuffed tube. Administration of a small dose of a nondepolarizing muscle relaxant before succinylcholine is often used to prevent skeletal muscle fasciculations. Nevertheless, fasciculations are not prominent in parturients, causing some to question the need for prior administration of a nondepolarizing muscle relaxant. The fetal brain will not be exposed to high concentrations of thiopental if the maternal dose is limited to about 5 $mg \cdot kg^{-1}$, reflecting clearance of the drug by the fetal liver and dilution by blood from the viscera and lower extremities.

Difficult (failed) intubation of the parturient's trachea is an important cause of anesthetic-related morbidity and mortality. A management plan is useful when failed tracheal intubation occurs, keeping in mind that the principal goal is oxygenation without aspiration.[14]

Maintenance of anesthesia until delivery of the fetus is often achieved with nitrous oxide (50% to 60% inspired) in oxygen plus intermittent injections or continuous infusion of succinylcholine for skeletal muscle paralysis. The major disadvantage of using only nitrous oxide is parturient awareness during the surgery. Maternal unconsciousness can be ensured by the administration of about 0.5 MAC of a volatile anesthetic plus nitrous oxide. This low dose of a volatile anesthetic does not increase maternal blood loss, alter the response of the uterus to oxytocin, or produce neonatal depression. Nitrous oxide supplemented with volatile anesthetics is associated with decreased autonomic nervous system responses to surgical stimulation and better maintenance of uterine blood flow. This response is presumed to reflect inhibition of endogenous norepi-

Suggested Approach for Management of a Difficult Airway in the Parturient

- Glottic opening cannot be visualized
  - Maintain cricoid pressure
  - Summon help
  - Repeat direct laryngoscopy
    - Optimal head position
    - Suction pharynx
    - Smaller tracheal tube with stylet
    - Temporarily reduce cricoid pressure
- If tracheal intubation still unsuccessful reapply cricoid pressure and select the appropriate following option
  - Ventilation possible—elective case
    - Maintain cricoid pressure
    - Allow patient to awaken
    - Select an alternative form of anesthesia
      - Regional
      - Awake tracheal intubation followed by general anesthesia
  - Ventilation possible—emergency case
    - Maintain cricoid pressure
    - Add an inhalation anesthetic during spontaneous or controlled ventilation
    - Expedite delivery and avoid fundal pressure
  - Ventilation impossible
    - Maintain cricoid pressure
    - Insert an oropharyngeal and/or nasopharyngeal airway
    - Summon surgical help
    - Cricothyrotomy
    - Tracheostomy

(Adapted from Davies et al.,[14] with permission.)

nephrine secretion by the volatile anesthetics. Excessive hyperventilation of the lungs must be avoided since the effects of positive pressure can decrease uterine blood flow.

There is controversy regarding the optimal time for delivery when a general anesthetic is used for cesarean section. More important than the duration of anesthesia before delivery is the time to delivery after incision into the uterus. Apgar scores are often decreased when the uterine incision-to-delivery time is longer than 90 seconds, presumably reflecting impaired uteroplacental blood flow.

After delivery, anesthesia can be supplemented with additional volatile drugs or opioids. It may be useful to pass an oral tube into the stomach to evacuate gastric fluid before the conclusion of surgery. The cuffed tube should not be removed from the trachea until it is certain that maternal laryngeal reflexes have returned.

Spinal Anesthesia

Spinal anesthesia as used for cesarean section must provide a sensory level of T4 to T6. A convenient guide for judging the appropriate dose of local anesthetic to be injected into the subarachnoid space is based on the height of the parturient (Table 25-5). Conversely, there are also data suggesting that the level of sensory anesthesia achieved in the parturient is not influenced by vertebral column length and thus a standard local anesthetic dose for spinal anesthesia may be acceptable.[15] Addition of morphine (0.2 to 0.25 mg) to the local anesthetic solution provides postoperative pain relief for about 24 hours.[16] After injection of the local anesthetic solution into the subarachnoid space, the parturient is placed supine with leftward displacement of the uterus.

Table 25-5. Dose of Local Anesthetic for Spinal Anesthesia Before Cesarean Section

	Lidocaine (5%, mg)	Tetracaine (1%, mg)	Bupivacaine (0.75%, mg)
Dose determined by height (cm)			
<160	65	8	10
160–182	70	9	13
>182	75	10	15
Onset (min)	1–3	3–5	2–4
Duration of action (min)	45–75	120–180	120–180

The T4 to T6 sensory level necessary for cesarean section is associated with significant peripheral sympathetic nervous system blockade and the likelihood of maternal hypotension. Hypotension is hazardous because a decrease in maternal blood pressure is associated with comparable decreases in uterine blood flow and placental perfusion, leading to fetal hypoxemia and acidosis. The incidence and magnitude of hypotension may be minimized by continuous left uterine displacement and intravenous hydration with lactated Ringer's solution (500 to 1000 ml) 15 to 30 minutes before performing the spinal anesthetic. On occasion, the anethesiologist may also prefer to inject ephedrine (25 to 50 mg IM) approximately 15 minutes before performing the spinal anesthetic. If hypotension occurs (systolic blood pressure lower than 100 mmHg or more than a 30% decrease in a previously hypertensive parturient) despite these measures, ephedrine (5 to 10 mg IV) is indicated. Backache is a frequent complaint in parturients, and the incidence does not increase after regional anesthesia. Nerve damage is not a risk of spinal anesthesia, with the most common neurologic dysfunction in the postpartum period being caused by compression of the lumbosacral trunk between the descending fetal head and the sacrum. Lumbosacral trunk injuries are characterized by foot drop combined with sensory loss.

Lumbar Epidural Anesthesia

Compared with spinal anesthesia, the sensory level necessary for a cesarean section is more controllable and hypotension is less precipitous with a continuous lumbar epidural anesthetic. Presumably, the slower onset of peripheral sympathetic nervous system blockade is responsible for the more gradual decrease in blood pressure. Unlike a spinal anesthetic, anesthesia provided with a lumbar epidural anesthetic requires doses of local anesthetics that are associated with significant systemic absorption of the drug. Technically, a lumbar epidural anesthetic is more difficult to perform than a spinal anesthetic. However, postoperative lumbar puncture headache does not occur because the dura is not punctured. Although rare, the most likely adverse effects of epidural anesthesia administered to the parturient are a transient neuropathy involving a single nerve (relation to anesthetic technique unproven) and seizures due to accidental intravascular injection of the local anesthetic solution (reason to perform an initial test dose).[17]

Bupivacaine concentrations must be at least 0.5% to ensure adequate anesthesia for the surgical stimulus associated with cesarean section. This contrasts with adequate analgesia for vaginal delivery produced by 0.25% bupivacaine. Limitation of the concentration of bupivacaine to 0.5% is recommended to minimize the likelihood of cardiotoxicity should this local anesthetic be accidentally injected intravenously (see Chapter 6). An initial 3-ml test dose of local anesthetic solution containing 1:200,000 epinephrine usually produces maternal tachycardia (beta effect of epinephrine) if administered intravenously and signs of spinal anesthesia if it enters the subarachnoid space. Assuming the absence of evidence of spinal anesthesia 3 minutes after the test dose, an additional amount (about 15 to 20 ml) of local anesthetic solution containing bupivacaine is injected through the lumbar epidural catheter so as to produce a T4 to T6 sensory level. When a rapid onset of analgesia is necessary, 3% 2-chloroprocaine can be used. When chloroprocaine is used, it is imperative that subarachnoid injection be avoided since permanent neurologic damage has occurred after accidental subarachnoid injection of large volumes of this local anesthetic. Lidocaine (2%) is an acceptable alternative to either bupivacaine or chloroprocaine. Analgesia can be extended 12 to 24 hours into the postoperative period by injection of opioids (morphine 3 to 5 mg) into the epidural space.[16] Side effects that may accompany the epidural administration of morphine to the parturient include pruritus, nausea and vomiting, and, rarely, delayed depression of ventilation (see Chapter 32).

ABNORMAL PRESENTATIONS AND MULTIPLE BIRTHS

Description of fetal position is based on the relationship of the fetal occiput, chin, or sacrum to the left or right side of the parturient. Approximately 90% of the deliveries are cephalic presentation in either the occiput transverse or occiput anterior position. All other presentations and positions are considered abnormal.

Persistent Occiput Posterior

During active labor, the occiput undergoes internal rotation to the occiput anterior position. If this rotation does not occur, the persistent occiput posterior position results in prolonged and painful labor. For example, severe back pain reflects pressure on the posterior sacral nerves by the fetal occiput. Regional anesthetic techniques that relax the maternal perineal muscles are often avoided until spontaneous internal rotation of the fetal head occurs.

Breech Presentation

Breech deliveries are associated with increased maternal (cervical lacerations, retained placenta, hemorrhage) and neonatal (intracranial hemorrhage, prolapse of the umbilical cord) morbidity. There is a tendency to deliver breech presentations by elective cesarean section. If cesarean section is planned, either a regional or general anesthetic may be selected. It should be appreciated that during a regional anesthetic, there may be difficultly in extracting the infant through the uterine incision. If uterine hypertonus is the cause, it will be necessary to rapidly induce general anesthesia, intubate the trachea, and administer a volatile anesthetic to relax the uterus.

When vaginal delivery is planned for a breech presentation, a frequent approach is infiltration of the perineum with a local anesthetic solution plus inhalation analgesia. Rapid induction of general anesthesia and intubation of the trachea may be necessary to permit administration of a volatile anesthetic if perineal muscle relaxation is inadequate for delivery of the aftercoming fetal head or if the lower uterine segment contracts and traps the fetal head. An alternative to infiltration and inhalation analgesia is the use of a continuous lumbar epidural anesthetic. For example, a lumbar epidural anesthetic provides analgesia and maximal perineal relaxation for delivery of the fetal head. The ability of parturients to push during delivery can be preserved by using low concentrations of local anesthetics (0.25% bupivacaine) and providing constant maternal encouragement. However, if uterine relaxation is required for facilitation of a breech extraction during vaginal delivery, it will be necessary to induce general anesthesia.

Multiple Gestations

The choice of anesthesia in the presence of multiple gestations must consider the frequent occurrence of prematurity and breech presentation. Inhalation analgesia plus local infiltration or a continuous lumbar epidural anesthetic is an acceptable method of anesthesia in these patients. Systemic medications, such as opioids, should be minimized, particularly if the fetus is premature.

PREGNANCY AND HEART DISEASE

Detection and evaluation of heart disease in parturients is crucial for planning management of anesthesia during labor and delivery. Increased cardiac output during pregnancy and after delivery may result in congestive heart failure in parturients with coexisting heart disease. For example, each uterine contraction increases cardiac output and central blood volume 10% to 25%. Subsequent delivery of the fetus and emptying of the uterus relieves compression of the inferior vena cava and aorta, resulting in marked increases in blood volume.

For most types of heart disease, no single technique of anesthesia is specifically indicated or contraindicated. Nevertheless, analgesia produced by a continuous lumbar epidural anesthetic can minimize the adverse effects of increased cardiac output, particularly when this increase is exaggerated by pain or anxiety. Inhalation analgesia is usually selected when sudden decreases in systemic vascular resistance and arterial blood pressure would be detrimental.

PREGNANCY-INDUCED HYPERTENSION

Pregnancy-induced hypertension (PIH) encompasses a range of disorders (gestational proteinuric hypertension, pre-eclampsia, eclampsia) formerly known as toxemia of pregnancy. Occurring in 5% to 15% of all pregnancies, PIH is a major cause of obstetric and perinatal morbidity and mortality. The pathophysiology of PIH involves nearly every organ system.

Pre-eclampsia is a syndrome manifesting after the 20th week of gestation characterized by hypertension (higher than 140/90 mmHg), proteinuria (more than 2 $g \cdot d^{-1}$), generalized edema, and complaints of headache. Manifestations of pre-eclampsia usually abate within 48 hours following delivery. Hemolysis (H), elevated liver enzymes (EL), and low platelet count (LP) make up the HELLP syndrome, which represents a severe form of pre-eclampsia. Eclampsia is present when seizures are superimposed on pre-eclampsia. Eclampsia occurs in about 5% of parturients who develop pre-eclampsia and is associated with a maternal mortality of about 10%. Causes of maternal mortality from eclampsia include congestive heart failure and cerebral hemorrhage.

Pathophysiology of Pregnancy-Induced Hypertension

- Cardiovascular system
  - Generalized vasoconstriction
  - Increased vascular responsiveness to sympathetic nervous system stimulation
  - Decreased uteroplacental perfusion
- Hepatorenal system
  - Decreased hepatic blood flow
  - Decreased glomerular filtration rate
  - Decreased renal blood flow
  - Retention of sodium and water
- Pulmonary system
  - Interstitial accumulation of fluid
  - Decreased PaO_2
  - Exaggerated edema of upper airway and larynx
- Central nervous system
  - Hyperreflexia
  - Cerebral edema
  - Seizure activity
- Intravascular fluid volume
  - Hypovolemia
- Coagulation
  - Decreased platelet count
  - Increased fibrin split products
- Uterus
  - Hyperactive
  - Premature labor

Treatment

Definitive treatment of PIH is delivery of the fetus and placenta. In the interim, magnesium and antihypertensive drugs may be required. A general or regional anesthetic should not be used in attempts to lower blood pressure.

Magnesium

Magnesium is effective in parturients with PIH by decreasing the irritability of the central nervous system, which decreases the likelihood of seizures. Magnesium also decreases hyperactivity at the neuromuscular junction, presumably by decreasing the presynaptic release of acetylcholine as well as by decreasing the sensitivity of postjunctional membranes to acetylcholine. In addition, magnesium relaxes uterine and vascular smooth muscle, which contributes to an increase in uterine blood flow.

Clinically, the therapeutic effects of magnesium therapy are estimated by the responsiveness of deep tendon reflexes. Marked depression of these reflexes is an indication of impending magnesium toxicity. Periodic determination of serum magnesium concentrations is also helpful in adjusting supplemental doses of magnesium so as to keep the level in a therapeutic range of 4 to 6 mEq·L^{-1}. Serum magnesium levels in excess of this range can lead to severe skeletal muscle weakness, hypoventilation, and cardiac arrest. Intravenous administration of calcium is the antidote for toxic effects of magnesium. Magnesium is excreted by the kidneys and must be used with caution when renal function is impaired.

Magnesium inhibits the release of acetylcholine from motor nerve terminals, thus enhancing the neuromuscular blocking properties of nondepolarizing muscle relaxants. Furthermore, PIH may be associated with decreases in plasma cholinesterase activity that are greater than those normally associated with pregnancy, resulting in potentiation of the effects of succinylcholine and mivacurium independent of magnesium therapy. This introduces the need for careful titration of the doses of muscle relaxants and monitoring of the effects produced by these drugs at the neuromuscular junction. Likewise, doses of sedatives and opioids should be decreased as magnesium can also enhance their effects. Because magnesium readily crosses the placenta, neonatal muscle tone can be decreased at birth.

Antihypertensives

Antihypertensive drugs are likely to be administered when the maternal diastolic blood pressure is higher than 110 mmHg. Hydralazine is frequently selected because of its rapid onset and ability to maintain or even increase renal blood flow. The presence of tachycardia may dictate the simultaneous administration of an adrenergic blocking drug such as labetalol. Nitroprusside is not a likely choice because cyanide resulting from the degradation of this vasodilator can cross the placenta and this could theoretically produce adverse effects on the fetus. The goal is to decrease diastolic blood pressure to about 100 mmHg. Fetal heart rate should be monitored continuously during drug-induced decreases of maternal blood pressure to ensure an early warning should uteroplacental circulation be jeopardized by decreased perfusion pressures.

Management of Anesthesia

Continuous lumbar epidural anesthesia is acceptable for vaginal delivery of the pre-eclamptic parturient in good medical control. Epidural anesthesia negates the need for administration of parenteral opioids to the parturient and possible adverse effects of these drugs on a premature fetus. The absence of the maternal urge to bear down decreases the likelihood of associated blood pressure increases. Before the lumbar epidural anesthetic is instituted, the parturient is often hydrated with intravenous fluids (1 to 2 L of lactated Ringer's solution) as guided by central venous pressure monitoring. More aggressive fluid administration may produce pulmonary edema, especially in the postoperative period. Coagulation studies are generally performed before the placement of the lumbar epidural catheter since both a quantitative and qualitative platelet defect can occur. Furthermore, low doses of aspirin may have been administered as prophylaxis against the development of PIH.

Initially, a segmental band of anesthesia (T10–L1) will provide analgesia for uterine contractions. As the second stage of labor is entered, the lumbar epidural anesthetic can be extended to provide perineal anesthesia. If hypotension occurs, the hypersensitivity of the maternal vasculature to catecholamines must be considered and decreased doses of ephedrine (2.5 mg IV) administered.

Cesarean section is necessary when fetal distress, reflecting deterioration of uteroplacental circulation, accompanies PIH. A general anesthetic is usually selected because a regional anesthetic would be associated with extensive peripheral sympathetic nervous system blockade. Before induction of anesthesia, an attempt must be made to restore intravascular fluid volume. Continuous monitoring of intra-arterial pressure, cardiac filling pressures, urine output, and fetal heart rate is useful. Induction of anesthesia is often performed with thiopental (3 to 5 mg·kg^{-1} IV) plus succinylcholine (1 to 1.5 mg·kg^{-1}

IV) to facilitate rapid intubation of the trachea. The use of a defasciculating dose of a nondepolarizing muscle relaxant before the administration of succinylcholine may not be necessary because magnesium therapy is likely to attenuate skeletal muscle fasciculations produced by the depolarizing muscle relaxant. Exaggerated edema of the upper airway structures may require the use of smaller tracheal tubes than anticipated. The blood pressure increase elicited by direct laryngoscopy and intubation of the trachea is predictably exaggerated in these parturients. A short duration of direct laryngoscopy is helpful for minimizing the magnitude and duration of the blood pressure increases. Hydralazine (5 to 10 mg IV) administered 10 to 15 minutes before the induction of anesthesia or nitroglycerin (1 to 2 $\mu g \cdot kg^{-1}$ IV) just before starting direct laryngoscopy has also been recommended for attenuating these blood pressure responses. A volatile anesthetic can be used to control intraoperative hypertension. The enhancement of the effects of all muscle relaxants by magnesium must be remembered and a peripheral nerve stimulator used to monitor the effect of decreased doses of muscle relaxants at the neuromuscular junction.

HEMORRHAGE IN THE PARTURIENT

Hemorrhage in the parturient is the leading cause of maternal mortality. Placenta previa and abruptio placentae are the major causes of bleeding during the third trimester. Uterine rupture can be responsible for uncontrolled hemorrhage that manifests during labor. Postpartum hemorrhage occurs in 3% to 5% of all vaginal deliveries and is typically due to retained placenta, uterine atony, or cervical or vaginal lacerations.

Hemorrhage in the Parturient

- Placenta previa
  - Painless vaginal bleeding
  - Advanced age and/or multiple parity
- Abruptio placentae
  - Abdominal pain
  - Bleeding partially or wholly concealed
  - Hemorrhagic shock
  - Disseminated intravascular coagulation
  - Acute renal failure
  - Fetal distress
- Uterine rupture
  - Abdominal pain
  - Hypotension
  - Disappearance of fetal heart tones
  - Associated with excessive uterine stimulation and/or rapid spontaneous delivery
- Retained placenta
  - Necessitates manual exploration of uterus
  - May require general anesthesia with a volatile anesthetic
- Uterine atony
  - Often associated with retained placenta
  - Oxytocin

Placenta Previa

Placenta previa is the abnormally low implantation of the placenta in the uterus. The cardinal symptom of placenta previa is painless vaginal bleeding that typically manifests around the 32nd week of gestation, when the lower uterine segment is beginning to form. When this diagnosis is suspected, the position of the placenta should be confirmed by ultrasonography or radioisotope scan. If these tests are not conclusive and vaginal bleeding persists, the diagnosis is made by direct examination of the cervical os. This examination should be done in the delivery room, only after preparations have been taken to replace acute blood loss and to proceed with an emergency cesarean section. Specifically, one and possibly two large-gauge intravenous cannulae should be inserted and cross-matched blood should be available. Ketamine (1 to 1.5 $mg \cdot kg^{-1}$ IV) is a useful drug for induction of anesthesia in the presence of acute hemorrhage due to placenta previa. Maintenance of anesthesia before delivery is typically with inhalation of 50% nitrous oxide plus intermittent intravenous injections or continuous infusion of succinylcholine to produce skeletal muscle relaxation. Neonates delivered from parturients in hemorrhagic shock are likely to be acidotic and hypovolemic.

Abruptio Placentae

Abruptio placentae is the separation of a normally implanted placenta after 20 weeks of gestation.

When the separation involves only the placental margin, the escaping blood can appear as vaginal bleeding. Alternatively, large volumes of blood loss can remain entirely concealed in the uterus. The definitive treatment of abruptio placentae is to empty the uterus. If there are no signs of maternal hypovolemia, clotting abnormalities, or fetal distress, a continuous lumbar epidural anesthetic can be used to provide anesthesia for labor and vaginal delivery. However, severe hemorrhage necessitates an emergency cesarean section involving a general anesthetic with ketamine for induction of anesthesia and nitrous oxide for maintenance of anesthesia. It is predictable that neonates born under these circumstances will be acidotic and hypovolemic.

Uterine Rupture

Uterine rupture can be associated with separation of a previous uterine scar, rapid spontaneous delivery, or excessive oxytocin stimulation. Overall, however, more than 80% of uterine ruptures are spontaneous without an obvious explanation.

Retained Placenta

Retained placenta occurs in about 1% of all vaginal deliveries and usually necessitates manual exploration of the uterus. If a lumbar epidural or spinal anesthetic was not used for vaginal delivery, manual removal of the placenta may be initially attempted under continuous inhalation analgesia. Induction of general anesthesia with intubation of the trachea and administration of a volatile drug to provide uterine relaxation will be necessary if the uterus remains firmly contracted around the placenta.

Uterine Atony

Uterine atony as a cause of postpartum hemorrhage can occur immediately after delivery or manifest several hours later. Retained placenta is a common accompaniment of uterine atony. It is treated with synthetic oxytocins (Pitocin, Syntocinon), which do not contain vasopressin. Dilute solutions of synthetic oxytocins exert no cardiovascular effects, but rapid intravenous injections may be associated with tachycardia, vasodilation, and hypotension. These cardiovascular effects are avoided by intravenous infusion of 10 to 15 units of synthetic oxytocin in 500 ml of balanced salt solution until uterine contraction is adequate. Synthetic oxytocins lack vasopressin and therefore do not produce exaggerated blood pressure increases in parturients who have been previously treated with sympathomimetics.

AMNIOTIC FLUID EMBOLISM

Amniotic fluid embolism is signaled by the sudden onset of respiratory distress, hypotension, and arterial hypoxemia, reflecting the cardiopulmonary effects of entrance of amniotic fluid into the circulation. Multiparous parturients who experience a tumultuous labor are most likely to experience an amniotic fluid embolism. Definitive diagnosis is made by demonstrating amniotic fluid material in maternal blood that has been aspirated from a central venous catheter. Treatment is directed toward cardiopulmonary resuscitation and correction of arterial hypoxemia. Conditions that can mimic an amniotic fluid embolism include inhalation of gastric contents and pulmonary embolus.

ANESTHESIA FOR NONOBSTETRIC SURGERY DURING PREGNANCY

The objectives for management of anesthesia in parturients undergoing nonobstetric surgery, such as excision of an ovarian cyst or appendectomy, are avoidance of teratogenic drugs, avoidance of intrauterine fetal hypoxia and acidosis, and prevention of premature labor. There is always the possibility that anesthesia will be unknowingly administered in early undiagnosed pregnancy.

Avoidance of Teratogenic Drugs

Most drugs, including anesthetics, have been demonstrated to be teratogenic in at least one animal species. In humans, the critical period of organogenesis is between 15 and 56 days of gestation. Nevertheless, there is no evidence that anesthetics administered during pregnancy are teratogenic. Sufficient circumstantial evidence exists, however, to warrant caution in the administration of nitrous oxide to parturients.[18] There is no evidence in humans that drugs administered to produce analgesia during labor and vaginal delivery adversely affect later mental and neurologic development of the offspring.

Avoidance of Intrauterine Fetal Hypoxia and Acidosis

Intrauterine fetal hypoxia and acidosis are prevented by avoiding maternal hypotension, arterial hypoxemia, and excessive changes in the $PaCO_2$. High inspired concentrations of oxygen do not produce in utero retrolental fibroplasia because the high oxygen consumption of the placenta plus uneven distribution of the maternal and fetal blood flow in the placenta prevent fetal PaO from exceeding about 45 mmHg.

Prevention of Premature Labor

The underlying pathology necessitating the surgery and not the anesthetic technique determines the onset of premature labor. After successful completion of surgery, it is advisable to continue monitoring the fetal heart rate and maternal uterine activity. Premature labor can be treated with beta-2 agonists such as terbutaline or ritodrine. These drugs relax uterine smooth muscle, resulting in inhibition of uterine contractions and improved uteroplacental blood flow. Side effects that may accompany beta-2 agonist therapy include maternal hypokalemia and cardiac dysrhythmias and fetal tachycardia and hypoglycemia. In the absence of surgery, premature labor is considered to be present when a parturient between 20 and 35 weeks of gestation experiences at least eight uterine contractions every hour combined with cervical effacement greater than 75%.

Management of Anesthesia

Elective surgery in the parturient should always be deferred until after delivery. When surgery is necessary, it is best to delay the operation until the second or third trimester. Emergency surgery in the first trimester is often performed with lumbar epidural anesthesia or spinal anesthesia. Spinal anesthesia is uniquely advantageous since it limits fetal drug exposure to a minimum. Continuous intraoperative monitoring of fetal heart rate, after about the 16th week of gestation, is helpful in providing early warning of fetal distress due to impaired uteroplacental perfusion (see the section *Diagnosis and Management of Fetal Distress*). When a general anesthetic is chosen, it should be appreciated that low concentrations of volatile drugs are not associated with significant decreases in uterine blood flow. Regardless of the technique of anesthesia selected, it is recommended that inhaled concentrations of oxygen be at least 50%.

SUBSTANCE ABUSE

Substance abuse, most often with cocaine and/or opioids, may be present in the parturient. The newborn is often premature and depressed. These parturients pose an added risk to the anesthesiologist owing to the possible presence of hepatitis or acquired immunodeficiency syndrome. Regional anesthesia may be the preferred anesthetic technique in these parturients, considering possible adverse drug reactions between the abused drug and those likely to be administered during general anesthesia.

DIAGNOSIS AND MANAGEMENT OF FETAL DISTRESS

Fetal well-being is often determined by evaluation of beat-to-beat variability in fetal heart rate as computed from R wave intervals on the fetal electrocardiogram. The fetal electrocardiogram is obtained via an electrode placed on the presenting fetal part or indirectly via ultrasound using a sensor placed on the maternal abdomen. Another useful method for monitoring fetal well-being is evaluation of fetal heart rate decelerations associated with contractions of the uterus. Fetal heart rate decelerations are classified as early, late, and variable (Figs. 25-8 to 25-10).[19] Fetal scalp blood sampling for determination of pH is indicated when abnormal fetal heart rate patterns occur. It has been observed that the fetus is usually depressed when one or more fetal scalp pH values are near 7.0.

Beat-to-Beat Variability

The fetal heart rate varies 5 to 20 beats·min^{-1}, with a normal heart rate ranging between 120 and 160 beats·min^{-1}. This normal variability is thought to reflect the integrity of the neural pathway from the fetal cerebral cortex through the medulla, vagus nerves, and cardiac conduction system. Fetal well-being is ensured when beat-to-beat variability is present. Conversely, fetal distress due to arterial hypoxemia, acidosis, or central nervous system damage is associated with minimal to absent variability of the

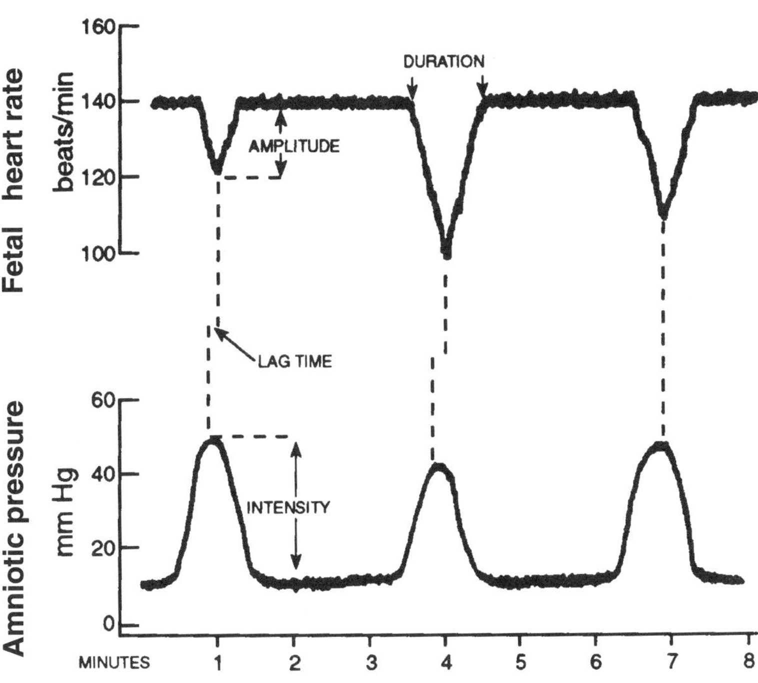

Figure 25-8. Early decelerations of the fetal heart rate are characterized by a short lag time between the onset of the uterine contraction and the beginning of heart rate slowing. The maximum fetal heart rate slowing occurs at the peak intensity of the contraction. Fetal heart rate returns to normal by the time the contraction has ceased. The most likely explanation for this fetal heart rate slowing is vagal stimulation due to compression of the fetal head. (From Shnider,[19] with permission.)

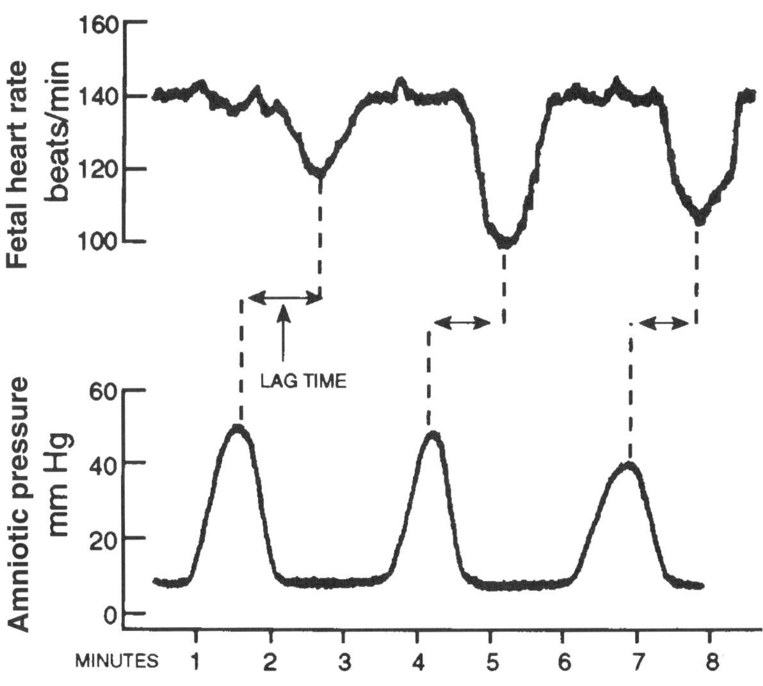

Figure 25-9. Late decelerations of the fetal heart rate are characterized by a delay between the onset of the uterine contraction and the beginning of fetal heart rate slowing. The fetal heart rate does not return to normal until after the contraction has ceased. Late decelerations indicate uteroplacental insufficiency. (From Shnider,[19] with permission.)

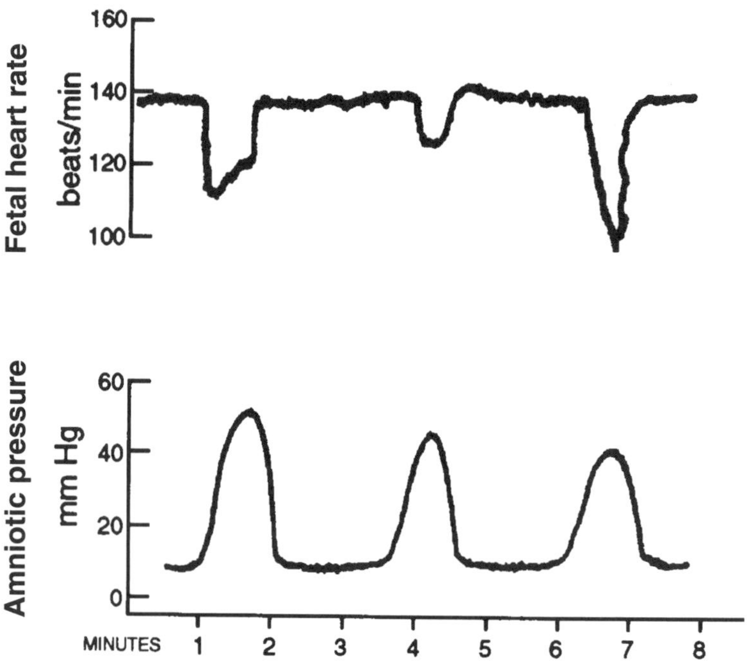

Figure 25-10. Variable decelerations of fetal heart rate are characterized by varying magnitudes and times of onset of heart rate slowing. This pattern is usually benign but if persistent may reflect compression of the umbilical cord. (From Shnider,[19] with permission.)

fetal heart rate. Drugs (local anesthetics used for continuous lumbar epidural anesthesia, benzodiazepines, opioids, anticholinergics) administered to parturients may eliminate fetal heart rate variability even in the absence of fetal distress. This drug-induced effect does not appear to be deleterious but may cause difficulty in the interpretation of fetal heart rate monitoring.

Early Decelerations

Early decelerations are characterized by slowing of the fetal heart rate that begins with the onset of the uterine contraction (Fig. 25-8).[19] This deceleration pattern is thought to be caused by vagal stimulation secondary to compression of the fetal head and is not indicative of fetal distress.

Late Decelerations

Late decelerations are characterized by slowing of the fetal heart rate that begins 10 to 30 seconds after the onset of the uterine contraction (Fig. 25-9).[19] This deceleration pattern is associated with fetal distress, most likely reflecting myocardial hypoxia secondary to uteroplacental insufficiency as produced by maternal hypotension. Determination of the fetal scalp pH is generally recommended when this pattern persists.

Variable Decelerations

As the designation indicates, these deceleration patterns are variable in magnitude, duration, and time of onset (Fig. 25-10).[19] Variable decelerations are thought to be caused by umbilical cord compression. Unless prolonged beyond 30 seconds or associated with fetal bradycardia (slower than 70 beats·min^{-1}), they are usually benign. Changing maternal position often lessens or abolishes this pattern.

EVALUATION OF THE NEONATE AND NEONATAL RESUSCITATION

The importance of assessment of the neonate immediately after birth is to promptly identify depressed infants who require active resuscitation. In this regard, the Apgar score, which assigns a numerical value to five vital signs measured or observed 1 and

5 minutes after delivery, has not been surpassed as a method of facilitating recognition of the newborn who requires active resuscitation (Table 25-6). Indeed, the Apgar score can be used to guide the extent to which resuscitation is necessary (Table 25-7) (see Chapter 35).

Apgar Score 8 to 10

Most newborns fall into this category, which requires little treatment other than suctioning the nose and mouth and placement in a radiantly heated bed.

Apgar Score 5 to 7

These newborns have likely suffered mild asphyxia before birth. They usually respond to external stimulation and delivery of supplemental oxygen over the face. If they do not respond in 1 to 2 minutes and the heart rate is slower than 100 beats·min^{-1}, ventilation of the newborn's lungs with oxygen should be instituted via a bag and mask.

Apgar Score 3 to 6

These newborns are moderately depressed, are cyanotic, and have poor breathing efforts. It may be necessary to control ventilation of the lungs with oxygen via a bag and mask. Ventilation of the newborn's lungs may be difficult because airway resistance is increased, which may cause gas to enter the stomach, leading to gastric distension and vomiting. If breathing has not started spontaneously, the trachea should be intubated and blood obtained from a doubly clamped segment of the umbilical cord for analysis of arterial blood gases and pH.

Table 25-6. Evaluation of the Neonate Using the Apgar Score

	Score		
	Zero	One	Two
Heart rate (beats·min^{-1})	Absent	<100	>100
Breathing	Absent	Slow	Irregular crying
Reflex irritability	No response	Grimace	Cry
Muscle tone	Limp	Flexion of extremities	Active
Color	Cyanotic	Body pink Extremities cyanotic	Pink

Table 25-7. Apgar Score as a Guide to Newborn Resuscitation

Apgar Score	Treatment
>8	Suction pharynx Place in a warm environment
5–7	External stimulation Oxygen by mask Mechanical ventilation by mask if no response
3–6	Initial mechanical ventilation by mask Intubation of the trachea if spontaneous ventilation does not occur promptly Analysis of arterial blood gases from a doubly clamped segment of the umbilical cord
<2	Intubation of the trachea and mechanical ventilation of the lungs with oxygen External cardiac compressions if heart rate <60 beats·min^{-1}

Apgar Score 0 to 2

These newborns are severely asphyxiated and require prompt resuscitative efforts. The trachea should be promptly intubated and ventilation of the lungs controlled at a rate of 30 to 60 breaths·min^{-1}. An occasional breath should be held for 2 to 3 seconds to expand atelectatic areas. Also, a positive end-expiratory pressure to 1 to 3 mmHg is often useful. The adequacy of ventilation of the newborn's lungs is best determined by physical examination and analysis of arterial blood gases. Both sides of the chest should rise equally and simultaneously. If one side rises before the other, the tip of the tracheal tube may have entered the bronchus or pneumothorax or a diaphragmatic hernia (rarely) may be present. Airway pressure higher than 25 cmH$_2$O should not be used. If the heart rate is slower than 60 beats·min^{-1}, external cardiac compressions are instituted. Epinephrine (0.005 mg·kg^{-1} IV) is indicated in the newborn who is severely hypotensive and bradycardic. Because asphyxiated newborns are often hypoglycemic, glucose administration may be required. Although these newborns are usually acidotic, the need for bicarbonate therapy is controversial (see Chapter 35).

The trachea should be suctioned before ventilation of the newborn's lungs is attempted, especially in infants born with meconium staining of the amniotic fluid. If meconium is distributed into the periphery of the lungs, a substantial number of these infants will develop pulmonary dysfunction in the first few days of life.

Vascular Resuscitation

If the response to ventilation of the lungs and stimulation is not immediate, an umbilical artery catheter should be inserted to permit analysis of arterial blood gases, pH, and blood pressure; to expand blood volume; and to administer drugs. The umbilical cord stump should be held straight up with a clamp and the abdomen and cord sterilized with an iodine-containing solution. The stump can then be tied near the base and the cord cleanly cut with a scalpel, leaving 1 to 2 cm of stump. The umbilical artery can then be dilated with a curved forcep. A 3.5- to 5.0-gauge French umbilical artery catheter is advanced into the dilated vessel and connected to a three-way stopcock. Before anything is injected, blood must be withdrawn to clear air from the catheter. Hypovolemic newborns are usually hypotensive (mean arterial pressure lower than 50 mmHg) and pale and have poor capillary filling and perfusion. Their extremities are cold and their pulses weak or absent. Hypovolemia is treated with blood, plasma, or crystalloid solutions. At times, the volume of fluid required may exceed 50% of the blood volume. On the other hand, care must be taken not to overexpand the intravascular fluid volume and cause hypertension.

NEUROBEHAVIORAL TESTING

Neurobehavioral testing is able to detect subtle or delayed effects of drugs administered during labor and delivery that are not appreciated by the Apgar score. This testing evaluates the neonate's state of wakefulness, reflex responses, skeletal muscle tone, and responses to sound. Studies of local anesthetics used to provide epidural anesthesia have not revealed differences in neurobehavioral scores in neonates exposed to lidocaine or bupivacaine.[20] Compared with spinal anesthesia, the use of general anesthesia for elective cesarean sections is associated with depression of neurobehavioral testing despite similar Apgar scores in both groups. Despite this difference, there is no evidence of prolonged adverse effects.[20]

POSTPARTUM TUBAL LIGATION

Postpartum tubal ligation is the most common type of surgery performed in the early postpartum period. Residual epidural anesthesia from the preceding delivery may be used to perform the intra-abdominal procedure, which necessitates a T5 sensory level to ensure patient comfort. When epidural or spinal anesthesia was not used for delivery, it is common to wait 8 to 12 hours postpartum before inducing general anesthesia for tubal ligation in hopes of improving the likelihood of gastric emptying. Nevertheless, there is no demonstrable difference in gastric fluid volume and pH when parturients are studied 1 to 8 hours following vaginal delivery.

REFERENCES

1. Clark SL, Cotton DB, Pivarnik JM, et al. Position change and central hemodynamic profile during normal third-trimester pregnancy and postpartum. Am J Obstet Gynecol 1991;64:883–7.
2. Gare DJ, Shime J, Paul WM, Hoskins M. Oxygen administration during labor. Am J Obstet Gynecol 1969;105:954–61.
3. Palahaniuk RJ, Shnider SM, Eger EI II. Pregnancy decreases the requirement of inhaled anesthetic agents. Anesthesiology 1974;41:82–3.
4. Fagraeus L, Urban BJ, Bromage PR. Spread of epidural analgesia in early pregnancy. Anesthesiology 1983;58:184–7.
5. Grundy EM, Zamora AM, Winnie AP. Comparison of spread of epidural anesthesia in pregnant and nonpregnant women. Anesth Analg 1979;57:544–6.
6. O'Sullivan GM, Bullingham RE. Noninvasive assignment by radiotelemetry of antacid effect during labor. Anesth Analg 1985;64:95–100.
7. Ormezzano X, Francois TP, Viaud J-Y, et al. Aspiration pneumonitis prophylaxis in obstetric anaesthesia: Comparison of effervescent cimetidine-sodium citrate mixture and sodium citrate. Br J Anaesth 1990;64:503–6.
8. Ralston DH, Shnider SM, deLorimier AA. Effects of equipotent ephedrine, metaraminol, mephentermine, and methoxamine on uterine blood flow in the pregnant ewe. Anesthesiology 1974;40:354–70.
9. Shnider SM, Wright RG, Levinson G, et al. Uterine blood flow and plasma norepinephrine changes during maternal stress in the pregnant ewe. Anesthesiology 1979;50:524–7.
10. Biehl D, Shnider SM, Levinson G, Callender K. Placental transfer of lidocaine. Effects of fetal acidosis. Anesthesiology 1978;48:409–12.

11. Friedman EA. Primigravid labor. A graphicostatistical analysis. Obstet Gynecol 1955;6:567–89.
12. Chestnut DH, Laszewski LJ, Pollack KL, et al. Continuous epidural infusion of 0.0625% bupivacaine-0.0002% of fentanyl during second stage of labor. Anesthesiology 1990;72:613–8.
13. Fong J, Gadalla F, Druzin M. Venous emboli occurring during cesarean section: The effect of patient position. Can J Anaesth 1991;38:191–6.
14. Davies JM, Weeks S, Crone LA, Pavlin E. Difficult intubation in the parturient. Can J Anaesth 1989;36: 668–74.
15. Norris MC. Patient variables and the subarachnoid spread of hyperbaric bupivacaine in the term parturient. Anesthesiology 1990;72:478–82.
16. Rosen MA, Hughes SC, Shnider SM, et al. Epidural morphine for the relief of postoperative pain after cesarean delivery. Anesth Analg 1983;62:666–72.
17. Scott DB, Hibbard BM. Serious non-fatal complications associated with extradural block in obstetric practice. Br J Anaesth 1990;64:537–41.
18. David AG, Moier DD. Anaesthesia during pregnancy. In: Ostheimer GN, ed. Clinics in Anaesthesiology. London, WB Saunders 1986;4:233–46.
19. Shnider SM. Diagnosis of fetal distress: Fetal heart rate. In: Shnider SM, ed. Obstetrical Anesthesia: Current Concepts and Practice. Baltimore, Williams & Wilkins 1970;197–203.
20. Corke BC. Neonatal neurobehavior II: Current clinical status. In: Ostheimer GW, ed. Clinics in Anaesthesiology. London, WB Saunders 1986;4:219–27.

26

Pediatrics

Understanding the physiologic and pharmacologic differences among neonates, infants, children, and adults permits principles used in adult anesthesia to be adapted to pediatric anesthesia. Neonates are defined as being 1 to 28 days of age, infants are 1 to 12 months of age, and children are 1 year to puberty. Neonates and infants are the age groups in which differences from adult patients are most marked.

PHYSIOLOGIC DIFFERENCES

One of the most important differences that physiologically separates neonates and infants from adults is oxygen consumption. Oxygen consumption in neonates may be higher than 6 $ml{\cdot}kg^{-1}{\cdot}min^{-1}$, which is about twice that in adults. To meet this increased demand, there are compensatory changes in the cardiovascular and pulmonary systems that distinguish pediatric from adult patients (Tables 26-1 and 26-2).

Cardiovascular

Cardiac output is increased 30% to 60% in neonates to help meet the increased oxygen requirements of this age group. Furthermore, the oxyhemoglobin dissociation curve is shifted to the left, reflecting the presence of fetal hemoglobin. In this regard, both an increased cardiac output and high hemoglobin concentration (average 17 $g{\cdot}dl^{-1}$) are important to offset the decreased release of oxygen from fetal hemoglobin to tissues. By 4 to 6 months of age, oxyhemoglobin dissociation curves approximate those of adults. This change is reflected by an increase in the P_{50} (arterial partial pressure of oxygen at which 50% of hemoglobin is saturated with oxygen) from 19 mmHg to about 26 mmHg and is preceded at 2 to 3 months of age by a decrease in hemoglobin concentrations to about 11 $g{\cdot}dl^{-1}$ (physiologic anemia) as fetal hemoglobin is replaced by adult hemoglobin. Anemia sufficient to jeopardize the oxygen carrying capacity of the blood is possible when hemoglobin concentrations are lower than 13 $g{\cdot}dl^{-1}$ in the newborn or lower than 10 $g{\cdot}dl^{-1}$ in infants older than 6 months of age.

Lack of distensibility of the neonate's left ventricle impairs diastolic filling and limits the significance of increasing the stroke volume as a means of increasing cardiac output. As a result, cardiac output in infants is, to a large extent, heart rate dependent.

Arterial blood pressure increases with increasing age. Anatomic closure of the foramen ovale occurs between 3 and 12 months of age, although 20% to 30% of adults have a probe-patent foramen ovale. Vasoconstrictive responses of neonates to hemorrhage are lower than those of adults.

Pulmonary

Alveolar ventilation is doubled in neonates compared with adults to help meet increased oxygen requirements of this age group. Carbon dioxide production is also increased in neonates, but increased alveolar ventilation maintains a near normal $PaCO_2$. Because tidal volume on a weight basis is similar for both neonates and adults, increased alveolar ventilation is achieved by increasing the fre-

Table 26-1. Comparison of Cardiovascular Variables

	Neonate	Infant	5 Years of Age	Adult
Weight (kg)	3	6–10	18	70
Oxygen consumption ($ml \cdot kg^{-1} \cdot min^{-1}$)	6	5	6	3
Systolic arterial blood pressure (mmHg)	65	90–95	95	120
Heart rate ($beats \cdot min^{-1}$)	130	120	90	80
Blood volume ($ml \cdot kg^{-1}$)	85	80	75	65
Hemoglobin ($g \cdot dl^{-1}$)	17	11–12	13	14

quency of breathing. The PaO_2 increases rapidly after birth, but several days are required to achieve levels comparable to those in older children. Central nervous system regulation of ventilation is immature in neonates, contributing to less predictable responses than those of adults when hypoxic gas mixtures are inhaled.

Extracellular Fluid Volume

Extracellular fluid volume is equivalent to about 40% of the body weight of neonates compared with about 20% in adults. By 18 to 24 months of age, the proportion of extracellular fluid volume relative to body weight is similar to that in adults. The increased metabolic rate characteristic of neonates results in accelerated turnover of extracellular fluid and dictates meticulous attention to intraoperative fluid replacement.

Table 26-2. Comparison of Pulmonary Variables

	Neonate	Infant	5 Years of Age	Adult
Weight (kg)	3	6–10	18	70
Breathing frequency ($breaths \cdot min^{-1}$)	35	24–30	20	15
Tidal volume ($ml \cdot kg^{-1}$)	6	6	6	6
Vital capacity ($ml \cdot kg^{-1}$)	35			70
Alveolar ventilation ($ml \cdot kg^{-1} \cdot min^{-1}$)	130			60
Carbon dioxide production ($ml \cdot kg^{-1} \cdot min^{-1}$)	6			3
Functional residual capacity ($ml \cdot kg^{-1}$)	25	25	35	40

Temperature Regulation

To maintain normal body temperature, infants and children create heat by metabolizing brown fat, crying, and moving more vigorously but, unlike adults, rarely by shivering. Maintaining normal body temperature is more difficult in neonates and infants than in adults because of a larger surface-to-volume ratio, increased metabolic rate, and lack of sufficient body fat for insulation. Therefore, the neonate or infant is more likely than the adult to experience adverse decreases in body temperature when anesthetized in cold operating rooms.

Renal

The kidneys at birth are characterized by decreased glomerular filtration rate, decreased sodium excretion, and decreased concentrating ability. Over the first 3 months of life, glomerular filtration rate increases twofold to threefold. Thereafter, the rate of increase is slower until adult values are reached by 12 to 24 months of age. After fluid restriction, maximum urine osmolarity for term neonates is about 525 $mOsm \cdot kg^{-1}$. By 15 to 30 days of age, maximum urine osmolarity may be as high as 950 $mOsm \cdot kg^{-1}$. Still, it takes 6 to 12 months before infants are able to concentrate urine as well as adults, emphasizing that this young age group is less able to compensate for extremes of fluid balance.

PHARMACOLOGIC DIFFERENCES

Pharmacologic differences between responses of pediatric and adult patients to drugs (especially muscle relaxants) is often predictable considering differences in extracellular fluid volume, metabolic rate, renal function, and receptor maturity.

Inhaled Anesthetics

The uptake, distribution, and potency of inhaled anesthetics differ in neonates and infants as compared with adults.[1–3] In general, the rate of induction of inhalation anesthesia is shortened in neonates as compared with adults. This is probably because of a smaller functional residual capacity per unit of body weight and a greater tissue blood flow, especially to vessel-rich group tissues (brain, heart, liver, kidneys). For example, vessel-rich group tissues compose approximately 10% of total body volume in adults but 22% of total body volume in neonates.[1]

Full-term neonates require lower concentrations of volatile anesthetics than infants. For example, the MAC of halothane in neonates is 0.87% compared with 1.20% in infants (Fig. 26-1).[2] Furthermore, MAC in preterm neonates is less than MAC in full-term neonates (Fig. 26-2).[3] MAC steadily increases until 2 to 3 months of age. After 3 months of age, it progressively declines with aging, although there are slight increases at the time of puberty.

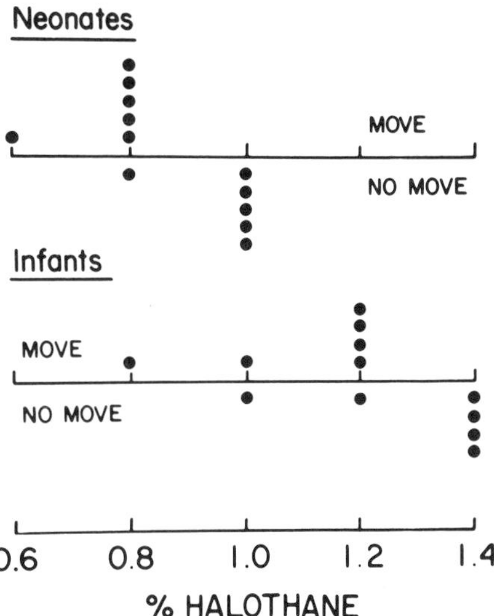

Figure 26-1. Halothane anesthetic requirements are decreased in neonates compared with infants. Each circle represents the response (move or no move) of an individual neonate or infant. (From Lerman et al.,[2] with permission.)

Injected Anesthetics

An immature blood-brain barrier and decreased ability to metabolize drugs could increase the sensi-

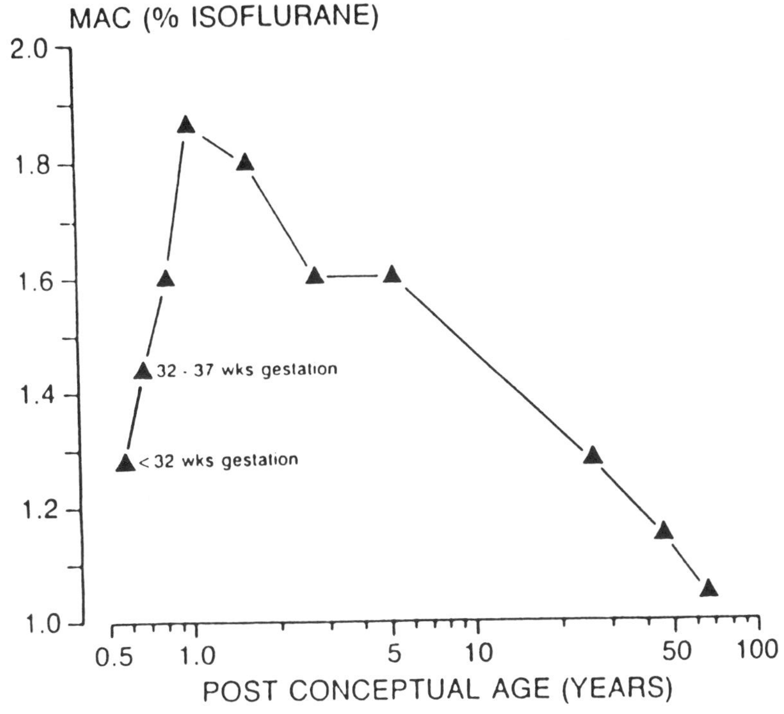

Figure 26-2. The MAC of isoflurane in preterm neonates (younger than 32 weeks of gestation) and after 32 to 37 weeks of gestation is lower ($P < 0.05$) than in full-term neonates and infants 1 to 6 months of age. Values for postconceptual age were obtained by adding 40 weeks to the mean postnatal age for each age group. (From LeDez and Lerman,[3] with permission.)

tivity of neonates to effects of injected anesthetics. As a result, neonates might require lower doses of these drugs to produce desired pharmacologic effects. Nevertheless, the dose of thiopental required to produce loss of the lid and corneal reflexes is similar in infants, children, and adults (Table 26-3).[4] Furthermore, the induction dose of propofol may be higher in infants than children.[5] Opioids, including morphine (high hepatic extraction) and alfentanil (low hepatic extraction), have a decreased rate of plasma clearance in neonates. Nevertheless, differences in the intensity and duration of opioid effect are difficult to determine in neonates versus children and adults.

Table 26-3. Thiopental Dose Response

	Dose that Produces Loss of Reflex (mg·kg^{-1}) in 90% of Patients
Lid reflex	
Infants[a]	6.4
Young children	5.3
Adults	6.0
Corneal reflex	
Infants	7.0
Young children	6.9
Adults	6.1

[a]Infants, 1 to 11 months; young children, 1 to 4 years; adults, 18 to 42 years

(Data from Brett and Fisher.[4])

Muscle Relaxants and Their Antagonists

Neonates and infants are more sensitive (lower plasma concentrations required to produce pharmacologic effects) than adults to nondepolarizing muscle relaxants. Nevertheless, initial doses of these drugs are similar in both age groups because less drug actually reaches the neuromuscular junction, reflecting the impact of increased extracellular fluid volume and volume of distribution in younger patients (Fig. 26-3).[6] Immaturity of hepatic or renal function could prolong the duration of action of muscle relaxants that are highly dependent on these mechanisms for their clearance (Fig. 26-4).[6,7] The dose of neostigmine required to antagonize nondepolarizing muscle relaxants is actually smaller in pediatric patients (Fig. 26-5).[8] In clinical practice, however, it is not necessary to alter the doses of neostigmine administered to infants and children compared with adults.

Neonates and infants require more succinylcholine on a body weight basis (2 mg·kg^{-1} IV) than do older children and adults (1 mg·kg^{-1} IV) to produce comparable degrees of skeletal muscle paralysis and intubating conditions. Presumably, this increased dose requirement reflects dilutional effects of the increased extracellular fluid volume and volume of distribution characteristic of younger patients.

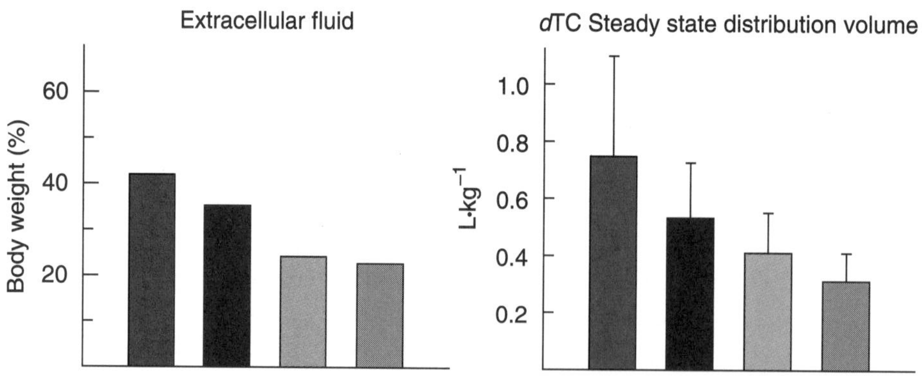

Figure 26-3. The steady state distribution volume for *d*-tubocurarine (*d*TC) parallels the extracellular fluid volume in neonates (dark red bars), infants (black bars), children (light red bars), and adults (12 to 30 years) (gray bars). The increased dilutional volume in neonates and infants masks an increased sensitivity of these age groups to nondepolarizing muscle relaxants. (From Fisher et al.,[6] with permission.)

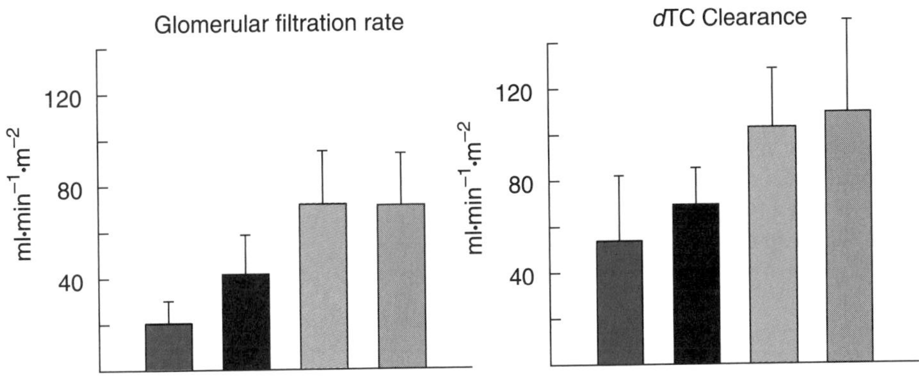

Figure 26-4. Clearance of *d*-tubocurarine (*d*TC) parallels the glomerular filtration rate in different age groups. Dark red bars, neonates; black bars, infants; light red bars, children; gray bars, adults. (From Fisher et al.,[6] with permission.)

IMMEDIATE PREOPERATIVE PERIOD

Preoperative Evaluation

The purpose of the preoperative evaluation is to obtain the history, perform a physical examination, evaluate laboratory data, and establish rapport with the child and parents. Pediatric anesthesia differs from adult anesthesia in that the history frequently must be obtained from the parent rather than the patient. The history should elicit congenital anomalies, allergies, bleeding tendencies, and any recent exposure to a communicable disease. The medications the child is taking should be determined. Experiences with previous anesthetics should be sought.

Physical examination includes evaluation of the heart, lungs, and a search for evidence of upper respiratory infections (fever, coryza). Although chronic rhinitis may not be a problem, recent upper respiratory infections, especially with associated leukocytosis, can be reasons for delaying elective surgery because of secretions and increased airway reactivity. The presence of loose teeth should be determined and dangerously loose teeth removed if necessary.

Laboratory data should seek evidence of hypoglycemia, hypocalcemia, or clotting disorders, which frequently occur in preterm infants or infants who have undergone asphyxia during birth. Also, if a history of vomiting or excessive fluid losses from diarrhea is evident, serum electrolytes, pH, and extracellular fluid volume should be measured. If the hemoglobin concentration is lower than 10 $g \cdot dl^{-1}$, the reason should be determined. Although hemoglobin concentrations lower than 10 $g \cdot dl^{-1}$ per se are not reasons for delaying elective operations, previously unknown abnormalities are often detected. A previously unrecognized cardiac murmur should be evaluated before anesthesia. In some cases, prophylactic antibiotic therapy is indicated.

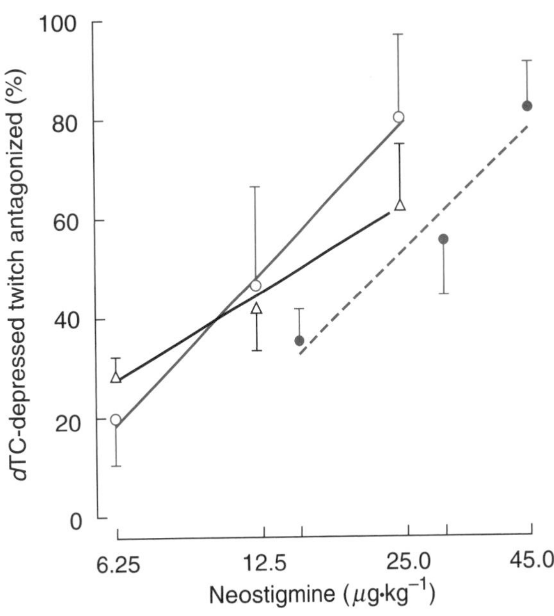

Figure 26-5. Dose-response curves demonstrate that infants (solid red line) and children (black line) require less neostigmine than adults (dashed red line) to antagonize nondepolarizing neuromuscular blockade produced by *d*-tubocurarine (*d*TC). (From Fisher et al.,[8] with permission.)

Preoperative Medication

The best preoperative medication is a friendly, reassuring visit from the anesthesiologist. By answering questions and describing the operative procedure (sometimes with animated illustrations), the need for preoperative medication may be decreased. Milk or solids can be ingested 4, 6, and 8 hours preoperatively by those 0 to 6 months old, 6 to 36 months old, and older than 3 years of age, respectively. Allowing pediatric patients independent of age to drink clear liquids until 2 hours before elective surgery decreases preoperative irritability and does not increase the gastric fluid volume present at the time of induction of anesthesia (see Fig. 9-6).[9] Oral administration of drugs such as midazolam in a flavored diluent is usually preferred by children, who predictably dislike drugs intended for preoperative medication that are delivered by intramuscular injection (see Chapter 9). Other routes of administration include nasal (sufentanil, midazolam) or transmucosal (fentanyl) delivery systems.

INDUCTION AND MAINTENANCE OF ANESTHESIA

The presence of the parents during induction of anesthesia may decrease the child's anxiety. An inhalation induction of anesthesia is very common for elective procedures in children and is especially easy to perform with halothane as compared with enflurane or desflurane because the former has a less pungent odor. Sometimes, the induction of anesthesia can be facilitated by initially breathing 70% nitrous oxide with the gradual introduction of halothane. Rapid increases in the concentration of the volatile anesthetic should be avoided because they can be irritating to the respiratory tract, resulting in coughing and even laryngospasm. A constant monotone conversation by the anesthesiologist is conducive to a rapid induction of anesthesia. If an intravenous catheter is in place, anesthesia can be induced by conventional induction drugs. If an intravenous catheter is not in place and an inhalation induction of anesthesia is not acceptable, ketamine can be given intramuscularly. It is recommended that heated and humidified gases be administered to children undergoing prolonged operations so as to decrease intraoperative heat loss and the development of undesirable decreases in body temperature.

Succinylcholine has been commonly (routinely) administered to pediatric patients to facilitate intubation of the trachea. Despite a long history of perceived safety, there is increasing concern that side effects of this drug (masseter muscle rigidity that may signal impending malignant hyperthermia, cardiac arrest from hyperkalemia in patients with undiagnosed myopathies) may contraindicate its routine use in pediatric patients.[10,11] The most likely nondepolarizing muscle relaxant alternatives to succinylcholine are mivacurium and rocuronium. Succinylcholine remains the recommended muscle relaxant when rapid onset of skeletal muscle paralysis is needed, as for treatment of laryngospasm or to facilitate tracheal intubation when the patient is judged to be at increased risk of aspiration of gastric contents. Appreciation of anatomic differences between pediatric and adult patients is essential in performance of direct laryngoscopy for intubation of the trachea and selection of appropriately sized tracheal tubes (see Chapter 11). Indeed, postintubation laryngeal edema is unlikely if the size of the tube placed in the trachea is such that an audible air leak occurs around it during positive airway pressures equivalent to 15 to 25 cmH_2O. Postintubation laryngeal edema is treated with humidification of inspired gases and aerosolized racemic epinephrine.

Anesthesia is often maintained with concentrations of volatile anesthetics, which cause the fewest physiologic changes and still offer adequate surgical conditions (usually in the range of 1.1 to 1.4 MAC). The signs of anesthesia (blood pressure, heart rate, skeletal muscle movement) required for adequate surgical conditions of neonates, infants, and children are similar to those of adults. Hypotension that accompanies administration of volatile anesthetics to neonates and infants most likely reflects unrecognized hypovolemia.

When and How Should an Intravenous Infusion Be Started?

Other than for very short surgical procedures, an intravenous infusion should be initiated in all children who are to be anesthetized. In many instances, an intravenous infusion is difficult to start preoperatively. After induction of anesthesia, however, especially with volatile anesthetics such as halothane, the peripheral veins dilate and movement of the child ceases, making placement of intravenous catheters much easier. Intravenous fluids are ideally delivered from a calibrated drip chamber to ensure that an excessive amount of fluid is not accidentally administered.

Monitoring

Monitoring of pediatric patients should be the same as for adult patients undergoing comparable types of surgery (see Chapter 15). Arterial blood pressure, electrocardiogram, heart and breath sounds with an esophageal or precordial stethoscope, body temperature, and systemic oxygenation (most often using pulse oximetry) should be monitored routinely in all infants and children undergoing surgery. Monitoring end-tidal carbon dioxide concentrations is useful, but falsely low readings may occur because of small tidal volumes and relatively high inspired gas flows. Selection of the proper width of blood pressure cuff (greater than one-third of the circumference of the limb) is important. For example, a cuff that is too small will produce an artificially high blood pressure, whereas one that is too large will produce a falsely low reading.

In seriously ill children who may be undergoing more extensive surgery, especially when hemorrhage or large shifts in extracellular fluid are expected, blood pressure probably should be monitored continuously via a catheter inserted into a peripheral artery. Monitoring of central venous pressure may aid in determining the adequacy of intravascular fluid volume. Central venous pressure can be measured via an umbilical vein catheter in neonates and either the internal jugular, external jugular, or subclavian vein in infants or children. Catheterization of the bladder and monitoring of urinary output also are helpful when blood loss or shifts in extracellular fluid volume are expected. A reasonable goal is a urinary output higher than 0.5 $ml \cdot kg^{-1} \cdot h^{-1}$ with a specific gravity lower than 1.010. Analysis of arterial blood gases and pH is often helpful during extensive surgery. Acidosis is not uncommon during pediatric anesthesia.

Fluid Maintenance and Replacement

It is often recommended that prior to induction of anesthesia, patients younger than 3 years of age receive 20 to 25 $ml \cdot kg^{-1}$ and those older than 3 years of age receive 10 to 15 $ml \cdot kg^{-1}$ of lactated Ringer's solution intravenously. Thereafter, intraoperative fluid replacement may be considered to be maintenance and replacement fluids (Table 26-4). Glucose administration is probably not necessary during the intraoperative period except for patients at risk of hypoglycemia (hyperalimentation, newborns of diabetic mothers).

Maintenance fluids are best correlated with metabolic rate; replacement fluid requirements should be based on the underlying disease process, extent of surgery, and anticipated fluid translocation. The hematocrit at which acute blood loss should be replaced is influenced by the age of the patient (Table 26-5). The following formula can be used to estimate the acceptable blood loss before replacement may be necessary.[12]

Table 26-4. Guidelines for Intraoperative Fluid Infusion Rates

	Lactated Ringer's Solution ($ml \cdot kg^{-1} \cdot h^{-1}$)		
	Maintenance	Replacement	Total
Minor surgery (herniorrhaphy)	4	2	6
Moderate surgery (pyloromyotomy)	4	4	8
Extensive surgery (bowel resection)	4	6	10

Acceptable blood loss = estimated erythrocyte mass – estimated erythrocyte mass when hematocrit is 30%

where erythrocyte mass = blood volume (80 $ml \cdot kg^{-1}$) × hematocrit.

For example, if a 4-kg infant has a preoperative hematocrit of 35%, approximately 16 ml of blood could be lost before the hematocrit would decrease to 30%. This formula, however, does not consider the dilutional aspect of crystalloid solution administration. If blood loss is to be replaced by crystalloid solutions, a volume of three times the estimated blood loss must be given, usually in the form of lactated Ringer's solution.

REGIONAL ANESTHESIA

Regional anesthesia is becoming increasingly popular in pediatric anesthesia. Peripheral nerve blocks used for pediatric anesthesia include penile block (circumcision, hypospadias repair), ilio-inguinal and iliohypogastric block (inguinal hernia repair), fascia

Table 26-5. Normal and Acceptable Hematocrits

Age	Normal Range (%)	Acceptable Range (%)
Premature	40–47	32–37
Newborn	47–63	30–35
6 months	33–40	26–30
1–10 years	36–43	21–26

iliaca compartment block (femur surgery), and brachial plexus block (arm and wrist surgery). Intravenous regional neural anesthesia can be used for repair of tendon lacerations or treatment of extremity fractures. Caudal anesthesia (bupivacaine 0.17% to 0.25% at a volume of 1 ml·kg^{-1} up to a maximum of 25 ml) can provide 3 to 6 hours of anesthesia for surgical procedures below the level of the diaphragm. Placement of an opioid in the local anesthetic solution is useful for providing prolonged postoperative analgesia (see Chapter 32). Identification of the caudal epidural space is technically easy in the pediatric patient, but it is also important to remember that the dural sac extends more caudad in children than in adults. Lumbar epidural anesthesia and spinal anesthesia can be used as alternatives to caudal anesthesia in pediatric patients.

MEDICAL AND SURGICAL DISEASES THAT AFFECT PEDIATRIC PATIENTS

Medical and surgical diseases that affect pediatric patients are often of greatest concern in the neonate, in whom incomplete adaptation to the extrauterine environment may further complicate perioperative management.

Medical and Surgical Diseases that Affect Pediatric Patients

- Medical diseases
  - Respiratory distress syndrome
  - Bronchopulmonary dysplasia
  - Intracranial hemorrhage
  - Retinopathy of prematurity
  - Apnea spells
  - Sudden infant death syndrome
  - Kernicterus
  - Hypoglycemia
  - Hypocalcemia
  - Sepsis
  - Trisomy 21 (Down syndrome)
  - Thermal (burn) injuries
  - Epiglottitis
  - Malignant hyperthermia
- Surgical diseases
  - Diaphragmatic hernia
  - Tracheoesophageal fistula
  - Abdominal wall defects
    - Omphalocele
    - Gastroschisis
  - Pyloric stenosis
  - Necrotizing enterocolitis

Respiratory Distress Syndrome

Respiratory distress syndrome ([RDS] hyaline membrane disease) is responsible for more than 50% of deaths that occur in preterm neonates. This syndrome is caused by a deficiency in the alveoli of a surface active phospholipid (surfactant) that is necessary to maintain alveolar stability. Without surfactant, alveoli collapse, leading to right-to-left intrapulmonary shunting, arterial hypoxemia, and metabolic acidosis. During anesthesia in the presence of RDS, the PaO_2 should be maintained at its preoperative level. Ideally, the PaO_2 is monitored from a preductal artery. For a brief surgical procedure or when arterial blood sampling is not feasible, monitoring of oxygenation using pulse oximetry is acceptable. Pneumothorax is an ever present danger and should be considered if oxygenation deteriorates abruptly in a neonate being treated for RDS.

Bronchopulmonary Dysplasia

Bronchopulmonary dysplasia is a chronic pulmonary disorder that typically afflicts infants and children who required increased concentrations of oxygen and mechanical ventilation of the lungs at birth to treat RDS. Characteristic findings include increased airway reactivity, decreased arterial oxygenation due to ventilation-to-perfusion mismatch, and recurrent pulmonary infections. Pulmonary dysfunction in these patients is most marked in the first year of life.

Retinopathy of Prematurity

Retinopathy of prematurity (retrolental fibroplasia) reflects neovascularization and scarring of retinal vasculature that may result in visual impairment. Arterial hyperoxia is an important risk factor in development of neovascularization, but prematurity (especially birth weights lower than 1500 g) must also be present. The risk of developing retinopathy is negligible after 44 weeks postconception. In this regard a preterm neonate born at 36 weeks of gestation would remain at risk until 8 weeks of age. It is generally recommended that during anesthesia, inhaled concentrations of oxygen be adjusted so as to maintain PaO_2 between 60 and 80 mmHg.

Apnea Spells

Apnea spells (cessation of breathing lasting at least 20 seconds and resulting in cyanosis and bradycardia) occur in 20% to 30% of premature neonates in the first month of life.[13] Since inhaled and injected anesthetics affect control of breathing, it is likely that the risk of apnea spells will be increased during the postoperative period, especially in preterm infants younger than 60 weeks postconceptual age.[14] For this reason, it has been recommended that apnea monitoring be used for at least 12 hours after surgery in infants younger than 60 weeks postconceptual age. The risk of apnea spells precludes outpatient surgery in susceptible patients (see Chapter 29).

Hypoglycemia

The neonate, in contrast to the adult, has a poorly developed system for maintenance of an adequate plasma glucose concentration and therefore is susceptible to the development of hypoglycemia. Manifestations of hypoglycemia in the neonate (irritability, seizures, apnea) are masked by general anesthesia, emphasizing the need for maintaining a high index of suspicion in susceptible patients. The immediate treatment of hypoglycemia is infusion of glucose (0.5 to 1 $g \cdot kg^{-1}$ IV).

Hypocalcemia

Preterm neonates are prone to development of hypocalcemia since fetal calcium stores are largely achieved during the last trimester of gestation. Hypocalcemia can occur with the rapid intraoperative infusion of citrate, as may occur during an exchange transfusion or infusion of citrated blood. The hypotensive effect of citrate-induced hypocalcemia can be minimized by administration of calcium gluconate (1 to 2 mg IV) for every 1 ml of blood transfused.

Sepsis

Sepsis in neonates is associated with a high mortality rate, presumably reflecting the presence of an immature immune system. Signs of sepsis are nonspecific but often include lethargy and tachypnea. Fever and leukocytosis, in contrast to adults, may not be present in septic neonates.

Trisomy 21 (Down Syndrome)

Trisomy 21 occurs in about 0.15% of all live births. Correction of associated congenital anomalies (atrial or ventricular septal defects, duodenal atresia) or the need to provide dental care may be the reason these patients undergo surgery. In this regard, the need to decrease excessive upper airway secretions with an anticholinergic drug and provide sedation for an often uncooperative patient must be considered in the preoperative medication. Patency of the upper airway may be difficult to maintain after the onset of unconsciousness, reflecting the short neck, small mouth, and large tongue characteristic of these patients. Intubation of the trachea, however, is usually not difficult. Movement of the head and neck during intubation of the trachea must be performed cautiously, as many of these patients have asymptomatic atlantoaxial instability.

Thermal (Burn) Injuries

About one-half of all thermal injuries occur in children, and one-third of burn-related deaths occur in children younger than 15 years of age. Associated pathophysiologic responses include catecholamine release, acute hypovolemia, ileus, and myocardial depression. After the initial 24 hours of fluid resuscitation, the circulatory system enters a hyperdynamic state often accompanied by hypertension. Urine output is a useful guide to the adequacy of fluid replacement. Thermal injuries of the upper airway manifesting as hoarseness and tachypnea may require emergency intubation of the trachea. An increase in serum potassium concentrations due to tissue necrosis and hemolysis is common during the early postburn period. Carbon monoxide poisoning often complicates burns that occur in closed spaces and is the most common immediate cause of death from fire. Management of anesthesia in these patients may be complicated by absence of access sites for placement of intravascular catheters or monitors due to thermal injury, perioral scarring and contractures, increased dose requirements for intravenous induction drugs, potassium release after administration of succinylcholine, and resistance to the effects of nondepolarizing muscle relaxants (see

Fig. 7-6). The mechanism for increased dose requirements for drugs in burn patients is most likely a pharmacodynamic rather than a pharmacokinetic response.

Epiglottitis

Epiglottitis typically manifests as an acute onset of difficulty in swallowing, high fever, and inspiratory stridor in children 2 to 6 years old. Since the inflammatory response involves tissues other than the epiglottis, a more correct designation may be supraglottitis. Differentiation of epiglottitis from laryngotracheobronchitis (croup) may be difficult; however, characteristically the latter occurs in younger patients, the onset is slower, the fever is lower, and airway obstruction less severe (Table 26-6). It is mandatory that children with suspected epiglottitis be admitted to the hospital, since sudden total upper airway obstruction can occur at any time. Epiglottitis is treated with antibiotics, such as ampicillin (causative bacterium is *Haemophilus influenzae*), and intubation of the trachea. Visualization of the epiglottis should not be attempted until the child is in the operating room and preparations are completed for intubation of the trachea and possible emergency tracheostomy. Induction and maintenance of anesthesia for intubation of the trachea are achieved with a volatile anesthetic, most often halothane, in oxygen. Muscle relaxants are not administered because onset of skeletal muscle paralysis in the presence of upper airway obstruction may result in total airway obstruction. Resolution of epiglottitis usually requires 48 to 96 hours. Extubation of the trachea is performed in the operating room only after direct laryngoscopy has confirmed the resolution of the swelling of the epiglottis.

Malignant Hyperthermia

Malignant hyperthermia is an inherited disease that manifests most often, but not exclusively, in children. The incidence of this syndrome is approximately 1 in 12,000 pediatric anesthetics and 1 in 40,000 adult anesthetics. The gene for malignant hyperthermia is also the genetic coding site for the calcium release channel of skeletal muscle sarcoplasmic reticulum (ryanodine receptor). It is presumed that a defect in the calcium release channel permits sustained higher concentrations of calcium in the myoplasm and persistent skeletal muscle contraction when susceptible patients are exposed to triggering drugs such as succinylcholine or volatile anesthetics, or both. Susceptible patients may develop spasm of the masseter muscles after administration of succinylcholine, making it impossible to

Table 26-6. Comparison of Epiglottitis and Laryngotracheobronchitis

	Epiglottitis (Supraglottitis)	Laryngotracheobronchitis
Age	2–6 years	2 years or less
Incidence	Accounts for 5% of children with stridor	Accounts for about 80% of children with stridor
Cause	Bacterial	Viral
Onset	Rapid over 24 hours	Gradual over 24–72 hours
Signs and symptoms	Inspiratory stridor Pharyngitis Drooling Fever (>39°C) Lethargic to restless Tachypnea Insist on sitting up and leaning forward	Inspiratory stridor Croupy cough Rhinorrhea Fever (<39°C)
Lateral radiograph of the neck	Swollen epiglottis	Narrowing of the subglottic area
Treatment	Oxygen Urgent intubation of the trachea Antibiotics	Oxygen Aerosolized racemic epinephrine Humidity

open the mouth to perform direct laryngoscopy for intubation of the trachea.[10] Sustained skeletal muscle contraction results in signs of hypermetabolism, including tachycardia, arterial hypoxemia, metabolic and respiratory acidosis, and profound increases in body temperature. Unexplained tachycardia or increases in the exhaled concentration of carbon dioxide are early manifestations of malignant hyperthermia, whereas increases in body temperature may be a late sign. Dantrolene (up to 10 $mg \cdot kg^{-1}$ IV) is the drug of choice for the treatment of malignant hyperthermia.

Identification of malignant hyperthermia-susceptible patients before anesthesia has obvious advantages. In this regard, a detailed medical and family history, with particular reference to previous anesthetic experiences, should be obtained. Prior uneventful anesthetics, however, do not necessarily indicate that individuals are not susceptible. Only about 70% of malignant hyperthermia-susceptible patients have increases of resting concentrations of creatine kinase. The absence of such an increase, therefore, does not rule out susceptibility to malignant hyperthermia. The definitive diagnosis of susceptibility to malignant hyperthermia requires skeletal muscle biopsy and in vitro isometric contracture testing in the presence of caffeine or halothane, or both.

No anesthetic regimen has been shown to be reliably safe for the patient who is susceptible to malignant hyperthermia. Prophylaxis in a susceptible patient may be provided with dantrolene (5 $mg \cdot kg^{-1}$ PO) administered in three or four divided doses every 6 hours with the last dose 4 hours preoperatively.[15] Alternatively, dantrolene (2.4 mg kg^{-1} IV) may be administered over 10 to 30 minutes as prophylaxis just prior to the induction of anesthesia. In the absence of evidence of malignant hyperthermia intraoperatively, it is probably not necessary to continue administration of dantrolene into the postoperative period. Despite prophylaxis with dantrolene, an occasional susceptible patient may still develop malignant hyperthermia. For this reason, plus the potential adverse effects associated with dantrolene prophylaxis therapy (skeletal muscle weakness, nausea, diarrhea), it has been suggested by some that prophylactic use of dantrolene is not necessary if susceptible patients do not receive known triggering drugs (especially succinylcholine) during anesthesia.[16] Regional anesthesia is an attractive selection in malignant hyperthermia susceptible patients.

Treatment of Malignant Hyperthermia

- Dantrolene (2–3 $mg \cdot kg^{-1}$ IV; repeat every 5–10 minutes until symptoms are controlled)
- Immediate termination of inhaled anesthetics
- Hyperventilate the lungs with oxygen
- Initiate active cooling
  - Cold saline (15 $ml \cdot kg^{-1}$ IV every 10 minutes)
  - Gastric lavage with cold saline
  - Surface cooling
- Sodium bicarbonate (1–2 $mEq \cdot kg^{-1}$ IV as guided by arterial pH)
- Induce diuresis
  - Hydration
  - Mannitol
  - Furosemide

Diaphragmatic Hernia

Diaphragmatic hernia results from incomplete embryologic closure of the diaphragm such that intestinal contents occupy the chest (most often the left thorax) with associated hypoplasia of the lung on that side. The incidence of this defect is about 1 in every 5000 live births. Approximately 30% of cases of diaphragmatic hernia are associated with

Drugs that Do Not Trigger Malignant Hyperthermia

- Barbiturates
- Opioids
- Benzodiazepines
- Propofol
- Etomidate
- Nitrous oxide
- Local anesthetics
- Nondepolarizing muscle relaxants

polyhydramnios. Manifestations at birth include a scaphoid abdomen and profound arterial hypoxemia. Radiographs of the chest demonstrate loops of intestine in the thorax and a shift of the mediastinum to the opposite side. Pulmonary hypertension and congenital heart disease are common.

Immediate treatment of the neonate is decompression of the stomach via a gastric tube and administration of oxygen, most often via a tracheal tube. Positive pressure ventilation of the lungs via a mask could further compromise pulmonary function if any gas passes via the esophagus to further increase gastric volume. Pneumothorax on the side opposite the hernia is a hazard if airway pressures exceed 25 to 30 cmH_2O during controlled ventilation of the lungs. Nitrous oxide is generally avoided during anesthesia for surgical correction, as this gas could diffuse into the loops of intestine in the chest (see Chapter 2). Arterial oxygenation is generally monitored, because these neonates may be at risk of developing retinopathy of prematurity. After reduction of the diaphragmatic hernia, attempts to expand the hypoplastic lung are not recommended, as damage to the normal lung can occur from excessive positive airway pressure. An alternative to prompt surgical intervention in selected patients is extracorporeal membrane oxygenation. Also, correction of the diaphragmatic hernia has been performed antenatally by intrauterine fetal surgery.

Tracheoesophageal Fistula

Tracheoesophageal fistula is often first suspected soon after birth, when an oral catheter cannot be passed into the stomach or when infants develop cyanosis and coughing during oral feedings. Pulmonary aspiration is likely to occur. Initial treatment is a gastrostomy under local anesthesia. This provides a vent for excess gas that may enter the stomach through the fistula as during mechanical ventilation of the lungs. During corrective surgery, it is important to place the tracheal tube below the level of the fistula while guarding against endobronchial intubation. There is an increased incidence of congenital heart disease in these neonates, and the incidence of prematurity approaches 40%.

Pyloric Stenosis

Pyloric stenosis occurs in about 1 in every 500 live births and usually manifests in a male infant at 2 to 5 weeks of age. Persistent vomiting results in loss of hydrogen ions, with compensatory attempts by the kidneys to maintain a normal pH by exchanging potassium for hydrogen. The result is a dehydrated infant with hypokalemic, hypochloremic metabolic alkalosis. Surgery is performed electively (not as an emergency) after 24 to 48 hours of intravenous fluid therapy that includes sodium and potassium chloride.

The likelihood of aspiration of gastric fluid may be increased in these patients during induction of anesthesia. Therefore, the stomach is often emptied as completely as possible with a large-bore catheter before induction of anesthesia. Postoperative depression of ventilation (possibly due to cerebrospinal fluid alkalosis) is common in these patients, emphasizing the need for close monitoring in the early hours after surgery.

REFERENCES

1. Eger EI II, Bahlman SH, Munson ES. The effect of age on the rate of increase of the alveolar anesthesia concentration. Anesthesiology 1971;35:365–72.
2. Lerman J, Robinson S, Willis MM, Gregory GA. Anesthetic requirements for halothane in young children 0–1 month and 1–6 months of age. Anesthesiology 1983;59:421–4.
3. LeDez KM, Lerman J. The minimum alveolar concentration (MAC) of isoflurane in preterm neonates. Anesthesiology 1987;67:301–7.
4. Brett CM, Fisher DM. Thiopental dose-response relations in unpremedicated infants, children and adults. Anesth Analg 1987;66:1024–7.
5. Westrin P. The induction dose of propofol in infants 1–6 months of age and in children 10–16 years of age. Anesthesiology 1991;74:455–8.
6. Fisher DM, O'Keefe C, Stanski DR, Cronnelly R, Miller RD, Gregory GA. Pharmacokinetics and pharmacodynamics of *d*-tubocurarine in infants, children and adults. Anesthesiology 1982;57:203–8.
7. Fisher DM, Miller RD. Neuromuscular effects of vecuronium (ORG NC45) in infants and children during N_2O, halothane anesthesia. Anesthesiology 1983;58:519–23.
8. Fisher DM, Cronnelly R, Miller RD, Sharma M. The neuromuscular pharmacology of neostigmine in infants and children. Anesthesiology 1983;59:220–5.
9. Crawford M, Lerman J, Christensen S, Farrow-Gillespie A. Effects of duration of fasting on gastric fluid pH and volume in healthy children. Anesth Analg 1990;71:400–3.
10. Littleford JA, Patel LR, Bose D, et al. Masseter spasm in children: Implication of continuing the triggering anesthetic. Anesth Analg 1991;72:151–60.
11. Rosenberg H, Gronert GA. Intractable cardiac arrest in children given succinylcholine. Anesthesiology 1992;77:1054.
12. Furman EB, Roman DG, Lemmer LAS, Hairabet J, Jasinski M, Laver MB. Specific therapy in water, elec-

trolye and blood-volume replacement during pediatric surgery. Anesthesiolgy 1975;42:187–93.
13. Gregory GA, Steward DJ. Life-threatening perioperative apnea in the "ex-premie." Anesthesiology 1983; 59:495–98.
14. Kurth CD, Spitzer AR, Broennle AM, Downes JJ. Postoperative apnea in preterm infants. Anesthesiology 1987;66:483–8.
15. Allen GC, Cattrain CB, Peterson RG, Lakende M. Plasma levels of dantrolene following oral administration in malignant hyperthermia-susceptible patients. Anesthesiology 1988;67:900–4.
16. Hackl W, Mauritiz W, Winkler M, Sporn P, Steinbereithner K. Anaesthesia in malignant hyperthermia susceptible patients without dantrolene prophylaxis: A report of 30 cases. Acta Anaesthesiol Scand 1990;34:534–7.

27
Elderly Patients

Elderly patients, who are arbitrarily defined as older than 65 years of age (a chronologic rather than biologic distinction), are becoming an increasingly larger segment of society, accounting for more than 12% of the population in the United States. Approximately one-half of patients who reach 65 years of age will require surgery before they die. Compared with younger patients, elderly patients may be at greater risk of perioperative complications because of age-related concomitant diseases and a generalized decline in organ function, which may manifest only with the added stress of the perioperative period (Fig. 27-1).[1–3] For example, cardiac function sufficient for a sedentary life style may become inadequate with the stress of intraoperative blood loss or postoperative infection. Psychological, physiologic, and pharmacologic changes that must be taken into account when anesthetizing elderly patients must be considered along with the concomitant disease processes that may also exist. Although morbidity and mortality of surgery in elderly patients are higher following surgery than that for their younger counterparts, these problems are usually due to concomitant disease processes, such as heart disease, diabetes mellitus, or renal failure, rather than aging per se.[2] It is likely that age-related diseases play a more important role than age itself in increasing the risk of anesthesia in elderly patients. Emergency surgery, which allows little time for control of co-existing diseases, may be particularly hazardous in elderly patients.

PSYCHOLOGICAL FACTORS

All patients, independent of age, have psychological concerns about upcoming surgery. In this respect, elderly patients do not differ from other surgical patients who have a variety of concerns about a proposed surgical experience. However, certain stresses, including the fear of the loss of function and independence, concerns about the possibility of impending death, and the fear that their current illness may result in long-term institutionalization and dependency, impinge on the elderly to a greater extent. In addition, especially with respect to elderly patients, there is the impact of social and sensory isolation. Before surgery, it is important to identify the existence of depressive illness and to distinguish between long-term endogenous and short-term reactive depression. The patient with endogenous depression is more likely to have a poor appetite, weight loss, agitation, lack of energy, and recurrent thoughts of suicide. Elderly patients, especially the very old, are prone to delirium as a consequence of almost any physical illness (pneumonia, myocardial infarction) or intoxication with therapeutic doses of prescribed or self-administered drugs. Delirium is characterized by acute and usually transient mental confusion with a sudden onset, often occurring at night. It is important to distinguish delirium from dementia (Alzheimer's disease), which is the only other syndrome characterized by global cognitive impairment. Unlike delirium, dementia is chronic and progressive.

Age-Related Concomitant Diseases in Elderly Patients

Systemic hypertension
Coronary artery disease
Congestive heart failure
Peripheral vascular disease
Chronic obstructive pulmonary disease
Anemia
Renal disease
Diabetes mellitus
Subclinical hypothyroidism
Arthritis
Dementia

PHYSIOLOGY

The generalized decline in organ function that accompanies aging may be characterized as a decreased margin of reserve for adaptation, especially with the introduction of acute stresses such as accompany the perioperative period (Fig. 27-1).[1]

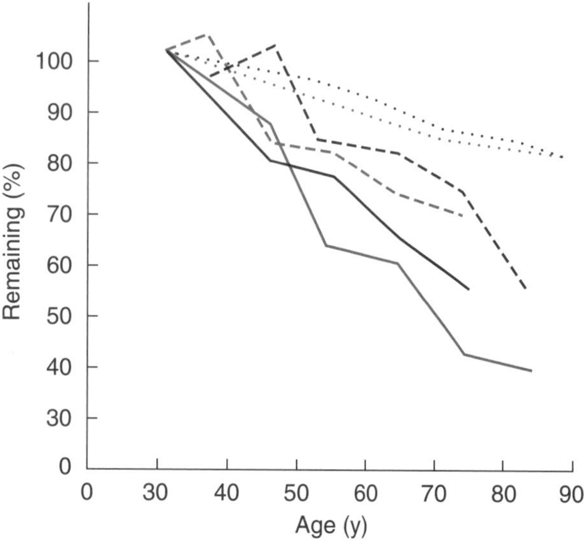

Figure 27-1. Aging is associated with progressive decreases (1% to 1.5% annually) in function of major organ systems. Solid red line, maximal breathing capacity; solid black line, vital capacity; dashed red line, cardiac index; dashed black line, glomerular filtration rate; dotted red line, standard cell water; dotted black line, basal metabolic rate. (From Evans,[1] with permission.)

Central Nervous System

Progressive declines in central nervous system activity and loss of neurons, especially in the cerebral cortex, accompany aging. Conduction velocity in peripheral nerves decreases, and there may be decreased numbers of fibers in spinal cord tracts. These changes may manifest as decreased dose requirements for drugs that act on the central nervous system (MAC) or peripheral nervous system (see the section *Pharmacology*).

Cardiovascular System

Systolic blood pressure increases with aging, reflecting development of poorly compliant arterial walls. Heart rate decreases with advancing age, suggesting an increase in activity of the parasympathetic nervous system. Furthermore, degenerative changes that accompany aging can involve the sinus node or cardiac conduction systems, or both, resulting in atrioventricular heart block. Drug-induced heart rate changes (atropine, isoproterenol, propranolol) are smaller and reflex-induced increases via the carotid sinus in response to hypotension (hypovolemia, anesthetic drug overdose) are attenuated in elderly patients. Decreases in cardiac output previously thought to be an unavoidable accompaniment of aging are more likely to be manifestations of age-related diseases or a sedentary lifestyle, resulting in prolonged deconditioning. Indeed, elderly patients who maintain physical fitness are likely to maintain a normal cardiac output.[2,3] Stroke volume is relatively unaffected by aging, although the ability to increase myocardial contractility in response to stress is impaired. Conceivably, drug-induced myocardial depression may be exaggerated in elderly patients. Cerebral, coronary, and skeletal muscle blood flows are relatively unchanged during aging.

Pulmonary System

Pulmonary system changes that accompany aging are characterized by deterioration of gas exchange and changes in the mechanics of breathing. For example, PaO_2 decreases about 0.5 mmHg per year after 20 years of age and the A-aDO_2 increases (Fig. 27-2).[4] These changes reflect mismatching of ventilation to perfusion, most likely paralleling degenerative changes (loss of alveolar septa) in the lungs. Aging alone does not alter the $PaCO_2$, although

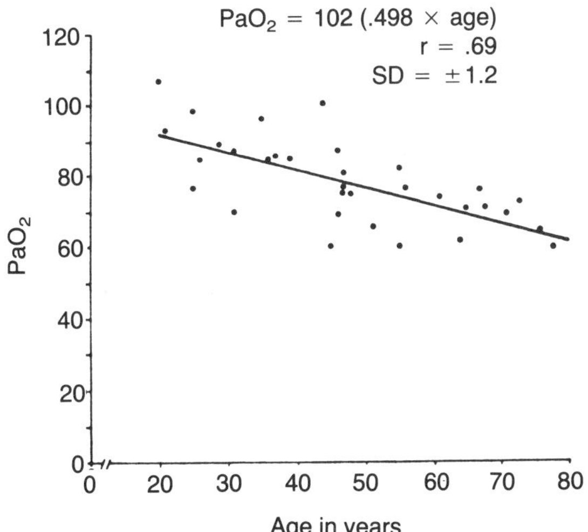

Figure 27-2. Increasing age is associated with progressive decreases in the resting awake PaO_2. Note, the formula should show that (0.498 x age) is subtracted from 102. (From Wahba,[4] with permission.)

the $A\text{-}aDCO_2$ may increase owing to ventilation of unperfused alveoli (increased physiologic deadspace). The ventilatory response to hypoxemia or hypercapnia in elderly patients is about one-half that in younger patients. This response is further impaired by opioid premedication and inhaled anesthetics.

Mechanical ventilatory function is impaired because of decreased elasticity of the lungs and increased stiffness of the thorax. Vital capacity and forced exhaled volume in 1 second decrease with aging whereas residual volume and functional residual capacity increase. Maximum breathing capacity is decreased as much as 50% in elderly patients. Pneumonia occurs with increased frequency in elderly patients, reflecting decreased pulmonary reserve and an increased incidence of aspiration of pharyngeal secretions. Indeed, laryngeal, pharyngeal, and airway cough reflexes are less active in elderly patients, making pulmonary aspiration more likely. Bacterial colonization in the pharynx because of poor oral hygiene and general depression of the immune system may further increase the risk of pneumonia.

Renal System

Aging is associated with decreases in renal blood flow (parallels decreases in cardiac output and the size of the renal vascular bed), glomerular filtration rate, and urine-concentrating ability. These changes combined with decreased cardiac function make elderly patients more vulnerable to fluid overload. Conversely, decreased urine-concentrating ability means that elderly patients are less able to concentrate urine after fluid deprivation. Prolonged and exaggerated responses to certain drugs (digoxin, antibiotics) are predictable in the presence of decreased renal clearance characteristic of aging (see the section *Pharmacology*). The ability to conserve sodium is decreased, making elderly patients vulnerable to hyponatremia. Despite decreased renal function, plasma concentrations of creatinine do not increase, reflecting decreased skeletal muscle mass and accompanying decreases in production of creatinine.

Hepatic System

Hepatic blood flow decreases with aging in proportion to decreases in cardiac output. Decreased activity of hepatic microsomal enzymes is predictable, but it is likely that decreased hepatic blood flow is more important in delayed drug clearance observed in elderly patients. Production of albumin is also decreased, resulting in decreased plasma protein binding of some drugs.

Gastrointestinal System

There is a general decrease in esophageal and intestinal motility, which may result in delayed gastric emptying. Also, gastroesophageal sphincter tone is frequently decreased. As a result of these changes, elderly patients could represent an increased risk of pulmonary aspiration when rendered unconscious by general anesthesia.

Endocrine System

Diabetes mellitus and hypothyroidism are potential accompaniments of increased aging (see Chapter 22). Subclinical hypothyroidism manifesting only as an increase in the plasma concentration of thyroid stimulating hormone is present in more than 13% of otherwise healthy elderly patients, especially females.[5]

Skin and Musculoskeletal Systems

Atrophy of the epidermis, with loss of collagen and decreases in elasticity, makes elderly patients more vulnerable to decubitus ulcers or skin damage during surgery. Removal of tape or monitoring electrodes may result in unexpected injury to the underlying skin. Osteoarthritis, rheumatoid arthritis, and osteoporosis have obvious implications for upper airway management and for positioning of elderly patients during surgery. Skeletal muscle atrophy predictably accompanies aging.

PHARMACOLOGY

Age-related changes in pharmacokinetics most often manifest as prolongation of elimination half-times of drugs, making elderly patients particularly vulnerable to cumulative drug effects and adverse drug interactions (Fig. 27-3). Increased elimination half-times of drugs can reflect decreased renal clearance (pancuronium, doxacurium, pipecuronium, digoxin, antibiotics), decreased hepatic clearance (vecuronium, lidocaine, propofol, propranolol), or increased volume of distribution (diazepam). For example, the hepatic clearance rate for propofol may be decreased in elderly patients, leading to a recommendation that both the induction dose and maintenance infusion rate be decreased. The dose of thiopental or etomidate required to induce anesthesia in elderly patients is decreased, most likely reflecting a decreased rate of clearance of drug from the central compartment (circulation) to peripheral compartments (Fig. 27-4).[6,7] This slowed rate of intercompartmental clearance can result in unexpected high plasma concentrations of these drugs if conventional doses are administered. Decreasing the dose administered offsets this effect of slowed intercompartmental clearance on the plasma concentration achieved. Prolonged elimination half-times of diazepam in elderly patients are consistent with increased tissue storage of this lipid-soluble drug in the greater fraction of adipose tissue relative to body weight that accompanies aging. Aging influences the pharmacokinetics of inhaled anesthetics as reflected by a delayed rate of elimination and increased volume of distribution.[8] These changes for inhaled drugs are compatible with age-induced decreases in tissue perfusion and an increase in the ratio of fat to lean body weight.

Causes of Increased Elimination Half-Times of Drugs

Decreased clearance
- Renal blood flow
- Glomerular filtration rate
- Hepatic blood flow
- Hepatic microsomal enzyme activity

Increased volume of distribution
- Body fat content
- Protein binding

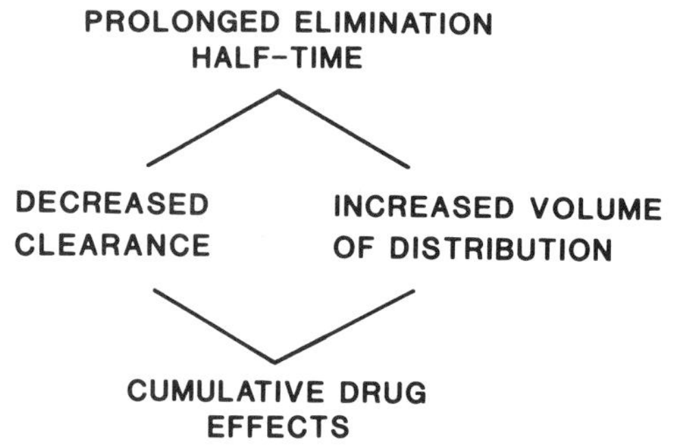

Figure 27-3. Age-related changes in pharmacokinetics most often manifest as a prolonged elimination half-time due to decreased clearance or increased volume of distribution of drugs. Cumulative drug effects are likely to occur with repeated doses.

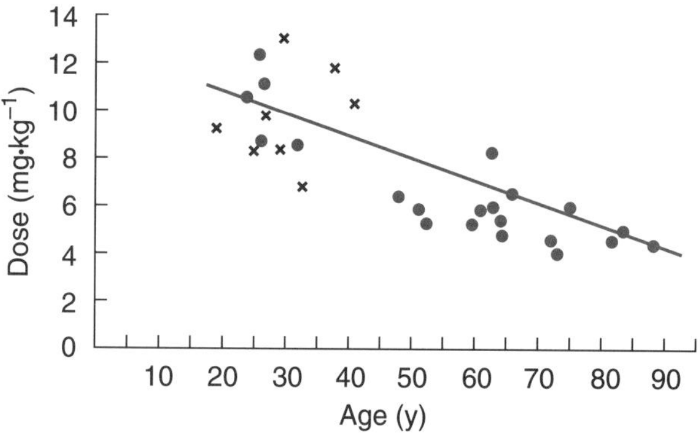

Figure 27-4. The dose of thiopental administered as a continuous intravenous infusion to produce burst suppression on the electroencephalogram decreases progressively with increasing age. (From Homer and Stanski,[6] with permission.)

Pharmacodynamics

Confirmation of pharmacodynamic changes is evidenced by demonstration of increases or decreases in plasma concentrations of drugs required to produce specific pharmacologic effects. For example, age-related decreases in anesthetic requirements for inhaled drugs (MAC) and opioids most likely reflect pharmacodynamic changes (Fig. 27-5).[9] Conversely, plasma concentrations of nondepolarizing muscle relaxants necessary to produce comparable degrees of twitch response suppression are similar in young and elderly adults, suggesting that changes in the neuromuscular junction do not accompany aging (Fig. 27-6).[10] Likewise, plasma concentrations of thiopental or etomidate necessary to produce equivalent pharmacologic effects are not changed with aging (Fig. 27-7).[6,7] A speculated decrease in numbers of receptors with aging is not supported by demonstrations that the density of beta receptors does not change in elderly patients.[11] Instead, the affinity of these receptors for adrenergic agonists decreases with aging, explaining the decreased responsiveness of the cardiovascular system to drugs acting on the autonomic nervous system.

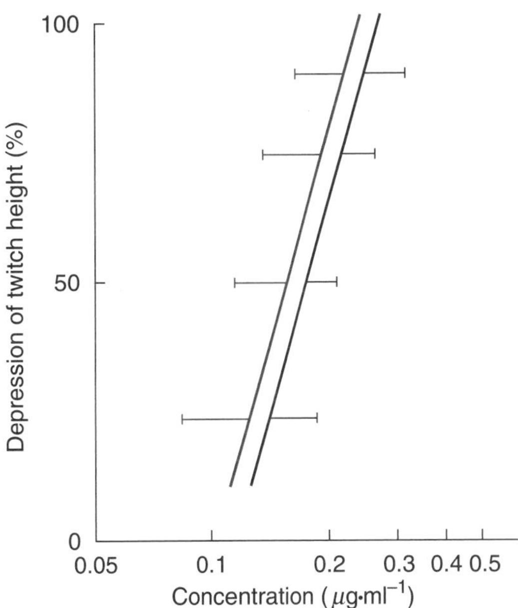

Figure 27-6. Absence of age-related changes in the responsiveness of the neuromuscular junction (pharmacodynamics) to long-acting muscle relaxants such as pancuronium is confirmed by the similarity of the plasma concentrations necessary to produce comparable twitch height depression in elderly (red line) and young (black line) adults. (From Duvaldestin et al.,[10] with permission.)

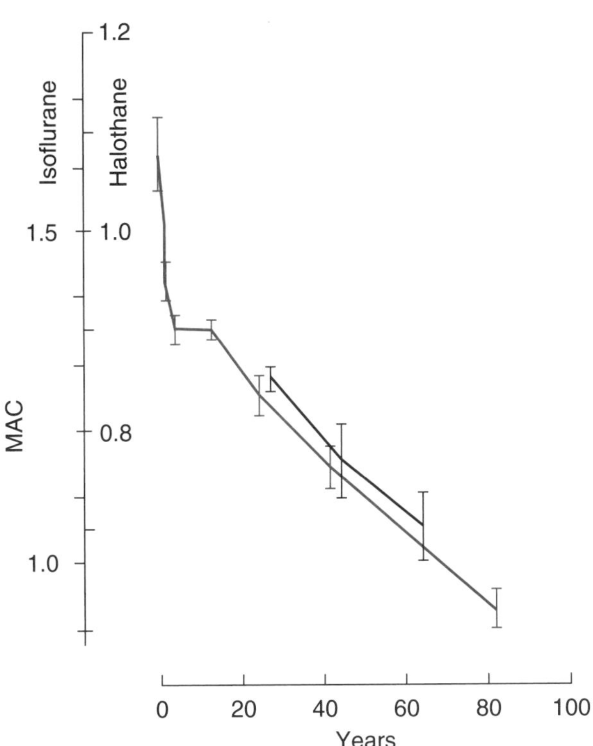

Figure 27-5. MAC for isoflurane (black line) and halothane (red line) (also true for other volatile anesthetics) decrease with increasing age. This decrease in MAC parallels concomitant decreases in the cerebral metabolic requirements for oxygen. (From Quasha et al.,[9] with permission.)

MANAGEMENT OF ANESTHESIA

Preoperative Evaluation and Preparation

Preoperative evaluation of elderly patients must consider the likely presence of co-existing diseases and decreases in major organ function that accompany aging independent of the reason for surgery (Fig. 27-1.)[1] Alcoholism may be an unexpected finding in elderly patients. A recent change in mental function should not be attributed to aging until cardiac or pulmonary disease has been considered. Even in the absence of symptoms, it is likely that many elderly patients have coronary artery disease. The likeli-

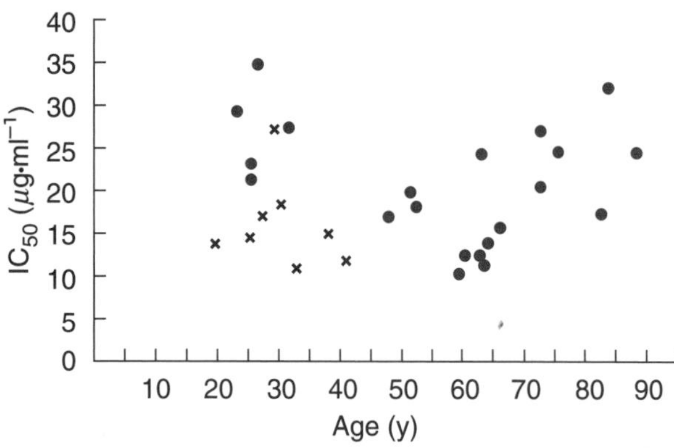

Figure 27-7. Plasma concentrations of thiopental that produce burst suppression on the electroencephalogram do not change with age, although the dose infused to produce this plasma concentration does decrease with age (see Fig. 27-4). (From Homer and Stanski,[6] with permission.)

hood of adverse drug interactions is increased by known alterations in pharmacokinetics and pharmacodynamics characteristic of aging. Furthermore, elderly patients are likely to be taking several different drugs (Table 27-1) that may contribute to adverse drug interactions. A drug history is particularly important because of the numerous abnormalities and drug interactions that may occur in elderly patients. Unfortunately, elderly patients can become confused and forget not only what drugs they are taking but also how much and when the last dose was taken. Close consultation with the family and primary physician is essential in these patients. Often, merely asking the patient to show you which drugs they are taking and how frequently they take them can alleviate some of the problems in taking an accurate history.

Table 27-1. Drugs Often Taken By Elderly Patients that May Contribute to Adverse Effects or Drug Interactions

Drug	Response
Diuretics	Hypokalemia Hypovolemia
Centrally acting antihypertensives	Decreased autonomic nervous system activity Decreased anesthetic requirements
Beta antagonists	Decreased autonomic nervous system activity Bronchospasm Bradycardia
Cardiac antidysrhythmics	Potentiation of muscle relaxants
Digitalis	Cardiac dysrhythmias Cardiac conduction disturbances
Tricyclic antidepressants	Anticholinergic effects
Antibiotics	Potentiation of muscle relaxants
Oral hypoglycemics	Hypoglycemia
Alcohol	Increased anesthetic requirements Delirium tremens

In awake elderly patients, orthostatic hypotension associated with increases in heart rate suggests decreased intravascular fluid volume. Conversely, orthostatic hypotension not accompanied by increases in heart rate is suggestive of a sympathetic nervous system that is not functioning properly owing to aging or drugs (antihypertensives). Changes in mental status that occur with extension and rotation of the head may reflect vertebrobasilar arterial insufficiency or cervical osteoarthritis. If maintenance of anesthesia with a face mask is anticipated, edentulous patients can keep their dentures in place. Careful preoperative evaluation and correction of electrolyte derangements (diuretics and hypokalemia) and pulmonary dysfunction may decrease the likelihood of perioperative complications. Preoperative medication with drugs is used sparingly in elderly patients, with a detailed explanation of events to anticipate in the perioperative period serving as a useful substitute for drug-induced anxiety relief and sedation. The possibility of increased sensitivity of elderly patients to sedative effects of drugs, especially midazolam, must be considered. Glycopyrrolate, which does not easily cross the blood-brain barrier, is probably less likely to cause undesirable central nervous system effects if an anticholinergic drug is included in the preoperative medication of elderly patients. Attempts to increase gastric fluid pH and decrease gastric fluid volume in selected elderly patients may be useful, considering the potential vulnerability to aspiration produced by changes (delayed gastric emptying, decreased glottic reactivity) associated with aging.

General Anesthesia

Changes associated with aging can cause mechanical problems during general anesthesia. In the

> **Mechanical Changes Associated with Aging**
>
> Edentulous or poor dental hygiene
> Arthritis
> Weak posterior membranous portion of trachea
> Senile atrophy of skin
> Decreased airway reactivity
> Decreased gastroesophageal sphincter tone

edentulous elderly patient or the patient with poor dental hygiene, it is difficult to obtain a proper mask fit and the chance of dislodging a loose tooth is enhanced. The presence of arthritis, especially in the cervical vertebrae, may make intubation of the trachea difficult. Senile atrophy makes the skin more sensitive to injury from adhesive tape and monitoring pads as used for the electrocardiogram. The combination of arthritis, osteoporosis, and sensitive skin makes the problems associated with positioning the elderly patient particularly important so as to avoid pressure necrosis of the skin and peripheral neuropathies. Progressive decreases in reactivity of protective upper airway reflexes with aging plus the high incidence of hiatal hernia in elderly patients may increase the importance of protecting the lungs from aspiration by placement of a cuffed tube in the trachea. The possible change in pharmacokinetics of drugs induced by aging is the basis for the recommendation that initial doses of drugs administered intravenously for the induction of anesthesia be decreased (see the section *Pharmacology*). There is no evidence that a specific inhaled or injected drug is preferable for maintenance of anesthesia in elderly patients. An increase in heart rate associated with administration of isoflurane is less likely to occur in elderly patients than in young adults. In contrast to long-acting muscle relaxants, intermediate-acting (atracurium, vecuronium) and short-acting (mivacurium) muscle relaxants are less dependent on renal or hepatic clearance mechanisms and thus are less likely to be influenced by age-related pharmacokinetic changes. Reversal of nondepolarizing muscle relaxants with anticholinesterase drugs does not seem to introduce any unique risks in elderly patients. Monitoring does not require special considerations, although vascular complications could be more likely from insertion of catheters into peripheral atherosclerotic arteries. Considering predictable decreases in organ function, monitoring cardiac filling pressures, electrocardiogram readings, urine output, and body temperature may assume increased importance in elderly patients. Mechanical ventilation of the lungs with supplemental oxygen is useful considering the predictable changes in the pulmonary system that accompany aging.

In the postoperative period, attention to the development of arterial hypoxemia or myocardial ischemia is important. Early ambulation is a goal so as to decrease the likelihood of pneumonia or the development of deep vein thrombosis. Postoperative confusion and memory loss may contribute to morbidity in elderly patients.

Regional Anesthesia

Regional anesthesia is an acceptable alternative to general anesthesia in alert and cooperative elderly patients, especially those undergoing transurethral resection of the prostate, gynecologic procedures, inguinal herniorrhaphy, or treatment of hip fractures. A T8 sensory level is desirable for these operative procedures. Maintenance of consciousness during surgery permits prompt recognition of acute changes in cerebral function or the onset of angina pectoris. Apprehension despite adequate anesthesia may require intravenous administration of a drug such as midazolam, keeping in mind that elderly patients may require low doses of this drug to achieve the desired effect. Regional anesthesia for hip surgery in elderly patients may decrease the magnitude of perioperative blood loss and decrease the incidence of postoperative deep vein thrombosis.[12] Furthermore, regional anesthesia may be associated with less postoperative confusion compared with patients receiving general anesthesia.

Elderly patients may be more sensitive to spinal anesthesia than younger patients; this manifests as prolonged duration of action (perhaps reflecting decreased vascular absorption and shortened vertebral column length) and exaggerated decreases in blood pressure (perhaps reflecting decreased reflex compensatory responses via the sympathetic nervous system). Some anesthesiologists administer a prophylactic intramuscular dose of ephedrine before institution of spinal anesthesia in an attempt to attenuate subsequent hypotensive effects of sympathetic nervous system blockade; however, this practice is debatable. Epidural anesthesia is an acceptable alternative to spinal anesthesia, since it has the possible advantage of a more gradual decrease in blood pressure than that which accompanies spinal anesthesia. The dose of local anesthetic required to achieve a given sensory level during epidural anesthesia is often perceived to be lower with aging, although not all reports support this notion.

REFERENCES

1. Evans TI. The physiological basis of geriatric anaesthesia. Anaesth Intensive Care 1973;1:319–28.
2. Wei JY. Age and the cardiovascular system. N Engl J Med 1992;327:1735–9.
3. Craig DB, McLeskey CH, Mitenko PA, Thomson IR, Janis KM. Geriatric anaesthesia. Can J Anaesth 1987;34:156–67.
4. Wahba W. Body build (age) and preoperative arterial oxygen tension. Can Anaesth Soc J 1975;22:653–8.
5. Cooper DS. Subclinical hypothyroidism. JAMA 1987; 158:246–7.
6. Homer TD, Stanski DR. The effect of increasing age on thiopental disposition and anesthetic requirement. Anesthesiology 1985;62:714–24.
7. Arden JR, Holley FO, Stanski DR. Increased sensitivity to etomidate in the elderly: Initial distribution versus altered brain response. Anesthesiology 1986;65:19–27.
8. Strum DP, Eger EI, Unadkat JD, Johnson BH, Carpenter RL. Age affects the pharmacokinetics of inhaled anesthetics in humans. Anesth Analg 1991; 73:310–8.
9. Quasha AL, Eger EI II, Tinker JH. Determination and applications of MAC. Anesthesiology 1980;53:315–34.
10. Duvaldestin P, Saada J, Berger JL, D'Hollander A, Desmonts JM. Pharmacokinetics, pharmacodynamics, and dose-response relationship of pancuronium in control and elderly subjects. Anesthesiology 1982; 56:36–40.
11. Feldman RD, Limbird LE, Nadeau J, Robertson D, Wood AJJ. Alterations in leukocyte beta-receptor affinity with aging. A potential explanation for altered beta-adrenergic sensitivity in the elderly. N Engl J Med 1984;310:815–9.
12. Covert CR, Fox GS. Anaesthesia for hip surgery in the elderly. Can J Anaesth 1989;36:311–9.

28

Organ Transplantation

Organ transplantation is the only therapeutic option for selected patients with end-stage disease of the kidneys, liver, heart, or lungs. Certain forms of cancer may be treated with bone marrow transplantation. Transplantation of the pancreas may be considered for patients with severe diabetes mellitus. Improvement in immunosuppressive regimens (corticosteroids, cyclosporine) and better tissue typing (human leukocyte antigens) have contributed to the increasing success of organ transplantation. Infection due to chronic immunosuppresion is the most common cause of death in transplant recipients, emphasizing the importance of strict asepsis during the management of anesthesia. Bacterial infections (pneumonia) are most likely, but fungal, viral (cytomegalovirus, Epstein Barr virus), and parasitic (*Pneumocystis carinii*) infections are also possible. The frequency of cancer is dramatically higher in transplant patients, perhaps reflecting the loss of the protective effect of an active immune system.

RENAL TRANSPLANTATION

Candidates for renal transplantation are selected from patients with end-stage renal disease who are on an established program of chronic hemodialysis. In adults, a common cause of end-stage renal disease is diabetes mellitus. The kidney must be removed from the donor and transplanted into the recipient promptly to minimize the potential for ischemic damage to the donor organ. Kidneys from cadaver donors can be preserved by perfusion at low temperatures for 24 to 36 hours. The donor kidney is placed in the lower abdomen and derives its vascular supply from the iliac vessels. The ureter is anastomosed directly to the bladder.

Management of Anesthesia

Management of anesthesia for renal transplantation invokes the same principles as described for patients with chronic renal failure, including hemodialysis before surgery to optimize coagulation and hydration and to improve electrolyte and acid-base balance (see Chapter 21).[1] Many of these patients are diabetics, emphasizing the value of monitoring blood glucose concentrations during the perioperative period.

Both regional and general anesthesia have been successfully used during renal transplantation. Advantages of regional anesthesia include elimination of the need for intubation of the trachea in immunosuppressed patients, as well as the absence of the need for muscle relaxants. Many of these advantages are negated, however, if regional anesthesia must be extensively supplemented with injected or inhaled drugs. Furthermore, blockade of the peripheral sympathetic nervous system, as produced by regional anesthesia, can complicate the control of blood pressure, especially considering the unpredictable intravascular fluid volume status of these patients. The use of regional anesthesia, particularly epidural anesthesia, is controversial in the presence of abnormal coagulation. For these reasons, general anesthesia is often the preferred approach for the management of patients undergoing renal transplantation.

Side Effects of Immunosuppressive Therapy

- Corticosteroids
  - Glucose intolerance
  - Decreased resistance to infection
  - Osteoporosis
  - Suppression of the pituitary-adrenal axis
- Cyclosporine
  - Nephrotoxicity
  - Hypertension
  - Hepatotoxicity
  - Seizures
  - Confusion
- Azathioprine
  - Anemia
  - Thrombocytopenia
  - Hepatitis
  - Decreased nondepolarizing muscle relaxant requirements
- Antilymphocyte globulin
  - Leukopenia
  - Thrombocytopenia

When general anesthesia is selected, a useful approach is administration of nitrous oxide combined with a volatile anesthetic or short-acting opioid. Disadvantages of opioids used during anesthesia for renal transplantation are their lack of skeletal muscle relaxant effects and the excessive increases in blood pressure that cannot be reliably prevented or treated with these drugs. Decreased cardiac output due to negative inotropic effects of volatile anesthetics must be minimized to avoid jeopardizing the adequacy of tissue oxygen delivery, especially if anemia is present. All factors considered, the skeletal muscle relaxant effects of isoflurane or desflurane plus their minimal metabolism make these volatile anesthetics an attractive choice. Selection of a nondepolarizing muscle relaxant that is not highly dependent on renal clearance (mivacurium, atracurium) is often recommended. Nevertheless, a newly transplanted but functioning kidney is able to clear muscle relaxants, as well as anticholinesterase drugs, used in their reversal at the same rate as in normal patients.[2]

Optimal hydration (avoiding potassium-containing crystalloid solutions) during the intraoperative period improves the early function of the transplanted kidney. Low-dose dopamine (about 3 $\mu g \cdot kg^{-1} \cdot min^{-1}$) may be administered in hopes of improving renal blood flow. Monitoring central venous pressure is a useful guide to the optimal rate of intravenous fluid infusion. An osmotic diuretic such as mannitol is often administered to facilitate urine formation by the newly transplanted kidney. Cardiac arrest has been described after completion of the renal artery anastomosis to the transplanted kidney, presumably owing to sudden hyperkalemia from washout of the potassium-containing solution used to preserve the kidney before transplantation.[3] Unclamping may also be followed by hypotension and is appropriately treated with the intravenous infusion of fluids.

Acute immunologic rejection of the newly transplanted kidney can occur. This rejection is manifested in the vasculature of the transplanted kidney. The only treatment for this acute rejection is removal of the transplanted kidney, especially if the rejection process is accompanied by disseminated intravascular coagulation. Postoperative hematoma may arise in the graft, causing vascular or ureteral obstruction.

LIVER TRANSPLANTATION

Liver transplantation may be considered for patients in hepatic failure and for the treatment of hepatoma, biliary tract tumor, or genetically determined metabolic disturbances. The urgent nature of the operation and the severity of the hepatic dysfunction often limit the time available to optimize preoperative disturbances before proceeding with surgery. Only cadaver livers are used for transplantation, but perfusion techniques permit procurement from long distances.

Management of Anesthesia

Management of anesthesia for liver transplantation includes invasive monitoring of arterial blood pressure and cardiac filling pressures (pulmonary artery catheter) as well as placement of large-bore intravenous catheters to optimize fluid replacement.[1]

Physiologic Disturbances Often Present Before Liver Transplantation

Encephalopathy (confusion to coma)
Congestive heart failure
Arterial hypoxemia
Anemia
Thrombocytopenia
Disseminated intravascular coagulation
Hypokalemia
Hypocalcemia
Glucose intolerance
Oliguria
Ascites

Monitoring arterial blood pressure via the radial artery is preferred over infradiaphragmatic sites because the abdominal aorta may be cross-clamped during hepatic arterial anastomosis. Clamping of the suprahepatic inferior vena cava dictates placement of venous access catheters above the diaphragm. Massive blood and fluid requirements require the use of cell-saver devices. Calcium administration is often required to treat citrate-induced hypocalcemia and myocardial depression. This is one of the rare clinical situations in which the intravenous administration of calcium is indicated. Decreased venous return when the inferior vena cava is clamped may necessitate the use of cardiac inotropic (dopamine) or sympathomimetic drugs. Venovenous bypass to decompress venous congestion when the inferior vena cava is clamped may be considered. Hypothermia must be guarded against by warming inhaled gases and infused fluids. Multiple types of coagulopathies can occur (thrombocytopenia, decreased levels of coagulation factors, fibrinolysis), requiring complex monitoring (thrombelastography) and appropriate blood component therapy (see Chapter 17). Metabolic acidosis during surgery is predictable and, when combined with electrolyte disturbances and hypothermia, may result in cardiac dysrhythmias. Hyperkalemia may accompany unclamping of previously clamped vessels or escape of potassium-rich perfusate from the newly transplanted liver. Blood glucose concentrations are monitored as hypoglycemia and hyperglycemia are potential problems. Oliguria may reflect co-existing renal dysfunction or hypovolemia.

Ketamine is a useful drug for induction of anesthesia. Prolongation of the action of succinylcholine or mivacurium administered to facilitate intubation of the trachea is offset by the prolonged duration of surgery and the presence of cholinesterase enzyme in the subsequently administered blood transfusions. Maintenance of anesthesia is often achieved with a volatile anesthetic such as isoflurane. Nitrous oxide is usually not administered, because of possible bowel distension and the risk of venous air embolism (nitrous oxide would increase the air bubble size) at the time of revascularization of the liver, reflecting the presence of air previously trapped in the liver. In addition, the effect of nitrous oxide on pulmonary vascular resistance is a consideration as these patients may have co-existing pulmonary hypertension (see Chapter 4). Hepatic and renal routes of elimination are considered in the selection of opioids and muscle relaxants during the maintenance of anesthesia. Atracurium is often selected because of its independence from renal or hepatic clearance mechanisms, keeping in mind that the principal metabolite of this muscle relaxant, laudanosine, is dependent on hepatic clearance.[4] It is likely that mechanical support of ventilation will be required during the early postoperative period. Postoperative rejection of the newly transplanted liver is signaled by abnormalities in liver function tests, which must be distinguished from mechanical factors, infection, and effects of hepatotoxic drugs, including cyclosporine.

HEART TRANSPLANTATION

Heart transplantation is the only available treatment for patients with end-stage heart disease most often due to coronary artery disease or cardiomyopathy. Preoperatively, the ejection fraction is generally less than 0.2. Heart-lung transplantation will be necessary if irreversible pulmonary hypertension is present.

Management of Anesthesia

Management of anesthesia for cardiac transplantation may include ketamine or a benzodiazepine, or both, for induction of anesthesia plus an opioid to provide analgesia during surgery.[1,5] Alternatively, an opioid may be used for induction and maintenance of anesthesia. A volatile anesthetic, especially in high doses, may produce an unacceptable amount of myocardial depression or vasodilation, or both. Nitrous oxide is seldom selected because of concern related to additive depressant effects in the presence of opioids and the possibility of venous air embolism (nitrous oxide would increase the air bubble size) since large blood vessels are opened during the operation. A long-acting muscle relaxant devoid of blood pressure lowering effects (pancuronium, doxacurium, pipecuronium) may be a useful selection.

The operative technique consists of cardiopulmonary bypass and anastomosis of the aorta, pulmonary artery, and left and right atria. It will be necessary to withdraw a central venous catheter or pulmonary artery catheter back into the internal jugular vein when the recipient's heart is removed. The catheter is then repositioned when the donor heart is in place. Use of the left internal jugular vein for placement of these catheters leaves the right internal jugular vein available as an access site to perform endomyocardial biopsies for evidence of acute allograft rejection in the postoperative period. A cardiac inotropic drug such as isoproterenol may be needed briefly to maintain myocardial contractility and heart rate of the denervated donor heart during cardiopulmonary bypass. Therapeutic attempts to lower pulmonary vascular resistance may be necessary and include administration of isoproterenol and vasodilating prostaglandin preparations.[6] The transplanted heart responds to direct-acting catecholamines, but drugs that act by an indirect mechanism (ephedrine) have a less intense effect. Heart rate responses do not accompany the administration of anticholinergic or anticholinesterase drugs. The most common cause of death after heart transplantation is opportunistic infection reflecting immunosuppressive therapy. Cyclosporine-induced hypertension is present in more than 90% of heart transplant patients.[7] It is estimated that coronary artery disease develops in up to 40% of patients within 3 years of heart transplantation.

LUNG TRANSPLANTATION

Single-lung transplantation is a consideration for patients experiencing end-stage respiratory failure, especially if the diagnosis is chronic interstitial pulmonary fibrosis.[8] Double-lung transplantation is a more likely selection for patients with chronic obstructive pulmonary disease or cystic fibrosis. Prompt transplantation of the donor lung is necessary as the ischemic time is relatively brief.

Management of Anesthesia

Management of anesthesia for lung transplantation includes the use of a double-lumen endobronchial tube and monitoring with a pulmonary artery catheter.[1] Intraoperative problems may include arterial hypoxemia, especially when one-lung anesthesia is initiated, and pulmonary hypertension when the pulmonary artery is clamped. Bronchoscopy may be required to facilitate reinflation of the allograft. Mechanical support of ventilation is maintained into the postoperative period. The denervated donor lung deprives the patient of a normal cough reflex from the lower airways and predisposes to the development of pneumonia.

PANCREAS TRANSPLANTATION

Pancreas transplantation (whole grafts, segmental grafts, processed islet cells) when successful results in return of blood glucose concentrations to normal within hours. Management of anesthesia for pancreas transplantation requires frequent monitoring for hypoglycemia or hyperglycemia and consideration of the impact of immunosuppressant drugs.[1]

BONE MARROW TRANSPLANTATION

Bone marrow transplantation offers the opportunity for cure of otherwise fatal leukemias. Bone marrow ablation in the recipient is achieved by combinations of chemotherapy and total body radiation. Donor bone marrow (up to 1500 ml) is harvested by multiple aspirations obtained from the superior iliac spines and iliac crests.

Management of Anesthesia

General anesthesia or regional anesthesia and placement of the patient in the supine position are required for the harvest.[1] Brief heparinization before removal of bone marrow may influence the selection of spinal or epidural anesthesia. Nitrous

Manifestations of Graft-versus-Host Disease

Oral ulcers and mucositis
Esophageal ulcers
Fluid and electrolyte loss due to diarrhea
Hepatic failure
Coagulopathy
Pancytopenia
Acute respiratory failure
Renal failure

oxide may be avoided because of potential bone marrow depression associated with use of this drug. There is no evidence, however, that bone marrow engraftment and subsequent function are adversely affected by nitrous oxide administered during the harvest procedure. Peripheral blood loss parallels the volume of bone marrow harvested, emphasizing that substantial fluid loss may accompany this procedure. Postoperative complications other than pain at the harvest puncture sites are rare. Graft-versus-host disease is a life-threatening complication in bone marrow transplant recipients.[9]

REFERENCES

1. Borland LM, Cook DR. Anesthesia for organ transplantation. In: Stoelting RK, Barash PG, Gallagher TJ, eds. Advances in Anesthesia. Chicago, Year Book Medical Publishers 1986:1–28.
2. Cronnelly R, Stanski DR, Miller RD, Sheiner LB. Pyridostigmine kinetics with and without renal function. Clin Pharmacol Ther 1980;28:78–81.
3. Hirshman CA, Leon D, Edelstine G, et al. Risk of hyperkalemia in recipients of kidneys preserved with intracellular electrolyte solution. Anesth Analg 1980; 59:283–6.
4. Pittett J-F, Tassonyi E, Schopfer C, et al. Plasma concentrations of laudanosine, but not atracurium, are increased during the anhepatic phase of orthotopic liver transplantation in pigs. Anesthesiology 1990; 72:145–52.
5. Demas K, Wyner J, Mihm FG, Samuels S. Anaesthesia for heart transplantation. A retrospective study and review. Br J Anaesth 1986;58:1357–64.
6. Cassella ES, Humphrey LS. Bronchospasm after cardiopulmonary bypass in a heart-lung transplant recipient. Anesthesiology 1988;69:135–8.
7. Scherrer U, Vissing SF, Morgan BJ, et al. Cyclosporine-induced sympathetic activation and hypertension after heart transplantation. N Engl J Med 1990;323:693–9.
8. Conacher ID. Isolated lung transplantation. A review of problems and guide to anaesthesia. Br J Anaesth 1988;61:468–74.
9. Stein RA, Messino MJ, Hessel EA. Anaesthetic implications for bone marrow transplant recipients. Can J Anaesth 1990;37:571–8.

29
Outpatient Surgery

Outpatient (ambulatory) surgery offers an alternative to the traditional sequence of hospitalization before elective operations requiring anesthesia. It is likely that more than 50% of all operations will someday be performed as outpatient surgery. Compared with inpatient surgery, advantages of performing the same operation as an outpatient procedure include a decrease in medical costs, increased availability of beds for patients who require hospitalization, protection from hospital-acquired infections, and avoidance of disruption of the family unit attendant on hospitalization. Cost savings extend beyond the actual medical expenses as patients can return to daily activity sooner, decreasing financial loss due to absence from work or need to provide for outside child care. Another cost saving results from the decreased need to build expensive hospital facilities, as existing beds become available for inpatients. The short separation time from family provided by outpatient surgery is especially important for children, as this decreases the number of postoperative psychological problems caused by separation-induced anxiety, which may persist long after completion of surgery.

An alternative to the same-day admission and discharge outpatient surgery concept is a prospectively planned overnight admission to the hospital following surgery. This approach, which has been designated *AM admit,* preserves the advantages of the same-day admission but eliminates any physician concerns regarding the ability to optimally manage potential anesthetic or operative complications in the early postoperative period.

FACILITIES

Outpatient surgical facilities are in either a hospital or a free-standing clinic (Surgicenter). The free-standing clinic must have a transfer and admission agreement with a nearby hospital should unexpected hospitalization be required after surgery. Nevertheless, unanticipated admission rates after outpatient surgery are usually lower than 3%.[1]

The operating rooms, monitors, anesthetic equipment, and postoperative recovery room facilities used for outpatient surgery should not differ from those used for inpatients. The recovery room must be large enough to permit patients to remain for several hours after surgery without overtaxing the facilities. Outpatient surgical facilities should have a physician director, usually an anesthesiologist, who is responsible for the daily administrative decisions, including the final judgments regarding whether a given procedure should be performed on an outpatient basis.

SELECTION

Selection of individuals for outpatient surgery is determined by the characteristics of the patient and the type of operation.

Characteristics of the Patient

The patient must desire to have surgery performed as an outpatient and be in otherwise good general health or have a systemic disease (diabetes mellitus, seizure disorder, essential hypertension, congenital heart disease) that is medically controlled. The patient or a responsible adult must be reasonably intelligent and reliable to ensure compliance with preoperative and postoperative instructions. Patients with a history of prolonged postoperative nausea and vomiting or in whom it is unlikely that pain will be relieved by oral analgesics are not likely candidates for outpatient surgery. Ideally, the driving distance to the outpatient facility should not exceed 1 hour in order to ensure rapid return to the hospital should serious postoperative complications develop.

Patients prone to hospital-acquired infections (infants, immunosuppressed patients) may benefit from having their surgery performed as outpatients. For example, about one in five infants admitted as inpatients for elective inguinal hernia repair develop an upper respiratory tract or enteric infection. The incidence of these types of infections is substantially lower when the surgery is performed on an outpatient basis.

Age is usually not a factor in the selection of patients for outpatient surgery. Nevertheless, pediatric patients probably benefit most from outpatient surgery. Premature neonates may be at increased risk of outpatient surgery because of the frequent presence of anemia in these patients plus the potential for immaturity of the respiratory center and apnea spells in the postoperative period.[2,3] The risk of postoperative apnea spells seems to be decreased by 60 weeks postconception, leading some to recommend postponement of nonessential surgery in a preterm infant to after this age. Other infants who may be at increased risk of outpatient surgery are those who required treatment of respiratory distress syndrome after birth. These infants may develop bronchopulmonary dysplasia associated with abnormal blood gases and an increased incidence of pulmonary infections in the first 6 to 12 months after termination of ventilatory therapy. In the presence of a family history of sudden infant death syndrome, it is unlikely that outpatient surgery will be selected. Despite these qualifications, performance of infant inguinal hernia repair is a well-accepted outpatient surgical procedure. In elderly patients, acceptability for outpatient surgery is influenced by physical status and the ability to be cared for by a competent adult at home.

Types of Operations

Types of operations acceptable as outpatient procedures are often established on an evolutionary basis.[4] Traditionally, operations of short duration (less than 2 hours) that are associated with minimal bleeding, postoperative pain, or physiologic derangement are considered suitable for outpatient surgery. Nevertheless, there is no evidence that recovery time parallels anesthesia time. This suggests that arbitrary limits placed on the type of outpatient surgery permitted based on the anticipated duration of the procedure are unwarranted.[4] Surgery should not be associated with the risk of airway obstruction or interfere with early postoperative ambulation. These recommendations, however, are only guidelines, as emphasized by the frequent performance as outpatient procedures of (1) tonsillectomy and adenoidectomy, which may be accompanied by postoperative hemorrhage, and (2) laparoscopy, which invades the peritoneal cavity. The need for blood transfusion is not a contraindication to outpatient surgery.

Operations that require a major intervention into the cranium, thorax, or abdomen are not considered acceptable for outpatient surgery. Infected cases are rarely considered for outpatient surgery because of the need for separate operative and recovery facilities. Likewise, emergency surgery is not likely to be an outpatient procedure, as this would disrupt the elective schedule. Furthermore, it is difficult to adequately evaluate patients requiring emergency surgery as outpatients.

PREOPERATIVE PREPARATION AND INSTRUCTIONS TO THE PATIENT

The surgeon is responsible for scheduling outpatient surgery, obtaining a medical history, performing a physical examination, initiating the necessary preoperative laboratory studies, and providing instructions to the patient or responsible parent. A preadmission anesthesia clinic is useful as this allows patients to be seen by an anesthesiologist prior to the day of scheduled outpatient surgery. The adequacy of the patient's preparation for anesthesia and specific details regarding management of anesthesia are discussed at this time. Pertinent areas to be pursued by the anesthesiologist include questioning regarding previous anesthetics, current drug therapy, allergies, and previous adverse responses such as postoperative vomiting. An examination of the upper airway, including dentition and evaluation of the peripheral nervous system if regional anesthesia is anticipated, is performed. When this evaluation cannot be performed before the scheduled surgery, it is satisfactory for the anesthesiologist to perform the preanesthetic evaluation on the day of surgery.

Laboratory Data Required Preoperatively

The laboratory data required preoperatively will depend on the patient's age, history, physical examination, and current drug therapy (see Chapter 8). Most guidelines for outpatient surgery require a recent (within 30 days of surgery) hemoglobin determination. The hemoglobin concentration should probably be higher than 10 $g \cdot dl^{-1}$. This minimum hemoglobin requirement is based on the concept that anemia is associated with medical diseases that could influence postoperative outcome. For patients older than 40 years of age, it may be appropriate to determine blood glucose concentrations and blood urea nitrogen concentrations preoperatively. Determination of liver aminotransferase concentrations as a routine screening test for the detection of unsuspected liver disease may be considered for adult patients. Serum potassium concentrations are usually measured if patients are being treated with potassium-losing diuretics. A pregnancy test may be indicated in premenopausal patients. Routine urinalysis offers little or no new information and in many respects only duplicates the blood chemistry measurements. In the absence of positive findings on the history or physical examination, it is not necessary to obtain routine preoperative electrocardiograms or radiographs of the chest in patients younger than 40 years of age.

Written Instructions

Written instructions describing outpatient surgery requirements should be given to the patient or parents by the surgeon at the time of scheduling the surgical procedure. The surgeon should verbally explain to the patient the reasons for these requirements, and the patient or parents should then sign the written instructions. Explaining the reasons for not eating or drinking before surgery is particularly important. Nevertheless, there is compelling evidence that ingestion of clear liquids up to 2 hours before the induction of anesthesia does not increase gastric fluid volume or place the patient at increased risk of acid pneumonitis (see Chapter 9). For this reason, many anesthesiologists are liberalizing their preoperative fluid guidelines and now permitting their patients to ingest clear liquids (water, coffee,

Information Often Provided on Written Instruction Sheet Given to Patients when Outpatient Surgery is Scheduled

- Verify requested laboratory tests are completed.
- Nothing to eat up to 8 hours before surgery (traditionally nothing by mouth after midnight).
- Clear fluids may be ingested up to 2 hours before scheduled surgery if approved by the anesthesiologist. Otherwise, the same fasting guidelines described for solids apply to clear liquids.
- Wear minimal to no cosmetics or jewelry.
- Where and when to report for surgery and estimate of discharge time.
- Must be accompanied by an adult to provide transportation home.
- Notify surgeon if there is a change in the patient's medical condition before surgery.
- After surgery resume eating when hungry, starting with clear liquids and progressing to soups and then regular diet.
- Do not drive an automobile (or other mechanized equipment), make important decisions, or ingest alcohol or depressant drugs for at least 24 to 48 hours after anesthesia.
- Telephone number to contact physician regarding postoperative complications.

pulp-free juices) up to 2 hours before induction of anesthesia. The permissible volume of fluid is often in the range of 1 to 2 $ml \cdot kg^{-1}$, although unrestricted clear liquid intake has not been shown to be hazardous (see Chapter 9). Solid food intake remains strictly forbidden (nothing by mouth after midnight) in the 8 hours preceding surgery.

ARRIVAL ON THE DAY OF SURGERY

After the patient arrives for outpatient surgery, compliance with the written instructions is verified. It is especially important that clandestine food intake by pediatric patients be considered and confirmed not to have occurred. The anesthesiologist should review the patient's medical record and laboratory data at this time. It is important to elicit any change in the medical condition (fever, cough, sputum production, diarrhea) that may have developed since the outpatient surgery was scheduled. Pediatric patients must be thoroughly evaluated for evidence of an upper respiratory tract infection that has manifested since scheduling. Indeed, rhinorrhea poses an enigma in pediatric patients scheduled for outpatient surgery. Benign rhinorrhea is usually an allergic rhinitis that does not contraindicate elective surgery, assuming there is no associated history of asthma. If there is any doubt, rhinorrhea should be assumed to be an upper respiratory infection and consideration given to delaying elective surgery. In this regard, the temperature pattern can be useful in differentiating between an infectious and noninfectious process. For example, a temperature higher than 38°C and leukocytosis in children is highly suggestive of an upper respiratory infection.

PREOPERATIVE MEDICATION

Preoperative medication with drugs to decrease anxiety or produce sedation before outpatient surgery is often avoided for fear of delaying the return to wakefulness after anesthesia and surgery (see Chapter 9). Opioids may be avoided in attempts to minimize drug-induced vomiting. A prophylactic antiemetic may be useful for outpatients undergoing operations associated with a high incidence of postoperative nausea and vomiting. Reassurance by the anesthesiologist and surgeon is a potent antidote to preoperative anxiety in most patients. Nevertheless, pharmacologic premedication may be desirable in mentally retarded or hyperactive patients. Barbiturates or benzodiazepines can be administered orally to these patients before they leave home. If this is not possible, the patient should arrive at the outpatient facility at least 2 hours before scheduled surgery to allow administration (ideally orally) of the preoperative medication and production of desirable effects before induction of anesthesia. Alternatively, intravenous administration of short-acting opioids (alfentanil, fentanyl, sufentanil) before induction of anesthesia may be useful as preoperative medication. The trend in the preoperative medication of young children is the oral administration of midazolam (0.5 $mg \cdot kg^{-1}$ dissolved in a flavored syrup) to provide preinduction sedation. Attempts to pharmacologically manipulate gastric fluid pH (antacids, H_2 antagonists) or volume (metoclopramide), or both, are not indicated on a routine basis.

Routine intramuscular administration of an anticholinergic drug as preoperative medication is not necessary, with the possible exception of patients scheduled for oral endoscopies. In these patients, excessive oral secretions may interfere with the production of topical anesthesia. Otherwise, the discomfort of a dry mouth and throat and the possibility of residual mydriasis and difficulty focusing are undesirable in adult outpatients. Furthermore, pediatric patients may be susceptible to increases in body temperature secondary to anticholinergic effects on sweating. If bradycardia develops intraoperatively, atropine can be administered intravenously.

TECHNIQUE OF ANESTHESIA

All techniques of anesthesia and drugs used to produce anesthesia for inpatients can be considered for use in outpatients. However, the use of techniques or drugs, or both, that permit a prompt and nearly complete recovery with minimal side effects (absence of sedation, nausea, vomiting, and orthostatic hypotension) is important for optimal safety of patients who will be discharged from the hospital within a few hours after surgery. Local infiltration anesthesia is preferable when the planned operative procedure permits. Alternatives to local anesthesia are general anesthesia, regional anesthesia, or peripheral nerve block anesthesia. Regardless of the technique of anesthesia selected, a catheter should probably be inserted into a peripheral vein before the institution of anesthesia. This catheter is necessary to allow administration of fluids (5 to 7 $ml \cdot kg^{-1}$

of lactated Ringer's solution with 5% glucose) to offset dehydration associated with preoperative fasting. The other important reason for placing an intravenous catheter is administration of drugs to produce anesthesia or to treat adverse intraoperative events such as bradycardia, cardiac dysrhythmias, or hypotension. Nevertheless, placement of an intravenous catheter in every patient may be unnecessary when technical difficulties outweigh the advantages of having an intravenous infusion site or when the surgery will be very short (less than 15 minutes) and only superficial tissues are involved.

General Anesthesia

General anesthesia is most frequently selected for outpatient surgery. Induction of anesthesia is pleasantly achieved with the intravenous administration of conventional induction drugs. Propofol (2.5 mg·kg^{-1} IV) produces a rapid onset of unconsciousness followed by a prompt and complete psychomotor recovery. There is a virtual absence of postoperative side effects such as nausea, vomiting, and dizziness. Thiopental and methohexital are also acceptable for the induction of anesthesia in outpatients, keeping in mind that repeated injections of any barbiturate can lead to cumulative effects and delayed postoperative awakening. Psychomotor recovery is more rapid after administration of methohexital than after thiopental. Etomidate, like methohexital, is associated with rapid awakening, but the increased incidence of myoclonic movements, nausea, and vomiting detracts from its use for outpatients.

Pediatric patients may prefer an inhalation induction to the needle stick required for an intravenous induction of anesthesia, but even this alternative should be discouraged as a small-gauge catheter can be placed with minimal discomfort. Furthermore, the discomfort associated with local infiltration can be obviated by using a topical local anesthetic preparation or by selecting a 30-gauge needle and wiping the alcohol preparation solution from the site with a dry gauze before puncturing the skin. When an inhalation induction of anesthesia is planned, however, the most frequently selected drug is halothane. Compared with halothane, induction of anesthesia with enflurane, isoflurane, or desflurane is associated with more patient excitement, breath-holding, coughing, and laryngospasm. Sevoflurane, like halothane, does not cause airway irritation, and its poor solubility in blood permits a more rapid achievement of an anesthetizing concentration than is possible with halothane. In uncontrollable patients, induction of anesthesia can be achieved with administration of rectal methohexital (10 to 25 mg·kg^{-1}), which usually produces unconsciousness in 7 to 10 minutes. The disadvantage of rectal methohexital is delayed awakening after surgery.

Placement of a tube in the trachea is often facilitated by skeletal muscle relaxation produced by intravenous administration of succinylcholine or short-acting nondepolarizing muscle relaxants. A significant disadvantage of succinylcholine for use in outpatients is the occasional occurrence of postoperative myalgia. This problem does not occur with nondepolarizing muscle relaxants and is a reason to consider the use of mivacurium. Spontaneous recovery to 95% twitch height occurs about 30 minutes after administration of a dose of mivacurium sufficient to facilitate tracheal intubation. Furthermore, pharmacologically enhanced antagonism of residual neuromuscular blockade is easily accomplished prior to spontaneous disappearance of the muscle relaxant's effects. Atracurium, vecuronium and rocuronium are somewhat longer-acting alternatives to mivacurium.

Intubation of the trachea should not be avoided because the surgery is being performed as an outpatient procedure. However, use of a small diameter tube and care to avoid trauma during direct laryngoscopy are particularly important for outpatients. Pediatric patients are probably the most vulnerable to airway edema after intubation of the trachea because of the small diameter of their glottic opening.

Maintenance of anesthesia is often achieved with nitrous oxide and a volatile anesthetic or short-acting opioid. Intravenous administration of short-acting opioids (fentanyl 1 to 3 mg·kg^{-1} IV or its equivalent dose) decreases anesthetic requirements for volatile drugs and may decrease the need for postoperative analgesics. The incidence of postoperative nausea and vomiting, however, may be greater after administration of opioids. The low blood and tissue solubility of desflurane and sevoflurane manifests as rapid recovery from the effects of these drugs (see Chapter 2). Indeed, awakening after intravenous induction of anesthesia and maintenance with nitrous oxide and desflurane is predictably more rapid than awakening when isoflurane is the volatile anesthetic (Fig. 29-1).[5] Likewise, recovery after

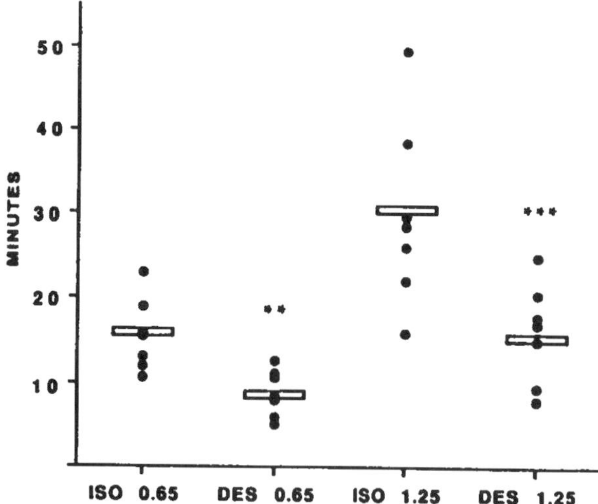

Figure 29-1. Individual emergence times (eye opening or hand grip on request) after discontinuation of 60% nitrous oxide and desflurane (DES, 0.65 MAC and 1.25 MAC) were more rapid than after comparable concentrations of nitrous oxide and isoflurane (ISO). ***P* <0.01 versus ISO 0.65. ****P* <0.05 versus ISO 1.25. (From Smiley et al.,[5] with permission.)

maintenance of anesthesia with sevoflurane is more rapid than after isoflurane, and this recovery is not influenced by the prior administration of propofol for the induction of anesthesia (Fig. 29-2).[6] There is probably no significant difference in awakening times after administration of halothane, enflurane, or isoflurane.

At the conclusion of surgery, infiltration of the incision with a long-acting local anesthetic, such as bupivacaine, may decrease the need for postoperative analgesics. Severe postoperative pain may be treated by intravenous administration of a short-acting opioid. Nausea, vomiting, and sedation may accompany administration of opioids for this purpose. Conversely, nausea and vomiting often accompany pain and can be relieved when analgesia is provided by intravenous administration of opioids. Droperidol or ondansetron may be useful for treatment of patients with persistent postoperative nausea and vomiting, remembering that high doses of droperidol may cause sedation and delay discharge from the postanesthesia care unit (see Chapters 9 and 31).

Regional Anesthesia

A disadvantage of regional anesthesia (lumbar epidural or spinal anesthesia) for outpatient surgery is residual sympathetic nervous system blockade that produces orthostatic hypotension and prevents early postoperative ambulation. The possibility of headache after spinal anesthesia further detracts from the use of this technique of anesthesia for outpatient surgery. Despite these disadvantages, regional anesthesia can be successfully used for outpatient surgery in selected patients. Furthermore, there is no evidence that early ambulation increases the incidence of postspinal headache. In younger patients or those in whom the potential for postspinal headache may be unacceptably high, epidural anesthesia is a suitable alternative to spinal anesthesia.

Peripheral Nerve Block

Peripheral nerve block anesthesia is useful for operations on the extremities. An intravenous regional neural block is appropriate for superficial surgery on the extremities. Brachial plexus block is necessary when procedures other than superficial surgery are performed on the arm.

DISCHARGE FROM THE OUTPATIENT FACILITY

Discharge from the outpatient facility postanesthesia care unit is based on documentation that residual effects of anesthesia have dissipated (see Chapter 31). Recovery from anesthesia is evidenced by the presence of stable and normal vital signs, a level of consciousness similar to preoperative status, and the ability to ambulate without assistance. If regional anesthesia was used, it is important to document complete return of both sensory and motor function. Nausea, vomiting, vertigo, and bleeding should be absent, and the patient should not be in excessive pain. Hoarseness or stridor in a patient in whom a tracheal tube was inserted must be watched carefully. Significant laryngeal edema typically manifests within the first hour after tracheal intubation. Most of these patients respond to conservative measures and can be discharged without overnight hospitalization. As a precaution, however, these patients should be observed for 3 to 4 hours after extubation of the trachea to ensure that symptoms are not progressing. Otherwise, most patients are ready for discharge from the outpatient facility to an adult escort within 1.5 hours after surgery. Even this time may be shortened in the future as more experience is gained with shorter-acting intravenous and inhaled anesthetic drugs.[7] The decision to discharge patients is often the responsibility of the anesthesiol-

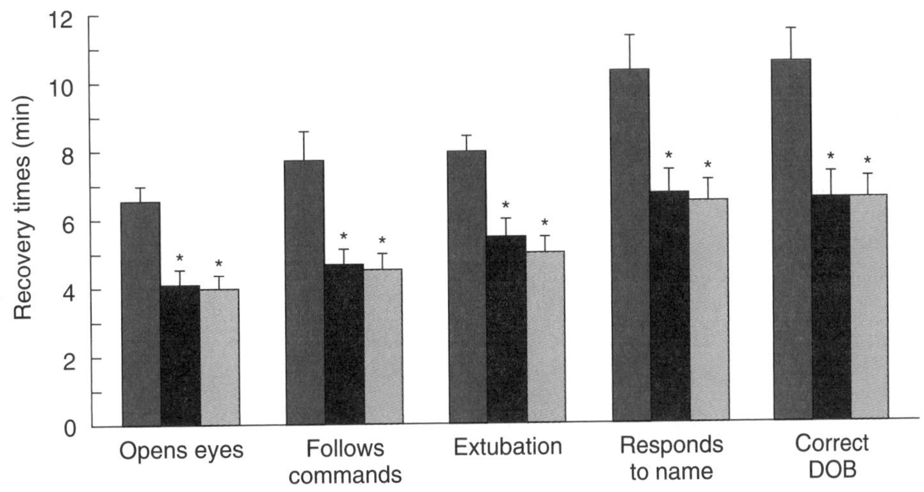

Figure 29-2. Recovery times to various end points were more rapid after propofol-sevoflurane (black bars) and sevoflurane alone (light red bars) than after propofol-isoflurane (dark red bars). DOB, date of birth. Mean values ± SEM. $*P < 0.05$ versus propofol-isoflurane. (From Smith et al.,[6] with permission.)

ogist in consultation, when appropriate, with the surgeon. Persistent nausea and vomiting or excessive postoperative pain may require an unanticipated admission to the hospital.

Patients should be reminded that mental clarity and dexterity may remain impaired for as long as 24 to 48 hours despite an overall feeling of well-being. Therefore, important decisions, driving an automobile, or operation of complex equipment should not be attempted during this period. Ingestion of alcohol or depressant drugs should be discouraged, as additive responses with residual anesthetic effects are possible. Diet should initially consist of clear liquids progressing to soups and then regular diet as tolerated. Oral analgesics, such as acetaminophen, should be provided for those likely to require such medication. Patients should be provided with the telephone number of a physician familiar with their case, as well as instructions for symptoms (bleeding, difficulty breathing, fever) that should be reported to the doctor and a list of possible complications (sore throat, myalgia, incisional pain, headache) that do not require physician consultation. A nurse or physician at the outpatient facility should call the patient the next day to ensure that recovery is proceeding without complications.

REFERENCES

1. Natof HE. Complications associated with ambulatory surgery. JAMA 1980;244:1116–8.
2. Kurth CD, LeBard SE. Association of postoperative apnea, airway obstruction, and hypoxemia in former premature infants. Anesthesiology 1991;75:22–6.
3. Welborn LG, Rice LJ, Hannallah RS, Broadman LM, Ruttimann UE, Fink R. Postoperative apnea in former preterm infants: Prospective comparison of spinal and general anesthesia. Anesthesiology 1990;72: 838–42.
4. Meridy HW. Criteria for selection of ambulatory surgical patients and guidelines for anesthetic management: A retrospective study of 1553 cases. Anesth Analg 1982;61:921–6.
5. Smiley RM, Ornstein E, Matteo RS, Pantuck EJ, Pantuck CB. Desflurane and isoflurane in surgical patients. Comparison of emergence time. Anesthesiology 1991;74:425–8.
6. Smith I, Dingy Y, White PF. Comparison of induction, maintenance, and recovery characteristics of sevoflurane-N_2O and propofol-sevoflurane-N_2O with propofol-isoflurane-N_2O anesthesia. Anesth Analg 1992; 74:253–9.
7. White PF. Studies of desflurane in outpatient anesthesia. Anesth Analg 1992;75:S47–54.

30

Procedures Performed Outside the Operating Room

The increasing number of diagnostic and therapeutic procedures, often based on equipment requiring specialized environments, has led to the need for delivery of anesthesia care outside the traditional confines of the operating rooms.[1] Fundamental anesthetic principles (monitoring capabilities, ability to deliver supplemental oxygen and mechanically ventilate the lungs, availability of anesthetic drugs and equipment, accessibility of suction) are not different from those applied in the operating room. Nevertheless, the often remote location of nonoperative areas (ease of summoning help and obtaining emergency equipment or drugs may be limited) combined with the unique needs of the procedure (access to the patient's airway may be limited, darkness may be required) introduces special challenges. In this regard, it is particularly important for the anesthesiologist to become familiar with these areas and to assess the function and availability of necessary equipment and drugs prior to the induction of anesthesia. The possibility of increased exposure to radiation and the adequacy of scavenging of waste anesthetic gases assumes special importance. At the conclusion of the procedure, transport of the patient to the postanesthesia care unit may require traveling a greater distance than usual, emphasizing the possible increased need for continued monitoring, administration of supplemental oxygen, and support of ventilation often with a self-inflating bag attached to a supply of oxygen.

EXTRACORPOREAL SHOCK WAVE LITHOTRIPSY

Extracorporeal shock wave lithotripsy (ESWL) is used principally as a noninvasive destruction of renal stones by shock waves. Patients undergoing ESWL are placed in a hydraulically operated chair-lift support device and submerged in water (electrohydraulic lithotripsy) from the clavicles down in a large immersion tub. In the future, nonimmersion techniques for ESWL may replace immersion techniques.

Management of Anesthesia

The impact of shock waves at the water-skin interface is painful and necessitates general or regional anesthesia or alternatively intravenous sedation and analgesia.[2,3] Immobilization is important as any movement may displace stones from the predetermined focus sites for shock waves. The method of ventilation of the lungs during general anesthesia is a consideration as movement of the diaphragm and abdominal contents could interfere with precise localization of the shock wave. There is no evidence, however, that high-frequency jet ventilation offers advantages over conventional methods of ventilation (especially a slow breathing rate ensuring a long expiratory pause during which time the stone is stationary) in patients undergoing ESWL. Patients may prefer general anesthesia because of the discomfort of submersion and exposure to the loud noise (in the range of 110 decibels or higher) associated with the procedure. When regional anesthesia is selected, a T6 sensory level is recommended. Sedation and plugging of the external auditory canals may be beneficial in these patients.

Side Effects

The head-up position during anesthesia can be associated with peripheral pooling of blood, but this effect is usually offset by the hydrostatic pressure of

Examples of Procedures Requiring Anesthesia Outside the Operating Room

Extracorporeal shock wave lithotripsy
Diagnostic and therapeutic radiology
- Contrast angiography
- Angiographic embolization
- Computed tomography
- Magnetic resonance imaging
- Radiation therapy
- Angioplasty
- Cardiac catheterization

Cardioversion
Electroconvulsive therapy
Dental surgery

water on submerged portions of the body. This hydrostatic pressure can displace blood centrally, causing acute congestive heart failure in patients with limited cardiac reserves. Likewise, hydrostatic forces on the thorax may decrease functional residual capacity and aggravate mismatching of ventilation to perfusion. Intravenous fluid administration is designed to maintain an adequate urine output so as to facilitate passage of disintegrated stones and to maintain blood pressure during anesthesia. Sudden and exaggerated peripheral vasodilation and hypotension may occur when the patient is transferred out of the bath. During immersion or emersion, cardiac dysrhythmias may occur, presumably reflecting abrupt changes in right atrial pressure as a result of rapid changes in venous return to the heart. To minimize the risk of initiating cardiac dysrhythmias, shock waves are triggered by the R wave of the electrocardiogram and delivered to the kidney during the absolute refractory period of the heart. The immersion bath is warmed to avoid hypothermia. Monitors, epidural catheter insertion sites, and vascular access sites must be protected with water-impermeable dressings.

DIAGNOSTIC AND THERAPEUTIC RADIOLOGY

Diagnostic and therapeutic radiology constitute the major requirement for anesthesia outside the operating room.[4] Most adult patients can tolerate noninvasive radiologic procedures without anesthesia. Children and adults who cannot cooperate and remain motionless are likely to require sedation or general anesthesia, or both. Most radiologic procedures, especially fluoroscopy, expose physicians and other health care workers to radiation. Wearing a lead apron and remaining at least 1 to 2 m from the radiation source should limit the radiation dose to an acceptable level. Contrast agents that may evoke allergic reactions in sensitive patients are routinely used during angiographic and other radiologic procedures. The anesthesiologist may be asked to monitor or care for patients at risk of adverse reactions to contrast media. Prophylaxis with diphenhydramine (25 to 50 mg IV) or steroids (methylpredinosolone 100 to 1000 mg IV), or both, may be of benefit in these patients. Patients undergoing contrast procedures usually have an induced diuresis from the osmotic load. In this regard, adequate hydration of these patients is important to prevent aggravation of co-existing azotemia. Nausea and vomiting are common after administration of contrast dye.

Computed Tomography

Computed tomography (CT) is essentially noninvasive and painless, such that adult patients rarely require more than emotional support. Sedation or general anesthesia is usually required only for children and adults who have difficulty remaining motionless, especially trauma patients. When sedation or general anesthesia is required, the primary concerns of the anesthesiologist are airway management and oxygenation. Positioning and movement of the gantry during CT may result in kinking or disconnection of the anesthesia circuit. The exposure of the anesthesiologist and other personnel to ionizing radiation from CT scanners is relatively low because the radiation is highly focused. Increased intracranial pressure is a concern in patients requiring CT for suspected head injury.

Magnetic Resonance Imaging

Magnetic resonance imaging (MRI) involves the use of high-strength magnetic fields to provide digitalized tomographic imaging of the body.[5] The imaging capabilities of MRI are similar to those of CT, although MRI is considered superior for neurologic and soft tissue examination. MRI is useful for mediastinal and pericardial examinations because it can easily distinguish between fat, vessels, and tumor. Like CT, this imaging technique is noninvasive and has the advantage of producing no ionizing radiation. MRI is not recommended for patients with artificial cardiac pacemakers, aneurysm clips, or intravascular wires. Patients with large metal implants (artificial joints) should be monitored for implant heating.

Management of Anesthesia

Most adult patients will tolerate MRI scanning with little or no sedation. Anesthesia is required to maintain patient immobility and for children. The patient environment is different from that of CT scanning. During MRI, the patient is positioned on a long thin table and then placed in the scanner (Fig. 30-1).[6] Claustrophobia may be severe, and the patient may require reassurance and sedation. Furthermore, once the patient is placed in the scanner, access is difficult, emphasizing the importance of prior planning and attention to the position of monitoring devices and anesthetic circuitry. As the magnetic field is not dangerous, the anesthesiologist can remain close to the patient. The noise from the MRI scanner makes communication difficult and renders assessment of cardiopulmonary function from acoustic precordial or esophageal stethoscopes impossible. Monitoring includes the electrocardiogram, blood pressure, and pulse oximetry. Appropriate extensions must be attached to these monitors. Burns from heating of the pulse oximeter probe during MRI are a risk. With awake, alert patients, monitoring is usually performed from a distance. In this regard, electrocardiogram telemetry and capnography systems have been used.

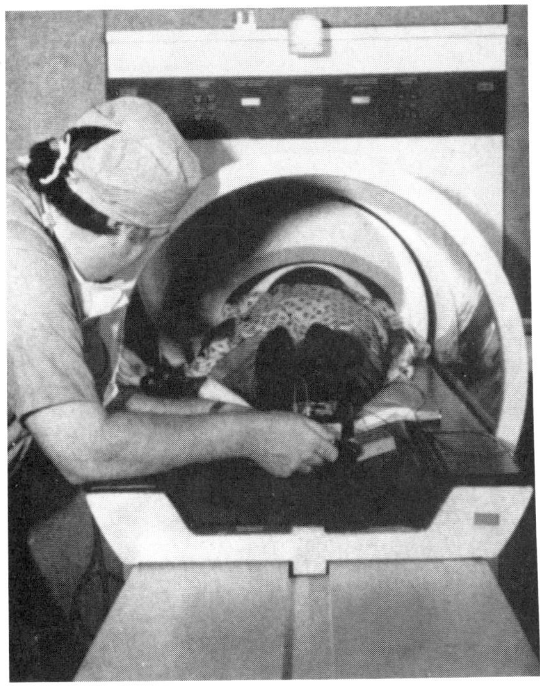

Figure 30-1. The patient is inaccessible after placement in the scanner during magnetic resonance imaging. (From Roth et al.,[6] with permission.)

General anesthesia for MRI requires the use of specially modified anesthetic machines, equipment, and ventilators in which ferromagnetic components have been replaced by aluminum, nonmagnetic steel, or plastic (Fig. 30-2).[5,7] Otherwise, activation of the magnetic field would cause forceful and sudden movement of the equipment with possible injury to personnel. Likewise, any other material that contains a magnetic strip (credit cards) should not be brought near the scanner, as they can become demagnetized. Plastic laryngoscopes modified to operate from an independent power source with a long nonmagnetic cable (batteries in a conventional laryngoscope handle would be attracted by the magnetic field) have been recommended. The use of a Bain circuit is a logical selection because of its length and light weight. Intravenous infusion pumps must be supported on nonferromagnetic poles. If accidental tracheal extubation occurs, it will probably be necessary to discontinue the scan and remove the patient from the scanner. Air flow through the scanner increases heat loss from the patient and introduces the risk of hypothermia, especially in pediatric patients. Nonferromagnetic devices to monitor body temperature may be indicated in certain patients.

Radiation Therapy

Radiation therapy may require sedation or general anesthesia to ensure patient immobility as large doses of radiation must be precisely focused to minimize damage to surrounding tissue. Patients are often children scheduled for a series of treatments extended over several weeks. All personnel must leave the area during the treatment period as the high doses of radiation may pose a hazard. For this

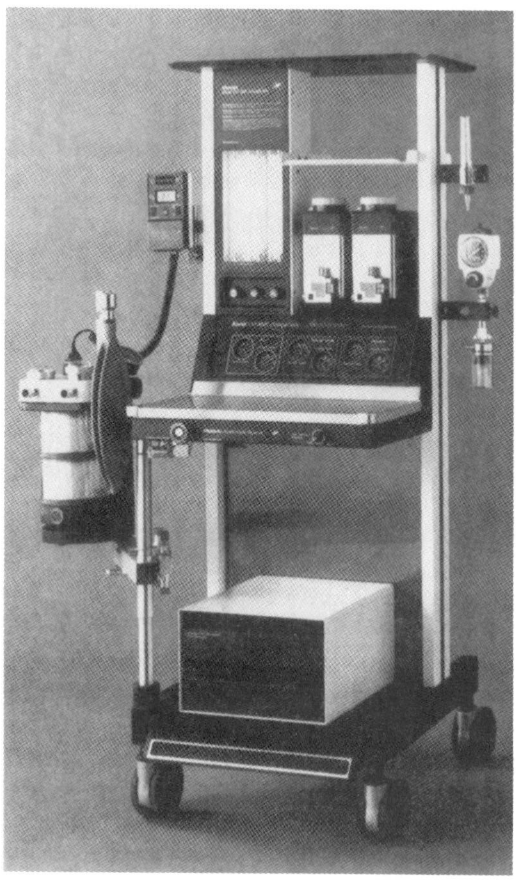

Figure 30-2. Commercially available, magnetic resonance imaging-compatible (all ferromagnetic components removed) Ohmeda Excel 210 anesthesia machine. (From Rao et al.,[7] with permission.)

reason, the anesthesiologist is required to be dependent on remote monitoring techniques that may include closed-circuit television.[8] General anesthesia with drugs appropriate for the brief duration of the procedure is recommended, keeping in mind these patients will likely require repeated anesthetics.

Cardiac Catheterization

Cardiac catheterization in children is usually performed for diagnosis and evaluation of congenital heart disease. Intravenous sedation or general anesthesia must not substantially interfere with existing intracardiac shunts (excess myocardial depression or changes in preload due to fluid balance) as reflected by arterial blood gas measurements. Normocapnia is a goal of ventilation during anesthesia for cardiac catheterization. A high hematocrit may be associated with an increased risk of thrombosis, whereas lowering the hematocrit may jeopardize tissue oxygen delivery. Cardiac dysrhythmias and heart block are important causes of morbidity, emphasizing the need for prompt access to a defibrillator and resuscitation drugs. A lead apron must be worn by the anesthesiologist for protection from the scatter ionizing radiation characteristic of fluoroscopy.

Premedication and sedation (often combinations of a benzodiazepine and short-acting opioid) may be sufficient to allay anxiety that could exacerbate co-existing cardiopulmonary problems. Atropine premedication may be especially useful in children, particularly those with cyanotic congenital heart disease. The onset of action of injected or inhaled drugs, or both, may be influenced by the presence of left-to-right or right-to-left intracardiac shunts as well as co-existing congestive heart failure. Monitoring of the patient during cardiac catheterization is likely to be supplemented by information derived from measurement of blood gases. Access to the patient may be limited by fluoroscopy equipment required during performance of the cardiac catheterization.

CARDIOVERSION

Elective cardioversion requires a brief period of sedation and amnesia for the discomfort produced by the electric shock. Following preoxygenation, a drug such as methohexital, thiopental, or propofol is generally injected intravenously. Etomidate-induced myoclonus may preclude the use of this drug for cardioversion as interpretation of the electrocardiogram may be difficult. The appropriate synchronized electrical charge is delivered once adequate central nervous system depression has occurred. The patient's airway is maintained manually, and ventilation of the lungs is supported with supplemental oxygen using a bag and mask until consciousness has returned. Monitoring includes blood pressure, pulse oximetry, and the electrocardiogram. Equipment for the unexpected need for intubation of the trachea is readily available.

ELECTROCONVULSIVE THERAPY

Electroconvulsive therapy (ECT) is indicated for the treatment of severe mental depression in a patient who is unresponsive to drugs or who becomes acutely suicidal. The electrical stimulus produces a grand mal seizure consisting of a brief tonic phase followed by a more prolonged clonic phase. Typically, about eight treatments are necessary, with 75% of treated patients showing a favorable response.

Side Effects

The side effects of ECT are manifested principally on the cardiovascular and central nervous systems.[9] An initial bradycardia and hypotension (parasympathetic nervous system stimulation) followed by increased heart rate and blood pressure (sympathetic nervous system stimulation) may be particularly undesirable in patients with coronary artery disease. Indeed, the most common cause of mortality after ECT is myocardial infarction and cardiac dysrhythmias. Cerebral blood flow increases dramatically during ECT and may produce detrimental increases in intracranial pressure in patients with a space-occupying lesion. Indeed, the only contraindication to ECT is co-existing intracranial hypertension. Increased intragastric pressure is likely to accompany ECT. Transient apnea plus postictal confusion may follow cessation of seizure activity.

Side Effects of Electroconvulsive Therapy

- Parasympathetic nervous system stimulation
  - Bradycardia
  - Hypotension
- Sympathetic nervous system stimulation
  - Tachycardia
  - Hypertension
  - Cardiac dysrhythmias
- Increased cerebral blood flow
- Increased intragastric pressure
- Apnea

Management of Anesthesia

The patient is fasted, but preoperative medication is not recommended as drug-produced sedation could delay recovery after ECT. Administration of an anticholinergic drug intravenously 1 to 2 minutes before induction of anesthesia may be helpful in preventing the initial bradycardia that may accompany ECT. Methohexital (0.5 to 1 $mg{\cdot}kg^{-1}$ IV; thiopental 1.5 to 3 $mg{\cdot}kg^{-1}$ and propofol 1 to 1.5 $mg{\cdot}kg^{-1}$ IV are alternatives) is a frequent choice for the induction of anesthesia before ECT.[9] Following the onset of unconsciousness, succinylcholine (0.3 to 1.0 $mg{\cdot}kg^{-1}$ IV) is administered to attenuate contraction of skeletal muscles, which otherwise might produce bone fractures. A low dose of succinylcholine is more likely to permit visual confirmation of seizure activity. Isolation of an upper extremity with a tourniquet prior to injection of succinylcholine also permits confirmation of seizure activity in the isolated arm that might otherwise be masked by skeletal muscle paralysis. Support of ventilation of the lungs with supplemental oxygen using a bag and mask is recommended both before the production of the seizure and until the effects of succinylcholine have dissipated. Denitrogenation of the lungs with oxygen before ECT decreases the likelihood that arterial hypoxemia will develop if it becomes difficult to support ventilation of the lungs in the presence of seizure-induced skeletal muscle contractions. Furthermore, it is important to recognize that apnea may follow ECT even in the absence of succinylcholine. Although tracheal intubation is not required, it is important to have all necessary equipment, including suction, should unexpected airway problems arise.

Monitoring with a pulse oximeter guides the need for continued administration of supplemental oxygen. The use of a peripheral nerve stimulator will confirm the degree of neuromuscular blockade produced by succinylcholine and will also identify the patient with previously unrecognized atypical cholinesterase enzyme. Since repeated anesthetics will be necessary, it is possible to establish a dose of anesthetic induction drug and succinylcholine that produces the most predictable and desirable effects in each patient. The electrocardiogram is a necessary monitor as cardiac dysrhythmias may accompany ECT. In some situations, the electroencephalogram is monitored to confirm the occurrence of a grand mal seizure.

DENTAL SURGERY

Anesthesia for dental surgery is most likely to be required for the mentally retarded or very young patient. Mentally retarded patients may have coexisting medical problems (congenital heart disease as in patients with Down syndrome) of importance to the anesthesiologist.

Management of Anesthesia

Goals for the management of anesthesia for dental surgery include rapid induction and prompt emergence.[10] A properly functioning suction apparatus is crucial to prevent aspiration of blood even in the presence of a cuffed tracheal tube. Inclusion of atropine in the preoperative medication may provide useful antisialagogue effects for intraoral surgery. Ketamine is a commonly selected drug for induction of anesthesia in uncooperative patients as this drug is effective intramuscularly. When intravenous access can be established before induction of anesthesia, other acceptable induction drugs include methohexital, thiopental, etomidate, and propofol. Tracheal intubation, usually through the nose, is recommended for lengthy or unusually bloody procedures. Maintenance of anesthesia is influenced by the likely duration of the planned dental surgery and may include combinations of injected and inhaled drugs. Bleeding and use of oropharyngeal packing during dental procedures emphasize the need for close observation of airway patency during emergence and the availability of appropriate personnel and equipment (airways, drugs, suction).

REFERENCES

1. Gallagher TJ. Anesthesia outside the operating room. In Stoelting RK, Barash PG, Gallagher TJ, eds. Advances in Anesthesia. Chicago, Year Book Medical Publishers 1987;4:25–46.
2. Zeitlin GL, Roth RA. Effect of three anesthetic techniques on the success of extracorporeal shock wave lithotripsy. Anesthesiology 1988;68:272–6.
3. Monk TG, Boure B, White PF, et al. Comparison of intravenous sedative-analgesic techniques for outpatient immersion lithotripsy. Anesth Analg 1991;72: 616–21.
4. Weston G, Strunin L, Amundson G. Imagery for anaesthetists: A review of the methods and anaesthetic implications of diagnostic imagery techniques. Can Anaesth Soc J 1985;32:552-61.
5. Patteson SK, Chesney JT. Anesthetic management for magnetic resonance imaging: Problems and solutions. Anesth Analg 1992;74:121–8.
6. Roth J, Nugent M, Gray J, et al. Patient monitoring during magnetic resonance imaging. Anesthesiology 1985;62:80–3.
7. Rao C, Krishna G, Emhardt J. Anesthesia machine for use during magnetic resonance imagery. Anesthesiology 1990;1054–5.
8. Bashein G, Russell A, Momil S. Anesthesia and remote monitoring for intraoperative radiation therapy. Anesthesiology 1986;64:804–7.
9. Selvin BL. Electroconvulsive therapy—1987. Anesthesiology 1987;67:367–85.
10. Klein SL. Anesthesia dental complications. In: Stoelting RK, Barash PG, Gallagher TJ, eds. Advances in Anesthesia. Chicago, Mosby-Year Book 1992; 9:269–88.

Section V
Recovery Period

31

Postanesthesia Care Unit

The postanesthesia care unit (PACU, recovery room) is the area designated for the monitoring and care of patients who are recovering from the immediate physiologic derangements produced by anesthesia and surgery. Standards for postanesthesia care have been endorsed by the American Society of Anesthesiologists and include the use of pulse oximetry (see Appendix 3). The PACU should be staffed with specially trained nurses skilled in the prompt recognition of postoperative complications. Location of the PACU in close proximity to the operating rooms facilitates rapid access to physician consultation and assistance. Specifically, an anesthesiologist should be readily available and responsible for ensuring safe recovery from anesthesia. Equipment and drugs must be available to provide routine care (supplemental oxygen, suction, monitoring of vital signs, pulse oximeter, electrocardiogram) and advanced organ support (ventilators, transducers to monitor intravascular pressures, devices for continuous infusion of drugs). An electrical defibrillator and appropriate drugs to assist in the optimal provision of cardiopulmonary resuscitation must be available. The PACU should have good access to radiographic and arterial blood gas services. The size of the PACU is determined by the number and type of operative procedures, with approximately 1.5 recovery room beds being necessary for every operating room. Discharge of patients from the PACU is the responsibility of a physician, most often an anesthesiologist. Administratively, an anesthesiologist usually serves as the medical director of the PACU.

RECOVERY FROM ANESTHESIA

Recovery from anesthesia is usually uneventful and routine, beginning with discontinuation of the administration of anesthetic drugs and extubation of the trachea while the patient is still in the operating room. The rate of decrease in the alveolar concentration (partial pressure) of an inhaled anesthetic as a reflection of recovery is dependent on the patient's alveolar ventilation, the blood and lipid solubility of the anesthetic drug, the magnitude of metabolism of the anesthetic drug, and the duration of anesthesia (see Chapter 2).[1] Patients are likely to begin responding to verbal stimuli when alveolar anesthetic concentrations are decreased to about one-half the MAC for the volatile anesthetic drug.[2] This value is designated MAC awake. Recovery from the anesthetic effects of injected drugs depends on the dose administered; the time since the last injection; and the drug's lipid solubility, hepatic inactivation, and/or renal excretion (see the section *Delayed Awakening*). If muscle relaxants have been administered, it is important to assess the residual activity of these drugs (see Chapter 7). This assessment is most often made in the operating room before allowing the return of spontaneous ventilation or considering extubation of the trachea.

ADMISSION TO THE POSTANESTHESIA CARE UNIT

On arrival in the PACU, the anesthesiologist provides the nurse with pertinent details of the patient's

Information Often Given to the Nurse at the Time of Admission to the Postanesthesia Care Unit

Patient's name and age
Surgical procedure and type of anesthetic, including drugs used
Other intraoperative drugs (antagonists, antibiotics, diuretics, vasopressors, antidysrhythmics)
Preoperative vital signs
Co-existing medical diseases
Preoperative drug therapy, including preoperative medication
Allergies
Intraoperative estimated blood loss and measured urine output
Intraoperative fluid and blood replacement
Anesthetic and surgical complications
Special medications or procedures that will be necessary in the postanesthesia care unit, including pain management (see Chapter 32), arterial blood gases, and radiographs

POSTANESTHESIA CARE UNIT RECORD

Anesthesia: General ☐ Spinal ☐ Epidural ☐ Other Regional ☐
Anesthesiologist: ______
Surgeon: ______
Procedure: ______
Received in PACU by: ______
Time In: ______ Time Out: ______

VITAL SIGNS

○ RESP • PULSE > < BLOOD PRESSURE
250 240 230 220 210 200 190 180 170 160 150 140 130 120 110 100 90 80 70 60 50 40 30 20 10 0
TEMP

Pre-Op BP
OR BP
O²
Begun:
Ended:
Method

INTAKE/OUTPUT		IN	OUT
Emesis			
Gastric Suction			
Voided			
Urinary Catheter			
Chest Drainage			
Wound Drainage			
Recovery Room Blood Given			
PO Fluid			
IV Fluid			
TOTAL			

O_2: Mask: ____ Ventilator: ____ Croupette: ____
Cannula: ____ Trach Collar: ____ T-Piece ____
Airways: NETT ____ TRACH ____ NASAL ____
OETT ____ ORAL ____

POST ANESTHESIA RECOVERY SCORE		IN	MINUTES 30	60	90	OUT	SCORING INTERPRETATION
Able to move 4 extremities voluntarily or on command = 2 Able to move 2 extremities voluntarily or on command = 1 Able to move 0 extremities voluntarily or on command = 0	ACTIVITY						A MINIMUM TOTAL SCORE OF 8 IS REQUIRED FOR DISCHARGE. EXCEPTIONS TO THIS ARE TO BE EXPLAINED IN THE SPACE BELOW BY THE DISCHARGING PHYSICIAN.
Able to deep breathe & cough freely = 2 Dyspnea or limited breathing = 1 Apneic = 0	RESPIRATION						
BP ± 20 of Preanesthetic level = 2 BP ± 20-50 of Preanesthetic level = 1 BP ± 50 of Preanesthetic level = 0	CIRCULATION						
Fully awake = 2 Arousable on calling = 1 Not responding = 0	CONSCIOUSNESS						
Pink = 2 Pale, dusky, blotchy, jaundiced, other = 1 Cyanotic = 0	COLOR						
	TOTALS						

DATE & TIME	MEDICATIONS (Drug Dosage, Route)	MD	NURSE'S NOTES

Evaluated and (M.D.) ______ Transferred to Unit by: ______
Discharged by: (R.N.) ______ Received on Unit by: ______
80-6000 Rev 1/87

Figure 31-1. Example of a postanesthesia care unit record.

history, medical condition, anesthetic, and surgery. Often, the PACU nurse is responsible for the care of only one patient. Particular attention should be given to monitoring oxygenation (pulse oximetry), ventilation (breathing frequency, airway patency), and circulation (blood pressure, heart rate, electrocardiogram). Vital signs should be recorded at least every 15 minutes while the patient is in the PACU. The vital signs and other pertinent information are recorded on a separate sheet that becomes part of the patient's medical record (Fig. 31-1). While in the PACU, the patient is encouraged by the nurse to cough, breathe deeply, and change position. Before discharge from the PACU, the patient is evaluated by a physician (usually an anesthesiologist), who writes a note in the patient's medical record describing pertinent aspects of the anesthetic and PACU period. This note serves as a source of information to anesthesiologists who may be responsible for administration of anesthesia to this patient in the future. Although criteria for discharge from the PACU are not standardized, they typically include an assessment of the patient's (1) activity (movement of extremities in response to a request), (2) breathing, (3) blood pressure, (4) consciousness, and (5) color (Fig. 31-1). The PACU nurse should give a full description of the patient's intraoperative and immediate postoperative course to the ward nurse at the time the patient is returned to the ward. Before an ambulatory patient is discharged to the care of a responsible adult, it is important to ensure that the patient can ambulate without dizziness or hypotension and that significant postoperative pain, nausea, and vomiting are absent.

EARLY POSTOPERATIVE PHYSIOLOGIC DISORDERS

A variety of physiologic disorders affecting multiple organ systems must be diagnosed and treated in the PACU during emergence from the effects of anesthesia and surgery.

Upper Airway Obstruction

Upper airway obstruction in the PACU is most often due to occlusion of the pharynx by the tongue.

Physiologic Disorders that May Manifest in the Postanesthesia Care Unit

Upper airway obstruction
Arterial hypoxemia
Hypoventilation
Hypotension
Hypertension
Cardiac dysrhythmias
Oliguria
Bleeding
Decreased body temperature
Agitation (emergence delirium)
Delayed awakening
Nausea and vomiting
Pain (see Chapter 32)

Laryngeal obstruction is less common but can occur secondary to laryngospasm or can be caused by edema, reflecting direct airway injury. Obstruction of the pharynx or larynx can occur after head and neck surgery when the head cannot be positioned optimally to maintain a patent upper airway.

Physical examination of patients with upper airway obstruction reveals flaring of the nares, retraction at the suprasternal notch (tracheal tug) and intercostal spaces, and vigorous diaphragmatic and abdominal contractions. The most effective method of eliminating upper airway obstruction due to occlusion of the pharynx by the tongue is extension of the head with or without anterior displacement of the mandible (head tilt-jaw thrust method) (see Chapter 35). This maneuver stretches muscles attached to the tongue, serving to pull the tongue away from the posterior pharyngeal wall. If upper airway obstruction is not promptly reversible by this maneuver, a nasopharyngeal or oropharyngeal airway can be inserted. A nasopharyngeal airway is better tolerated by patients awakening from general anesthesia and thus may be the preferred initial selection. An oropharyngeal airway placed in the semiconscious patient may stimulate gagging and vomiting, as well as laryngospasm.

Laryngospasm is initially treated by extension of the head and anterior displacement of the mandible plus application of positive airway pressure with a bag and mask delivering pure oxygen. If laryngospasm is incomplete, this treatment is satisfactory until the spasm spontaneously dissipates. Complete laryngospasm that persists despite these maneuvers should be promptly treated with the intravenous administration of succinylcholine. Direct laryngoscopy and intubation of the trachea with a cuffed tube is indicated when upper airway obstruction persists despite proper head positioning and use of an artificial airway. Should intubation of the trachea be technically impossible, the placement of a 12- to 14-gauge extracath needle (catheter over needle) through the cricothyroid membrane (cricothyrotomy) will provide temporary oxygenation until a more definitive procedure, such as tracheostomy, can be performed (see Fig. 35-11).

Upper airway obstruction due to laryngeal edema as may follow tracheal intubation may be treated by humidifying the inhaled gases and administering nebulized racemic epinephrine (0.25 to 0.5 ml of 2.25% epinephrine in 5 ml water or normal saline). Administration of dexamethasone (0.15 $mg \cdot kg^{-1}$ IV) has been used for treatment of laryngeal edema, but the efficacy of this therapy has not been confirmed. In children, laryngeal edema can rapidly progress to complete upper airway obstruction, emphasizing the importance of close surveillance in the PACU. Prolonged upper airway obstruction can lead to sustained decreases in interstitial hydrostatic pressure with resultant noncardiogenic pulmonary edema.

Arterial Hypoxemia

Arterial hypoxemia (PaO_2 lower than 60 mmHg) in the immediate postoperative period most likely reflects the impact of anesthetic drugs or surgery. The incidence of arterial hypoxemia may exceed 50% in the first 3 hours postoperatively. Decreases in the PaO_2 are common, particularly following upper abdominal or thoracic surgery.[3] For example, the PaO_2 decreases about 20 mmHg following upper abdominal or thoracic surgery. The decrease in PaO_2 is much smaller following lower abdominal (about 10 mmHg) or peripheral (about 6 mmHg) surgery.

Etiology

Factors leading to postoperative arterial hypoxemia are multiple. Advanced age, obesity, smoking histo-

Factors Leading to Postoperative Arterial Hypoxemia

Right-to-left intrapulmonary shunt (atelectasis)
Mismatching of ventilation to perfusion (decreased functional residual capacity)
Decreased cardiac output
Alveolar hypoventilation (residual effects of anesthetics and/or muscle relaxants)
Inhalation of gastric contents (aspiration)
Pulmonary embolus
Pulmonary edema
Pneumothorax
Posthyperventilation hypoxia
Increased oxygen consumption (shivering)
Advanced age
Obesity

ry, and co-existing lung disease are likely to be associated with postoperative arterial hypoxemia. Probably the most common cause of postoperative arterial hypoxemia is an increase in right-to-left intrapulmonary shunting due to atelectasis. Atelectasis may be segmental, reflecting bronchial obstruction with secretions, or diffuse, reflecting decreased lung volumes. Ventilation-to-perfusion mismatching is accentuated by mechanical abnormalities of the lungs such as decreases in the functional residual capacity (FRC). Decreases in cardiac output can contribute to decreases in the PaO_2 in patients with ventilation-to-perfusion mismatching or intrapulmonary shunts. In the absence of supplemental inspired oxygen, the accumulation of carbon dioxide in the alveoli due to drug-induced hypoventilation may lead to arterial hypoxemia. Inhalation of acidic gastric fluid may result in the rapid onset of profound arterial hypoxemia due to (1) reflex airway closure, (2) loss of surfactant activity leading to atelectasis, and (3) loss of capillary integrity manifesting as noncardiogenic pulmonary edema. A pulmonary embolus in the immediate postoperative period can cause profound arterial hypoxemia, although the exact physiologic explanation for the hypoxemia is unclear. This diagnosis should be suspected in any patient who develops acute dyspnea and tachypnea in the recovery room. Pulmonary edema due to left ventricular failure is usually preceded by systemic hypertension and typically occurs in the first hour after surgery.[4] Arterial hypoxemia due to a pneumothorax reflects compression of alveoli, producing a right-to-left intrapulmonary shunt. Patients undergoing radical neck dissection, mastectomy, or nephrectomy are particularly vulnerable to the development of a pneumothorax. Insertion of a chest tube is likely to be recommended for the treatment of a pneumothorax larger than 20% in spontaneously breathing patients. Any degree of pneumothorax in the presence of mechanical ventilation of the lungs is likely to be treated by insertion of a chest tube. If circulatory depression accompanies a tension pneumothorax, emergency treatment is placement of a 12- to 14-gauge extracath needle (catheter over needle) into the second anterior intercostal space. Posthyperventilation hypoxia reflects compensatory hypoventilation in attempts to replenish body stores of carbon dioxide that have been depleted by intraoperative hyperventilation. Arterial hypoxemia due to this compensatory hypoventilation is prevented by increasing the inhaled concentration of oxygen. Diffusion hypoxia as a cause of arterial hypoxemia in the PACU is unlikely because the early dilutional effect of nitrous oxide on the alveolar partial pressure of oxygen is prevented by only a few breaths of oxygen at the conclusion of the anesthetic. Postoperative shivering can result in substantial increases in oxygen consumption but only rarely contributes to arterial hypoxemia.[5]

Diagnosis

Diagnosis of arterial hypoxemia (PaO_2 lower than 60 mmHg) in the PACU requires measurement of the PaO_2. Monitoring arterial hemoglobin oxygen saturation with a pulse oximeter is useful for facilitating early recognition of decreases in PaO_2. Clinical signs of arterial hypoxemia (hypertension, hypotension, tachycardia, bradycardia, cardiac dysrhythmias, agitation) are nonspecific. A decreased hemoglobin concentration may impair detection of cyanosis. Furthermore, circulatory and ventilatory responses to arterial hypoxemia may be attenuated by the effects of residual anesthetics.[6] Thus, arterial hypoxemia may not stimulate ventilation in postoperative patients who have received a volatile anesthetic.

Treatment

Arterial hypoxemia in the PACU is treated with supplemental oxygen (see the section *Postoperative Respiratory Therapy, Oxygen Therapy*). Supplemental oxygen does not eliminate the cause of hypoxemia but may symptomatically alleviate it while concomitant corrective measures are employed. For example, if arterial hypoxemia is due to hypoventilation from excessive residual effects of opioids, specific pharmacologic antagonism with naloxone is a consideration. If arterial hypoxemia persists despite administration of 100% oxygen, or if hypercapnia accompanies supplemental oxygen therapy, the patient's trachea should be intubated and the lungs mechanically ventilated. In such patients, ventilation of the lungs using positive end-expiratory pressure (PEEP) will increase the FRC and result in an increased PaO_2. Furthermore, ventilation of the lungs using PEEP often allows a decrease in the inspired concentrations of oxygen without decreases in the PaO_2.

It is not clear how long supplemental oxygen should be continued in the PACU. A guideline is that if supplemental oxygen is to be discontinued, the patient should be able to maintain an acceptable arterial hemoglobin oxygen saturation as measured by pulse oximetry for about 30 minutes prior to discharge from the PACU. The acceptable pulse oximetry reading will need to be individualized for each patient but generally should be higher than 95%. If a patient does not meet these criteria, it would seem logical to continue administration of supplemental oxygen into the postoperative period following the patient's discharge from the PACU.

Hypoventilation

Hypoventilation leading to hypercarbia is a possibility in the early postoperative period.

Etiology

Factors leading to postoperative hypoventlation are multiple. A frequent cause, however, is inadequate central nervous stimulation to ventilation due to residual effects of inhaled or injected anesthetic drugs, or both. Anesthetic-induced depression of ventilation is evidenced by a shift of the carbon dioxide response curve to the right with or without a concomitant increase in the $PaCO_2$. Ventilatory depression produced by inhaled anesthetics decreases with time. By contrast, opioids, such as fentanyl, can produce biphasic ventilatory depression. For example, drug-induced depression may dissipate with the increased external stimulation provided by the transport and admission to the PACU only to be followed by a second period of ventilatory depression as external stimulation wanes (Fig. 31-2).[7] Residual effects of muscle relaxants may interfere with optimal activity of respiratory muscles leading to accumulation of carbon dioxide. Persistent neu-

Factors Leading to Postoperative Hypoventilation

- Drug-induced central nervous system depression (volatile anesthetics, opioids)
- Residual effects of muscle relaxants
- Suboptimal ventilatory muscle mechanics
- Increased production of carbon dioxide
- Co-existing chronic obstructive pulmonary disease

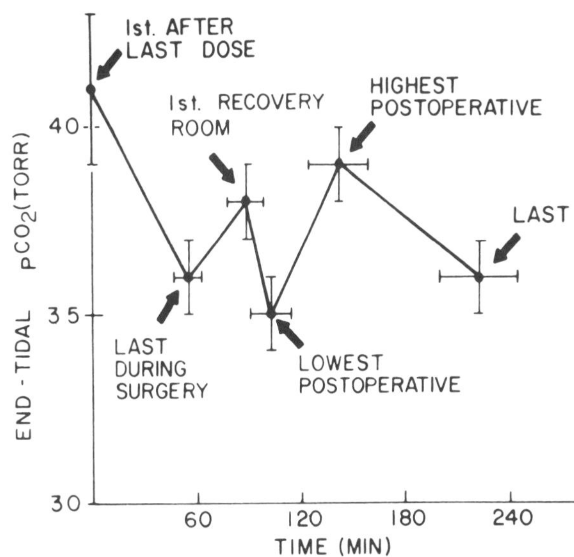

Figure 31-2. Recurrent fentanyl-induced depression of ventilation is evidenced by increases of the end-tidal PCO_2 after arrival in the postanesthesia care unit. (From Becker et al.,[7] with permission.)

romuscular blockade may reflect (1) prior inadequate pharmacologic antagonism, (2) delayed excretion of the muscle relaxant owing to renal disease, or the (3) potentiation of these drugs by other mechanisms (aminoglycoside antibiotics, hypermagnesemia, hypothermia). It should be appreciated that both respiratory acidosis and hypokalemia inhibit reversal of neuromuscular blockade with anticholinesterase drugs. Conceivably, alveolar hypoventilation in the PACU could lead to respiratory acidosis and an unmasking of residual neuromuscular blockade, leading to further carbon dioxide retention. Evidence of residual neuromuscular blockade is often detected with a peripheral nerve stimulator, although subtle degrees of residual drug effect may not be detected with this monitor. In addition, the ability to sustain head lift for at least 5 seconds, vigorous hand grasp, tongue protrusion for several seconds, and vital capacity (VC) can be used as evidence of recovery from the effects of the muscle relaxant (see Chapter 7). Residual effects of muscle relaxants (train-of-four less than 0.7, double vision, difficulty swallowing) in the PACU are more likely to occur in patients who received long-acting (pancuronium) rather than intermediate- or short-acting muscle relaxants even after long operations.[8]

Suboptimal ventilatory mechanics may be related to the patient's position, obesity, gastric dilation, and the site of the surgical incision. For example, the site of surgical incision affects the ability to take a deep breath as measured by VC. Patients undergoing thoracic or upper abdominal surgery have the greatest decrease in VC, showing as much as a 60% decrease on the day of surgery. Postoperative pain can limit tidal volume. Increased production of carbon dioxide is rare but may be a consideration when hyperalimentation solutions are being administered or body temperature is increased. Chronic obstructive pulmonary disease associated with preoperative hypercarbia is predictably accompanied by a similar finding postoperatively.

Diagnosis

Diagnosis of hypoventilation ($PaCO_2$ higher than 44 mmHg) in the PACU requires measurement of the $PaCO_2$. Signs of carbon dioxide retention, such as tachycardia and hypertension, are nonspecific and not reliably present in postoperative patients. Indeed, spontaneous ventilation after surgery is often rapid and shallow. This restrictive pattern of breathing is accentuated by pain and the surgical incision, which may interfere with normal chest and abdominal wall function. All these changes lead to the accumulation of secretions in the alveoli and the early development of atelectasis. For these reasons, postoperative mechanical ventilation of the lungs through a tracheal tube in selected at-risk patients (especially those with co-existing chronic obstructive pulmonary disease undergoing upper abdominal or thoracic operations) may serve to decrease the likelihood of significant pulmonary complications. Equally important is provision of adequate postoperative analgesia (see the section *Pain* and Chapter 32).

Treatment

If hypoventilation is due to residual effects of inhaled anesthetics but the patient remains capable of maintaining a patent upper airway, it is permissible to allow spontaneous emergence from anesthesia combined with a regimen to keep the patient alert. If not, controlled ventilation of the lungs via a cuffed tube in the trachea will be necessary to maintain normocarbia and accelerate elimination of the inhaled drugs. If hypoventilation is due to residual effects of opioids, the administration of incremental doses of naloxone (40 μg IV every 2 minutes up to 200 μg) is an appropriate consideration. Careful titration of a dose of naloxone is important to avoid precipitous reversal of opioid-induced analgesia and abrupt activation of the sympathetic nervous system. Indeed, naloxone administration resulting in abrupt reversal of opioid effects has been associated with pulmonary edema, hypertension, and cardiac dysrhythmias, including ventricular fibrillation, particularly when a tracheal tube is in place.[9] It must also be appreciated that the duration of naloxone is brief (shorter than 45 minutes), such that hypoventilation due to opioids may recur. Naloxone administration may also be associated with nausea and vomiting. When residual neuromuscular blockade is responsible for alveolar hypoventilation, treatment is either administration of additional anticholinesterase drugs or mechanical ventilation of the lungs until the effects of the muscle relaxants dissipate spontaneously.

Criteria for extubation of the trachea after surgery must be individualized. Useful criteria include (1) state of consciousness, (2) VC greater than 15 $ml \cdot kg^{-1}$, (3) inspiratory force greater than −20

cmH_2O, and (4) acceptable arterial blood gases and pH (see Chapter 33). The directional change of these measurements is more important than a single value. Extubation of the trachea is performed after suctioning the patient's pharynx and trachea. The patient then inhales deeply or the lungs are passively expanded with oxygen, the cuff on the tracheal tube is deflated, and the tube is removed from the trachea at maximum lung inflation. This sequence ensures that the initial gas flow is outward and permits secretions to be forcefully exhaled rather than inhaled as the tracheal tube is removed.

Hypotension

Etiology

Multiple causes must be considered in the differential diagnosis of hypotension in the recovery room. The most likely cause of hypotension, however, is decreased venous return and decreased cardiac output due to hypovolemia. Indeed, residual effects of anesthetic drugs are likely to attenuate peripheral vasoconstrictor responses, leading to hypotension as an early manifestation of hypovolemia. Hypovolemia is usually a reflection of inadequately replaced blood loss or third-space loss during surgery. Unrecognized continuing hemorrhage as a cause of hypovolemia and hypotension must also be considered. Decreases in myocardial contractility as a cause of hypotension in the PACU may be due to residual effects of anesthetics, co-existing cardiac dysfunction, or an acute myocardial infarction. Indeed, many patients with confirmed postoperative myocardial infarction are found to have experienced a period of unexplained hypotension with or without ventricular premature contractions in the PACU. Angina pectoris occurs in only about one-fourth of these patients, possibly reflecting masking of pain by residual analgesic effects of anesthetics. Patients most likely to experience a postoperative myocardial infarction include those with left ventricular hypertrophy, history of hypertension, diabetes mellitus, or co-existing coronary artery disease.[10] Sepsis leading to vasodilation and capillary fluid leakage may be responsible for hypotension, particularly after surgery on the genitourinary tract.

Factors Leading to Postoperative Hypotension

- Arterial hypoxemia
- Hypovolemia (most common cause)
- Decreased myocardial contractility (myocardial ischemia, pulmonary edema)
- Decreased systemic vascular resistance (residual effects of anesthetics, sepsis)
- Cardiac dysrhythmias
- Pulmonary embolus
- Pneumothorax
- Cardiac tamponade

Diagnosis and Treatment

Before any therapy of hypotension is instituted, it is important to confirm the accuracy of the blood pressure measurement. Artifactual blood pressure readings can be due to an improperly placed or sized blood pressure cuff, an inaccurately calibrated transducer, or positioning of the transducer above the level of the right atrium (midaxillary line). For example, the measured blood pressure is falsely decreased about 0.7 mmHg for every 1 cm the transducer is elevated above heart level in supine patients.

Oliguria (less than 0.5 $ml{\cdot}kg^{-1}{\cdot}h^{-1}$) is a useful guide to the presence of hypovolemia or decreased myocardial contractility. Increased urine output after a fluid challenge with 3 to 6 $ml{\cdot}kg^{-1}$ IV of lactated Ringer's solution suggests the presence of hypovolemia rather than decreased myocardial contractility. A low hematocrit plus evidence of bleeding at the operative site should suggest inadequate surgical hemostasis. Elevation of the legs and administration of a sympathomimetic drug to maintain perfusion pressure until hypovolemia can be corrected is prudent treatment.

If hypotension persists despite intravenous fluid replacement, an estimate of right atrial pressure is indicated. In the presence of normal left ventricular function, central venous pressure will be a reasonable reflection of intravascular fluid volume. In the presence of selective left ventricular dysfunction or co-existing chronic obstructive pulmonary disease, the central venous pressure may not be a reliable guide and pressures measured via a pulmonary artery catheter are necessary for an accurate diagnosis. Hypovolemia as a cause of hypotension is suggested by a low pulmonary artery occlusion pressure (lower than 10 mmHg), a low cardiac index (lower than 2.5 $L \cdot min^{-1} \cdot m^{-2}$), and an increased calculated systemic vascular resistance (normal 900 to 1400 $dynes \cdot s \cdot cm^{-5}$). Decreased myocardial contractility as the etiology of hypotension is characterized by high pulmonary artery occlusion pressures (higher than 15 mmHg) and a low cardiac output. After intravascular fluid volume has been optimized, hypotension due to decreased myocardial contractility is treated with inotropic drugs (see Chapter 3). Sepsis as a cause of hypotension is characterized by a low pulmonary artery occlusion pressure, increased cardiac output, and decreased systemic vascular resistance. Replacement of fluid loss with crystalloid or colloid solutions and maintenance of coronary perfusion pressure with an alpha agonist, such as phenylephrine, are indicated in the immediate treatment of hypotension due to sepsis.

Hypertension

Etiology

Hypertension that develops in the immediate postoperative period is most often due to the stimulation provided by the sensation of pain during emergence from anesthesia. When hypertension does develop during recovery from anesthesia, it usually manifests in the first 30 minutes after surgery.[11] Preoperative hypertension is present in over one-half of patients who develop hypertension in the PACU. Postoperative hypertension can be exaggerated if antihypertensive drugs were withdrawn preoperatively. Other causes to consider when hypertension occurs in the PACU include excessive intravenous fluid administration, arterial hypoxemia, and hypercarbia. Excessive and sustained increases in arterial blood pressure can lead to left ventricular failure with pulmonary edema, myocardial ischemia due to increased myocardial oxygen requirements, cardiac dysrhythmias, and cerebral hemorrhage.

Factors Leading to Postoperative Hypertension

- Arterial hypoxemia
- Enhanced sympathetic nervous system activity (pain, bladder distension)
- Preoperative hypertension
- Hypervolemia

Diagnosis and Treatment

Before any therapy of hypertension is initiated, it is important to confirm the accuracy of the blood pressure measurement (see the section *Hypotension, Diagnosis and Treatment*). Management of acute hypertension begins with identification and correction of the initiating cause. When pain is the etiology of acute hypertension, the immediate treatment is the administration of an opioid (morphine 15 to 40 $\mu g \cdot kg^{-1}$ IV) or a nonsteroidal anti-inflammatory drug (ketorolac 0.4 $mg \cdot kg^{-1}$ IM or IV) until adequate pain relief is achieved (see the section *Pain* and Chapter 32). Hypertension that persists in the absence of a known etiology is often managed by the continuous infusion of a vasodilator such as nitroprusside. The arterial blood pressure is titrated to a desired level by adjusting the infusion rate of nitroprusside (up to 10 $\mu g \cdot kg^{-1} \cdot min^{-1}$ IV or a total dose of 1.5 $mg \cdot kg^{-1}$ IV for a 1- to 3-hour administration). Even when these dose recommendations are followed, it is important to measure the arterial pH approximately every hour to detect the appearance of acidosis caused by the metabolism of nitroprusside to cyanide. Should metabolic acidosis appear, nitroprusside must be discontinued immediately. Alternative drugs to nitroprusside include labetalol (5 to 10 mg IV) or hydralazine (2.5 to 5 mg IV). Disadvantages of hydralazine include a delayed onset (5 to 15 minutes) and baroreceptor-mediated tachycardia when the blood pressure decreases. Regardless of the drug selected to produce normotension, it is important to accurately monitor blood pressure often via a catheter in a peripheral artery.

Cardiac Dysrhythmias

Etiology

Cardiac dysrhythmias in the immediate postoperative period have multiple causes. Arterial hypoxemia should be the first cause considered when cardiac

Factors Leading to Postoperative Cardiac Dysrhythmias

Arterial hypoxemia
Hypovolemia
Pain
Hypothermia
Anticholinesterases
Myocardial ischemia
Electrolyte abnormalities
 Hypokalemia
 Hypocalcemia
Respiratory acidosis
Hypertension
Digitalis intoxication
Preoperative cardiac dysrhythmias

dysrhythmias manifest initially in the PACU. Sinus tachycardia, which is a common occurrence in the early postoperative period, suggests the presence of arterial hypoxemia, hypovolemia, or pain. Sinus bradycardia accompanies arterial hypoxemia and decreases in body temperature and may reflect effects of anitcholinesterase drugs administered earlier to reverse nondepolarizing muscle relaxants. The appearance of ventricular premature contractions suggests the presence of arterial hypoxemia, myocardial ischemia, electrolyte abnormalities, or respiratory acidosis. Hypertension may increase myocardial irritability, leading to ventricular premature contractions. The appearance of cardiac dysrhythmias in patients receiving digitalis preparations should arouse suspicion of digitalis toxicity.

Treatment

Most cardiac dysrhythmias occurring in the PACU do not require treatment other than correction of the underlying cause. Regardless of the type of cardiac dysrhythmia, the first priority is to ensure the patency of the upper airway and the adequacy of arterial oxygenation. Specific drug therapies to treat hemodynamically significant cardiac dysrhythmias include administration of atropine (3 to 6 $\mu g \cdot kg^{-1}$ IV) to increase heart rate, verapamil (75 to 150 $\mu g \cdot kg^{-1}$ IV infused over 1 to 3 minutes) to decrease heart rate, and lidocaine (1 to 1.5 $mg \cdot kg^{-1}$ IV) to suppress ventricular premature contractions. Electrical cardioversion is necessary to treat hemodynamically significant atrial or ventricular tachydysrhythmias that are unresponsive to drug therapy.

Renal Dysfunction

Oliguria (less than 0.5 $ml \cdot kg^{-1} \cdot h^{-1}$) that manifests in the PACU most likely reflects decreased renal blood flow due to hypovolemia or decreased cardiac output (see the section *Hypotension*). An indwelling urinary catheter is important for the early recognition of oliguria in postoperative patients at high risk of renal failure.

Patients at High Risk of Postoperative Renal Dysfunction

Co-existing renal disease
Major trauma
Sepsis
Advanced age
Multiple intraoperative blood transfusions
Prolonged intraoperative hypotension
Cardiac or vascular operations
Biliary tract surgery in presence of obstructive jaundice

Bleeding Abnormalities

Bleeding abnormalities in the postoperative period most often reflect hemorrhage secondary to inadequate surgical hemostasis. Alternatively, postoperative bleeding may be due to coagulopathies, which can be diagnosed using specific laboratory tests (Table 31-1). While awaiting the results of laboratory tests, it may be helpful to perform a whole-blood clotting test at the bedside to evaluate both clot formation (forms in less than 12 minutes), retraction (platelet function), and lysis.

A platelet count is useful in evaluation of bleeding after massive transfusions of blood. A qualitative platelet defect may be due to drugs ingested preoperatively, such as aspirin. This problem is recognized

Table 31-1. Laboratory Tests for Evaluation of Postoperative Bleeding Abnormalities

Test	Normal Value	Abnormality Detected
Platelet count	>150,000 cells·mm^{-3}	Dilutional thrombocytopenia DIC
Bleeding time	3–10 min	Platelet-inhibiting (acetylsalicyclic acid-containing) drug
Prothrombin time	12–14 s	DIC Vitamin K deficiency Liver disease Warfarin
Partial thromboplastin time	25–35 s	Factor V and/or VIII deficiencies Heparin Hemophilia
Fibrinogen	200–400 mg·dl^{-1}	DIC
Fibrin split products	<4 μg·ml^{-1}	DIC
Thrombelastography		Platelet and clotting factor deficiencies

DIC, disseminated intravascular coagulation.

by demonstration of prolonged bleeding times despite normal platelet counts. In these situations, the administration of platelets will reverse thrombocytopenia and also return bleeding times to normal. Disseminated intravascular coagulation is suggested by thrombocytopenia, prolonged prothrombin time, decreased serum concentrations of fibrinogen, and increased circulating levels of fibrin split products. Dilution of factors V and VIII by massive transfusions of whole blood or inadequate reversal of heparin will manifest as a prolonged partial thromboplastin time. Fresh frozen plasma will reverse prolongation of the prothrombin time and partial thromboplastin time when due to liver disease or factor V or VIII deficiency. Protamine reverses heparin-induced prolongation of the partial thromboplastin time.

Decreased Body Temperature

Decreased body temperature is a complication of operations performed in cold operating rooms. Compensatory mechanisms to offset heat loss (peripheral vasoconstriction, shivering) are prevented by anesthetics and muscle relaxants. Loss of body heat intraoperatively is minimized by maintaining the operating room temperature near 21°C and warming the inhaled gases. When shivering develops in postoperative patients, it is important to provide supplemental inspired oxygen to offset the marked increases (300% to 400%) in oxygen consumption that accompany increased skeletal muscle activity. Postoperative shivering can be treated with skin surface warming (Bair Huggar system) and drugs (meperidine 25 mg IV).[12]

Agitation (Emergence Delirium)

A small number of patients awaken from anesthesia in an agitated state, which may require physical restraint. The incidence of this behavior seems to be increased in young patients who are apprehensive about the findings at operation as well as in individuals who fear pain. Arterial hypoxemia or hypercapnia, or both, as the cause of agitation must be initially considered. The perception of pain by patients who have not regained full consciousness and self-control may manifest as agitation. Other causes of agitation include unrecognized gastric dilation and urinary retention. The incidence of postoperative agitation is increased in patients who have received scopolamine as preoperative medication, particularly when this drug is administered in the absence of opioids (see Chapter 9). Agitation can also follow the administration of atropine, but the incidence is lower than that associated with scopolamine. Administration of physostigmine (15 to 45 $\mu g \cdot kg^{-1}$ IV) will attenuate or reverse agitation associated with anticholinergic drugs. Presumably, physostigmine (a tertiary amine anticholinesterase) crosses the blood-brain barrier and increases the level of acetylcholine, which then displaces anticholinergic drugs from central receptor sites.

Delayed Awakening

Even after prolonged surgery and anesthesia, it is reasonable to expect a response to stimulation within 60 to 90 minutes. When delayed awakening occurs, it is important to evaluate vital signs (arterial blood pressure, arterial hemoglobin oxygen saturation, electrocardiogram, body temperature) and perform a neurologic examination (patients may be hyperreflexic in the early postoperative period). Analysis of arterial blood gases detects problems of oxygenation, ventilation, electrolyte imbalance, and metabolic disturbances (blood glucose concentration). Radiographic procedures may be indicated for evaluation of possible intracranial or intrathoracic abnormalities.

Possible Explanations for Delayed Awakening in the Postanesthesia Care Unit

- Residual drug effects
  - Opioids
  - Benzodiazepines
  - Anticholinergics
- Hypothermia
- Hypoglycemia
- Electrolyte disturbances
- Arterial hypoxemia
- Increased intracranial pressure (cerebral hemorrhage)
- Air embolism
- Hysteria

Treatment

Residual sedation from drugs used during anesthesia is the most frequent cause of delayed awakening in the PACU. If residual effects of opioids are a possible cause of delayed awakening, it is appropriate to administer naloxone (see the section *Hypoventilation, Treatment*). Physostigmine (15 to 45 $\mu g \cdot kg^{-1}$ IV) may be effective in reversing central nervous system effects of anticholinergic drugs (especially scopolamine) that are contributing to sedation. Flumazenil (8 to 15 $\mu g \cdot kg^{-1}$ IV) is a specific antagonist for residual depressant effects of benzodiazepines. In the absence of pharmacologic effects to explain delayed awakening, it is important to consider other causes such as hypothermia (especially lower than 33°C), hypoglycemia, and increased intracranial pressure. An empirical trial of 50% glucose administered intravenously is indicated if hypoglycemia is a consideration.

Nausea and Vomiting

Nausea and vomiting, along with pain, are the most common postoperative problems encountered by patients. The incidence of nausea and vomiting is dependent on many factors and is likely to affect 20% to 30% of postoperative patients.[13] Although rarely a cause of serious morbidity, persistent vomiting can delay discharge from the PACU.

Factors Associated with an Increased Incidence of Postoperative Nausea and Vomiting

- History of postoperative emesis
- Female gender
- Obesity
- Postoperative pain
- Type of surgery (eye muscle surgery, middle ear surgery, laparoscopic surgery)
- Anesthetic drugs (opioids, nitrous oxide?)
- Gastric distension

Treatment

Administration of a prophylactic antiemetic (droperidol 10 to 20 μg·kg^{-1} IV; ondansetron 4 to 8 mg IV) may be indicated for patients considered to be at increased risk of adverse events should postoperative nausea and vomiting occur[14,15] (see Chapter 9). Larger doses of droperidol may produce sedation that delays discharge from the PACU. The efficacy of metoclopramide (10 to 20 mg IV) seems to be less than that of droperidol.[14] Transdermal scopolamine may be an effective prophylactic treatment for decreasing the postoperative incidence of nausea and vomiting, especially following laparoscopic procedures. Should postoperative nausea and vomiting be deemed sufficient to merit pharmacologic therapy, it is important to first rule out causes such as arterial hypoxemia, hypotension, hypoglycemia, and increased intracranial pressure. The most commonly administered antiemetic in the PACU is droperidol.

Pain

Pain is a predictable response as the effects of anesthetic drugs wane in the early postoperative period.

Etiology

Many factors influence the incidence and severity of postoperative pain. Infants and elderly patients seem to experience less pain than do middle-aged patients. The need for postoperative pain medication is decreased when the anesthesiologist visits patients preoperatively and provides detailed explanations of postoperative events, including the occurrence of pain (Fig. 31-3).[16] Inclusion of opioids in the preoperative medication or administration of an opioid with the induction of anesthesia usually delays the first postoperative request for pain medication. It is presumed that administration of an opioid prior to a painful stimulus (preemptive analgesia) decreases the subsequent intensity of pain by producing C-fiber inhibition and subsequent development of any "memory" of the pain stimulus in the nervous system (see Chapter 9). Preoperative traits such as a neurotic personality or fear of pain tend to increase postoperative pain. The site of operation influences the severity of postoperative pain, with thoracic, upper abdominal, and orthopaedic surgery being the most painful.

Treatment

Evolution of effective pain management techniques, especially continuous or intermittent (patient controlled analgesia) infusion of opioids and neuraxial administration of opioids has led to the development of anesthesiology-based Acute Pain Management Services, which may assume complete responsibility for postoperative pain relief (see Chapter 32).

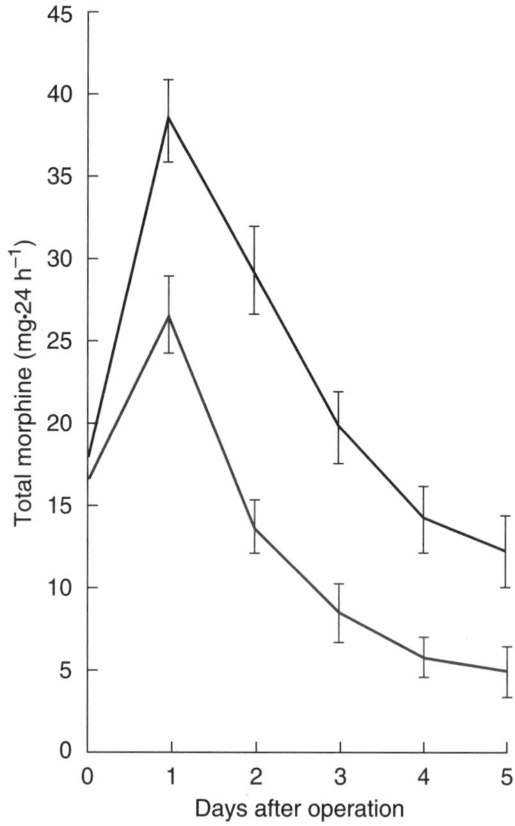

Figure 31-3. Adult patients (n = 97) undergoing abdominal surgery were divided into two groups. Both groups were visited preoperatively by the anesthesiologist, but only the special care group (red line) received a detailed explanation of the character, intensity, and management of pain in the postoperative period. The normal occurrence of postoperative pain was stressed to these patients. The value of this explanation was evidenced by the decreased total dose of morphine administered to the special care patients compared with the control group (black line). (From Egbert et al.,[6] with permission.)

POSTOPERATIVE RESPIRATORY THERAPY

Postoperative respiratory therapy is designed to prevent pulmonary complications that are most often characterized as pneumonia and arterial hypoxemia (Fig. 31-4). The frequency of postoperative pul-

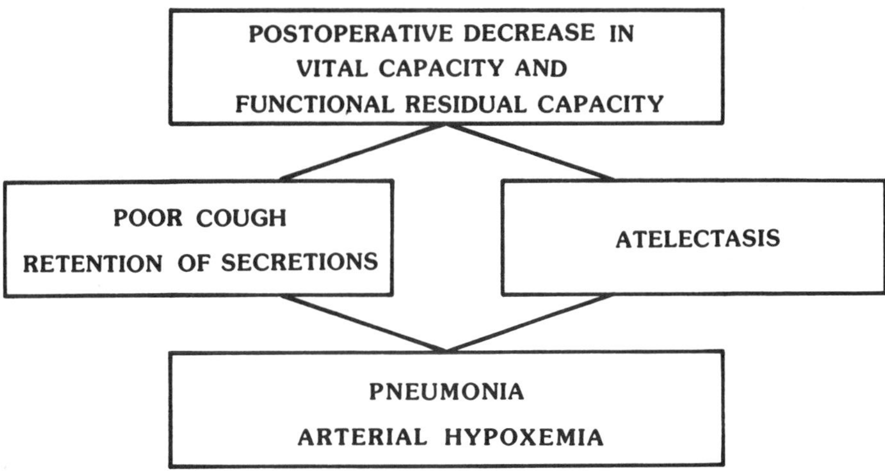

Figure 31-4. Pathogenesis of postoperative pulmonary infections.

monary complications is greatest after thoracic and upper abdominal surgery.[17] For example, significant postoperative atelectasis occurs in 20% to 40% of patients undergoing these types of surgery. Lower abdominal surgery is associated with a lower incidence of postoperative pulmonary complications. In addition to the site of surgery and an associated decrease in lung volumes (FRC, VC), other factors that influence the incidence of postoperative pulmonary complications include co-existing pulmonary disease, a history of cigarette smoking, obesity, and increasing age. The choice of drugs or techniques used to produce anesthesia does not seem to alter predictably the incidence of postoperative pulmonary infections. A vertical versus transverse upper abdominal incision, as for a cholecystectomy, probably does not alter the incidence of postoperative pulmonary complications.[18]

Factors that Influence the Incidence of Postoperative Pulmonary Complications

Site of surgery
Co-existing pulmonary disease
Cigarette smoking
Obesity
Advanced age

Respiratory therapy includes oxygen therapy, humidification and aerosol therapy, bronchial hygiene, and interventions designed to increase resting lung volumes, especially FRC and VC. These treatments may be initiated as the patient recovers from anesthesia in the PACU for continuation into the subsequent postoperative period as necessary.

Oxygen Therapy

Oxygen therapy administered as increased inhaled concentrations of oxygen (supplemental oxygen) is indicated for a PaO_2 lower than 60 mmHg. Indeed, supplemental inspired oxygen is often routinely provided in the PACU regardless of the duration or type of surgery, since almost every patient demonstrates a decrease in PaO_2 after anesthesia and surgery. Supplemental oxygen should never be withheld in the postoperative period for fear of abolishing the hypoxic drive to ventilation that may be present in patients with chronic obstructive pulmonary disease. In the presence of chronic obstructive pulmonary disease associated with carbon dioxide retention, graded doses of supplemental oxygen administered via an air-entrainment (Venturi) mask increase the patient's PaO_2 to acceptable levels (Table 31-2) (see the section *Face Mask*). Oxygen therapy is usually delivered by a nasal cannula or face mask.

Nasal Cannula

Supplemental oxygen can be administered through a nasal cannula with minimal patient discomfort. A

Table 31-2. Air-Entrainment (Venturi) Face Masks

Inhaled Concentration of Oxygen (%)	Oxygen Flows ($L \cdot min^{-1}$)	Air Entrainment ($L \cdot min^{-1}$)
24	2–4	50–100
28	4–6	40–60
31	6–8	56
35	8	40
40	8–12	24–36

nasal cannula incorporates two prongs that extend about 1 cm into the patient's nares and is held in place by an adjustable elastic head strap. Inspired oxygen concentrations achieved with a nasal cannula depend on the flow rate of oxygen ($L \cdot min^{-1}$) as well as the patient's tidal volume, breathing frequency, inspiratory flow rate, and volume of the nasopharynx. As a guideline, the inhaled oxygen concentration is increased about 4% for each 1 $L \cdot min^{-1}$ of oxygen delivered. Oxygen flow rates higher than 6 $L \cdot min^{-1}$ (inhaled oxygen concentrations about 44%) do not predictably increase further the inhaled concentrations of oxygen because the volume of the nasopharynx is already filled. Excessive flow rates of oxygen may result in air swallowing and gastric distension. Mouth breathing does not decrease the effectiveness of oxygen therapy delivered by nasal cannula because inspiratory airflow through the posterior pharynx entrains (Bernoulli effect) oxygen from the nose.

Face Mask

Face masks used for oxygen therapy are categorized as simple, partial rebreathing, nonrebreathing, and air-entrainment (Fig. 31-5).[19]

Simple. A simple face mask does not include a valve or oxygen reservoir bag. This mask can provide inhaled concentrations of oxygen between 35% and 60% with oxygen flow rates of 5 to 8 $L \cdot min^{-1}$ (Fig. 31-5A).[19] Variations in the patient's ventilatory parameters alter the inhaled concentrations of oxygen. In adults, the oxygen flow rate should be at least 5 $L \cdot min^{-1}$ to ensure the absence of rebreathing of carbon dioxide. A simple face mask affords little, if any, advantage over a nasal cannula in terms of delivering constant inhaled concentrations of oxygen.

Partial Rebreathing. A partial rebreathing face mask is a valveless system that includes an oxygen reservoir bag (Fig. 31-5B).[19] With oxygen flows higher than 10 $L \cdot min^{-1}$, the inhaled concentrations of oxygen are between 50% and 65%.

Nonrebreathing. A nonrebreathing face mask includes a unidirectional valve plus an oxygen reservoir bag (Fig. 31-5C).[19] Inhaled concentrations of oxygen can be increased to near 100% using this face mask. It is difficult, however, to provide a sufficiently tight mask fit to completely eliminate entrainment of room air. The flow rate of oxygen into this system should be sufficient to maintain an inflated reservoir bag.

Air-Entrainment. An air-entrainment (Venturi) face mask employs the Bernoulli principle to entrain large volumes of room air (up to 100 $L \cdot min^{-1}$) to mix with oxygen flowing through an injector (2 to 12 $L \cdot min^{-1}$) (Fig. 31-5D).[19] The resultant mixture of gases produces stable inhaled concentrations of oxygen between 24% and 40% depending on the bore of the oxygen injector (Table 31-2). Furthermore, the high flow of gas into the face mask results in constant inhaled concentrations of oxygen despite changes in the characteristics of the patient's ventilation.

Humidification and Aerosol Therapy

Inhaled gases are normally warmed, filtered, and humidified in the upper respiratory tract. When dry gases are inhaled or the natural conditioning system (nose) is bypassed by a tracheal tube or tracheostomy tube, the lower airways must provide the additional moisture. In these situations, artificial humidifying devices, such as humidifiers or nebulizers, are often considered. Humidifiers are commonly used when dry gases are inhaled through a natural airway in an attempt to provide a water content similar to that normally present in room air. When the upper airway is bypassed, a humidifier is often inadequate and the water deficit must be made up by the use of a more efficient device, the nebulizer. Nebulizers are devices that deliver a suspension of particles (aerosol) in a carrier gas. Sterile, pyrogen-free water should be used for all humidifiers and nebulizers to avoid the possibility of the water reservoir becoming a source of hospital-acquired (nosocomial) infections.

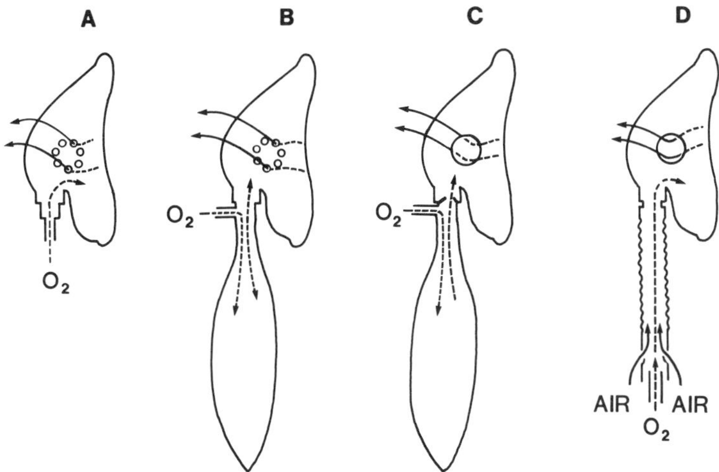

Figure 31-5. Examples of face masks used to provide supplemental oxygen. *(A)* Simple face mask. Oxygen flows directly into the mask, and exhaled gases leave through holes at the side of the mask. *(B)* Partial rebreathing face mask. Because there are no valves, the initial portion of the exhaled gases, which contains little or no carbon dioxide (deadspace gas), is free to mix with the oxygen in the reservoir bag. As the reservoir bag fills and the pressure in the bag increases, the gases exhaled during the last part of exhalation, which contain carbon dioxide (alveolar gas), are forced out through the holes at the side of the mask. This preferential loss of alveolar gas means that carbon dioxide rebreathing is less likely. *(C)* Nonrebreathing face mask. A unidirectional valve prevents dilution of inhaled gases containing oxygen with room air or rebreathing of exhaled gases containing carbon dioxide. *(D)* Air-entrainment face mask. Oxygen flow through an air injector entrains various volumes of room air, producing predictable (24% to 40%) and unchanging inhaled concentrations of oxygen. (From Dripps et al.,[19] with permission.)

Pass-Over Humidifiers

Pass-over humidifiers depend on evaporation to add water vapor to gases that pass over the water surface. The relative humidity of the effluent gases is dependent on gas flow and the temperature of both the water and gases. Inability to predictably deliver 90% to 100% relative humidity at 37°C limits the usefulness of these types of humidifiers.

Bubble-Through Humidifiers

Bubble-through humidifiers that break up the delivered gases into small bubbles as they pass through a heated water reservoir are frequently used to humidify inhaled gases delivered by mechanical ventilators. Heating the water is important because the capacity of gases to hold moisture is greatly increased when temperatures are increased. The water in the humidifier can be heated to body temperature, but as gases travel through the delivery tubing, they cool and water collects ("rains out") in the tubing. Increasing the water temperature above body temperature to ensure delivery of gases at body temperature is acceptable. The temperature of the inhaled gases, however, should be monitored at the proximal airway of the patient to provide an early warning should these gases reach a temperature capable of producing respiratory mucosa burn. Ideally, inhaled gases should be 36°C to 37°C to ensure a relative humidity near 100%.

Jet Nebulizers

Jet nebulizers are the most frequently used type of aerosol generators. High pressure gas enters the nebulizer chamber through a restricted orifice that produces a jet stream of high velocity. This jet stream is directed across one end of a small-diameter tube that is immersed in the liquid to be nebulized. Subambient pressure (Bernoulli effect) immediately adjacent to the tube is produced, resulting in pulling of surface liquid into the tube. When the liquid reaches the top of the tube, it is aerosolized by the jet stream to particles usually smaller than 30 μm in diameter.

Jet nebulizers are used in respiratory therapy to humidify inspired gases (more efficient than humidifiers), decrease the viscosity of airway secretions, and deliver bronchodilator drugs (racemic epinephrine, albuterol) directly to the airways.

Bronchial Hygiene

Bronchial hygiene depends on optimal removal of secretions from the lungs by mucociliary clearance, tracheal suctioning, and chest physiotherapy.

Mucociliary Clearance

Cilia located on epithelial cells lining the respiratory mucosa are responsible for moving respiratory tract secretions (10 to 100 ml per day) toward the glottic opening. Depression of ciliary activity and an associated retention of secretions are produced by inhaled anesthetics, tracheal tubes, inhalation of cold and dry gases, high inhaled concentrations of oxygen, and pulmonary infections.

Coughing

Coughing is a major mechanism for removal of secretions from large airways. High airflow velocities necessary to propel secretions from the upper airways are generated most effectively at large lung volumes. Rapid shallow breathing patterns and decreased lung volumes characteristic of postoperative patients with pain limit the effectiveness of coughing.

Tracheal Suctioning

Orotracheal or nasotracheal suctioning should be performed only when there is evidence during auscultation of the chest of retained secretions that do not clear with coughing. Tracheal suctioning should not be prophylactic or routine. For example, mechanical irritation by the catheter during tracheal suctioning may cause trauma to the respiratory mucosa and predispose to bacterial colonization. Mechanical stimulation of the trachea or carina by the catheter may evoke a vasovagal response with resultant bradycardia and hypotension. Tracheal suctioning also predisposes to significant arterial hypoxemia because of aspiration of pulmonary gases with associated small airway closure and alveolar collapse. Arterial hypoxemia during tracheal suctioning is minimized by (1) administration of oxygen before suctioning, (2) selection of a suction catheter that is no greater than one-half the internal diameter of the trachea, (3) limitation of the duration of suctioning to less than 15 seconds, and (4) manual inflation of the lungs with oxygen after suctioning.

Chest Physiotherapy

Chest physiotherapy consists of postural drainage, percussion, vibration, deep breathing, and assisted coughing. These maneuvers aid in the removal of airway secretions and improve inflation of poorly ventilated alveoli.

Interventions to Increase Resting Lung Volumes

The severity of postoperative pulmonary complications parallels the magnitude of decrease in lung volumes. Presumably decreases in the VC and FRC interfere with the generation of an effective cough and contribute to the collapse of alveoli. The net effect of these changes is a decreased clearance of secretions from the airways and atelectasis, leading to pneumonia and arterial hypoxemia (Fig. 31-4). Atelectasis is likely to accompany shallow breathing ("splinting") that is a result of postoperative incisional pain. Likewise, a cough may be excruciatingly painful. The inability to prevent the postoperative decrease in FRC by totally relieving incisional pain suggests that trauma from the surgical procedure also interferes with the optimal function of the chest wall by changing the normal relationship of the diaphragm, intercostal muscles, and abdominal muscles.[17] Nevertheless, relief of pain contributes to optimal performance of therapies designed to restore FRC.

The identification of FRC as the most important lung volume in the postoperative period provides a specific goal for respiratory therapy after surgery. Specific therapies designed to increase FRC include voluntary deep breathing and ambulation, intermittent positive pressure breathing, and incentive spirometry. Exhalation maneuvers (inflating balloons, using blow bottles) are not recommended, because their performance causes the patient to exhale below the FRC, leading to atelectasis and increased airway resistance.

Voluntary Deep Breathing and Ambulation

Voluntary deep breathing with maintenance of inspiration at peak inflation for 3 to 5 seconds creates a large transpulmonary pressure gradient and facilities re-expansion of collapsed alveoli and restoration of lung volumes. A motivated patient and adequate postoperative analgesia are necessary to ensure optimal deep breathing.

Ambulation and the associated changes in position have great therapeutic benefit in the prevention of postoperative pulmonary complications. Presumably, this therapeutic benefit reflects increased lung volumes, particularly FRC.

Intermittent Positive Pressure Breathing

Intermittent positive pressure breathing (IPPB) as a method to decrease the incidence of postoperative pulmonary complications is controversial.[20] Certainly, postoperative IPPB therapy does not need to be routine. In fact, there is no evidence that IPPB treatment is more efficacious than voluntary deep breathing and ambulation in altering the incidence and severity of postoperative pulmonary complications. When IPPB is prescribed, the emphasis should be an achievement of an optimal tidal volume rather than creation of a peak airway pressure.

Incentive Spirometry

Incentive spirometry is a form of voluntary deep breathing in which patients are given an inhaled volume as a goal to achieve. When the use of incentive spirometry is anticipated, it is helpful to measure preoperative inspiratory capacity and also to instruct the patient in the use of the device. The preoperative inspiratory capacity should be the postoperative goal. Incentive spirometry therapy also emphasizes holding the inhaled volume to provide a sustained inflation important for expanding collapsed alveoli. The major disadvantage of this therapy is the need for patient cooperation, which may be limited in the presence of postoperative pain.

REFERENCES

1. Carpenter RL, Eger EI II, Johnson BH, Unadkat JD, Sheiner LB. Pharmacokinetics of inhaled anesthetics in humans: Measurements during and after the simultaneous administration of enflurane, halothane, isoflurane, methoxyflurane, and nitrous oxide. Anesth Analg 1986;65:575–82.
2. Stoelting RK, Longnecker DE, Eger EI II. Minimum alveolar concentrations in man on awakening from methoxyflurane, halothane, ether and fluroxene anesthesia: MAC awake. Anesthesiology 1970;33:5–9.
3. Daley MD, Norman PH, Colmenares ME, Sandler AN. Hypoxaemia in adults in the post-anaesthetic unit. Can J Anaesth 1991;38:740–6.
4. Cooperman LH, Price HR. Pulmonary edema in the operative and postoperative period: Review of 40 cases. Ann Surg 1970;172:883–91.
5. Bay J, Nunn JF, Prys-Roberts C. Factors influencing arterial PO_2 during recovery from anaesthesia. Br J Anaesth 1968;40:398–407.
6. Knill RL, Gelb AW. Ventilatory responses to hypoxia and hypercapnia during halothane sedation and anesthesia in man. Anesthesiology 1978;49:244–51.
7. Becker LD, Paulson BA, Miller RD, Severinghaus JW, Eger EI II. Biphasic respiratory depression after fentanyl-droperidol or fentanyl alone used to supplement nitrous oxide anesthesia. Anesthesiology 1976; 44:291–6.
8. Bevan DR, Donati F, Kopman AF. Reversal of neuromuscular blockade. Anesthesiology 1992;77:785–92.
9. Andree RA. Sudden death following naloxone administration. Anesth Analg 1980;59:782–4.
10. Hollenberg M, Mangano DT, Browner WS, et al. Predictors of postoperative myocardial ischemia in patients undergoing noncardiac surgery. JAMA 1992; 268:205–9.
11. Gal TJ, Cooperman LH. Hypertension in the immediate postoperative period. Br J Anaesth 1975;47:70–4.
12. Lennon RL, Hosking MP, Conover MA, et al. Evaluation of forced-air system for warming hypothermic postoperative patients. Anesth Analg 1990;70: 424–7.
13. Watcha MF, White PF. Postoperative nausea and vomiting. Anesthesiology 1992;77:162–84.
14. Pandit SK, Kothary SP, Pandit UA, Randel G, Levy L. Dose-response study of droperidol and metoclopramide as antiemetics for outpatient anesthesia. Anesth Analg 1989;68:798–802.
15. McKenzie R, Kovac A, O'Connor T, et al. Comparison of ondansetron versus placebo to prevent postoperative nausea and vomiting in women undergoing ambulatory gynecologic surgery. Anesthesiology 1993; 78:21–8.
16. Ebgert LD, Battit GE, Welch CE, Bartlett MK. Reduction of postoperative pain by encouragement and instruction of patients. N Engl J Med 1964; 270:825–7.
17. Craig DB. Postoperative recovery of pulmonary function. Anesth Analg 1981;60:46–52.
18. Williams CD, Brenowitz JB. Ventilatory patterns after vertical and transverse upper abdominal incisions. Am J Surg 1975;130:725–8.
19. Dripps RD, Eckenhoff JE, Vandam LD, eds. Inhalation therapy and pulmonary physiotherapy. In: Introduction to Anesthesia. The Principles of Safe Practice. Philadelphia, WB Saunders 1988:469–76.
20. Inverson LIG, Ecker RR, Fox HE, May IA. A comparative study of IPPB, the incentive spirometer, and blow bottles: The prevention of atelectasis following cardiac surgery. Ann Thorac Surg 1978;25:197–200.

32

Acute Postoperative Pain Management

Acute postoperative pain is a complex physiologic reaction to tissue injury, visceral distension, or disease. Postoperative pain produces adverse physiologic effects with manifestations on multiple organ systems. For example, pain following upper abdominal or thoracic surgery often leads to hypoventilation from splinting. This change promotes atelectasis, which impairs ventilation-to-perfusion relationships and increases the likelihood of arterial hypoxemia and pneumonia. Pain that limits postoperative ambulation combined with a stress-induced hypercoagulable state may contribute to an increased incidence of deep vein thrombosis.[1,2] Catecholamines released in response to pain may result in tachycardia and hypertension, which may induce myocardial ischemia in susceptible patients.

With the development of expanding awareness of the epidemiology and pathophysiology of pain, more attention is being paid to the management of postoperative pain in an effort to improve patient comfort, decrease perioperative morbidity, and decrease cost by shortening the time spent in postanesthesia care units, intensive care units, and hospital rooms.[2] The natural progression of this expanding awareness of the importance of postoperative pain is the formation of acute pain management services, most often directed by anesthesiologists.[3,4] In this regard, the continuity of acute postoperative pain management is enhanced because the anesthesiologist is routinely involved in the preoperative assessment, intraoperative management, and postoperative follow-up of surgical patients.

The complexity of new analgesic techniques (neuraxial analgesia, patient controlled analgesia [PCA], peripheral nerve blocks) for the management of acute postoperative pain requires the adoption of written policies and procedures (medication protocols, algorithms, preprinted postoperative orders) to maximize efficacy while minimizing adverse effects (Figs. 32-1 and 32-2).[4] Ultimately, the goals of the acute pain management service are (1) evaluation and treatment of postoperative pain and (2) identification and management of undesirable side effects related to postoperative analgesic techniques. This is a 24 hour a day commitment to postoperative patients by the anesthesiologists responsible for the acute pain management service. In addition, there must be cooperation between anesthesiology, nursing, pharmacy, and surgery personnel.

NEUROPHYSIOLOGY OF PAIN

Understanding the mechanisms of pain and its pharmacologic modification are essential to optimal treatment of acute postoperative pain.

Nociception

Nociception describes the recognition and transmission of painful stimuli. Stimuli generated from thermal, mechanical, or chemical tissue damage may activate nociceptors, which are free afferent nerve endings of myelinated A-delta and unmyelinated C fibers (Fig. 32-3).[5] These peripheral afferent nerve endings send axonal projections into the dorsal

Adverse Physiologic Effects of Postoperative Pain

Pulmonary system (decreased lung volumes, increased skeletal muscle tension)
- Atelectasis
- Ventilation-to-perfusion mismatching
- Arterial hypoxemia
- Hypercarbia
- Pneumonia

Cardiovascular system (sympathetic nervous system stimulation)
- Hypertension
- Tachycardia
- Myocardial ischemia
- Cardiac dysrhythmias

Endocrine system
- Hyperglycemia
- Sodium and water retention
- Protein catabolism

Immune system (decreased immune function)

Coagulation system
- Increased platelet adhesiveness
- Decreased fibrinolysis
- Hypercoagulation
- Deep vein thrombosis

Gastrointestinal system
- Ileus

Genitourinary system
- Urinary retention

horn of the spinal cord, where they synapse with second order afferent neurons. Axonal projections of second order neurons cross to the contralateral hemisphere of the spinal cord and ascend as afferent sensory pathways (spinothalamic tract) to the level of the thalamus (Fig. 32-3).[5] Along the way, these neurons divide and send axonal branches to the reticular formation and the periaqueductal gray matter. In the thalamus, second order neurons synapse with third order neurons, which send axonal projections into the sensory cortex.

Modulation of Nociception

Modulation of nociception can occur at several levels of the afferent sensory pathway prior to perception of pain at the sensory cortex. For example, modula-

Patient Controlled Analgesia Standard Orders

1. Drug
   ___MORPHINE (1 mg·ml^{-1})
   ___MEPERIDINE (10 mg·ml^{-1})
   ___OTHER _____ Concentration _____
2. Loading dose (optional) _____ mg Time _____
3. Incremental dose _____ mg (i.e., _____ ml)
4. Lockout interval—8 minutes
5. Four-hour limit (ml) _____ (max = 30 ml·4 h^{-1})
6. If pain not controlled after 1 hour, increase incremental dose by _____ mg (i.e., _____ ml) one time only.
7. If pain still not controlled after 1 additional hour, reduce lockout interval by _____ minutes, one time only.
8. *No systemic opioids* to be given except by order of Acute Pain Management Service.
9. Monitoring:
   Respiratory rate, analgesic level, sedation level—q2h for 8 hours, then q4h.
10. Documentation:
    Record drug use on vital signs sheet at each monitoring interval and 8-hour totals on medication sheet.
11. Treatment of side effects:
    A. DROPERIDOL (0.25 mg IV) for nausea/vomiting. May repeat × 1.
    B. "In and out" bladder catheter prn for urinary retention.
    C. NALOXONE (0.1 mg IV stat) for respiratory rate <8. May repeat × 3. Call Acute Pain Management Service.
12. For inadequate analgesia or other problems related to PCA, call the Acute Pain Management Service.

Dr. ______________________________
of the Acute Pain Management Service was notified about this patient at ______ (hours).

Date ________ ______________________, M.D.

Figure 32-1. Standard order form for patient controlled analgesia. (Modified from Ready et al.,[4] with permission.)

Epidural Opioid Standard Orders

1. Initial dose:
   Drug ______ mg ______ Time ______
2. Drug for continuing analgesia:
   A. MORPHINE (1 mg·ml^{-1}), preservative free
   ______ mg q6–12h.
   B. FENTANYL (5 μg·ml^{-1}). Infuse ______ μg·h^{-1} (______ ml·h^{-1}) with infusion controller.
   C. OTHER: Drug/concentration______
   Dose______ Interval ______
3. Maintain IV access (drip, heparin lock) for 24 hours after last dose of epidural opioid.
4. NALOXONE 0.4 mg at bedside.
5. *No systemic opioids* to be given except as ordered by Acute Pain Management Service.
6. Monitoring:
   A. Respiratory rate and sedation scale q1h for first 24 hours. Sedation scale q1h for second 24 hours. After 48 hours, sedation scale q4h.
   B. Respiratory monitor for first 24 hours.
   Yes ______ No ______
7. Nausea/vomiting prophylaxis:
   METOCLOPRAMIDE (10 mg IV slowly) q8h x 3; then q8h prn for nausea/vomiting.
8. Treatment of side effects:
   A. RR <10 per minute, call Acute Pain Management Service.
   RR <8 per minute, NALOXONE 0.4 mg IV stat. May repeat prn.
   Call Acute Pain Management Service.
   B. NALOXONE (0.1 mg IV) for severe itching. May repeat q10min x 5.
   C. DROPERIDOL (0.25 mg IV) if metoclopramide ineffective for nausea/vomiting. May repeat x 1.
   D. NALOXONE (0.1 mg IV) for urinary retention. May repeat q10min x 5. If ineffective, "in and out" bladder catheter.
9. For inadequate analgesia or other problems related to epidural, call Acute Pain Management Service.

Dr.______________________________
of the Acute Pain Management Service was notified about this patient at _____ (hours).

Date________ ______________________, M.D.

Figure 32-2. Standard order form for epidural opioid analgesia. (Modified from Ready et al.,[4] with permission.)

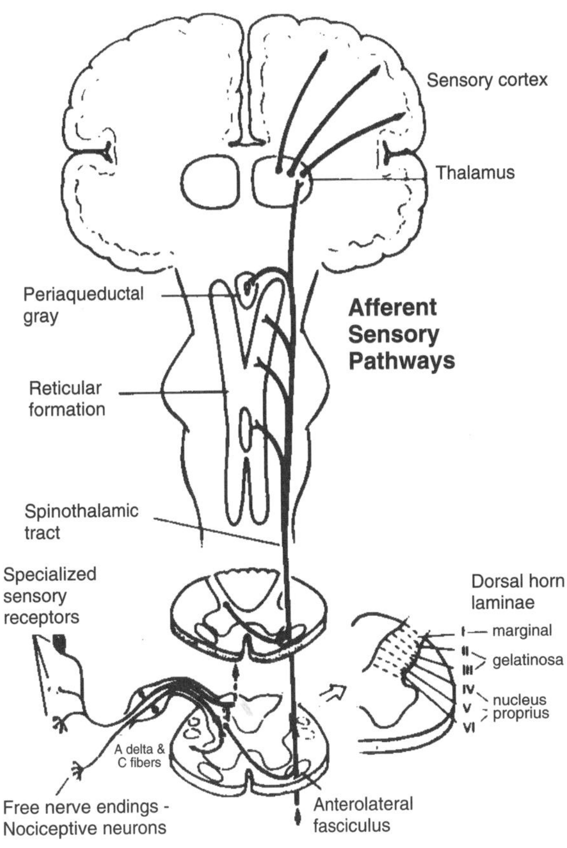

Figure 32-3. Afferent sensory pathways for recognition and transmission of painful stimuli. (From Lubenow et al.,[5] with permission.)

tion of the painful impulse may occur at the origin of the stimulus (nociceptor) or at any point in the ascending sensory afferent pathways where synaptic transmission occurs (Fig. 32-3).[5] Furthermore, modulation of nociception may occur through descending efferent inhibitory pathways that originate at the level of the brain stem (Fig. 32-4).[5]

Peripheral

Peripheral modulation of nociception occurs by either the liberation or elimination of endogenous mediators of inflammation in the vicinity of the nociceptor. These mediators sensitize (hyperalgesic effect) and excite nociceptors, especially in tissues that have been subjected to trauma and inflammation. Aspirin and nonsteroidal anti-inflammatory drugs (NSAIDs) such as ketorolac decrease the synthesis of prostaglandins by inhibiting the action of the enzyme cyclooxygenase, which is necessary for

Endogenous Mediators of Inflammation

Prostaglandins (PGE_1 > PGE_2)
Histamine
Bradykinin
Serotonin
Acetylcholine
Lactic acid
Hydrogen ions
Potassium ions

the conversion of arachidonic acid into prostaglandins. By decreasing prostaglandin synthesis, these NSAIDs modulate (block) nociception at peripheral sites.

Spinal Cord

Modulation of nociception in the spinal cord results from the effects of excitatory or inhibitory neurotransmitters in the dorsal horn or by spinal reflexes, which transmit efferent impulses back to peripheral nociceptors (Fig. 32-4).[5]

Examples of Pain-Modulating Neurotransmitters

Excitatory
- L-Glutamate
- Aspartate
- Vasoactive intestinal polypeptide
- Cholecystokinin
- Gastrin-releasing peptide
- Angiotensin
- Substance P

Inhibitory
- Enkephalins
- Endorphins
- Substance P
- Somatostatin

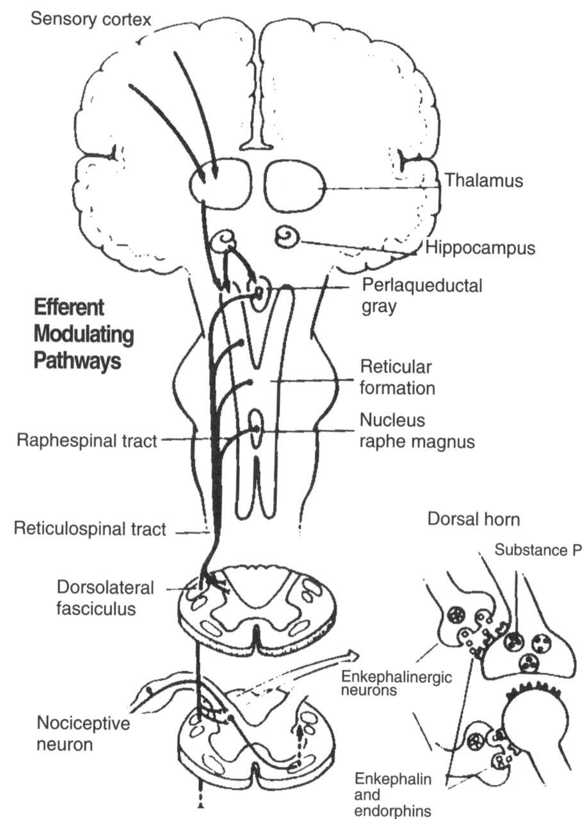

Figure 32-4. Descending efferent inhibitory (modulating) pathways involved in nociceptive regulation. (From Lubenow et al.,[5] with permission.)

Supraspinal

Modulation of nociception may occur through descending efferent inhibitory pathways that originate at the level of the brain stem and synapse in the substantia gelatinosa region of the dorsal horn (Fig. 32-4).[5] An opioid descending inhibitory pathway releases endorphins and enkephalins, which act presynaptically to hyperpolarize nerve fibers; this serves to negate the current (action potential) to the next synapse and subsequent release of neurotransmitter. Morphine and other exogenous opioids act as agonists at stereoselective membrane-bound receptors that are distributed throughout the central nervous system (see Table 5-3). In addition to the opioid descending inhibitory pathway, there is an alpha-adrenergic descending inhibitory pathway that terminates in the substantia gelatinosa region of the dorsal horn. Norepinephrine is released from these nerve terminals and produces hyperpolarization of nerve fibers, which serves to negate the current to the next synapse and subsequent release of neurotransmitter. Analgesic effects of clonidine most likely reflect its actions through this alpha-adrenergic inhibitory pathway.

ANALGESIA DELIVERY SYSTEMS

Traditional delivery systems for management of acute postoperative pain as represented by oral and parenteral on-demand administration of analgesics are being replaced by more efficacious techniques such as neuraxial analgesia or PCA. New drug delivery techniques are based on an improved understanding of the neurophysiology of pain and the potential deleterious effects of postoperative pain. The formation of an acute pain management service directed by anesthesiologists with expertise in regional anesthesia and the pharmacology of analgesics has facilitated the widespread application of these new analgesic delivery systems.

Routes of Delivery for Analgesic Drugs

- Oral
- Transmucosal
- Transdermal
- Intramuscular
- Intravenous
  - Intermittent
  - Continuous
  - Patient controlled
- Neuraxial
  - Epidural
  - Intrathecal
- Peripheral nerve block
- Intrapleural regional analgesia
- Transcutaneous electrical nerve stimulation

Oral Administration

Oral administration of analgesics is not considered optimal for management of moderate to severe acute postoperative pain, principally because of lack of titratability and prolonged time to peak effect. Traditionally, postoperative patients are switched to oral analgesics when pain has diminished to the extent that the need for rapid adjustments in the level of analgesia is unlikely. Nevertheless, with the increased complexity of outpatient surgical procedures, there is a growing need for oral analgesics that are efficacious in the treatment of moderate to severe acute postoperative pain. Transmucosal delivery of analgesics such as fentanyl may serve as an alternative to oral administration of NSAIDs, especially when a prompt drug effect is desirable.

Intramuscular Administration

Intramuscular administration of analgesics is the traditional method for treating moderate to severe postoperative pain, providing a more rapid onset and time to peak effect than oral analgesics. Nevertheless, plasma concentrations of opioids achieved after intramuscular administration may vary as much as three- to fivefold.[6] Plasma concentrations of opioids following intramuscular administration on a fixed time interval (typically every 3 to 4 hours) results in a cyclic period of sedation, analgesia, and, finally, inadequate analgesia.[7] It is estimated that plasma concentrations will exceed or equal analgesia concentrations only 35% of the time during such a fixed dosing interval. As a result, an estimated 75% of patients receiving intermittent intramuscular opioids postoperatively remain in moderate to severe pain.[3] Delivery of opioids by PCA circumvents many of the problems of intramuscular opioid administration and is predicted to provide more effective analgesia with fewer side effects by maintaining plasma concentrations in a more narrow but analgesic range (see the section *Patient Controlled Analgesia*). An alternative to intramuscular administration of opioids is the injection of ketorolac, an NSIAD with efficacy equal to that of moderate doses of opioids but lacking depressant effects on ventilation.

Intravenous Administration

Intermittent intravenous administration of small doses of opioids (morphine 0.5 to 3 mg, fentanyl 15 to 50 μg, sufentanil 3 to 15 μg) is commonly used to treat acute and severe pain in the postanesthesia care unit or intensive care unit where continuous nursing surveillance and monitoring (pulse oximetry) is available. With a small intravenous dose of an opioid, the time delay for analgesia and variability in plasma concentrations characteristic of intramuscular injections are minimized. Rapid redistribution of the opioid will shorten the duration of analgesia after a single intravenous administration compared with an intramuscular injection.

Patient Controlled Analgesia

Advances in computer technology have permitted the development of drug delivery systems that allow the patient to titrate analgesic needs by activating a switch (PCA) that delivers a small intravenous dose of an opioid. Limits can be placed on the number of activations per unit of time the patient is allowed and the minimum time that would have to elapse between activations (lockout interval) (Fig. 32-1 and Table 32-1).[4] It is also possible for these devices to record a profile of the drug administration, including the number and time of bolus delivery, number of activations that did not result in drug delivery, and total amounts of drug that were administered per unit time. Further refinement of these delivery systems permits the physician to administer a continuous background intravenous infusion of opioid superimposed on patient controlled boluses. Most patients tend to determine a level of pain at which they feel comfortable and taper their dosage requirements as they convalesce. Patient acceptance of PCA is high since patients feel that they have significant control of their therapy. Compared with traditional methods of intermittent intramuscular injections of opioids to manage acute postoperative pain, PCA has been shown to provide better analgesia with less total drug usage, less sedation, fewer nocturnal sleep disturbances, and a more rapid return to physical activity.[8]

Table 32-1. Guidelines for Delivery Systems Used in Patient Controlled Analgesia

	Bolus Dose (mg)	Lock-Out Interval (min)	Continuous Infusion ($mg \cdot h^{-1}$)
Morphine	0.5–3	5–20	1–10
Meperidine	5–15	5–15	5–40
Fentanyl	0.015–0.05	3–10	0.02–0.1
Sufentanil	0.003–0.015	3–10	0.004–0.03

Neuraxial Analgesia

Placement of an opioid in the intrathecal or epidural space (neuraxial placement) to manage acute postoperative pain is based on the knowledge that opioid receptors are present in the substantia gelatinosa of the spinal cord.[9] Presumably, opioids placed in the epidural space diffuse across the dura to gain access to opioid receptors on the spinal cord. Analgesia produced by neuraxial opioids, in contrast to intravenous administration of opioids or regional anesthesia with local anesthetics, is not associated with sympathetic nervous system denervation, skeletal muscle weakness, or loss of proprioception. As a result, it is possible to render postoperative patients pain free without interfering with their ability to ambulate. There is evidence that neuraxial analgesia improves postoperative pulmonary function, decreases cardiovascular and infectious complications, and decreases total hospital costs.[1,2]

Side effects associated with neuraxial opioids include (1) pruritus, (2) urinary retention, (3) nausea and vomiting, (4) sedation, and (5) early and delayed depression of ventilation. Early depression of ventilation reflects systemic absorption of opioid from its epidural placement site, whereas delayed depression of ventilation (6 to 24 hours after neuraxial administration) is due to cephalad spread of the opioid in cerebrospinal fluid to medullary centers in the area of the fourth cerebral ventricle. Opioids with high lipid solubility, such as fentanyl or sufentanil, attach to lipid components in the spinal cord; therefore, less drug is available to diffuse cephalad, making delayed depression of ventilation less likely than after injection of poorly lipid soluble morphine. Elderly patients and patients not tolerant to opioids (in contrast to cancer treatment patients) may be at increased risk of the development of delayed depression of ventilation.

Intrathecal Administration

Intrathecal administration of an opioid provides long-lasting postoperative analgesia after a single injection. The intrathecal route offers the advantage of precise and reliable placement of low concentrations of drug near its site of action.[10] The onset of analgesic effect following the intrathecal administration of an opioid is directly proportional to the lipid solubility of the drug, whereas the duration of effect is longer with more hydrophilic compounds. Morphine, for example, has been shown to produce peak analgesic effects in 20 to 60 minutes and provide postoperative analgesia for 12 to 36 hours. The onset of analgesic effect may be enhanced by adding a small dose of fentanyl to the morphine-containing opioid solution. For example, intrathecal placement of morphine (0.6 to 0.8 mg) plus fentanyl (0.025 mg) at the conclusion of a thoracotomy is likely to permit an early onset of analgesia. As a result, the patient is able to breathe deeply without pain and the trachea can often be extubated at the conclusion of surgery. This analgesia may also be supplemented by the intraoperative performance of intercostal nerve blocks by the surgeon. For lower abdominal procedures performed with spinal anesthesia (cesarean section, transurethral resection of the prostate), morphine (0.2 to 0.4 mg) may be added to the local anesthesia solution at the time the anesthetic is performed to ensure analgesia at the conclusion of surgery.

A clinical impression that the incidence of side effects, particularly delayed depression of ventilation, is higher after intrathecal than after epidural opioid injection is most likely the result of excessive intrathecal opioid doses.[10] For example, the analgesic effect of neuraxial opioids exerted through the receptors in the substantia gelatinosa should be the same regardless of whether the drug is placed in the epidural space and diffuses across the dura or is placed directly into the cerebrospinal fluid. On the basis of this logic, equally potent doses of opioids placed in the epidural or intrathecal space (dose about 1/10 the epidural dose) should produce similar effects at opioid receptors in the substantia gelatinosa and hence a comparable degree of analgesia and a similar incidence of side effects. The principal disadvantage of an intrathecal opioid injection is its lack of titratability and the need to either repeat the injection or consider other options when the analgesic effect of the initial dose wanes. Nevertheless, it is common clinical experience that after the analgesic effect of the initial intrathecal dose wanes, the intensity of postoperative pain is greatly diminished and can be satisfactorily managed with oral analgesics or PCA. The practical aspects of leaving a catheter in the intrathecal space for either continuous or repeated intermittent opioid injections is controversial, especially in view of reports of cauda equina syndrome following continuous spinal anesthesia with hyperbaric local anesthetic solutions injected through a small-diameter catheter.[11]

Epidural Administration

Epidural administration of an opioid as either an intermittent injection or a continuous epidural infusion through an epidural catheter is a common method for providing postoperative analgesia (Fig. 32-2 and Tables 32-2 and 32-3).[4] A low dose of local anesthetic may be added to the opioid-containing solution for injection into the epidural space. When an opioid is placed in the epidural space, it must cross the dura to reach opioid receptors in the substantia gelatinosa of the spinal cord. Besides the physical barrier presented by the dura, opioid is deposited in the fat and connective tissues present in the epidural space. The impact of these factors on the pharmacokinetics of drugs placed in the epidural space is evidenced by the estimated 10-fold increase in dose requirements for epidural opioids compared with intrathecal opioids required to produce a similar analgesic effect (Table 32-2). Furthermore, the epidural space is highly vascularized, and there is significant absorption of drug into the systemic circulation. In fact, plasma concentrations of fentanyl are similar after placement of this opioid into the epidural space compared with intravenous injection (Fig. 32-5).[12] Clearly, part of the analgesic effect as well as side effects (early depression of ventilation) reflects systemic absorption of the opioid from the epidural space.

It may take as long as 3 to 4 hours to provide effective analgesia when epidural opioids are admin-

Table 32-2. Comparison of Epidural Administration Techniques

Intermittent Epidural Injection	Continuous Epidural Injection
No need for infusion devices	Need sophisticated infusion devices
Requires personnel to inject catheter periodically	Removes need for personnel to inject catheter periodically
Limited number of suitable opioids	Allows use of shorter-acting opioids such as fentanyl or sufentanil
Difficult to titrate dose	Provides continuous analgesia, avoiding peaks and valleys in the plasma opioid concentration
Higher incidence of side effects	Less rostral spread so side effects are minimized

Table 32-3. Guidelines for Epidural Analgesia

	Bolus Dose (mg)	Onset (min)	Analgesic Peak Effect (min)	Duration (h)	Continuous Infusion Concentration (%)	Infusion Rate (ml·h^{-1})
Morphine	5	20	30–60	12–24	0.01	1–6
Meperidine	30–100	5–10	12–30	4–6		
Fentanyl	0.1	4–10	20	2–4[a]	0.001	4–12
Sufentanil	0.03–0.05	7	25	3[a]	0.0001	10
Bupivacaine		2.5–5			0.1	4–6

[a]Estimates.
[b]Combined with opioid.

istered by intermittent injection or continuous infusion. This delayed onset of effective analgesia can readily be overcome by adjusting the infusion rate to provide the equivalent of a small bolus (5 to 10 ml) prior to beginning the maintenance infusion. Alternatively, a short-acting opioid such as fentanyl may be added to the morphine-containing solution or the drug-containing analgesic solution can be injected preoperatively to ensure the presence of analgesia when the patient awakens at the conclusion of surgery. Bupivacaine (1 mg·ml^{-1}) may also be added to the opioid-containing solution. The synergy between the analgesic effects of opioids and local anesthetics may be the result of blockade of afferent impulses at two different sites in the spinal cord. Opioids produce analgesia by binding to opioid receptors in the substantia gelatinosa, whereas local anesthetics block transmission of afferent impulses at the nerve roots and dorsal root ganglia. Another benefit of these combinations is a decrease in dosage of individual drugs with a concomitant decrease in the incidence of side effects. Intermittent intravenous injections of an opioid may be necessary to treat "breakthrough" pain until epidural analgesia is adequate. Ketorolac administered parenterally may also be a useful nonopioid analgesic in these situations. A clear advantage of continuous epidural infusion compared with intermittent epidural injection is the ability to titrate the infusion rate to the desired level of analgesia. It is even possible to combine a continuous epidural infusion regimen with patient-activated intermittent boluses. Complications that can occur with a continuous epidural technique include accidental intrathecal administration of the drug, infection, and depression of breathing.

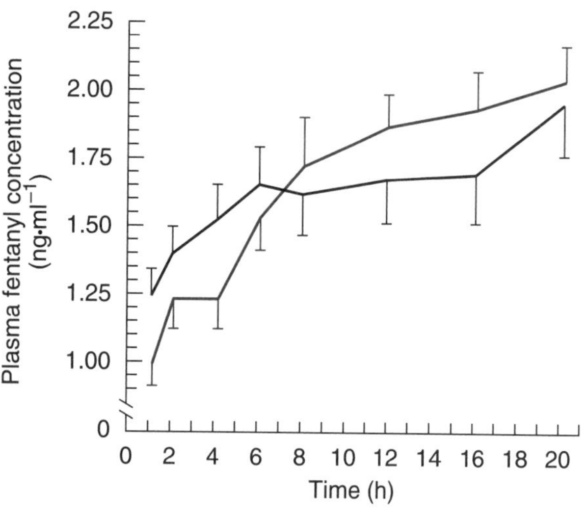

Figure 32-5. Plasma fentanyl concentrations postoperatively were similar in patients receiving lumbar epidural fentanyl infusions (red line) or intravenous fentanyl infusions (black line). (From Sandler et al.,[12] with permission.)

Hydrophilic opioids such as morphine, when injected into the epidural space, result in cerebrospinal fluid concentrations of the opioid that allow the drug to follow the rostral spread of cerebrospinal fluid and saturate the entire length of the spinal cord. Because of this property, epidural morphine may be infused at a lower lumbar level and still provide analgesia for surgical procedures performed on the upper abdomen and thorax. Lipophilic opioids such as fentanyl and sufentanil tend to provide more of a segmental analgesic effect, perhaps reflecting more intense drug binding to opioid receptors. The segmental nature of analgesia produced by these lipophilic opioids is the basis for the recommendation by some anesthesiologists that the epidural catheter be placed in a position to cover the dermatomes included in the surgical field.

Achievement of optimal results with continuous epidural analgesia techniques requires appropriate perioperative planning and assessment. This strategy includes identification of patients who may benefit from epidural analgesia and scheduling the epidural catheter placement as part of the anesthetic plan. This may include epidural catheter placement in the holding area before the patient is brought to the operating room, permitting the anesthesiologist to administer a test dose of the local anesthetic (usually bupivacaine) while the patient is still awake. This facilitates diagnosis of intrathecal or intravascular placement and allows confirmation of epidural catheter placement by virtue of segmental epidural analgesia when the test dose of local anesthetic is administered.

ALTERNATIVE APPROACHES TO MANAGEMENT OF ACUTE POSTOPERATIVE PAIN

Alternative approaches to analgesia delivery systems for treatment of acute postoperative pain include peripheral nerve blocks, intrapleural regional analgesia, and transcutaneous electrical nerve stimulation (TENS).

Peripheral Nerve Blocks

Peripheral nerve blocks may provide effective postoperative analgesia, but their relatively short duration of analgesia and their selective nature preclude their general application to all patient populations. Nevertheless, pain relief afforded by a regional nerve block may be superior to that achievable with systemic opioids. For example, intercostal nerve blocks may be useful for providing postoperative analgesia after abdominal or thoracic operations (see Chapter 13).

Intrapleural Regional Analgesia

Intrapleural regional analgesia is produced by injection of local anesthetic solution through a catheter placed percutaneously into the intrapleural space. The local anesthetic diffuses across the parietal pleura to the intercostal neurovascular bundle, producing a unilateral intercostal nerve block at multiple levels. Effective postoperative pain relief requires intermittent intrapleural injections approximately every 6 hours with approximately 20 ml of 0.25% to 0.5% bupivacaine. Pleural drainage tubes as placed following a thoracotomy may result in loss of the local anesthetic solution and inadequate analgesia.

Transcutaneous Electrical Nerve Stimulation

TENS is a simple conservative technique that utilizes electrical stimulation of the skin to provide pain relief (see Chapter 34). The mechanism by which TENS produces pain relief is presumed to involve the release of endogenous endorphins by the electrical stimulation of afferent cutaneous nerves. Endorphins exert an inhibitory effect on the dorsal horn and augment the descending inhibitory modulating pathways. The degree of acute pain relief provided by TENS is variable and less effective than that produced by neuraxial opioids or PCA.

REFERENCES

1. Tuman KJ, McCarthy RJ, March R, et al. Effects of epidural anesthesia and analgesia on coagulation and outcome after major vascular surgery. Anesth Analg 1991;73:696–704.
2. Yeager MP, Glass DD, Neff RK, et al. Epidural anesthesia and analgesia in high-risk surgical patients. Anesthesiology 1987;66:729–36.
3. Lubenow TR, Ivankovich AD. Organization of an acute pain management service. In: Stoelting RK, Barash PG, Gallagher TJ, eds. Advances in Anesthesia. Vol. 8. St. Louis, Mosby-Year Book 1991;1–28.
4. Ready LB, Oden R, Chadwick HS, et al. Development of an anesthesiology-based postoperative pain management service. Anesthesiology 1988;68:100–6.
5. Lubenow TR, McCarthy RJ, Ivankovich AD. Management of acute postoperative pain. In: Barash PG, Cullen BF, Stoelting RK, eds. Clinical Anesthesia. Philadelphia, JB Lippincott 1992;1547–77.
6. Rigy JR, Browne RA, Davis C, et al. Variation in the disposition of morphine after administration in surgical patients. Br J Anaesth 1978;50:1125–30.
7. Tuman KJ, McCarthy RJ, Ivankovich AD. Pain control in the postoperative cardiac surgery patient. Hosp Formul 1988;23:580–95.
8. Egbert AM, Parks LH, Short LM, et al. Randomized trial of postoperative patient-controlled analgesia vs. intramuscular narcotics in frail elderly men. Arch Intern Med 1990;150:1897–1903.
9. Cousins MJ, Mather LE. Intrathecal and epidural administration of opioids. Anesthesiology 1984; 61:276–310.

10. Stoelting RK. Intrathecal morphine—An underused combination for postoperative pain management. Anesth Analg 1989;68:707–9.
11. Rigler ML, Drasner K, Krejcie TC, et al. Cauda equina syndrome after spinal anesthesia. Anesth Analg 1991;72:275–81.
12. Sandler AN, Stringer D, Panos L, et al. A randomized, double-blind comparison of lumbar epidural and intravenous fentanyl infusions for postthoracotomy pain relief. Analgesic, pharmacokinetic, and respiratory effects. Anesthesiology 1992;77:626–34.

Section VI

Consultant Anesthetic Practice

33

Critical Care Medicine and Management of the Trauma Patient

The evolution of critical care medicine as a legitimate and important area of specialization reflects the contributions of many clinicians, particularly anesthesiologists. Indeed, 10 of the 28 founding members of the Society of Critical Care Medicine were anesthesiologists. A certificate of Special Qualifications in Anesthesiology Critical Care Medicine is available to diplomates of The American Board of Anesthesiology who spend 1 year of additional postgraduate training in critical care medicine beyond primary training requirements and subsequently achieve a passing score on a written examination administered by The American Board of Anesthesiology.

The training of anesthesiologists in the management of anesthesia is a useful beginning for subsequent development of additional skills required for the care of critically ill patients with multiple organ system dysfunction. For example, no other specialty provides day-to-day experience in airway management, ventilation of the lungs, intravenous administration of potent and rapidly acting drugs, blood and fluid administration, and both noninvasive and invasive monitoring of vital organ function.

Life-threatening injuries owing to trauma (commonly motor vehicle accidents) are a frequent cause of multiple organ system failure requiring treatment in an intensive care unit (ICU) by specialists in critical care medicine.[1] Ethical and legal considerations (definition of brain death, "do not resuscitate" orders) as well as cost effectiveness are important issues in management of patients in an ICU (see Chapter 35). Hospital ethics committees are useful to evaluate individual cases and make nonbinding recommendations to the primary physician regarding treatment.

LIFE-THREATENING TRAUMA

Trauma and associated life-threatening injuries account for 10% to 15% of all patients hospitalized because of injuries.[1] Prompt transport of a trauma victim to a regional trauma center rather than to the nearest hospital results in improved outcome for the victim. A level 1 trauma center is characterized by the immediate availability of personnel (trauma surgeons, anesthesiologists, nurses) and facilities (emergency room, operating rooms, ICU beds, radiology, stat laboratory, blood bank) 24 hours every day of the year. The anesthesiologist must have available and ready to use an assortment of supplies and equipment.

Initial Evaluation

On arrival to the hospital, the patient's airway, breathing, circulation, and neurologic status (computed tomography, magnetic resonance imaging, Glasgow Coma Scale) must be rapidly evaluated (Table 33-1)[2] (see the section *Head Injury*). The first priority is establishment of an airway and adminis-

Immediately Available Equipment for Care of the Trauma Victim

Anesthesia machine
Mechanical ventilator
Airway equipment (laryngoscopes, fiberscopes, tracheal tubes)
Monitoring devices
Blood pumps and primed infusion sets in blood warmers
Drugs in labeled syringes
Electrical defibrillator

tration of oxygen. Until the possibility of cervical spine injury (present in 1.5% to 3% of all major trauma victims) has been ruled out, orotracheal intubation should only be attempted with the patient's head stabilized in a neutral position (a rigid collar decreases flexion and extension to about 30% of normal and rotation and lateral movement to about 50% of normal).[3] Computed tomography is the best way to diagnose cervical spine injury, although two-thirds of all trauma victims have multiple injuries that may interfere with the ability or safety of performing routine computed tomography. Early tracheal intubation in selected patients has been a major factor in decreasing mortality from trauma. Nasotracheal intubation should not be attempted if there is the possibility of a basal skull fracture. If airway obstruction exists and tracheal intubation cannot be accomplished, emergency cricothyrotomy (see Fig. 35-11) or tracheostomy is indicated. All trauma victims are assumed to have full stomachs.

Indications for Tracheal Intubation After Life-Threatening Trauma

Protection against aspiration
Airway obstruction
Unconsciousness
Provision of positive pressure ventilation
Need for sedation or skeletal muscle paralysis, or both

Likely Presence of Cervical Spine Injury

No risk
- Alert patient without neck pain or tenderness

Moderate risk
- Motor vehicle accident
- Head injury
- Non-head-first fall
- Contact sport injury

High Risk
- Front-end motor vehicle accident without seat belt
- Head-first fall

Thoracic trauma may involve the lungs or cardiovascular system, or both. An upright inspiratory chest radiograph is preferred for visualization of a pneumothorax (high index of suspicion if rib fractures are present), although the more likely radiograph will be an anteroposterior supine film. Pneumothorax or hemothorax is treated with a tube thoracotomy (tube placed in the fourth or fifth interspace in the midaxillary line and directed

Table 33-1. Glasgow Coma Scale

Category	Score
Eyes open	
Never	1
To pain	2
To verbal stimuli	3
Spontaneously	4
Best verbal response	
None	1
Incomprehensible sounds	2
Inappropriate words	3
Patient disoriented and converses	4
Patient oriented and converses	5
Best motor response	
None	1
Extension (decerebrate rigidity)	2
Flexion abnormal (decorticate rigidity)	3
Flexion withdrawal	4
Patient localizes pain	5
Patient obeys	6

posteriorly and attached to suction). Intrathoracic vascular injury is suggested by a widening mediastinum, whereas lung contusion is predictable when flail chest is present.

Abdominal injuries in the presence of blunt trauma are most often splenic rupture or laceration of the liver, resulting in profound hemorrhage. Intra-abdominal hemorrhage is diagnosed by peritoneal lavage or computed tomography. Continued hematuria after placement of a bladder catheter indicates a possible bladder injury and the need for a cystogram or intravenous pyelogram. Evaluation of the extremities includes palpation of distal pulses and visual symmetry of the extremities for evidence of bleeding, especially in the thighs after femur fractures. Early immobilization of fractures is indicated.

Management of Anesthesia

General anesthesia is required for most trauma patients who require surgical intervention. There is no ideal anesthetic agent or technique for a trauma patient. If the patient's trachea has not already been intubated, a rapid sequence induction of anesthesia is indicated. In the presence of hypovolemia, ketamine (0.25 to 0.5 $mg \cdot kg^{-1}$ IV) is often selected for induction of anesthesia since this drug is usually a cardiovascular stimulant. In the presence of suspected or known cervical spine injury, avoidance of excessive head movement during direct laryngoscopy is more important than the technique (awake versus asleep) selected to accomplish tracheal intubation.[3] Maintenance of anesthesia is achieved with drugs titrated to a dose consistent with hemodynamic stability. Often the dose of anesthetic tolerated by the patient is too small to prevent movement, thus necessitating the production of skeletal muscle paralysis with a muscle relaxant. In this regard, some patients may experience recall of intraoperative events.

Hemodynamic stability results from control of surgical bleeding and restoration of the patient's blood volume. Initially, administration of a crystalloid solution such as lactated Ringer's solution restores intravascular fluid volume to help maintain venous return and cardiac output. When hemorrhage is extreme, it will be necessary to eventually administer blood (preferably whole blood less than 6 hours old). Dilutional thrombocytopenia may accompany massive blood transfusion necessary to re-establish

Treatment of Hypovolemia in the Trauma Victim

Crystalloid solutions (warmed) guided by measurements of adequacy of intravascular fluid volume replacement
Type O-negative blood in desperate situations
Use of autotransfusion (cell-saver) systems

Management of Anesthesia for Surgical Treatment of Life-Threatening Trauma

Induction of anesthesia
- Ketamine if hypovolemia present
- Succinylcholine acceptable in first few hours after trauma—nondepolarizing drugs are alternatives, keeping in mind the potential for hypotension with histamine release

Maintenance of anesthesia
- Low doses of a volatile anesthetic—ketamine or opioids are alternatives if unacceptable hypotension occurs, nitrous oxide avoided if possibility of pneumothorax or need to administer high concentrations of oxygen
- Invasive monitoring of blood pressure and cardiac filling pressures

Signs of Adequate Intravascular Fluid Volume Replacement

Heart rate <100 $beats \cdot min^{-1}$
Pulse pressure >30 mmHg
Urine output >0.5–1 $ml \cdot kg^{-1} \cdot h^{-1}$
Absence of metabolic acidosis
Minimal effects of positive pressure ventilation on blood pressure

intravascular fluid volume, whereas disseminated intravascular coagulation may accompany persistent hypotension. It is important to warm intravenous fluids to minimize the likelihood of hypothermia. A pressurized infusion device is helpful in selected patients. Unfortunately, assessment of blood loss and adequacy of replacement can be very difficult in the trauma victim. Arterial blood gases, pH, and hematocrit are measured at frequent intervals during anesthesia and surgery. On a less frequent basis, it may be useful to analyze blood for electrolytes, glucose, and coagulation factors (see Table 31-1).

Postoperative Care

Severely injured patients often require continued postoperative support of major organ function, especially mechanical ventilation of the lungs, in an ICU.

Examples of Organ System Failure Treated in the Intensive Care Unit

Acute respiratory failure
Congestive heart failure
Sepsis
Head injury
Acute renal failure
Acute hepatic failure
Malnutrition

THERMAL (BURN) INJURY

Initial treatment of the burn injury patient, like that of the trauma victim, is based on evaluation of the airway, breathing, and cardiovascular system. Tracheal intubation is indicated if the patient has stridor or is hoarse, since subsequent facial and glottic edema is predictable. Smoke inhalation with associated carbon monoxide inhalation may lead to inadequate oxygen carrying capacity despite a normal PaO_2. Carbon monoxide inhalation is treated with the administration of 100% oxygen. After the airway has been secured, the burn injury patient is resuscitated with large volumes of fluid (lactated Ringer's solution 4 $ml \cdot kg^{-1}$ for every 1% of body surface area burned). Fluid loss is greatest in the first 12 hours and subsides after about 24 hours. Urine output and hemodynamic variables ultimately determine the volume of fluid replacement required. Within a few hours after the burn injury, the patient becomes hypermetabolic (increased oxygen consumption, tachycardia, increased serum catecholamine concentrations).

Management of Anesthesia

Provision of anesthesia is most often required for excision and grafting of the burn injury area. In these patients, access for monitoring may be difficult, requiring use of needle electrodes for the electrocardiogram and peripheral nerve stimulator. A blood pressure cuff may be placed over a burned area, but an intra-arterial catheter is often recommended for patients with a large percentage of body surface area burn. Accurate measurement and maintenance of body temperature (warm intravenous fluids, heated humidifier) plus anticipation of significant blood loss are important considerations.

Induction and maintenance of anesthesia often include ketamine or opioids, or both, since intraoperative and postoperative pain is intense. Burn contractures around the mouth may interfere with direct laryngoscopy for tracheal intubation. Halothane may be avoided if it is anticipated that epinephrine-soaked sponges will be applied to control bleeding from excision and grafting sites. Succinylcholine is not recommended when the burn injury is older than 24 hours as drug-induced hyperkalemia may result in cardiac arrest. Conversely, burn injury patients are likely to manifest resistance to the effects of nondepolarizing muscle relaxants.

ACUTE RESPIRATORY FAILURE

Acute respiratory failure is not a single disease entity but instead is a combination of pathophysiologic derangements that can arise from a variety of etiologic insults. Nevertheless, manifestations of acute respiratory failure are sufficiently similar to be considered a single entity designated the adult respiratory distress syndrome (ARDS).

Diagnosis

Arterial hypoxemia (PaO_2 lower than 60 mmHg) despite supplemental inhaled oxygen is an invariable accompaniment of ARDS. Ventilation-to-perfu-

Etiology of Acute Respiratory Failure

Trauma with associated multiple organ system failure
Pulmonary dysfunction
- Obstructive pulmonary disease
- Restrictive pulmonary disease
- Pneumonia
- Inhaled toxins (gastric fluid, smoke, meconium)
- Oxygen toxicity
- Emboli (blood, fat, amniotic fluid)
- Lung contusion
- Near-drowning
- Hyaline membrane disease

Cardiac dysfunction
- Shock (hemorrhage, sepsis)
- Congestive heart failure
- Post-cardiopulmonary bypass

Central nervous system dysfunction
- Hypothalamic injury
- Depressant drug overdose

Neuromuscular dysfunction
- Myasthenia gravis
- Spinal cord transection
- Guillain-Barré syndrome
- Tetanus
- Drugs (muscle relaxants, antibiotics)

Miscellaneous
- Massive blood transfusion
- Disseminated intravascular coagulation
- Morbid obesity
- Uremia
- Acute pancreatitis

sion mismatching is the most likely cause for arterial hypoxemia. In its most extreme form, this mismatching may be right-to-left intrapulmonary shunting in which unventilated alveoli continue to be perfused. Also contributing to this mismatching is a decrease in functional residual capacity (FRC) and decreased pulmonary compliance. Loss of pulmonary capillary integrity is reflected by pulmonary edema despite pulmonary artery occlusion pressures lower than 15 mmHg. Increased pulmonary vascular resistance and pulmonary hypertension are likely to develop when ARDS persists.

Acute respiratory failure is often distinguished from chronic respiratory failure on the basis of the relationship of the $PaCO_2$ to the pH. For example, acute respiratory failure is associated with an abrupt increase in the $PaCO_2$ and a corresponding decrease in pH. Conversely, in the presence of chronic respiratory failure, the pH is near normal, reflecting compensation by virtue of renal tubular reabsorption of bicarbonate ions.

Serial measurement of arterial blood gases and pH is necessary to establish the diagnosis of ARDS, determine the need for mechanical support of ventilation, assess the effects of therapy, and confirm when the patient no longer needs mechanical support of ventilation.

Treatment

Treatment of ARDS is directed at supporting pulmonary function until the lungs can recover from the insult that initiated pulmonary dysfunction. In addition to administration of supplemental oxygen and maintenance of intravascular fluid volume, it is usually necessary to intubate the trachea and provide mechanical ventilation of the lungs, including the use of positive end-expiratory pressure (PEEP). Inhalation of nitric oxide (5 to 80 ppm) by patients with ARDS decreases pulmonary artery pressure and improves arterial oxygenation without producing systemic vasodilation.[4] More than 75% of patients dying of ARDS now die of multiple organ system failure rather than because of impaired gas exchange.[1]

Mechanical Ventilation of the Lungs

Mechanical ventilation of the lungs is provided by machines known as ventilators. Ventilators may be classified as pressure-cycled, volume-cycled, or time-cycled, depending on the mechanism responsible for terminating the inspiratory phase of the mechanical breath. Mechanical ventilators may change from the expiratory to inspiratory phase by being set to deliver assisted ventilation, controlled ventilation, assisted-controlled ventilation, or intermittent mandatory ventilation (IMV).

Pressure-cycled ventilators terminate the inspiratory phase of the mechanical breath when a preselected pressure is achieved in the ventilator circuit. Therefore, tidal volume and inspiratory time are directly related to pulmonary compliance and inversely related to airway resistance. Significant leaks in the delivery circuit may prevent development of sufficient airway pressure to cycle the ventilator to exhalation. Conversely, decreased pulmonary compliance or increased airway resistance may result in attainment of the predetermined airway pressure before a sufficient tidal volume has been delivered to the patient. Most pressure-cycled ventilators are incapable of providing the constant tidal volume and unchanging inhaled concentration of oxygen considered desirable for the management of critically ill patients.

Volume-cycled ventilators terminate the inspiratory phase of the mechanical breath after delivery of a preselected volume of gas to the delivery circuit. Flow generators maintain a uniform gas flow rate throughout the inspiratory phase that is independent of the airway pressure. Changes in pulmonary compliance or airway resistance are unlikely to alter the flow characteristics of the volume-cycled ventilator, ensuring a more constant tidal volume with changing clinical conditions. For this reason, most ventilators used for critical care are volume-cycled.

It is a common misconception that the tidal volume delivered by a volume-cycled ventilator is constant regardless of changes in the patient's pulmonary compliance and airway resistance. In fact, a portion of the tidal volume generated by the ventilator is compressed within the ventilator breathing circuit and does not reach the patient. This lost compression volume is dependent on the compliance of the entire ventilator-patient circuit and the peak inspiratory pressure. For most ventilators, the compression volume of the delivery circuit is 3 to 5 ml for every 1 cmH_2O airway pressure. For example, a volume-cycled ventilator (equally true for all other types of ventilators) with a preset tidal volume of 700 ml, a peak inspiratory pressure of 20 cmH_2O, and a compression factor of 4 ml will deliver 620 ml (700 ml minus compression volume) to the patient's lungs. If the patient's pulmonary compliance further decreases, the peak inflation pressure will increase and the delivered tidal volume will be further decreased. Compression volume is particularly important to consider in setting the tidal volume delivered to children. For example, a ventilator set to deliver a tidal volume of 10 $ml{\cdot}kg^{-1}$ to a 10-kg child would deliver only 20 ml, assuming a peak inspiratory pressure of 20 cmH_2O and a compression factor of 4 ml. Consideration of compression volume loss may indicate the need to measure exhaled tidal volume with a spirometer in selected patients.

Time-cycled ventilators terminate the inspiratory phase of the mechanical breath after a preselected time interval has elapsed. The tidal volume delivered by time-cycled ventilators is determined by the inspiratory time and inspiratory flow rate.

Assisted Ventilation. Ventilators capable of assisted (patient-triggered) mechanical ventilation of the lungs respond to a decrease in airway pressure caused by the patient's spontaneous breathing effort, which causes the ventilator to switch to the inspiratory mode. The magnitude of the decreased airway pressure necessary to trigger mechanical augmentation of a spontaneously initiated tidal volume is adjustable by means of a sensitivity control on the ventilator.

Controlled Ventilation. Controlled mechanical ventilation of the lungs provides automatic cycling of the ventilator at a preselected rate independent of the patient's effort to breathe. This mode of ventilation is used primarily to ensure delivery of a predictable minute ventilation to patients being treated for ARDS. Initiation or maintenance, or both, of controlled ventilation of the lungs may require depression of the patient's own spontaneous ventilatory effort by the administration of sedatives or opioids, muscle relaxants, or deliberate hyperventilation to lower the $PaCO_2$ below the apneic threshold.

The initial ventilator settings typically include a breathing rate of 6 to 10 $breaths{\cdot}min^{-1}$, a tidal volume 10 to 15 $ml{\cdot}kg^{-1}$, and an inhaled concentration of oxygen near 50%. A slow breathing rate combined with a large tidal volume optimizes the distribution of ventilation relative to perfusion, particularly in the presence of regional differences in airway resistance. Subsequent adjustments of the ventilator settings and the inhaled concentration of oxygen are based on the measurement of arterial blood gases and pH. The typical goal is to achieve a PaO_2 between 60 and 100 mmHg, $PaCO_2$ between 36 and 44 mmHg, and pH between 7.36 and 7.44.

Pressure Control Inverse Ratio Ventilation. This form of ventilation is characterized by an inspiratory phase equal to or longer than exhalation. The potential advantage of this mode of ventilation is the recruitment of collapsed alveoli by prolonged inspiratory times, which allow alveoli with slow rates of gas flow to fill. This may improve oxygenation and ventilation but, at the same time, result in overdistension of the alveoli if adequate exhalation cannot occur.

Assisted-Controlled Ventilation. A ventilator used to provide assisted-controlled ventilation is set such that the cycling frequency is slightly lower than the patient's spontaneous breathing frequency. If the patient stops breathing, the ventilator will convert to the controlled ventilation mode at the preset respiratory frequency.

IMV is a ventilation mode that may be incorporated into ventilators. This mode of ventilation finds its greatest use during weaning (see the section *Cessation of Mechanical Inflation of the Lungs*).

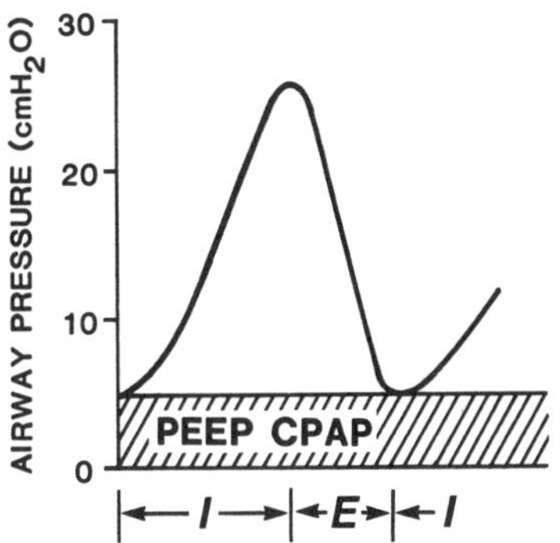

Figure 33-1. Schematic diagram of airway pressures during the inspiratory phase (I) and expiratory phase (E) of a mechanically delivered breath. Airway pressure does not decrease below 5 cmH_2O during I and E, reflecting positive end-expiratory pressure (PEEP). Spontaneous breathing during which airway pressure does not decrease to zero during I and E is commonly referred to as continuous positive airway pressure (CPAP).

Positive End-Expiratory Pressure

PEEP is produced by applying positive pressure to the exhalation valve at the conclusion of the mechanical exhalation phase (Fig. 33-1). Alternatively, the exhalation valve can be depressurized gradually to provide resistance (retard) to exhalation (Fig. 33-2). Retardation of expiratory gas flow rate serves to maintain the patency of peripheral airways.

Mechanism of Beneficial Effect. It is presumed that PEEP increases arterial oxygenation, pulmonary compliance, and FRC by expanding previously collapsed but perfused alveoli. As a result, the matching of ventilation to perfusion is improved and the magnitude of right-to-left intrapulmonary shunting of blood is decreased. PEEP is unlikely to improve the PaO_2 when arterial hypoxemia is due to hypoventilation or is associated with a normal or even increased FRC.

Institution of Positive End-Expiratory Pressure. Institution of PEEP is often recommended when the PaO_2 cannot be maintained higher than 60 mmHg despite inhaled concentrations of oxygen higher than 50%. Short-term administration of more than 50% oxygen to maintain adequate arterial oxygenation is acceptable, but it must be recognized that pulmonary oxygen toxicity is a potential hazard when inhaled concentrations of oxygen are higher than 50% for longer than 24 hours.

Initially, PEEP is added in 2.5- to 5-cmH_2O increments until the PaO_2 is higher than 60 mmHg while the patient is breathing less than 50% oxygen. The goal is to deliver the amount of PEEP that maximally improves the PaO_2 without substantially decreasing cardiac output or increasing the risk of pulmonary barotrauma. Typically, maximum improvement of PaO_2 is achieved with less than 15 cmH_2O of PEEP. Refractory arterial hypoxemia, however,

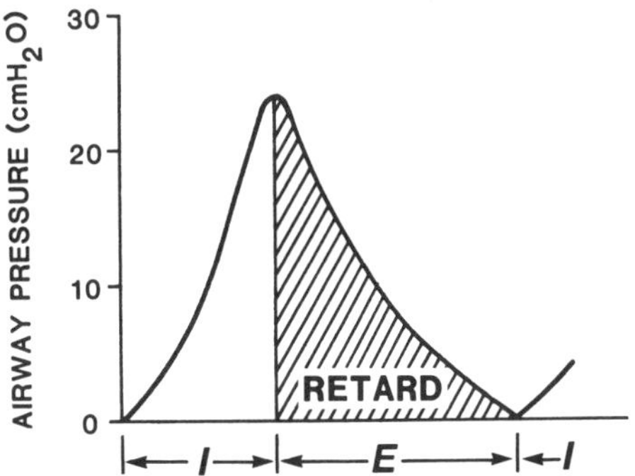

Figure 33-2. Schematic diagram of airway pressures during the inspiratory phase (I) and expiratory phase (E) of a mechanically delivered breath. The exhalation valve is depressurized slowly so as to "retard" or slow the rate at which airway pressure decreases towards zero during E.

may require PEEP higher than 30 cmH_2O before improvement in arterial oxygenation is produced.

Hazards of Positive End-Expiratory Pressure. Hazards of PEEP include (1) decreased cardiac output, (2) pulmonary barotrauma, (3) increased extravascular lung water, and (4) redistribution of pulmonary blood flow.

The decrease in cardiac output produced by PEEP is due to interference with venous return and a leftward displacement of the cardiac ventricular septum that restricts filling of the left ventricle. It is conceivable that improvements in PaO_2 produced by PEEP could be offset by decreases in cardiac output. The potential for PEEP to decrease cardiac output is exaggerated in the presence of decreased intravascular fluid volume or normal lungs, which permit maximal transmission of increased airway pressures. A pulmonary artery catheter is helpful in guiding fluid replacement and for monitoring the impact of PEEP on cardiac output. Levels of PEEP higher than 10 cmH_2O can interfere with the interpretation of the pulmonary artery occlusion pressure as a monitor of left atrial pressure. This reflects transmission of intra-alveolar pressure to the pulmonary capillaries, which is then measured as the pulmonary artery occlusion pressure.

Pneumothorax, pneumomediastinum, and subcutaneous emphysema are examples of barotrauma due to overdistension of alveoli by PEEP. An abrupt deterioration of PaO_2 and cardiovascular function during PEEP should arouse suspicion of pulmonary barotrauma, especially pneumothorax. Increased intravascular lung water associated with PEEP may reflect obstruction to pulmonary lymph flow as well as alterations in permeability characteristics of the pulmonary capillaries.

The adverse effects of PEEP on distribution of pulmonary blood flow are complex but presumably reflect, in part, overdistension of alveoli. When overdistension of alveoli occurs, pulmonary blood flow is likely to be shunted to areas with less resistance to flow, such as less distended or even collapsed alveoli. The net effect of this alveolar overdistension is increased ventilation-to-perfusion mismatching, manifesting as a decrease in PaO_2.

Monitoring of Treatment

Monitoring of treatment for ARDS depends on evaluation of pulmonary gas exchange and cardiac function. Measurements of arterial and venous blood gases, pH, cardiac output, cardiac filling pressures, and intrapulmonary shunt and calculation of systemic and pulmonary vascular resistance are used to monitor the adequacy of treatment for ARDS. A pulmonary artery catheter is useful for making many of the measurements and calculations.

Arterial Oxygenation

The adequacy of treatment for ARDS that is directed toward relieving arterial hypoxemia is reflected by the PaO_2 (normal 60 to 100 mmHg). The efficiency of the exchange of oxygen across the capillary membrane is reflected by the difference between the calculated alveolar partial pressure of oxygen (PAO_2) and the measured PaO_2. Calculation of the alveolar-to-arterial difference for oxygen ($A\text{-}aDO_2$) when patients are breathing oxygen provides an estimate of the magnitude of right-to-left intrapulmonary shunting of blood (see Chapter 16). One of the difficulties with the use of the $A\text{-}aDO_2$ is that the normal range changes with variations in the inhaled concentrations of oxygen. With this in mind, a more useful calculation may be the ratio of the PaO_2 to PAO2, which is less influenced by the inhaled concentrations of oxygen (see Chapter 16).

Ventilation

The adequacy of alveolar ventilation during treatment of ARDS is monitored by measurement of the $PaCO_2$ (normal 36 to 44 mmHg). The efficiency of the transfer of carbon dioxide across the alveolar capillary membrane is reflected by the ratio of deadspace ventilation to tidal volume (VD/VT) (see Chapter 16). Normally, the VD/VT is less than 0.3, but it may increase to greater than 0.6 in patients with ARDS.

Tissue Oxygenation

The mixed venous partial pressure of oxygen ($P\bar{v}O_2$), as measured in blood obtained from the pulmonary artery, reflects tissue extraction of oxygen (see Chapter 16). A $P\bar{v}O_2$ lower than 30 mmHg indicates the need to increase cardiac output so as to ensure adequate tissue oxygenation.

Acidemia

Measurement of pH is necessary to detect metabolic or respiratory acidosis, or both, that commonly accompanies ARDS. For example, metabolic acidosis predictably accompanies arterial hypoxemia and inadequate delivery of oxygen to the tissues. Respiratory acidosis reflects alveolar hypoventilation and the resulting acute increase of the $PaCO_2$. Cardiac dysrhythmias, increased pulmonary vascular resistance, and decreased responsiveness to catecholamines are adverse effects of acidosis.

Cardiac Output and Filling Pressures

Measurement and maintenance of a normal cardiac output (higher than 2.5 $L \cdot min^{-1} \cdot m^{-2}$) are essential for ensuring adequate delivery of oxygen to tissues during treatment of ARDS. Cardiac output is most frequently measured by the thermodilution technique with a pulmonary artery catheter. Measurement of left and right atrial filling pressures combined with the value for cardiac output permits construction of ventricular function curves for use in guiding fluid administration and drug therapy. Likewise, systemic and pulmonary vascular resistance can be calculated using appropriate pressure measurements and the cardiac output.

Guidelines that Suggest the Likelihood of Successful Cessation of Mechanical Ventilation of the Lungs

Vital capacity >15 $ml \cdot kg^{-1}$
Alveolar-to-arterial difference for oxygen <350 mmHg breathing 100% oxygen
Arterial-to-alveolar PO_2 ratio >0.75
PaO_2 >60 mmHg
pHa >7.3
$PaCO_2$ <50 mmHg
Maximum inspiratory pressure greater than −20 cmH_2O
Deadspace-to-tidal volume ratio <0.6
Conscious and oriented
Stable cardiac function
Optimal intravascular fluid volume and electrolyte status
Absence of infection
Good nutritional status

Cessation of Mechanical Support of Ventilation

Cessation of mechanical support of ventilation of the lungs in patients being treated for ARDS can be considered in the presence of (1) measurements that are compatible with spontaneous ventilation, (2) cardiovascular stability, and (3) a favorable clinical impression of the patient's condition. Weaning can be considered to occur in three stages: cessation of mechanical inflation of the lungs, followed by removal of the tracheal tube, and finally by elimination of the need for supplemental oxygen.

Cessation of Mechanical Inflation of the Lungs

Guidelines that suggest the likely success of weaning include serial measurements and calculations of several parameters. Ultimately, the decision to attempt weaning must be individualized, considering not only the status of pulmonary function but also the co-existence of other organ system abnormalities.

T-tube and IMV are the two methods used in weaning patients from mechanical support of ventilation of the lungs.

T-Tube. T-tube weaning is initiated by connecting the tube in the patient's trachea to a device (T-tube) through which humidified and oxygen-enriched gases are delivered. In addition, 2.5 to 5 cmH_2O of continuous positive airway pressure (CPAP) is often delivered via the T-tube to the airway. The use of CPAP prevents the decrease in FRC associated with cessation of positive pressure ventilation of the lungs.[5] Indeed, incompetence of the glottic opening produced by the presence of a tracheal tube seems to interfere with the maintenance of a normal FRC. Initially, the patient is allowed to breathe spontaneously for 5 to 10 minutes each hour. Tachycardia, tachypnea (more than 35 $breaths \cdot min^{-1}$), or alterations in the level of consciousness during the brief period of spontaneous ventilation confirm that weaning has been premature and mechanical support of ventilation is immediately reinstituted. When pulmonary function has recovered to the extent that weaning is appropriate, it will be possible to lengthen gradually the periods of spontaneous ventilation to 2 hours or longer.

Intermittent Mandatory Ventilation. Periodic mechanical inflation of the lungs during periods of spontaneous ventilation is described as IMV. The intermittent mechanical breath can be provided as a mandatory breath at a preset interval (nonsynchronous) or as a synchronized breath (SIMV) initiated by the spontaneous ventilatory effort of the patient. There is no evidence to substantiate any advantage of SIMV over IMV.

Weaning by IMV is initiated by gradually decreasing the number of mechanical breaths delivered each minute. Ideally, the IMV rate is sequentially decreased as long as the $PaCO_2$ remains near the patient's normal level, the pH is 7.36 to 7.44, and tachypnea is absent.

Removal of the Tracheal Tube

Extubation of the trachea should be considered when the patient tolerates 2 hours of spontaneous ventilation during T-tube weaning or an IMV rate of 1 to 2 breaths·min^{-1} without deterioration of (1) arterial blood gases, (2) pH, (3) consciousness, or (4) cardiac status. In addition, the patient should have active laryngeal reflexes and the ability to generate an effective cough so as to clear secretions from the airway.

Elimination of the Need for Supplemental Oxygen

Supplemental inhaled oxygen is often needed for a time despite recovery from ARDS sufficient to permit spontaneous ventilation. This need for supplemental oxygen most likely reflects persistence of ventilation-to-perfusion mismatching. Weaning from supplemental oxygen is accomplished by the gradual decrease in the inhaled concentration of oxygen, as guided by monitoring the PaO_2. It is probably not necessary to increase the PaO_2 to higher than 60 mmHg using supplemental inhaled oxygen. Furthermore, a PaO_2 higher than 60 mmHg can eliminate the hypoxic stimulus to ventilation in patients with chronic obstructive pulmonary disease associated with chronic carbon dioxide retention. This loss of hypoxic stimulation of ventilation in these patients could result in unacceptable hypercarbia despite an acceptable level of oxygenation.

CONGESTIVE HEART FAILURE

Congestive heart failure characterized by decreased cardiac output requires pharmacologic treatment with inotropic or vasodilator drugs, or both, guided by information obtained from a pulmonary artery catheter. Drug-induced increases in cardiac output are reflected as decreases in atrial filling pressures, improved arterial oxygenation, and increased $P\bar{v}O_2$.

Treatment

The present trend in the pharmacologic treatment of congestive heart failure is to optimize cardiac output by manipulating the peripheral circulation with a vasodilator (Table 33-2). Vasodilators increase cardiac output by decreasing impedance to the forward ejection of left ventricular stroke volume. Decreases in systemic blood pressure with associated decreases in coronary perfusion pressure, however, limit the usefulness of vasodilator therapy of congestive heart failure. Maintenance of an optimal intravascular fluid volume as guided by cardiac filling pressures will minimize decreases in blood pressure as produced by nitroprusside or nitroglycerin. Nitroglycerin is an alternative to nitroprusside and is particularly useful in patients with coronary artery disease, as it selectively redistributes coronary blood flow to subendocardial areas. Inotropic drugs (dopamine, dobutamine, epinephrine) that improve cardiac output by increasing myocardial contractility are reserved for treatment of congestive heart failure when afterload reduction with vasodilators yields less than optimal results.

Table 33-2. Vasodilator Therapy of Congestive Heart Failure

	Effect on Venous System	Effect on Arterial System	Usual Dose and Route
Nitroprusside	+++	+++	0.5–5 μg·kg^{-1}·min^{-1} IV
Nitroglycerin	+++	+	0.5–5 μg·kg^{-1}·min^{-1} IV
Hydralazine	0	+++	25–100 mg PO
Captopril	++	+++	25–75 mg PO

Intra-aortic Balloon Counterpulsation

Intra-aortic balloon counterpulsation may be helpful in some patients who develop cardiogenic shock after a myocardial infarction. The intra-aortic balloon is programmed to the electrocardiogram so as to deflate just before systole and to inflate during diastole. The presystolic deflation of the balloon diminishes systemic blood pressure and afterload, which decreases cardiac work and myocardial oxygen requirements. Inflation of the balloon during diastole increases diastolic blood pressure and thus improves coronary blood flow and myocardial oxygen delivery.

SEPSIS

Hospital-acquired (nosocomial) infections are an important cause of death of patients in an ICU. Common sources of infections in critically ill patients include the urinary tract, surgical wounds, pneumonia, intravascular devices, and sinusitis. Pneumonia is the leading cause of mortality from infections. Sinusitis may be an unexplained cause of fever, especially if a nasotracheal tube is in place.

Septic Shock

The presence of septic shock is suggested by the development of hypotension (systolic blood pressure lower than 90 mmHg) in the presence of peripheral vasodilation and oliguria. This diagnosis should be particularly suspected if these symptoms occur following operations or instrumentation of the genitourinary tract. Changes in the state of consciousness, including confusion and disorientation, can occur as manifestations of gram-negative bacteremia. Measurement of cardiac output and calculation of systemic vascular resistance are helpful in confirming the diagnosis in the early phase. A positive blood culture is diagnostic but is not always present.

Treatment

Septic shock is treated with intravenous antibiotics and repletion of intravascular fluid volume. Antibiotics should be started immediately after the drawing of blood for culture and sensitivity. Most often, two antibiotics are selected, with one (clindamycin) effective against gram-positive bacteria and the other (aminoglycoside derivative) effective against gram-negative bacteria. Antibiotics can be changed if necessary following the results of the blood culture. Immunologic therapy of septic shock with a human monoclonal antibody that binds to the lipid portion of the endotoxin may improve survival of patients with gram-negative sepsis. Fluid replacement must be aggressive and guided by measurement of right or left atrial filling pressures, or both, and urine output. Dopamine is an effective inotrope when pharmacologic support of both cardiac output and renal function is necessary. Administration of large doses of corticosteroids has not been shown to be beneficial in the treatment of septic shock.[6]

Surgical intervention may be necessary to treat the source of bacteremia. No anesthetic drug has been shown to be ideal in the presence of septic shock. Nevertheless, ketamine would seem an acceptable drug for induction of anesthesia in patients requiring emergency surgery in the presence of hypotension due to bacteremia.

HEAD INJURY

Brain damage resulting from head injury is the leading cause of death among individuals younger than 24 years of age.[7] The hallmark of closed head injury is a loss of consciousness. Computed tomography should be performed as the most important diagnostic test (evidence of increased intracranial pressure [ICP], subdural hematoma, epidural hematoma) and the level of consciousness classified according to the Glasgow Coma Scale (Table 33-1). Patients with a score of 8 or less by definition are in a coma, and about 50% of these patients die or remain in a vegetative state.

Critical care of the head-injured patient is based on the recognition and treatment of hazardous increases of ICP. Interventions designed to provide cerebral protection and resuscitation have been most successful in patients who experience head injury. Institution of deliberate hyperventilation of the lungs plus administration of diuretics and corticosteroids are the recommended initial interventions to decrease ICP. Administration of barbiturates is recommended when the ICP remains increased despite traditional therapy.

Intracranial Pressure

A catheter placed through a burr hole into a cerebral ventricle or a transducer placed on the surface of the brain is used to monitor ICP. High-risk patients, including those with head injury (comatose, cerebral edema on computed tomography), large brain tumors, cerebral aneurysms, and hydrocephalus, should probably have their ICP monitored.[7] A normal ICP pressure wave is pulsatile and varies with the cardiac impulse and breathing. The mean ICP should remain lower than 15 mmHg. An abrupt increase in the ICP observed during continuous monitoring is known as a plateau wave (Fig. 33-3). Painful stimulation in an otherwise unresponsive patient can initiate a plateau wave. Hence, the liberal use of analgesics to avoid pain is indicated even in unresponsive patients.

Treatment

Methods to decrease ICP include posture; deliberate hyperventilation; administration of osmotic or renal tubular diuretics (or both), corticosteroids, and barbiturates; and institution of cerebrospinal fluid drainage. A frequent recommendation is to treat sustained increases of ICP higher than 20 mmHg. Treatment may be indicated when ICP is lower than 20 mmHg if the appearance of an occasional plateau wave suggests a low intracranial compliance.

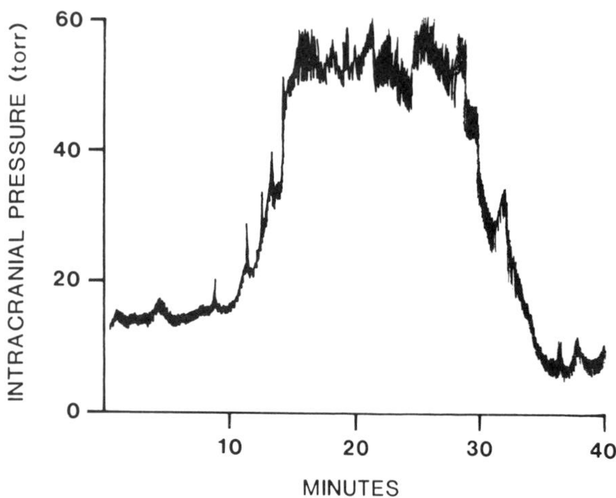

Figure 33-3. Schematic diagram of a plateau wave characterized by an abrupt and sustained (10 to 20 minutes) increase in intracranial pressure followed by a rapid decrease in intracranial pressure, often to a level lower than that present before the onset of the plateau wave.

Posture. Elevation of the head to about 30 degrees is useful in the care of head-injured patients to encourage venous outflow from the brain and thus lower ICP. It should also be appreciated that extreme flexion or rotation of the head can obstruct the jugular veins and restrict venous outflow from the brain. The head-down position as used to place central catheters via the external or internal jugular vein must be avoided, since this position can markedly increase ICP.

Hyperventilation. Deliberate hyperventilation of the adult patient's lungs to a $PaCO_2$ between 25 to 30 mmHg is an effective and rapid method to decrease ICP. Further decreases in the $PaCO_2$ in previously normocapnic patients do not provide additional benefits, and excessive alkalosis might result in cerebral ischemia. Presumably, beneficial effects of hyperventilation of the lungs on ICP reflect decreased cerebral blood flow and resulting decreases in intracranial blood volume. Children have higher cerebral blood flows than adults and are treated with more aggressive hyperventilation of the lungs to lower the $PaCO_2$ to between 20 and 25 mmHg. The duration of the efficacy of hyperventilation for decreasing ICP is unknown. In volunteers, however, the effect of hyperventilation wanes with time, as evidenced by a return of cerebral blood flow to normal after about 6 hours.[8] Furthermore, if the cerebral vessels are damaged (trauma) or diseased (tumor), their reactivity may be diminished.

Osmotic Diuretics. Administration of hyperosmotic drugs, such as mannitol (0.25 to 1 $g \cdot kg^{-1}$ IV over 15 to 30 minutes) decreases ICP by producing a transient increase in the osmolarity of plasma, which acts to draw water from tissues, including the brain. However, if the blood-brain barrier is disrupted, mannitol may pass into the brain and cause cerebral edema by drawing water into the brain. The duration of the hyperosmotic effect of mannitol is about 6 hours. It is important to note that mannitol is not associated with a high incidence of rebound increase in ICP after this time. The brain eventually adapts to sustained increases in plasma osmolarity such that chronic use of hyperosmotic drugs is likely to become less effective.

Diuresis induced by mannitol may result in acute hypovolemia and adverse electrolyte changes (hypokalemia, hyponatremia), emphasizing the need to replace intravascular fluid volume with infusions of crystalloid and colloid solutions. A rule of thumb is to replace urine output with an equivalent volume of crystalloids, most often lactated Ringer's solution. Glucose and water solutions are not recommended, because they are rapidly distributed in total body water, including the brain. If the blood glucose concentration decreases more rapidly than brain glucose, the brain water becomes relatively hyperosmolar, and water enters the central nervous system and exaggerates existing cerebral edema.

Tubular Diuretics. Rapid administration of furosemide (0.5 to 1 mg·kg^{-1} IV) is particularly useful in lowering an increased ICP that is associated with increased intravascular fluid volume.

Corticosteroids. Corticosteroids such as dexamethasone or methylprednisolone are effective in decreasing ICP. The mechanism for the beneficial effect of corticosteroids is not known but may involve stabilization of capillary membranes or decreases in the production of cerebrospinal fluid, or both.

Barbiturates. Administration of barbiturates may be recommended when the ICP remains increased despite deliberate hyperventilation of the lungs, drug-induced diuresis, and administration of corticosteroids. This recommendation is based on the predictable ability of these drugs to decrease ICP, presumably by decreasing cerebral blood volume secondary to cerebral vascular vasoconstriction and decreased cerebral blood flow. The goal of barbiturate therapy is to maintain the ICP lower than 20 mmHg without the occurrence of plateau waves. Discontinuation of the barbiturate infusion can be considered when the ICP has remained in a normal range for 48 hours. Failure of barbiturates to decrease the ICP is a grave prognostic sign. Even when barbiturates are effective, the overall morbidity and mortality in head-injured patients has not been shown to be improved by the use of these drugs compared with that of patients treated aggressively with deliberate hyperventilation of the lungs, drug-induced diuresis, and administration of corticosteroids.[9]

A hazard of barbiturate therapy as used to lower the ICP is hypotension, which can jeopardize the maintenance of an adequate cerebral perfusion pressure. Such hypotension is particularly likely in the presence of decreased intravascular fluid volume. Dopamine or dobutamine may be necessary if barbiturate-induced hypotension due to myocardial depression occurs.

ACUTE RENAL FAILURE

The best treatment of acute renal failure is prevention by maintenance of an optimal intravascular fluid volume and cardiac output (see Chapter 21). A pulmonary artery catheter is helpful in achieving these goals. A relative fluid overload, resulting in pulmonary edema, may be necessary to prevent oliguria and the risks of acute renal failure. Treatable iatrogenic pulmonary edema is an acceptable complication if the fluids responsible for this adverse response help prevent oliguric renal failure. When acute renal tubular necrosis develops, however, the only treatment is hemodialysis.

ACUTE HEPATIC FAILURE

Regardless of the etiology, acute hepatic failure is associated with a poor prognosis. Hyperventilation is a constant feature of early hepatic failure and most likely reflects stimulation of ventilation by ammonia. Hypoglycemia is common. Cardiac output tends to be increased, reflecting decreased systemic vascular resistance and increased arteriovenous shunting. Most patients with acute hepatic failure develop a bleeding diathesis resembling disseminated intravascular coagulation. Renal failure, arterial hypoxemia, hypotension, and hepatic encephalopathy accompanied by increased ICP are frequent terminal events. Treatment of acute hepatic failure is symptomatic and supportive, including the use of neomycin or lactulose, or both, to decrease the production of ammonia.

MALNUTRITION

Critically ill patients often experience malnutrition (negative caloric intake) complicated by hypermetabolic states due to increased caloric needs produced by trauma (multiple fractures increase energy about 25% and burns by as much as 100%), fever (every degree Celsius increases energy needs by about 15%), sepsis, and wound healing. Malnutrition is

Complications Associated with Total Parenteral Nutrition

Hyperglycemia
Hypoglycemia
Hyperchloremic metabolic acidosis
Increased carbon dioxide production
Electrolyte abnormalities
Catheter-related sepsis

treated by enteral nutrition (tube feedings) or total parenteral nutrition (usually delivered through a catheter placed in the subclavian vein). Potential complications of total parenteral nutrition are numerous (see Chapter 22).

REFERENCES

1. DeCamp MM, Demling RH. Posttraumatic multisystem organ failure. JAMA 1988;260:530–4.
2. Trunkey D. Initial treatment of patients with extensive trauma. N Engl J Med 1991;324:1259–63.
3. Hastings RH, Marks JD. Airway management for trauma patients with potential cervical spine injuries. Anesth Analg 1991;73:471–82.
4. Rossaint R, Falke KJ, Lopez F, Slama K, Pison U, Zapol WM. Inhaled nitric oxide for the adult respiratory distress syndrome. N Engl J Med 1993;328:399–405.
5. Annest SJ, Gottlieb M, Paloski WH, et al. Detrimental effects of removing end-expiratory pressure prior to endotracheal extubation. Ann Surg 1980;191:539–45.
6. Bone RC, Fisher CJ, Clemmer TP, et al. A controlled clinical trial of high-dose methylprednisolone in the treatment of severe sepsis and septic shock. N Engl J Med 1987;317:653–8.
7. White RJ, Likavec MJ. The diagnosis and initial management of head injury. N Engl J Med 1992;327:1507–11.
8. Raichle ME, Posner JB, Plum F. Cerebral blood flow during and after hyperventilation. Arch Neurol 1970;23:394–403.
9. Miller JD. Barbiturates and raised intracranial pressure. Ann Neurol 1979;6:189–93.

34

Chronic Pain Management

Ironically, chronic pain, which is one of the most common symptoms in medicine, remains difficult to treat and poorly understood.[1] Although cardiovascular disease and cancer are dramatic and life-threatening diseases, chronic pain can be the cause of months or years of discomfort with a resultant poor quality of life. Furthermore, chronic pain has the potential of interfering with an individual's livelihood and interaction with family members and colleagues. Although accurate statistics have not been accumulated, chronic pain probably costs society millions of dollars in medical services and loss of work productivity. Often patients are exposed to a high risk of iatrogenic complications from improper therapy, including opioid addiction and multiple and often unsuccessful surgical procedures.

Chronic pain may last weeks to years and persist in the absence of noxious stimulation that activates nociceptors. For example, psychological aspects of chronic pain can alter sensitivity to somatic stimuli. Complex central nervous system mechanisms such as memory may be required to sustain chronic pain. Autonomic nervous system dysfunction may accompany chronic pain disorders. The large number of therapeutic approaches available for the management of the patient with chronic pain is reflected by the establishment of pain clinics and recognition of pain management as a subspecialty of the practice of anesthesiology (see Chapter 1).

ROLE OF THE ANESTHESIOLOGIST IN THE DIAGNOSIS AND TREATMENT OF CHRONIC PAIN

Depending on the level of commitment, an anesthesiologist may be a full-time member of a pain clinic or, at the other extreme, may provide occasional diagnostic and therapeutic nerve blocks in the role of a consultant.

Pain Clinic

A pain clinic consists of a group of physicians from different specialties, including anesthesiology, who interact to solve the problem of chronic pain by evaluating the nociceptive and psychological aspects of the problem. Anesthesiologists are frequently directors of pain clinics. Patients are usually referred to the pain clinic by their primary physician. Comprehensive records should be collected that document the activities and pain levels of the patient. After arriving at the pain clinic, patients undergo medical and psychological examinations and evaluation by a social worker, who documents significant social problems. After this information has been collected, the multidisciplinary pain clinic physicians discuss the case and arrive at a diagnosis of the most likely origin of the pain. A decision is then reached as to what further evaluation or treatment is necessary, such as drug detoxification if drug dependency exists, referral to an orthopaedic or neurosurgical physician if neural deficits are pre-

Treatment Modalities for Management of Chronic Pain

Orally administered drugs (alternatively transdermal or transmucosal)
- Opioids (especially cancer pain)
- Nonsteroidal anti-inflammatory drugs
- Antidepressants
- Antipsychotics
- Anticonvulsants
- Alpha-2 agonists

Diagnostic and therapeutic nerve blocks (local anesthetics, neurolytics)
- Spinal block
- Epidural block
- Stellate ganglion block
- Brachial plexus block
- Intercostal nerve block
- Intravenous regional neural block
- Lumbar sympathetic block
- Celiac plexus block

Neuraxial (subarachnoid, epidural) opioids

Surgery (especially refractory chronic pain)
- Cordotomy
- Dorsal rhizotomy
- Neurostimulators (dorsal column, deep brain)

Transcutaneous electrical nerve stimulation

Biofeedback

Physical therapy

sent, or performance of a nerve block by an anesthesiologist. Patients in a multidisciplinary pain clinic may receive several treatment approaches simultaneously, which places emphasis on the value of participation of physicians from different medical specialties.

Consultant

The anesthesiologist whose primary commitment is in areas other than the diagnosis and treatment of chronic pain may be asked to perform diagnostic or therapeutic nerve blocks. Of prime importance is that the anesthesiologist recognize personal limitations. Expertise in performing a diagnostic or therapeutic nerve block does not imply an equivalent amount of expertise in the overall evaluation of chronic pain. For example, has a patient with chronic back pain undergone complete evaluation before the epidural injection of corticosteroids? Has a spinal cord tumor been ruled out? Diagnostic and therapeutic nerve blocks should only be performed after a thorough medical evaluation has been performed to ensure that an important disease process is not being overlooked.

APPROACH TO THE PATIENT WITH CHRONIC PAIN

The anesthesiologist's initial patient contact is an interview to determine whether a nerve block or other pain-removing procedure will be helpful in the diagnosis or treatment of chronic pain. The interview should be constructed to answer several types of questions. Certain guidelines indicate how satisfied a patient may be if the pain were removed. Patients who are socially happy with adequate family support may continue their occupation despite the pain. The same patients who are unhappy taking analgesics and who have had pain for several months, rather than years, are more likely to be motivated to want to remove their pain.

Psychological Tests

Chronic pain is often accompanied by psychological changes that may, with time, become more disabling than the somatic pain. Psychological testing such as the Minnesota Multiphasic Personality Inventory is helpful for detecting psychopathology that may initiate or aggravate pain complaints and for determining the psychological impact of chronic pain. Despite sophisticated psychological testing, the clinician must resist the temptation to label patients with chronic pain as malingerers. Patients with chronic

Psychological Aspects of Chronic Pain

- Mental depression
- Insomnia
- Avoidance of social and vocational obligations
- Dependence on analgesics
- Visits to multiple physicians

pain are often despairing, demoralized, and worried and are sometimes hostile. Neurotic behavior is a normal response to chronic pain. In fact, one may become suspicious of a patient who has chronic debilitating pain and yet appears to be a happy, well-adjusted individual. Patients should not be excluded from treatment because of their personality profiles. Neurotic patients are entitled to the same pain relief as "normal" patients.

Measurement of Pain

Although several methods of measuring pain exist, the "pain estimate" is probably the most useful method for the clinician who occasionally performs diagnostic or therapeutic nerve blocks. With the pain estimate, the patient assigns a number to the intensity of the pain. The patient is asked to rank the pain on a visual analog scale of 0 to 10 where "zero" refers to no pain and "10" refers to pain so severe that suicide may be considered. Several numbers may be assigned each day; for example, one number might be the average pain per day and another number might be the worse pain. Patients can record these numbers before and after a nerve block to assess the magnitude and duration of pain relief.

Physical Examination

A routine physical examination should be performed, with special emphasis on a thorough neurologic examination. In addition, the following areas require special attention during the physical examination.

Map Out the Painful Area

If the area is not too tender, the painful area can be outlined with a felt-tipped pen. If possible, the painful area should be identified according to the peripheral nerve or dermatome areas (see Fig. 12-3).

Skin

The characteristics of the skin often provide a clue to sympathetic nervous system function. Warm, dry, smooth skin with coarse hair is evidence of vasodilation. Vasoconstricted skin is blanched, clammy, cool, thin, and glistening, with thin or sparse hair.

Muscle and Joint

Evidence of guarding, wasting, deformity, swelling, and temperature changes should be noted and will give a clue to how active a painful area has been. For example, a muscular hand and arm with a preliminary diagnosis of causalgia should be highly suspect because the evidence is that the patient has been using that arm extensively.

Maneuvers that Alter Pain

An assessment of maneuvers that relieve and cause the pain may include locally applied pressure (especially on a trigger point), leg raising to elicit lumbar root irritation, and changes in temperature.

DIAGNOSTIC NERVE BLOCKS

Diagnostic nerve blocks can be used to (1) anatomically define the pain pathway, (2) differentiate pharmacologically the size of the fibers that mediate the pain, (3) differentiate central pain from peripheral pain, and (4) determine whether a neurolytic block or surgical resection of a nerve should be performed. If a specific pathway of pain can be localized, a neurolytic nerve block might be considered. Furthermore, the diagnostic block allows the patient to undergo a "trial run" without permanent change. Sometime, the numbness or lack of sensation is more unpleasant for the patient than is the pain itself. Also, by using different concentrations of local anesthetics, the size of the nerve fiber mediating the pain can be better defined (small-diameter sympathetic nerve fibers versus larger somatic nerve fibers).

Nerve blocks can sometimes be used to detect drug addiction. If a patient with chronic pain still requires a normal dose of opioid during the effective period of a successful nerve block, addiction should be suspected.

Placebo

Placebo injection is the administration of a solution without known analgesic action. For example, a small amount of saline may be injected rather than a local anesthetic for a diagnostic nerve block. An inexperienced clinician might assume that a patient does not have an organic basis for pain if a placebo relieves the discomfort. A placebo, however, may relieve pain (often very transiently) 30% to 40% of the time in any one patient.[2] Therefore, a patient may have an organic basis for pain but still achieve partial relief from a placebo injection.

Differential Nerve Block

Because fiber size is an important factor that governs susceptibility of a nerve to be blocked by local anesthetics, differential nerve blocks can be used to distinguish placebo, sympathetic, and somatic sensory sources of pain. The most commonly used differential nerve block is a graduated spinal anesthetic technique.[3] After a lumbar subarachnoid puncture is performed, the following solutions are injected in a four-step procedure:

1. Seven milliliters of "artificial cerebrospinal fluid" with no preservatives (placebo)
2. Seven milliliters of 0.2% procaine (sympathetic nerve blockade)
3. Seven milliliters of 0.5% procaine (sensory blockade)
4. Seven milliliters of 1.0% procaine (motor blockade)

Pain is judged to be psychogenic if relief occurs with the placebo injection. If relief occurs with a 0.2% procaine injection, a sympathetic nervous system pathway of transmission is usually assigned as the cause. If pain persists after 1.0% procaine has been administered, a more central origin or psychogenic pain should be considered.

Unfortunately, the differential spinal anesthetic approach has many drawbacks. A patient cannot move during a differential spinal anesthetic to perform the maneuvers that elicit the pain. Insertion of an epidural catheter may provide more flexibility in this regard. Also, the placebo may itself cause transient relief of pain of an organic basis. Hypotonic solutions injected into the cerebrospinal fluid have been known to result in blockade of pain conduction. Thus, a slow withdrawal of cerebrospinal fluid and then reinjection 5 minutes later is a preferable technique. Also, it is assumed that 0.2% procaine only blocks sympathetic nerves without sensory involvement. Although the dominant block probably is sympathetic, sensory fibers are undoubtedly blocked to a limited extent. Thus, if a sympathetic nervous system origin for the pain is suspected, a more specific stellate ganglion or lumbar sympathetic block can be performed (see Chapter 13).

THERAPEUTIC NERVE BLOCKS

Therapeutic nerve blocks may be performed with local anesthetics, neurolytics, or neuraxial placement of opioids.

Local Anesthetics

Although nerve blocks with local anesthetics can be very valuable diagnostically, they also can be used in a therapeutic manner in patients with chronic pain. For example, reflex sympathetic dystrophy and myofascial pain can be interrupted with local anesthetics. A temporary local anesthetic-induced nerve block may allow physical therapy to be performed in areas that are normally painful. The inflammatory response can be decreased by a local anesthetic nerve block, usually in combination with a corticosteroid injection. Occasionally, chronic pain can be relieved with one or more local anesthetic nerve blocks on a prolonged or even a permanent basis; however, these situations are very rare. By performing a sympathetic nerve block with a local anesthetic, the vascular supply in an ischemic area in patients with vascular disease can be improved.

Neurolytic Block

In patients with persistent chronic pain, nerve destruction with neurolytics such as alcohol or phenol may be useful. The use of alcohol or phenol probably should be restricted to anesthesiologists with special expertise and experience in the injection of these substances. Furthermore, the use of neurolytics usually is indicated only in patients with short life expectancy, such as those with pain from terminal cancer. The use of alcohol or phenol on peripheral nerves can be followed by the appearance of a denervation hypersensitivity type of pain, which may be worse than the original pain. For this reason, injection of alcohol and phenol probably should be restricted to the epidural or subarachnoid spaces. There is little difference in the efficacy between alcohol and phenol, although initial responses are very different (Table 34-1). For example, alcohol causes intense pain on injection and

Table 34-1. Characteristics of Drugs Used for Neurolytic Block

Alcohol	Phenol
Pain with injection	No pain with injection
Prompt neurolysis	Delayed onset of neurolysis
Hypobaric	Hyperbaric

produces neurolysis promptly. By contrast, phenol in glycerin produces no pain on injection but requires about 15 minutes to produce its neurolytic effects. It must be recognized that when used for intrathecal neurolysis, alcohol is hypobaric (it must be injected with the patient positioned so the affected sensory roots are uppermost) and phenol is hyperbaric. Patient movement during or shortly after the injection can result in unwanted spread of the neurolytic solutions. Indeed, the principal disadvantage of neurolytic nerve blocks is the difficulty in preventing the spread of destructive effects to surrounding normal tissues or impairment of bowel and bladder activity. For somatic nerve blocks, 100% alcohol is used. Blockade of small-diameter sympathetic nerve fibers is done with 50% alcohol. Phenol is used in concentrations ranging from 5% to 20% for peripheral nerves.

One problem with neurolytics is that alcohol or phenol rarely produces an analgesic state as intense as did the diagnostic local anesthetic block. Therefore, patients are frequently disappointed that the neurolytic block has not produced as much pain relief as did the diagnostic local anesthetic block. The patient should therefore be cautioned about the effectiveness of a neurolytic block. Furthermore, "permanent" neurolytic blocks are really not permanent, and recovery of sensation of pain occurs in a matter of weeks or months, emphasizing their usefulness in patients with a short life expectancy.

Neuraxial Opioids

Chronic pain, especially pain due to cancer, is effectively managed by neuraxial (subarachnoid or epidural) administration of opioids, most often morphine. Effectiveness of neuraxial opioids reflects the presence of opioid receptors in the substantia gelatinosa of the spinal cord. Advantages of neuraxial opioids for relief of pain include prolonged duration of action and absence of sympathetic nervous system blockade or skeletal muscle paralysis. Delayed depression of ventilation (6 to 12 hours after neuraxial administration) and other side effects of neuraxial opioids (pruritus, sedation, urinary retention, nausea, and vomiting) are less likely to occur after administration of neuraxial opioids for the treatment of cancer pain than when this approach is used to treat acute postoperative pain in patients who are not tolerant to opioids (see Chapter 32). Because the duration of pain relief is usually shorter than 36 hours, it is unrealistic to expect to repeat subarachnoid or epidural injections for prolonged periods. As a result, long-term subarachnoid or epidural catheters may be implanted surgically or percutaneously.[4] These catheters can remain indefinitely. In this regard, the use of an implanted infusion device, which consists of a percutaneously refillable reservoir for the opioid and a mechanism for pumping the drug from the reservoir through the catheter in the subarachnoid or epidural space, may be useful.[4] More than 50% of patients who receive these catheters experience excellent pain relief.[5] In 5% to 12% of patients, technical problems with the catheter (leakage, occlusion, infection) occur.[5] In about 10% of patients, injection of morphine causes pain, which may be attenuated by prior administration of a local anesthetic such as lidocaine. Tolerance to opioids develops in about 2% of patients. Abrupt discontinuation of chronic neuraxial opioid infusions may be followed by an opioid withdrawal syndrome.

EVALUATION OF A NERVE BLOCK

Evaluation of a patient's physiologic and psychological responses to a nerve block is often more difficult than the technical procedure required to produce the block. It is incorrect to assume that if the diagnostic block relieves the pain, a neurolytic block or a surgical resection certainly will be successful. For instance, local anesthetic blocks frequently produce a more intense relief of pain than neurolytics. Furthermore, if a surgical procedure is performed, the pain may return, because of either regeneration of the nerve or a denervation hypersensitivity type of reaction. Also, even though diagnostic nerve blocks allow the patient to experience the numbness and side effects that could be permanent from nerve ablation techniques, they are not always accurate predictors of long-term pain relief. In this regard, diagnostic nerve blocks provide little help in evaluating the influence of pain relief on psychological factors, such as family interactions and financial gain (litigation).

Evaluation of results from therapeutic nerve blocks requires more thorough questioning than "Is your pain gone?" For example, the frequency and intensity of the pain should be recorded, including the number of hours in bed and the number of hours spent standing and reclining daily. Patients should record their estimate of their ability to walk, bend, and work. The number of activities (making the bed, washing the car) that can be performed before versus after a nerve block may be useful information. Furthermore, the influence on recreational and social activity should be documented. Perhaps most important, an accurate list of medications taken daily should be made. Only after this type of evaluation can the true effectiveness of a therapeutic nerve block be evaluated.

TRANSCUTANEOUS ELECTRICAL NERVE STIMULATION

Transcutaneous electrical nerve stimulation (TENS) is the patient-activated delivery of pulsed electrical current to skin overlying the painful area. Presumably, this electrical current activates large afferent fibers, resulting in stimulation of inhibitory dorsal horn neurons or release of endorphins, or both. As such, TENS acts by activating the descending inhibitory system for the prevention of the transmission of pain. This represents a clinical application of the gate theory of pain, which presumes that stimulation of A-beta fibers inhibits transmission (closes the gate for transmission) of pain impulses via A-delta and C fibers.[6] Biochemical mechanisms may also be involved, since TENS increases cerebrospinal fluid levels of substance P and 5-hydroxytryptamine. Achievement of the maximally comfortable paresthesia at the site of pain is necessary to produce effective analgesia. Stimulation may be applied continuously or for intermittent periods of about 30 minutes. TENS is most commonly used for persistent pain following back surgery, peripheral nerve injury, phantom limb pain, and sometimes postherpetic neuralgia.[7] Biofeedback is another example of an attempt to use the gate theory in the management of chronic pain syndromes.

ORAL DRUG THERAPY

The use of opioids for the treatment of chronic pain that is not associated with cancer is controversial. When opioids are administered to treat the terminally ill patient with cancer pain, it is important to maintain adequate and sustained blood levels of the analgesic. In this regard, the use of adequate doses administered at regular intervals (not as needed when pain reappears) is recommended.[7] Now many other classes of drugs are used either alone or in combination with opioids.[1] In the presence of bone pain (arthritis) or any condition that includes an inflammatory response, the administration of aspirin or an alternative nonsteroidal anti-inflammatory drug is useful. Furthermore, combining a low potency opioid with a nonsteroidal anti-inflammatory drug may enhance the analgesic effect of the opioid. Antidepressants (no evidence exists that any single drug is superior to another) are useful in the treatment of some chronic pain syndromes. Benefits of these drugs in patients with chronic pain syndromes include normalization of sleep patterns (drug-induced sedation), a decrease in anxiety, and a decrease in the patient's perception of pain. Analgesia produced by antidepressant drug therapy is probably a result of enhancement of neurotransmitters acting on descending efferent inhibitory pain pathways (see Fig. 32-2).[8] Antipsychotic drugs (haloperidol, droperidol, chlorpromazine) are useful for treatment of neuropathic pain and neuralgias such as trigeminal neuralgia and glossopharyngeal neuralgia.

COMMON PAIN PROBLEMS

Although the clinician should refer most chronic pain problems to physicians who are involved with pain clinics, there are a few pain problems that all anesthesiologists should be capable of managing, at least in the initial stages of diagnosis or treatment, or both.

Causalgia and Reflex Sympathetic Dystrophy

Causalgia occurs after nerve injury, whereas reflex sympathetic dystrophy typically follows a trivial injury without apparent neurologic damage. Often, however, these terms are used interchangeably. Both are accompanied by similar manifestations, which include chronic severe burning pain, localized sympathetic nervous system dysfunction, and atrophic changes. In addition, the pain is characterized as aching, intense, and/or agonizing and is usually enhanced by mechanical stimulation, movement, and application of heat or cold. Initially, vascular changes, probably resulting from altered sympathetic nervous system activity, lead to a warm, erythematous, dry, swollen extremity. Later, the extremity will be cool, pale, and/or cyanotic, and there will be atrophy of skin and skeletal muscles and decreased density of bones.

Manifestations of Reflex Sympathetic Dystrophy

- Severe burning pain
- Hyperalgesia
- Warm and erythematous skin followed by vasoconstriction and edema
- Bone demineralization
- Joint stiffness

The diagnosis is traditionally established and treatment initiated by performing a stellate ganglion block for causalgia of the upper extremity or a lumbar sympathetic block for causalgia of the lower extremity (see Chapter 13). If sympathetic nerve blockade clearly produces relief of pain, the diagnosis of causalgia is established. Brachial plexus block will relieve pain of sympathetic nervous system origin, but it is likely that unnecessary blockade of sensory and even motor fibers may also occur. Once the diagnosis is confirmed, treatment consists of a series of blocks (up to seven) until symptoms become minimal. Physical therapy and occasionally TENS are performed following each sympathetic block. Early treatment (within 1 month) with sympathetic blocks is successful in about 90% of patients. Delay of treatment for longer than 6 months is associated with success rates of 50% or less.

Dramatic relief of pain and increase in skin temperature have been reported in several patients in whom sympathetic nerve blockade was performed in an extremity isolated from the general circulation by a tourniquet.[9,10] Specifically, guanethidine (10 to 20 mg) or phentolamine (5 to 15 mg) in 20 to 25 ml of normal saline is injected intravenously through an indwelling needle into the extremity. The extremity is isolated from the circulation for 10 minutes with a tourniquet to allow the binding of drug to the tissues. This intravenous regional sympathetic nerve block technique is used most often when stellate ganglion or lumbar sympathetic blocks have been ineffective. Furthermore, this approach appears to be useful in patients who show signs of returning sympathetic nervous system function despite apparently adequate surgical excision of the sympathetic ganglia. Presumably, drug-induced alpha blockade decreases sympathetic nervous system input to alpha receptors that may be present in injured nerves. This approach has been used with ketorolac, which decreases prostaglandin synthesis and subsequent alpha receptor stimulation and release of norepinephrine.[11]

Chronic Back Pain

Chronic back pain (lumbosacral radiculopathy) represents a significant health problem, with various conservative and surgical treatments frequently being ineffective. The result is chronic pain, loss of productivity, and occasionally disability. Patients who have a lumbosacral radiculopathy usually have pain as a result of inflammation of the nerve root or compression of the dorsal root ganglion. Pain arising from inflammation surrounding the nerve root is frequently responsive to the epidural administration of corticosteroids such as triamcinolone or methyprednisolone. Before proceeding with this treatment, it is mandatory to rule out the presence of infection or a space-occupying lesion. An epidural injection of corticosteroids should not be performed until a careful diagnostic evaluation (including consultation with a neurosurgeon or an orthopaedic surgeon) has been performed and the patient is advised of the possible benefits and complications of corticosteroid injections, including the distinct possibility that no relief from the injections may occur. All information given and received should be recorded in the patient's chart.

The patient is placed in the lateral position, and 3 to 4 ml of a solution containing 1% lidocaine (other local anesthetics could be used) is injected. The local anesthetic provides temporary relief of pain, confirming that the tip of the needle is in the epidural space. Methylprednisolone (80 mg) or triamcinolone (50 mg) is then injected into the epidural space as close to the affected nerve root as possible. Intrathecal injection of corticosteroids has been associated with symptoms consistent with aseptic meningitis. If symptoms are improved but still present 1 to 2 weeks after the initial epidural injection, it is acceptable to repeat the epidural injection. Few patients obtain relief from repeated injections if the first injection was of no help, radicular pain has been present for 6 months, or laminectomy has been previously performed. This is probably due to proliferation of scar and fibrous tissue around the damaged tissue surrounding the nerve root. If the decision is made to administer epidural corticosteroids on a repeated basis (more than two injections), they should not be given more frequently than every 6 weeks, because excessive steroid administration may cause Cushing syndrome.

Degeneration and inflammation of the lumbar facet joints and sacroiliac joints may produce low back pain that is difficult to distinguish from radicular pain. Diagnosis is confirmed by prolonged pain relief following injection of local anesthetic (1 ml) into the facet joint, often with fluoroscopy to guide needle placement. Nonsteroidal anti-inflammatory drugs may be of some help in these patients.

Intercostal Neuralgia

Intercostal neuralgia following thoracotomy or rib fracture is characterized by paresthesias and pain in response to touch or movement of the thorax. Although the pain usually subsides within 2 weeks, it can persist for several months or years, requiring active treatment. In most cases, destructive nerve blocks with alcohol or phenol, or surgical removal of a neuroma or rhizotomy offer little help. Alcohol or phenol injections are usually followed by a 10% to 50% incidence of postblock neuritis, in which the pain is worse than before the block was performed. One approach is to perform local anesthetic intercostal or paravertebral nerve blocks. During the pain-free time, physical therapy can be performed. Repeated efforts of this kind occasionally result in prolonged relief of pain.

Postherpetic Neuralgia

After an acute infection of herpes zoster, a syndrome called postherpetic neuralgia can exist for an extended period, especially in elderly or immunosuppressed patients. After the acute infective period, in which the cutaneous lesions (most often T1–T8 dermatomes) gradually disappear over 2 to 4 weeks, the pain usually subsides. Pain and scarring, however, may persist. Local anesthetic, alcohol, and phenol intercostal nerve blocks are not predictably effective in relieving the pain. Early cases (less than 3 months duration) sometimes can be effectively treated with sympathetic nerve blocks with local anesthetic. Institution of TENS or administration of a phenothiazine (fluphenazine) and a tricyclic antidepressant (amitriptyline) can occasionally relieve the pain. In elderly patients, however, complications such as orthostatic hypotension can occur after use of these drugs. Also, patients may become sleepy and lose their appetite, leading to increasing debilitation. Another approach has been the subcutaneous injection of a local anesthetic (bupivacaine 0.25%) and triamcinolone (2 $mg{\cdot}ml^{-1}$) under the painful skin area. The success of this treatment is not predictable. More recently, a continuous infusion of lidocaine (5 $mg{\cdot}kg^{-1}{\cdot}h^{-1}$ IV) for 1 to 2 hours has provided many days of pain relief not only for postherpetic neuralgia but also for diabetic neuropathy, low back pain with radiculopathy, and myofascial pain.[12]

Myofascial Pain

Myofascial pain is characterized by marked tenderness of discrete points (trigger points) within affected skeletal muscles and the appearance of tight, ropy bands of skeletal muscle. Precise neuroanatomic connections between the trigger point and the pain are not present. A positive "jump sign" has been described whereby the trigger area is palpated and the patient "jumps away" from the pain. There often are multiple trigger points in the same patient. The scapulocostal syndrome is characterized by a trigger point located medial and superior to the upper portion of the scapula. Pain may radiate to the occiput, shoulder, or anterior chest. Myofascial pain involving gluteal muscles produces pain referred to the posterior thigh and calf, mimicking S1 radiculopathy.

The most important aspect of treatment for myofascial pain is physical therapy designed to restore skeletal muscle strength and elasticity. Infiltration of local anesthetic solution (0.5% lidocaine, 0.25% bupivacaine), often with a small amount of corticosteroid (cortisol 25 mg), into the trigger point provides analgesia that confirms the diagnosis and permits initiation of physical therapy. These injections may be performed daily if necessary. Ultrasound therapy, TENS, or vapocoolant spray applied over the affected area may produce periods of analgesia during physical therapy.

MANAGEMENT OF PAIN IN THE CANCER PATIENT

It is estimated that as many as 40% of patients with cancer experience pain, especially if there is metastatic disease involving bone or compression of nerves.[13] Effective pain management has a profound beneficial impact on the quality of the cancer patient's life. Patients with cancer who suffer from pain frequently exhibit signs of depression and increased anxiety. Cancer pain may be subdivided into nociceptive (peripheral stimulation of nociceptors in somatic or visceral structures, producing aching or throbbing) and neuropathic (stimulation of afferent neural pathways or vascular structures, producing burning pain) categories. Nociceptive pain is usually responsive to nonopioid or opioid analgesics, whereas neuropathic pain is unlikely to be responsive to these drugs.

Causes of Pain in Patients with Cancer

- Tumor infiltration of bone
- Tumor infiltration of nerve or vascular structures
- Side effects of cancer therapy
  - Phantom limb syndrome
  - Peripheral neuropathy
  - Radiation fibrosis

Drug therapy (large doses of opioids such as morphine administered orally) is the cornerstone of cancer pain management. Fear of drug addiction in a patient who is dying of cancer is not an issue when rendering that patient as comfortable as possible. Tricyclic antidepressants are effective in treating depression associated with cancer, and, furthermore, these drugs potentiate opioid-induced analgesia. Anticonvulsant drugs (carbamazepine) suppress neuronal firing and may be effective for the management of neuropathic pain. Corticosteroids may be beneficial when administered to patients with pain as these drugs decrease pain perception, improve mood, and increase appetite.

Alternative routes of analgesic drug delivery (intravenous, neuraxial, transdermal, transmucosal) may be considerations when oral administration is not effective (see the section *Neuraxial Opioids*). Neurolytic procedures are typically reserved for patients with a limited life expectancy who are experiencing constant pain despite more conventional treatment modalities (see the section *Pancreatic Cancer*). Neurosurgical procedures such as cordotomy (open or percutaneous interruption of the spinothalamic tract) or dorsal rhizotomy (interruption of the sensory nerve root) are reserved for patients unresponsive to less invasive procedures. Neurostimulators and deep brain stimulation have limited usefulness for treating pain in the cancer patient.

Pancreatic Cancer

Neurolytic celiac plexus block is useful for relief of pain associated with pancreatic cancer and other upper abdominal malignancies. This reflects the fact that the celiac plexus carries sensory and autonomic nervous system fibers from all the abdominal viscera except the left colon and the pelvic organs. Typically, neurolytic block is performed with 30 to 50 ml of 50% alcohol or 6% phenol injected through needles whose proper position has been verified (by radiography or computed tomography) to minimize the risk of accidental subarachnoid injection.[14] Analgesics are necessary to offset the pain produced by injection of alcohol, and administration of fluids (10 to 15 ml·kg^{-1} IV) decreases the likelihood of symptomatic postblock orthostatic hypotension owing to splanchnic vasodilation. Neurolytic celiac plexus block should probably be performed only by those with experience in this technique.

REFERENCES

1. Forrest JB. Sympathetic mechanisms in postoperative pain. Can J Anaesth 1992;39:532–4.
2. Taub A. Factors in the diagnosis and treatment of chronic pain. J Autism Child Schizophr 1975;5:1–12.
3. Miller RD, Munger WL, Power PE. Chronic pain and

local anesthetic neural blockade. In: Cousins MJ, Bridenbaugh PO, eds. Neural Blockade. Philadelphia, JB Lippincott 1988;616-37.

4. Coombs DW, Saunders RL, Gaylor MS, Pageau MG. Epidural narcotic infusion reservoir: Implantation techniques and efficacy. Anesthesiology 1982;56:469–73.
5. Erdine S, Aldemir T. Long term results of peridural morphine in 225 patients. Pain 1991;45:155–9.
6. Melzack R, Wall PD. Pain mechanisms: A new theory. Science 1965;150:971–3.
7. Grond S, Zech D, Schug SA, et al. Validation of World Health Organization guidelines for cancer pain relief during the last days and hours of life. J Pain Symptom Management 1991;6:411–22.
8. Fields HL, Heinricher MM, Mason P. Neurotransmitters in nociceptive modulating circuits. Annu Rev Neuroscience 1991;14:219–45.
9. Hannington-Kiff G. Intravenous regional sympathetic block with guanethidine. Lancet 1974;1:1019–20.
10. Arner S. IV phentolamine test: Diagnostic and prognostic use in RDS. Pain 1991;45:17–22.
11. Vanos DN, Ramamurthy S, Hoffman J. Intravenous regional block using ketorolac: Preliminary results in the treatment of reflex sympathetic dystrophy. Anesth Analg 1992;74:138–41.
12. Robotham MC, Reisner-Keller LA, Fields HL. Both intravenous lidocaine and morphine reduce the pain of postherpetic neuralgia. Neurology 1991;41:1024–8.
13. Ashburn MA, Lipman AG. Management of pain in the cancer patient. Anesth Analg 1993;76:402–16.
14. Brown DL, Bulley CK, Quiel EL. Neurolytic celiac plexus block for pancreatic cancer pain. Anesth Analg 1987;66:869–73.

35

Cardiopulmonary Resuscitation

Cardiopulmonary arrest is the abrupt cessation of spontaneous and effective cardiac output and ventilation. Cardiopulmonary resuscitation (CPR) is intended to provide artificial circulation and ventilation until Advanced Cardiac Life Support (ACLS) can be instituted and spontaneous cardiopulmonary function restored.[1] Cardiopulmonary arrest is usually the result of a cardiac dysrhythmia. CPR applies many of the skills unique to the practice of anesthesiology (Table 35-1). Indeed, The American Board of Anesthesiology in its Booklet of Information and definition of the specialty, cites as tasks of the anesthesiologist the provision and teaching of CPR. In addition, CPR research and administrative functions are often part of the anesthesiologist's responsibilities. Administrative duties may include review of CPR equipment and its function and establishment of an organized response within the hospital when cardiopulmonary arrest occurs.

CPR is categorized as Basic Life Support (BLS), ACLS, and Postresuscitation Life Support. BLS consists of provision of a patent upper airway (A–airway), exhaled air ventilation (B–breathing), and circulation of blood by closed chest cardiac compressions (C–circulation). The ABCs of BLS may be instituted by trained lay persons, as well as by physicians, without the need for specialized equipment. ACLS includes use of specialized equipment to maintain the airway, external defibrillation, drug therapy, and postresuscitation life support. The highest survival rates and quality of survival are attained when BLS is initiated within 4 minutes from the time of cardiopulmonary arrest and when ACLS is initiated within 8 minutes.[1] Regardless of the time from cardiopulmonary arrest to initiation of CPR, more than 6 minutes of closed chest cardiac compression is associated with increased neurologic morbidity.[2]

Management of CPR is a team effort, and coordination of the team is the responsibility of the team leader, ideally a physician skilled in airway management. It is the responsibility of the team leader to (1) ensure the quality of BLS, (2) facilitate early use of electrical defibrillation, and (3) direct and monitor adequacy of drug therapy.[2] Ultimately, the team leader may also decide when resuscitation efforts should cease. In this regard, decisions to end CPR must consider cardiac and brain function and responsiveness to therapy. Often it is only by a trial of CPR that the heart can be diagnosed as irreversibly damaged and unresponsive to further therapy. A prospective diagnosis of irreversible brain damage is almost impossible to make. Studies of in-hospital cardiopulmonary arrest have demonstrated that CPR is not associated with the likelihood of survival in patients with pre-existing oliguria, metastatic cancer, sepsis, pneumonia, or acute stroke. In fact, after more than 30 years of widespread use of CPR, a re-evaluation of its benefits in terms of survival and quality of life shows CPR to be a desperate effort that will help only a limited number of patients.[1] Rates of survival to hospital discharge after CPR initiated in and outside the hospital are similar and generally range from 10% to 20%.

PROVISION OF A PATENT UPPER AIRWAY

Methods to provide a patent upper airway after a cardiopulmonary arrest are designed to relieve obstruction due to the tongue falling against the posterior pharynx. Extension of the head and displacement of the mandible anteriorly serves to stretch the muscles attached to the tongue and thus pull the tongue off the posterior pharynx. This maneuver is known as the head tilt-jaw thrust method and is identical to the recommended procedure for securing a patent airway in the patient rendered unconscious by anesthetic drugs (Fig. 35-1). The jaw thrust maneuver without head tilt is the recommended method for opening the airway in a victim with a suspected neck injury.

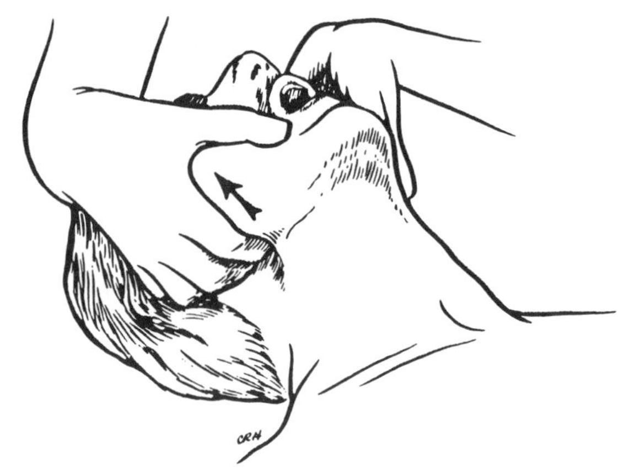

Figure 35-1. The head tilt-jaw thrust maneuver provides a patent upper airway by stretching muscles attached to the tongue, thus pulling the tongue away from the posterior pharynx. Forward displacement of the mandible is accomplished by grasping the angles of the mandible and lifting with both hands, serving to displace the mandible forward while tilting the head backward.

EXHALED AIR VENTILATION

Exhaled air ventilation (mouth-to-mouth ventilation), when performed properly, may provide adequate alveolar ventilation. However, delivered oxygen concentrations using this technique are only 16% to 17%, such that the maximum PAO_2 obtainable is about 80 mmHg. The PaO_2 will be even lower (arterial hypoxemia is predictable), reflecting increased venous admixture and low cardiac output present during CPR. Gastric distension often accom-

Table 35-1. Comparative Resuscitation Techniques

	Adult	Child (1–8 y)	Infant (<1 y)
Airway patency	Head tilt-jaw thrust	Head tilt-jaw thrust	Head tilt-jaw thrust
Ventilation method	Mouth-to-mouth	Mouth-to-mouth	Mouth-to-mouth and nose
Check for pulse	Carotid artery	Carotid artery	Brachial artery at midforearm
Sternal compression method	Depress sternum with heel of hand on lower one-third of sternum	Depress sternum with three fingers	Encircle chest with both hands and depress midsternum with thumbs
Sternal compression depth	3.8–5 cm	2.5–3.8 cm	1.25–2.5 cm
Sternal compression rate	80–100 per minute	80–100 per minute	At least 100 per minute
Sternal compression-to-ventilation ratio	15:2	5:1	5:1
Management of an obstructed upper airway	Give 6–10 subdiaphragmatic abdominal thrusts (Heimlich maneuver) Blind finger sweep if unconscious	Give 6–10 subdiaphramatic abdominal thrusts (Heimlich maneuver) Finger sweep only if foreign object is visible	Give 4 back blows Give 4 chest thrusts Finger sweep only if foreign object is visible

panies exhaled air ventilation, particularly if high airway pressures due to a partially obstructed upper airway are required. Even with a patent upper airway, some gas is likely to enter the stomach when inflation pressures are higher than 15 cmH_2O. Manual pressure applied over the victim's epigastrium to relieve gastric distension is not recommended, as this maneuver may produce regurgitation of gastric contents.[3] Nevertheless, gastric distension that impairs ventilation of the victim's lungs must be relieved by any method available, including manual pressure over the epigastrium. Concern about transmission of viral disease to the rescuer is a deterrent to provision of mouth-to-mouth ventilation (see the section *Specialized Equipment to Maintain the Airway*).

CLOSED CHEST (EXTERNAL) CARDIAC COMPRESSION

Optimal blood flow produced by closed chest cardiac compression is influenced by the proper placement of the rescuer's hands on the victim's sternum, the position of the rescuer's body in relationship to the victim, and the depth and rate of depression of the sternum.

The heel of the rescuer's hand is placed over and parallel to the lower one-third of the adult victim's sternum to provide maximum compression of the underlying cardiac ventricles (Fig. 35-2).[3] Pressure over the xiphoid process or rib cage must be avoided to minimize the likelihood of damage to abdominal organs, particularly the liver, or the production of rib fractures with resulting damage to the heart and lungs. The rescuer should kneel next to the victim so that the rescuer's upper body is over the victim's chest. The rescuer's elbows are kept straight and the shoulders positioned directly over the hands. This position enables the rescuer to use the weight of the upper body for compression, which must depress the sternum of an adult victim 3.8 to 5 cm.[3] Relaxation on the sternum must be complete at the end of each compression to permit the heart to fill. The rescuer's hands, however, must maintain contact with the victim's sternum, or correct hand position may be lost. The recommended minimum compression rate is 80 per minute, whereas the duration of each compression is ideally 50% of the cycle time. Achievement of the proper ratio of compression time to relaxation time requires a pause at the point of maximal sternal depression. This is the reason for avoidance of quick, bouncing compressions. When a single rescuer is present, external cardiac compression and exhaled air ventilation are provided at a compression-to-breath ratio of 15:2 each minute. When two rescuers are available, the compression rate is 80 to 100 per minute, and a breath is delivered during the upstroke of every fifth compression (a ratio of 5:1). The effectiveness of closed chest cardiac compressions should be verified by palpation of peripheral pulses.

The mechanism responsible for blood flow during closed chest cardiac compression is traditionally attributed to compression of the cardiac ventricles between the sternum and the spine, resulting in an increase in pressure within the ventricles and closure of the mitral and tricuspid valves (direct cardiac compression mechanism) (Fig. 35-3).[4] This pressure is thought to cause antegrade flow into the pulmonary artery and aorta. In addition, increases in intrathoracic pressure that accompany closed chest cardiac compressions are important for producing antegrade flow (thoracic pump mechanism). Conceptually, the heart is like a balloon in a closed box such that increases in intrathoracic pressure squeeze blood from the heart. Indirect evidence for the thoracic pump mechanism is the observation that patients who develop acute ventricular fibrillation remain conscious for several seconds if they cough vigorously.[3] Presumably, cough-induced increases in intrathoracic pressure provide antegrade blood flow. Patient-related factors (heart size, anterior-to-posterior chest distance, thoracic compliance) and technique-related variables (manual versus mechanical compression, compression duration and depth) may influence which mechanism is predominantly responsible for blood flow during closed chest cardiac compressions.

Closed chest cardiac compressions can produce systolic blood pressures that exceed 100 mmHg, but diastolic pressures are not more than 10 to 40 mmHg.[5] Carotid artery blood flow is usually less than one-third of normal at these pressures. As a result of low diastolic pressures, coronary artery blood flow during closed chest compression seldom exceeds 5% to 10% of normal values. Although these blood flows will temporarily sustain brain viability, prompt restoration of a spontaneous cardiac output and coronary artery blood flow by ACLS

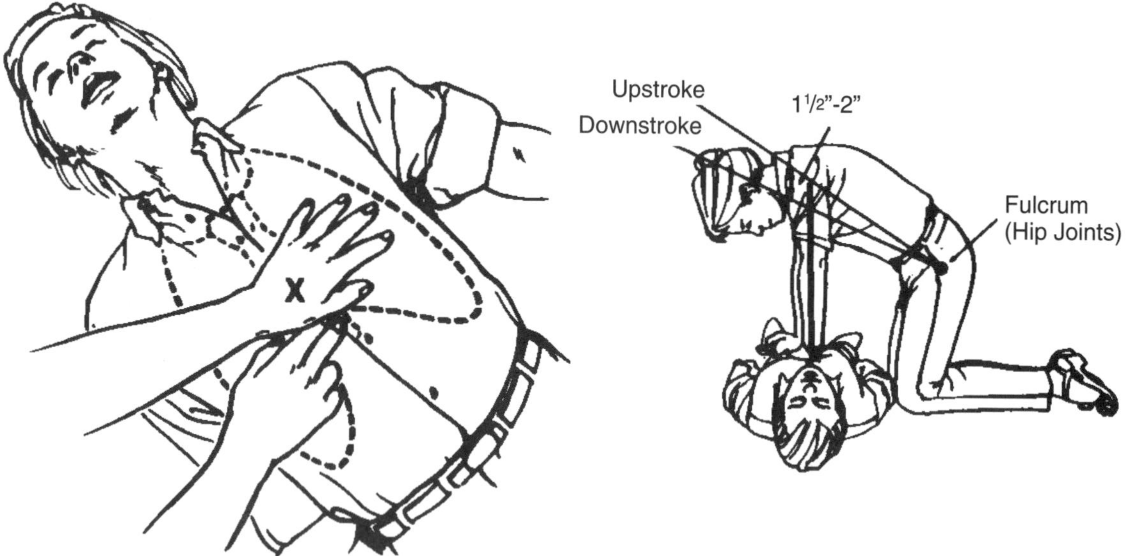

Figure 35-2. Proper hand and body position for performance of closed chest (external) cardiac compression in an adult. (From Guidelines for cardiopulmonary resuscitation and emergency cardiac care,[3] with permission.)

(epinephrine, electrical defibrillation) is critical for myocardial viability. Although irreversible brain damage is a feared complication of prolonged cardiac arrest, the most vulnerable organ for damage from severe arterial hypoxemia is the heart.[6] Intravenous administration of epinephrine is crucial to maximize the cardiac output and coronary and cerebral perfusion pressures generated by closed chest cardiac compression. External chest compression must always be accompanied by effective airway management and oxygenation because circulation of unoxygenated blood will not sustain cardiac or cerebral viability.

The effectiveness of closed chest cardiac compressions can be monitored by palpation of peripheral pulses. A pulse is generally not palpable when the systolic blood pressure is lower than 70 mmHg. In the rare instances when end-tidal carbon dioxide concentration can be monitored as a reflection of pulmonary blood flow (cardiac output), the presence of an end-tidal PCO_2 lower than 10 mmHg suggests a poor prognosis.[7]

SPECIALIZED EQUIPMENT TO MAINTAIN THE AIRWAY

Supplemental oxygen and adjuncts for airway management must be instituted as promptly as possible during CPR. Adjuncts for use in airway management are designed to ensure control of the airway, improve ventilation and oxygenation, and isolate the trachea from the gastrointestinal tract. A portable pocket face mask is the simplest advancement beyond mouth-to-mouth ventilation. Use of this mask circumvents the concern about transmission of viral diseases from the victim to the rescuer and the negative impact of vomitus on the willingness of a rescuer to provide mouth-to-mouth ventilation. Exhaled air ventilation may be provided via this mask. Alternatively, a reservoir bag with a one-way valve may be attached to this mask to permit manual ventilation of the victim's lungs. Another advantage of a reservoir bag is the ability to deliver oxygen for ventilation of the lungs. For example, a $10\text{-L}\cdot\text{min}^{-1}$ flow of oxygen will provide inhaled oxygen concentrations of about 50%. This mask should be transparent so that regurgitated gastric contents may be recognized promptly. Oropharyngeal or nasopharyngeal airways may be useful, remembering that oral airways may evoke vomiting or laryngospasm if introduced into conscious or semiconscious victims. Incorrect placement of an oral airway can displace the tongue back into the pharynx and result in airway obstruction.

The best method for maintenance of a patent upper airway is placement of a cuffed tube in the

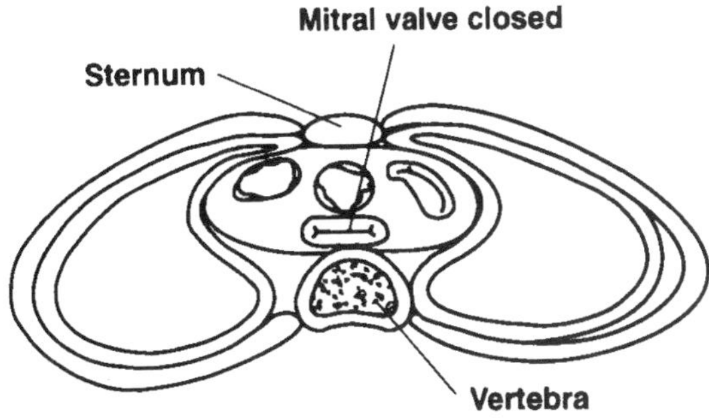

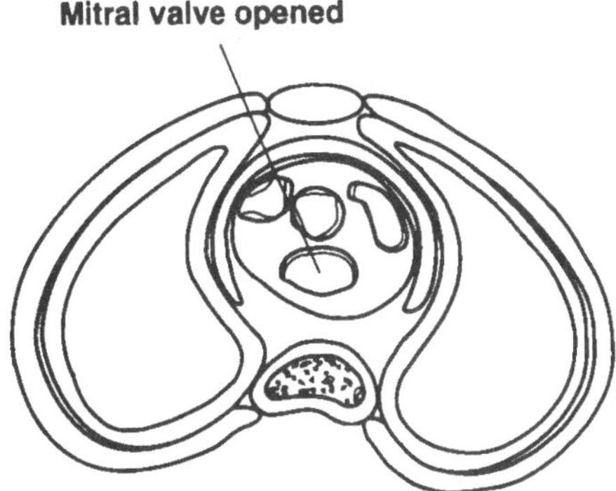

Figure 35-3. Possible mechanisms for blood flow during CPR. (From Schleien et al.,[4] with permission.)

trachea using direct laryngoscopy. This tracheal tube permits (1) optimal adjustment of tidal volume and breathing frequency, (2) reliable addition of supplemental oxygen to the inhaled gases, and (3) protection of the lungs from inhalation of gastric contents when the cuff is inflated with air to provide a seal against the tracheal mucosa. An alternative to placement of a cuffed tube in the trachea is blind insertion of a solid cuffed tube known as an esophageal obturator airway (EOA) into the esophagus.

Mechanical ventilators are not reliably effective during CPR. For example, pressure-cycled ventilators will prematurely cease to deliver gas flow when the sternum is depressed, whereas volume-cycled ventilators will not be able to deliver a reliable tidal volume during this time. Alternatively, manually triggered oxygen-powered breathing devices are available for ventilation of the lungs via a face mask, tracheal tube, or esophageal airway. Using these devices, the instantaneous development of a high flow rate of oxygen (100 L·min^{-1}) and maximum pressures (50 cmH_2O) by manual depression of the control button allows the rescuer to interpose breaths at the desired time during external cardiac compressions.

EXTERNAL DEFIBRILLATION AND TREATMENT OF VENTRICULAR FIBRILLATION

External defibrillation is the definitive treatment of ventricular fibrillation (Fig. 35-4).[3] The most important determinant of the success of external defibrillation and the survival of the victim is the length of the interval from cardiopulmonary arrest to application of countershock.[1] Prompt tracheal intubation is important, but external defibrillation should not be delayed to accomplish this goal if ventilation of the victim's lungs can be accomplished without intubation. Current recommendations are to apply external defibrillation as soon as ventricular fibrillation is identified and a defibrillator is available. An initial defibrillation setting of approximately 200 joules (watt·sec) is recommended for adult victims regardless of body weight. If this initial attempt is unsuccessful, a second attempt should be made using an energy setting of 200 to 300 joules, remembering that thoracic impedance decreases modestly after the first shock. As a result, a second attempt at the same energy level may deliver more current to the heart than with the first attempt. Should the first two shocks fail to defibrillate, a third shock not to

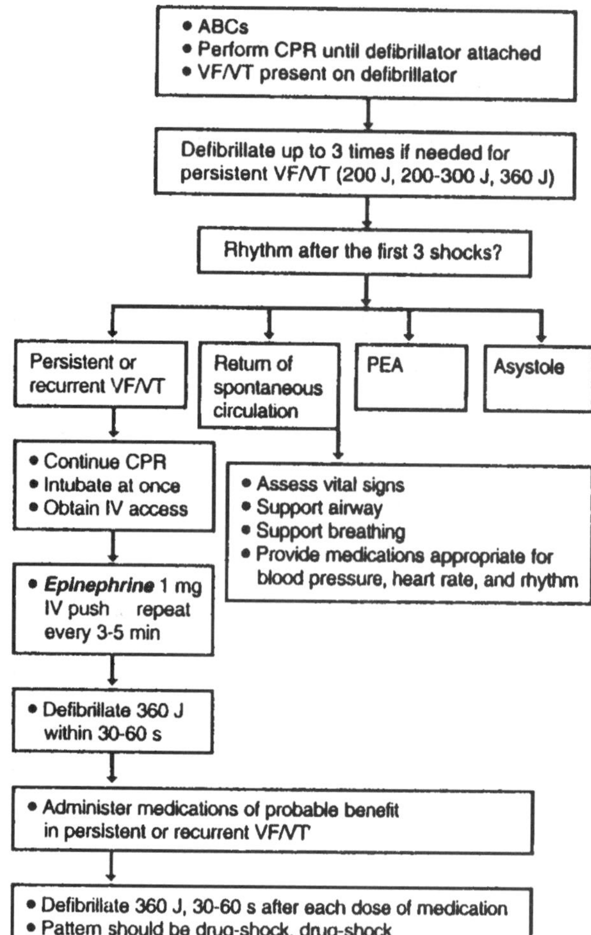
• ABCs
• Perform CPR until defibrillator attached
• VF/VT present on defibrillator
Defibrillate up to 3 times if needed for persistent VF/VT (200 J, 200-300 J, 360 J)
Rhythm after the first 3 shocks?
Persistent or recurrent VF/VT
Return of spontaneous circulation
PEA
Asystole
• Continue CPR
• Intubate at once
• Obtain IV access
• Assess vital signs
• Support airway
• Support breathing
• Provide medications appropriate for blood pressure, heart rate, and rhythm
• Epinephrine 1 mg IV push repeat every 3-5 min
• Defibrillate 360 J within 30-60 s
• Administer medications of probable benefit in persistent or recurrent VF/VT
• Defibrillate 360 J, 30-60 s after each dose of medication
• Pattern should be drug-shock, drug-shock

Figure 35-4. Algorithm for ventricular fibrillation (VF) and pulseless ventricular tachycardia (VT). Treatment of cardiac arrest due to VF or pulseless VT is based or prompt electrical defibrillation and intravenous administration of epinephrine. For management of asystole or pulseless electrical activity (PEA), refer to Figures 35-6 and 35-7, respectively. Medications of probable benefit in persistent or recurrent VF/VT include lidocaine, bretylium, procainamide, and sodium bicarbonate (Table 35-2). CPR, cardiopulmonary resuscitation. (Adapted from Guidelines for cardiopulmonary resuscitation and emergency cardiac care,[3] with permission.)

exceed 360 joules should be delivered immediately. If ventricular fibrillation recurs, defibrillation should be reinitiated at the energy level that had previously resulted in successful defibrillation. It is important to minimize the current delivered to the heart to decrease the likelihood of damage to the myocardium.

Paddle electrodes used to deliver current from the defibrillator must be placed in positions that will maximize current flow through the myocardium. Electrodes 8 to 10 cm in diameter are appropriate for adults, and electrodes 4.5 cm in diameter are adequate for infants and children. Standard placement is with one electrode to the right of the sternum below the clavicle and with the other electrode at the level of the apex of the heart in the midaxillary line (Fig. 35-5). The paddles for the electrodes should be applied to the chest with firm pressure equivalent to about 10 kg. In the presence of a permanent artificial cardiac pacemaker, care should be taken to avoid placing the electrodes too near (not closer than 10 to 12 cm) to the pacemaker generator, because defibrillation can cause artificial cardiac pacemaker malfunction.

DRUG THERAPY

An essential part of ACLS is prompt establishment of an intravenous infusion site for reliable delivery of drugs and fluids into the circulation (Table 35-2). Initial drug therapy during CPR is directed at correction of arterial hypoxemia and increasing coronary and cerebral perfusion pressures during closed chest cardiac compressions. In this regard, oxygen and epinephrine when combined with artificial ventilation and closed chest cardiac compressions are

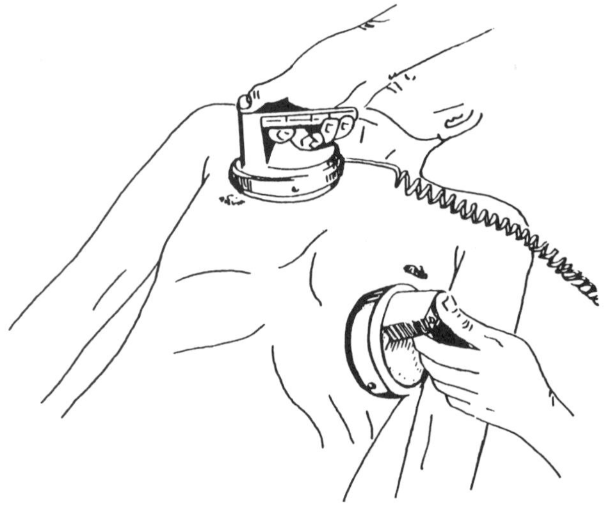

Figure 35-5. Schematic depiction of proper placement of paddle electrodes in an adult.

the mainstays of drug therapy during CPR. Prompt administration of epinephrine as soon as cardiac arrest is recognized is associated with improved rates of successful resuscitation in models of ventricular fibrillation and asystole.[8] The beneficial effects of epinephrine depend primarily on its alpha–1 effects, which include arterial vasoconstriction (increased cerebral and coronary perfusion pressure) and selective redistribution of cardiac output. It is unclear whether antidysrhythmic drugs (lidocaine, bretylium) are of value if repeated attempts at external defibrillation and administration of epinephrine fail to terminate ventricular fibrillation.

Peripheral venous injection sites are associated with delayed delivery of drugs to the heart during CPR, emphasizing the importance of administration of drugs via a centrally placed catheter (subclavian vein, internal jugular vein) when possible. A period of 1 to 2 minutes should be allowed for drugs to reach the central circulation when they are injected via a peripheral vein. Despite advantages of central venous placement, it is mandatory not to delay or

Table 35-2. Drug Therapy During Cardiopulmonary Resuscitation

	Indications	Dose
Oxygen	All cardiac arrests	100%
Epinephrine	All cardiac arrests	0.5–1 mg IV (10 $\mu g \cdot kg^{-1}$ in children) 1 mg in 10 ml through TT Repeat every 5 minutes Consider higher doses in refractory cardiac arrest
Sodium bicarbonate	Not recommended except in selected patients (hyperkalemia) Adequate alveolar ventilation is the most important factor in management of hypoxic lactic acidosis	1 $mEq \cdot kg^{-1}$ IV initially; 0.5 $mEq \cdot kg^{-1}$ IV every 10 minutes of continued CPR or as dictated by pH
Lidocaine	Recurrent ventricular fibrillation or ventricular tachycardia	1 $mg \cdot kg^{-1}$ IV or TT 1–4 $mg \cdot min^{-1}$ IV (adult)
Bretylium	When lidocaine is not effective	5 $mg \cdot kg^{-1}$ IV every 5 minutes; not to exceed 30 $mg \cdot kg^{-1}$ in an adult
Atropine	Bradycardia Heart block Asystole	70 $\mu g \cdot kg^{-1}$ IV or TT (20 $\mu g \cdot kg^{-1}$ children)
Isoproterenol	When atropine is not effective	0.03–0.3 $\mu g \cdot kg^{-1} \cdot min^{-1}$ IV (2–20 $\mu g \cdot min^{-1}$ IV in adults)
Adenosine	Paroxysmal atrial tachycardia	6–12 mg IV (may repeat once in 1–2 min)
Dopamine		5–20 $\mu g \cdot kg^{-1} \cdot min^{-1}$ IV
Calcium chloride	Not recommended except in selected patients for treatment of hypocalcemia or hyperkalemia	

TT, tracheal tube; CPR, cardiopulmonary resuscitation.

interrupt early resuscitation efforts to place a central catheter in preference to peripheral venous placement (antecubital vein), which can be accomplished without interruption of CPR. If a tracheal tube is in place and there is a delay in achieving venous access, it is useful to remember that epinephrine, lidocaine, and atropine are absorbed across tracheal and bronchial mucosa when injected through the tracheal tube (Table 35-2). Ideally, a catheter is passed beyond the tip of the tracheal tube, so the injected drug is reliably exposed to tracheal mucosa. Intraosseous infusion of drugs is an alternative when intravenous access is not readily available, particularly in pediatric patients.

CARDIAC ASYSTOLE

Cardiac asystole is a less frequent cause of cardiac arrest than ventricular fibrillation, and the prognosis for resuscitation is poor (survival to hospital discharge is less than 2%), often reflecting extensive myocardial ischemia from prolonged periods of inadequate coronary perfusion. It may be difficult to differentiate cardiac asystole from ventricular fibrillation on the electrocardiogram (ECG). If the cardiac rhythm is unclear, the recommendation is to apply electrical defibrillation (Fig. 35-4).[3] If cardiac asystole is present, the treatment is continued CPR, drug therapy, and consideration of transvenous artificial cardiac pacemaker insertion (Fig. 35-6).[3]

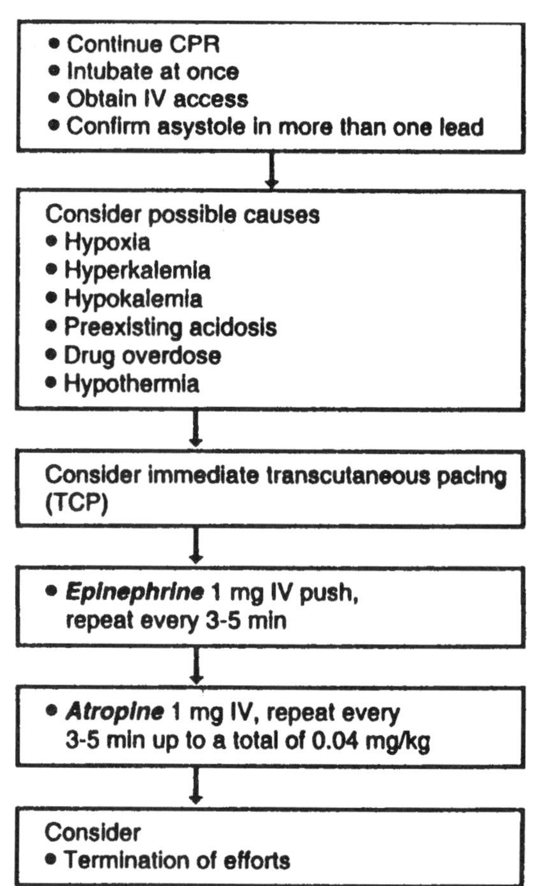

• Continue CPR
• Intubate at once
• Obtain IV access
• Confirm asystole in more than one lead
Consider possible causes
• Hypoxia
• Hyperkalemia
• Hypokalemia
• Preexisting acidosis
• Drug overdose
• Hypothermia
Consider immediate transcutaneous pacing (TCP)
• Epinephrine 1 mg IV push, repeat every 3-5 min
• Atropine 1 mg IV, repeat every 3-5 min up to a total of 0.04 mg/kg
Consider
• Termination of efforts

Figure 35-6. Algorithm for treatment of asystole. Treatment of cardiac arrest due to asystole is based on prompt intravenous administration of epinephrine and/or atropine. To be effective, transcutaneous pacing (TCP) must be performed early and simultaneously with drug therapy. Evidence, however, does not support routine use of TCP for treatment of asystole. In the absence of reversible causes, the persistence of asystole despite aggressive therapy may be an indication to terminate resuscitation efforts. (Adapted from Guidelines for cardiopulmonary resuscitation and emergency cardiac care,[3] with permission.)

PULSELESS ELECTRICAL ACTIVITY

Pulseless electrical activity (electromechanical dissociation) is present when a normal ECG persists in the absence of an effective stroke volume as evidenced by the disappearance of peripheral pulses and blood pressure. The prognosis is grave and mandates aggressive therapy and an intense search for correctable causes (Fig. 35-7).[3]

VENTRICULAR TACHYCARDIA

Treatment of ventricular tachycardia depends on the hemodynamic significance of the cardiac dysrhythmia (Fig. 35-8).[3] Cardioversion requires less electrical energy than defibrillation but must be synchronized to avoid delivering the shock during the relative refractory portion of the cardiac cycle, which could result in ventricular fibrillation.

PAROXYSMAL SUPRAVENTRICULAR TACHYCARDIA

Emergency treatment of paroxysmal supraventricular tachycardia (PSVT) depends on the hemodynamic stability of the patient and the presence of underlying disease (Fig. 35-9).[3] D istinction on the ECG between sinus tachycardia, ventricular tachycardia, and PSVT may be difficult.

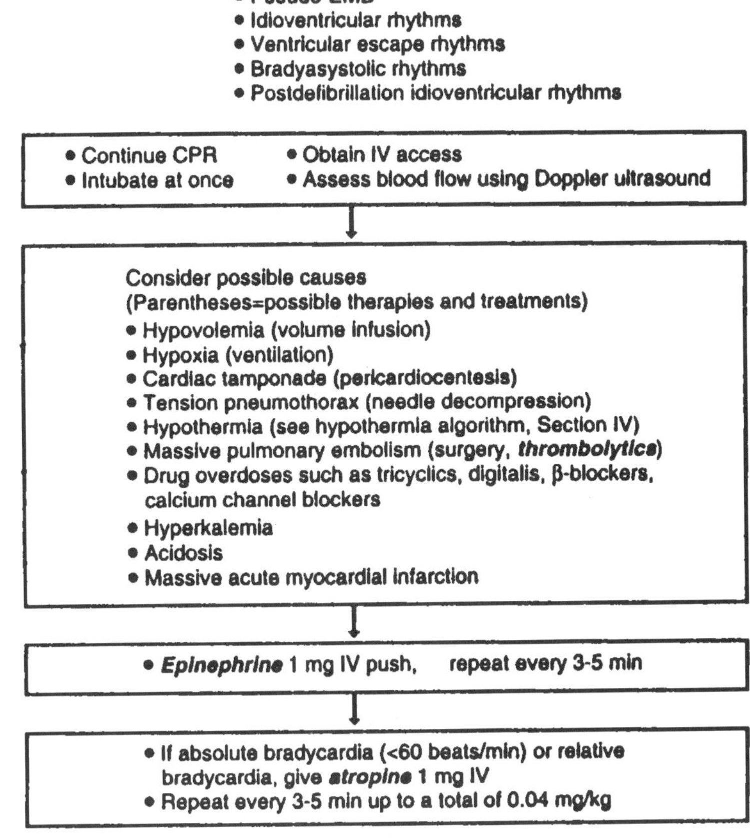

PEA includes
• Electromechanical dissociation (EMD)
• Pseudo-EMD
• Idioventricular rhythms
• Ventricular escape rhythms
• Bradyasystolic rhythms
• Postdefibrillation idioventricular rhythms
• Continue CPR
• Intubate at once
• Obtain IV access
• Assess blood flow using Doppler ultrasound
Consider possible causes
(Parentheses=possible therapies and treatments)
• Hypovolemia (volume infusion)
• Hypoxia (ventilation)
• Cardiac tamponade (pericardiocentesis)
• Tension pneumothorax (needle decompression)
• Hypothermia (see hypothermia algorithm, Section IV)
• Massive pulmonary embolism (surgery, thrombolytics)
• Drug overdoses such as tricyclics, digitalis, β-blockers, calcium channel blockers
• Hyperkalemia
• Acidosis
• Massive acute myocardial infarction
• Epinephrine 1 mg IV push, repeat every 3-5 min
• If absolute bradycardia (<60 beats/min) or relative bradycardia, give atropine 1 mg IV
• Repeat every 3-5 min up to a total of 0.04 mg/kg

Figure 35-7. Algorithm for treatment of pulseless electrical activity (PEA). Treatment of PEA is based on aggressive attempts to discover and reverse the cause of PEA plus intravenous administration of epinephrine and possibly atropine. (Adapted from Guidelines for cardiopulmonary resuscitation and emergency cardiac care,[3] with permission.)

MANAGEMENT OF THE OBSTRUCTED AIRWAY

An airway that is obstructed by the lodgement of a foreign body in the glottic opening will not be effectively managed by maneuvers, such as the head tilt-jaw thrust method, designed to pull the tongue away from the posterior pharynx (Fig. 35-1). In this situation, the recommended treatment in both conscious and unconscious victims is delivery of manual pressure to the abdomen or chest to increase airway pressures (Table 35-1). For example, manual inward and upward depression over the victim's epigastrium (abdominal thrust, external subdiaphragmatic compression, or Heimlich maneuver) forces the diaphragm cephalad, compressing the lungs and increasing airway pressures.[9] Increased airway pressures produced by the abdominal thrust forces ("pops") the obstructing particle out of the glottic opening into the pharynx. The abdominal thrust maneuver can be used in awake and unconscious victims and is equally effective with the victim in the supine or standing position (Fig. 35-10).[3] Complications of this maneuver include rib fractures and rupture or laceration of thoracic or abdominal viscera. The chest thrust (manual compression over the mid- or lower sternum) is an alternative to abdominal compression in morbidly obese or near-term parturients experiencing foreign body airway obstruction (Fig. 35-10).[3] In the unconscious adult

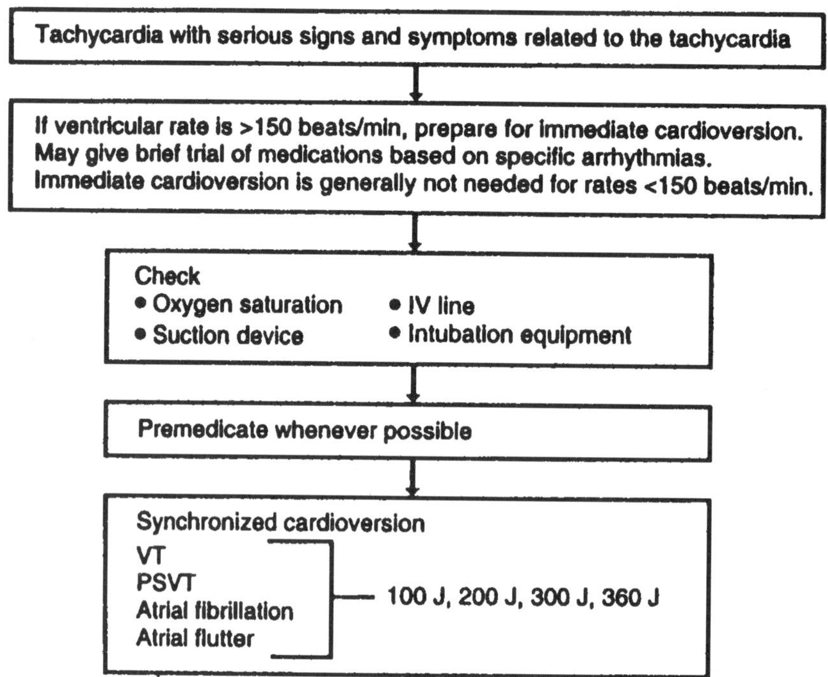

Figure 35-8. Algorithm for electrical cardioversion. Ventricular tachycardia that results in cardiovascular instability is treated with synchronized electrical cardioversion. When appropriate, patients may be sedated by the intravenous administration of short-acting central nervous system depressants such as methohexital. (Adapted from Guidelines for cardiopulmonary resuscitation and emergency cardiac care,[3] with permission.)

victim, delivery of a precordial thump (see the section *Precordial Thump*) or external cardiac compression creates airway pressures similar to those produced by a chest thrust. In the unconscious adult victim, a blind finger examination of the pharynx is indicated if these previous maneuvers have not been successful. Caution is necessary during blind probing of the pharynx to avoid impaction of an object deeper into the airway. Because this risk is greatest in the small mouths of infants and children, finger sweeps of the posterior pharynx are not recommended in these age groups unless the foreign object is visualized.

Cricothyrotomy

Cricothyrotomy is a method to provide emergency oxygenation when upper airway obstruction cannot be relieved by translaryngeal intubation of the trachea (Fig. 35-11). If the upper airway is obstructed, exhalation must occur through the ventilatory catheter that is intermittently disconnected from the oxygen source and opened to the atmosphere. In fact, elevated airway pressures may cause an obstructing foreign body to be expelled from the glottic opening into the pharynx. If passive exhalation cannot occur, hypercarbia as well as dangerously increased airway pressures may occur. A cricothyrotomy is most useful for maintaining oxygenation while a more definitive procedure such as tracheostomy is accomplished.

PRECORDIAL THUMP

Precordial thump is a forceful blow delivered with the fleshy part of the rescuer's fist to the midportion of the victim's sternum. A single precordial thump is recommended only for initial treatment of (1) monitored ventricular fibrillation or tachycardia and (2) cardiac asystole due to complete heart block. The precordial thump may serve as a mechanical defibrillation or cardioversion or as a mechanism to pro-

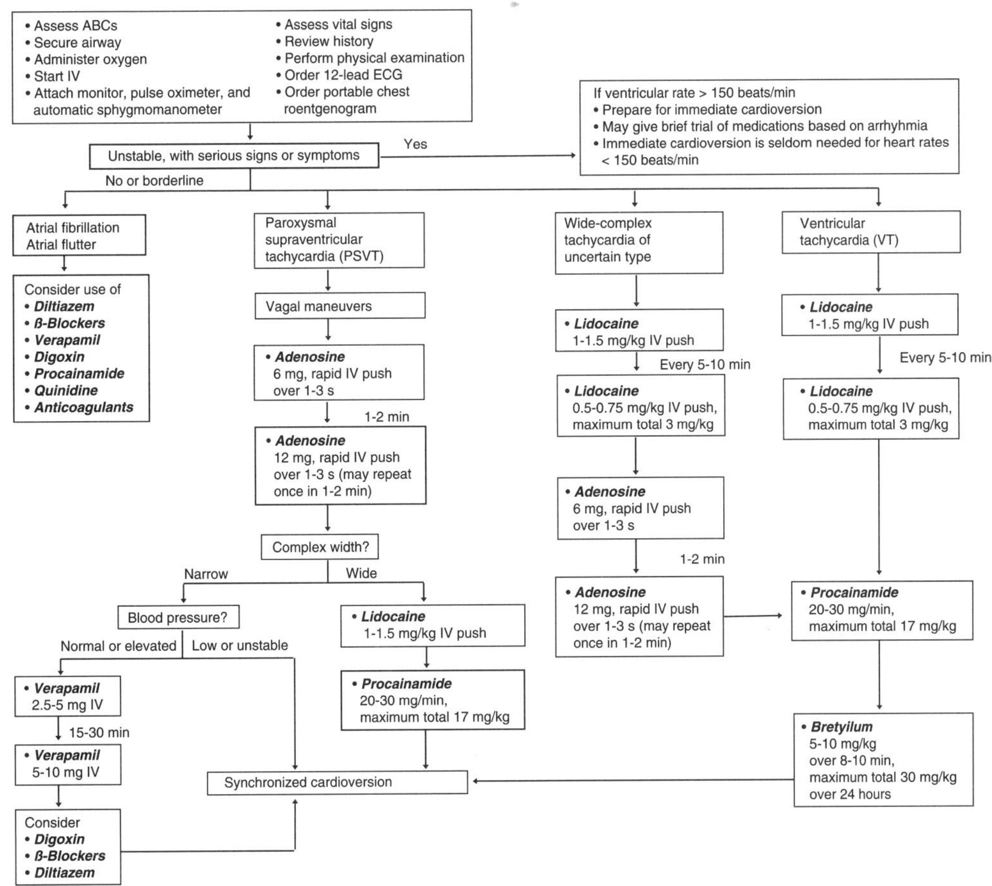

Figure 35-9. Algorithm for tachycardia. Paroxysmal supraventricular tachycardia or ventricular tachycardia that results in serious signs or symptoms (dyspnea, angina pectoris, hypotension, altered level of consciousness) requires prompt treatment with synchronized cardioversion (see Fig. 35-8). In the absence of associated symptoms, the tachycardia may be treated with intravenous administration of drugs based on the electrocardiographic characteristics of the cardiac dysrhythmia. Attempts to elicit a vagal response by carotid sinus massage are not recommended for patients with evidence of carotid artery disease (bruits). (Adapted from Guidelines for cardiopulmonary resuscitation and emergency cardiac care,[3] with permission.)

duce cardiac contraction until a transvenous artificial cardiac pacemaker can be inserted. Precordial thump is not recommended for pediatric patients.

RESUSCITATION OF INFANTS AND CHILDREN

Techniques of CPR as applied to infants (younger than 1 year of age) differ in some instances from those of children (1 year to puberty) or adults. These differences relate to airway management, ventilation of the lungs, closed chest cardiac compression, external defibrillation, and doses used for drug therapy (Tables 35-1 and 35-2). Furthermore, the most readily palpable pulse in infants up to 1 year of age is the brachial artery at the mid-upper arm, in contrast to the carotid artery in children and adults.

Airway Management and Ventilation of the Lungs

Excessive extension of the infant's head may obstruct the upper airway. The infant's tongue is large, however, in relation to the mouth, such that moder-

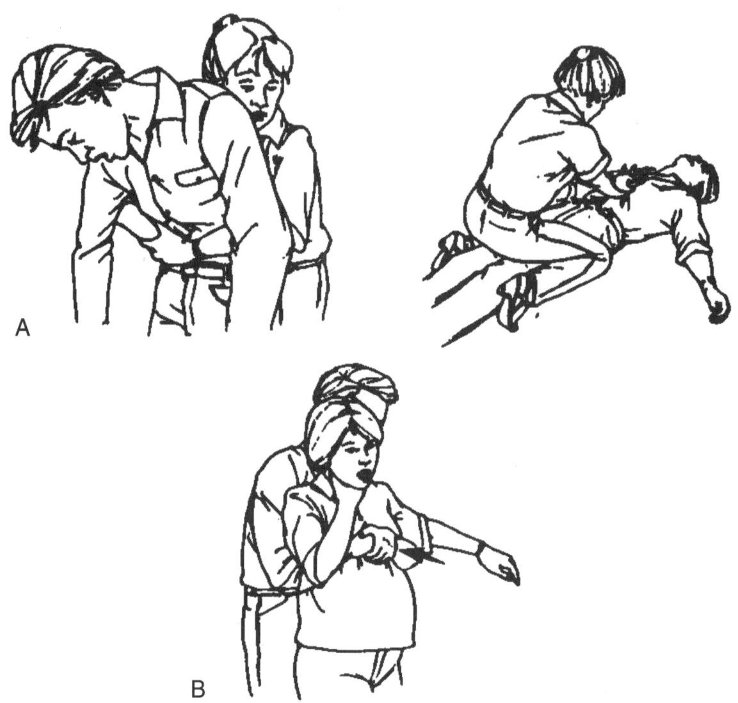

Figure 35-10. Manual thrust artificial cough techniques are recommended to treat an upper airway that is obstructed by a foreign object. *(A)* Rapid inward and upward subdiaphragmatic abdominal thrusts (Heimlich maneuver) forces the diaphragm in a cephalad direction, compressing the air volume trapped in the lungs below the obstruction. *(B)* In children and parturients, rapid manual thrusts applied to the lower chest (chest thrusts) produce the same increase in airway pressures as abdominal thrusts and may be associated with fewer complications. (Adapted from Guidelines for cardiopulmonary resuscitation and emergency cardiac care,[3] with permission.)

ate extension of the head is useful for opening the upper airway. The rescuer's mouth must be sealed over the infant's mouth and nose to provide exhaled air ventilation. This approach is easier than mouth-to-mouth ventilation because of the disparate sizes of the structures involved. In addition, the lungs of the infant younger than 9 months of age are more easily ventilated through the nose than through the mouth due to the cephalad position of the infant's larynx (C1–C3) and the proximity of the epiglottis to the palate. After 1 year of age, mouth-to-mouth ventilation is acceptable.

Closed Chest Cardiac Compression

Differences in size and anatomy of infants, children, and adults dictate differences in the technique of external cardiac compression for these various age groups. In infants, the cardiac ventricles are positioned more cephalad in the chest such that external compression is performed on the midsternum rather than the lower sternum. The recommended rate of sternal compression is a rate of at least 100 per minute and the depth of sternal depression is 1.25 to 2.5 cm.[3] The rescuer's hands should encircle the infant's chest, and the thumbs are used to depress the sternum against the heart. Depression of the sternum may be achieved with three fingers in young children and the heel of one hand in older children.

External Defibrillation and Drug Therapy

The energy setting for successful external defibrillation in children is directly related to body weight.[3] To avoid myocardial damage and cardiac dysrhythmias, the recommended initial energy setting is 2 joules·kg^{-1}. If this is unsuccessful, the dose is doubled until a satisfactory response is achieved.

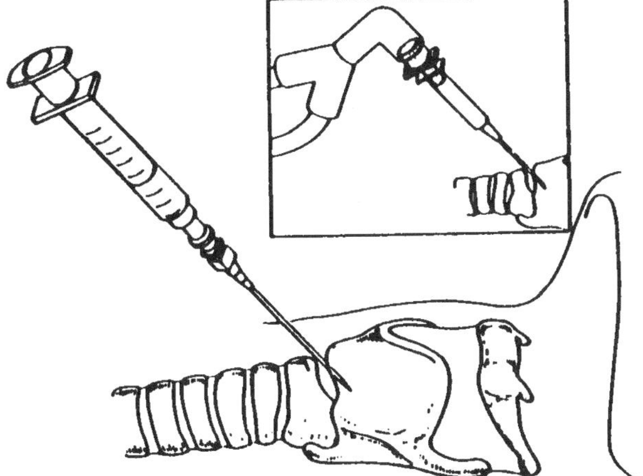

Figure 35-11. Cricothyrotomy (transtracheal oxygenation) is accomplished by placement of a 12- to 14-gauge catheter over needle (extracath) through the cricothyroid membrane into the trachea (recognized by aspiration of air from the trachea). The needle is removed and the catheter connected to a 3-ml syringe with the plunger removed. A 15-mm tracheal tube adapter fits into the barrel of the syringe and permits connection of an anesthetic breathing system, serving as a temporary method to provide oxygenation until more definitive steps can be taken to reverse total upper airway obstruction.

Table 35-3. Postresuscitation Life Support

Drug	Indications
Lidocaine	Cardiac ventricular irritability
Dopamine	Decreased myocardial contractility associated with oliguria
Dobutamine	Same as dopamine but not specific for increasing renal blood flow
Furosemide Barbiturates	Increased intracranial pressure
Barbiturates Diazepam Phenytoin	Central nervous system seizure activity
Nitroprusside	Systemic hypertension

POSTRESUSCITATION LIFE SUPPORT

Postresuscitation life support begins after establishment of a spontaneous cardiac output in the victim of a cardiopulmonary arrest. The patient who is awake and breathing spontaneously needs only to be monitored closely in an intensive care unit. Supplemental oxygen and a radiograph of the chest should be routine after CPR. Drug therapy may be necessary to optimize vital organ function and survival (Table 35-3). For example, a continuous intravenous infusion of lidocaine is often maintained for the first 24 hours. Optimal adjustment of the intravascular fluid volume and support of the circulation as facilitated by monitoring with a pulmonary artery catheter may be necessary. Renal failure may necessitate hemodialysis.

The early doctrine that 4 to 6 minutes of global cerebral ischemia produced by cardiac arrest results in irreversible brain injury is no longer tenable. Evidence suggests that central nervous system neurons can tolerate 20 to 60 minutes of complete anoxia without always sustaining irreversible damage.[2] Furthermore, events that follow cerebral ischemia (profound decreases in cerebral blood flow often to less than 10% of normal that occur 15 to 90 minutes after successful resuscitation) may be incompatible with neuronal viability. Administration of calcium during and after CPR is not recommended in view of the possible role of neuronal calcium overloading in small vessel vasoconstriction and postresuscitation cerebral hypoperfusion.[2]

The victim who remains unresponsive and apneic and has cardiovascular instability in the postresuscitation period is likely to have hypoxia-related multiple organ failure that requires stabilization of cardiac function and support of the postischemic central nervous system (Table 35-3). Although postresuscitation care of the central nervous system cannot alter damage produced by the primary ischemic episode, it can modify the degree of secondary injury occurring with postresuscitation cerebral hypoperfusion. Support of the central nervous system entails measures to control intracranial pressure (ICP), maintain cerebral oxygen delivery, and decrease cerebral metabolic oxygen requirements (Table 35-3). In this regard, the use of barbiturates in central nervous system protection after an ischemic insult is based on the ability of these drugs to decrease ICP and produce dose-dependent decreases (maximum about 50%) in cerebral metabolic oxygen requirements. This maximum decrease in oxygen requirements corresponds to an isoelectric electroencephalogram (reflects depression of mentation but not a change in oxygen needed to maintain cell viability) and is evidence that additional doses of barbiturates are not necessary. During cardiac arrest (global ischemia) the electroencephalogram becomes flat in 20 to 30 seconds, and subsequent administration of a barbiturate would not be expected to improve neurologic outcome. Indeed, administration of thiopental (30 $mg \cdot kg^{-1}$ IV) as a single injection to comatose survivors of cardiac arrest does not increase survival or improve neurologic outcome.[10] Possibly, the most beneficial effect of barbiturates or other drugs, such as diazepam or phenytoin, is to suppress seizure activity and associated increases in cerebral oxygen requirements in the postresuscitation period. There is no evidence that hypothermia or corticosteroids instituted after cardiac arrest improve survival or neurologic outcome. Mild hypothermia present at the time of cardiac arrest, however, may offer some degree of cerebral protection.

Patients with hyperglycemia at the time of cardiac arrest have a less favorable neurologic outcome than do patients who are normoglycemic. Presumably, this reflects lactate production and intracellular acidosis due to anaerobic glycolysis of glucose. It remains uncertain whether infusion of glucose-containing solutions should be avoided in the postresuscitation period.

Monitors specific for the central nervous system in the cardiac arrest victim with residual neurologic dysfunction include (1) ICP monitoring devices, (2) the electroencephalogram, (3) computed tomography of the cerebral ventricles, (4) cortical evoked potentials, (5) measurement of total and/or regional cerebral blood flow, and (6) frequent neurologic examination. Resuscitation and protection of the brain that has experienced potential ischemic damage includes maintenance of systemic blood pressure at normal levels and prevention of increased ICP (see Chapter 33).

Brain Death

The need to define and confirm irreversible central nervous system damage (brain death) following CPR is apparent. Diagnosis of brain death in the very young is difficult, as it is recognized that the immature brain is resistant to the damaging effects of arterial hypoxemia. Nevertheless, criteria for brain death in an adult in the absence of hypothermia (lower than 32°C) or depressant drug overdose, or both, have been established. Measurement of somatosensory evoked potentials may also be useful in confirming the presence of brain death.

DO NOT RESUSCITATE ORDERS

The Council on Ethical and Judicial Affairs of the American Medical Association has proposed guidelines for the appropriate use of do not resuscitate (DNR) orders.[11] It is recommended that efforts should not be made to resuscitate patients when circumstances indicate that administration of CPR would be futile (no hope of restoration to normal integrated functioning cognitive existence) or not in accord with the desires or best interests of the patient. If a patient is incapable of rendering the

Criteria for Brain Death in an Adult

- Coma persisting >12 hours in the presence of a known cause
- Absent brain stem function
  - Fixed and unreactive pupils
  - Apnea despite normal to increased $PaCO_2$
- Absent cortical function as reflected by a flat electroencephalogram (maximum gain for 60 minutes)
- Angiographic evidence of absent cerebral circulation

Treatment Modalities that May Require Discussion Before Delivery of Anesthesia Care to Patients with DNR Orders

- Blood product transfusion
- Maintenance of intravascular volume with nonblood products
- Supplemental oxygen
- Tracheal intubation
- External cardiac compressions, electrical defibrillation, artificial cardiac pacing
- Vasoactive drug administration
- Postoperative support of ventilation

decision regarding the use of CPR, a prospective decision may be made by a surrogate decision maker.

An obvious dilemma is created when the patient with a DNR order requires a surgical procedure that includes anesthesia. In that regard, guidelines adopted by the American Society of Anesthesiologists for the anesthetic care of patients with DNR orders emphasize the need for communication among involved parties (patient and/or legal representative, anesthesiologist, primary physician) and the need to document relevant aspects of this communication.[12] Policies automatically suspending DNR orders prior to procedures requiring anesthetic care may not sufficiently address a patient's right to self-determination. Prior to procedures requiring anesthetic care, any changes in existing directives that limit treatment should be discussed and documented in the patient's medical record, including any exceptions to directives against interventions should a recognized complication of the anesthesia occur. For this reason, the anesthesiologist should describe and discuss the appropriate use of commonly used and accepted therapies to correct cardiopulmonary changes predictably resulting from drugs or techniques (or both) needed for anesthetic care. Should the anesthesiologist find the DNR orders to be incompatible with the delivery of anesthetic care, it is permissible to withdraw from the case while providing an alternative for care in a timely fashion. If this is not possible within the time frame necessary to prevent further suffering or morbidity to the patient, then, in accordance with the American Medical Association's Principles of Medical Ethics, anesthetic care should proceed with reasonable adherence to the patient's directives.[11,12]

REFERENCES

1. Niemann JT. Cardiopulmonary resuscitation. N Engl J Med 1992;327:1075–80.
2. White BC, Wiegenstein JG, Winegar CD. Brain ischemic anoxia. Mechanisms of injury. JAMA 1984; 251:1586–90.
3. Guidelines for cardiopulmonary resuscitation and emergency cardiac care. JAMA 1992;268:2171–2295.
4. Schleien CL, Berkowitz ID, Traystman R, Rogers MC. Controversial issues in cardiopulmonary resuscitation. Anesthesiology 1989;71:133–49.
5. Roberts MC, Weisfeldt ML, Traystman RJ. Cerebral blood flow during cardiopulmonary resuscitation. (Editorial.) Anesth Analg 1981;60:73–5.
6. Plum F. Vulnerability of the brain and heart after cardiac arrest. N Engl J Med 1991;324:1278–80.
7. Sanders AB, Kern KB, Otto CW, Milander MM, Ewy GA. End-tidal carbon dioxide monitoring during cardiopulmonary resuscitation. A prognostic indicator for survival. JAMA 1989;262:1347–51.
8. Paradis NA, Koscove EM. Epinephrine in cardiac arrest: A critical review. Ann Emerg Med 1990; 19:1288–1301.
9. Heimlich HJ. A life-saving maneuver to prevent food-choking. JAMA 1975;234:398–401.
10. Brain Resuscitation Clinical Trial 1 Study Group. Randomized clinical study of thiopental loading in comatose survivors of cardiac arrest. N Engl J Med 1986;314:397–403.
11. Council on Ethical and Judicial Affairs, American Medical Association: Guidelines for the appropriate use of do-not-resuscitate orders. JAMA 1991;265: 1868–71.
12 Ethical Guidelines for the Anesthesiza Care of Patients with Do Not Resuscitate Orders or Other Directives that Limit Treatment. American Society of Anesthesiologists. October, 1993. Park Ridge, IL.

Section VII
Appendices

Appendix 1
Standards for Basic Anesthetic Monitoring

(Approved by House of Delegates on October 21, 1986 and last amended on October 13, 1993)

These standards apply to all anesthesia care, although, in emergency circumstances, appropriate life support measures take precedence. These standards may be exceeded at any time based on the judgment of the responsible anesthesiologist. They are intended to encourage quality patient care, but observing them cannot guarantee any specific patient outcome. They are subject to revision from time to time, as warranted by the evolution of technology and practice. This set of standards addresses only the issue of basic intraoperative monitoring, which is one component of anesthesia care. In certain rare or unusual circumstances, (1) some of these methods of monitoring may be clinically impractical and (2) appropriate use of the described monitoring methods may fail to detect untoward clinical developments. Brief interruptions of continual[†] monitoring may be unavoidable. *Under extenuating circumstances, the responsible anesthesiologist may waive the requirements marked with an asterisk (*); it is recommended that when this is done, it should be so stated (including the reasons) in a note in the patient's medical record.* These standards are not intended for application to the care of the obstetric patient in labor or in the conduct of pain management.

STANDARD I

Qualified anesthesia personnel shall be present in the room throughout the conduct of all general anesthetics, regional anesthetics, and monitored anesthesia care.

[†]Note that "continual" is defined as "repeated regularly and frequently in steady rapid succession," whereas "continuous" means "prolonged without any interruption at any time."

Objective

Because of the rapid changes in patient status during anesthesia, qualified anesthesia personnel shall be continuously present to monitor the patient and provide anesthesia care. In the event there is a direct known hazard (e.g., radiation) to the anesthesia personnel that might require intermittent remote observation of the patient, some provision for monitoring the patient must be made. In the event that an emergency requires the temporary absence of the person primarily responsible for the anesthetic, the best judgment of the anesthesiologist will be exercised in comparing the emergency with the anesthetized patient's condition and in the selection of the person left responsible for the anesthetic during the temporary absence.

STANDARD II

During all anesthetics, the patient's oxygenation, ventilation, circulation, and temperature shall be continually evaluated.

Oxygenation

Objective

To ensure adequate oxygen concentration in the inspired gas and the blood during all anesthetics.

Methods

1. Inspired gas: During every administration of general anesthesia using an anesthesia machine, the concentration of oxygen in the patient breathing system shall be measured by an oxygen analyzer with a low oxygen concentration limit alarm in use.*

2. Blood oxygenation: During all anesthetics, a quantitative method of assessing oxygenation such as pulse oximetry shall be employed.* Adequate illumination and exposure of the patient is necessary to assess color.*

Ventilation

Objective

To ensure adequate ventilation of the patient during all anesthetics.

Methods

1. Every patient receiving general anesthesia shall have the adequacy of ventilation continually evaluated. While qualitative clinical signs such as chest excursion, observation of the reservoir breathing bag, and auscultation of breath sounds may be adequate, quantitative monitoring of the CO_2 content and/or volume of expired gas is encouraged.
2. When an endotracheal tube is inserted, its correct positioning in the trachea must be verified by clinical assessment and by identification of carbon dioxide in the expired gas.* End-tidal CO_2 analysis, in use from the time of endotracheal tube placement, is strongly encouraged.
3. When ventilation is controlled by a mechanical ventilator, there shall be in continuous use a device that is capable of detecting disconnection of components of the breathing system. The device must give an audible signal when its alarm threshold is exceeded.
4. During regional anesthesia and monitored anesthesia care, the adequacy of ventilation shall be evaluated, at least, by continual observation of qualitative clinical signs.

Circulation

Objective

To ensure the adequacy of the patient's circulatory function during all anesthetics.

Methods

1. Every patient receiving anesthesia shall have the electrocardiogram continuously displayed from the beginning of anesthesia until preparing to leave the anesthetizing location.*
2. Every patient receiving anesthesia shall have arterial blood pressure and heart rate determined and evaluated at least every 5 minutes.*
3. Every patient receiving general anesthesia shall have, in addition to the above, circulatory function continually evaluated by at least one of the following: palpation of a pulse, auscultation of heart sounds, monitoring of a tracing of intra-arterial pressure, ultrasound peripheral pulse monitoring, or pulse plethysmography or oximetry.

Body Temperature

Objective

To aid in the maintenance of appropriate body temperature during all anesthetics.

Methods

There shall be readily available a means to continuously measure the patient's temperature. When changes in body temperature are intended, anticipated, or suspected, the temperatures shall be measured.

Appendix 2
Guidelines for Regional Anesthesia in Obstetrics

(Approved by House of Delegates on October 12, 1988 and last amended on October 30, 1991)

These guidelines apply to the use of regional anesthesia or analgesia in which local anesthetics are administered to the parturient during labor and delivery. They are intended to encourage quality patient care but cannot guarantee any specific patient outcome. Because the availability of anesthesia resources may vary, members are responsible for interpreting and establishing the guidelines for their own institutions and practices. These guidelines are subject to revision from time to time as warranted by the evolution of technology and practice.

GUIDELINE I

Regional anesthesia should be initiated and maintained only in locations in which appropriate resuscitation equipment and drugs are immediately available to manage procedurally related problems.

Resuscitation equipment shall include, but is not limited to, sources of oxygen and suction, equipment to maintain an airway and perform endotracheal intubation, a means to provide positive pressure ventilation, and drugs and equipment for cardiopulmonary resuscitation.

GUIDELINE II

Regional anesthesia should be initiated by a physician with appropriate privileges and maintained by or under the medical direction[1] of such an individual.

Physicians should be approved through the institutional credentialing process to initiate and direct the maintenance of obstetric anesthesia and to manage procedurally related complications.

GUIDELINE III

Regional anesthesia should not be administered until (1) the patient has been examined by a qualified individual[2] and (2) the maternal and fetal status and progress of labor have been evaluated by a physician with privileges in obstetrics who is readily available to supervise the labor and manage any obstetric complications that may arise.

Under circumstances defined by department protocol, qualified personnel may perform the initial pelvic examination. The physician responsible for the patient's obstetric care should be informed of her status so that a decision can be made regarding risk and further management.[2]

GUIDELINE IV

An intravenous infusion should be established before the initiation of regional anesthesia and maintained throughout the duration of the regional anesthetic.

GUIDELINE V

Regional anesthesia for labor and/or vaginal delivery requires that the parturient's vital signs and the fetal heart rate be monitored and documented by a qualified individual. Additional monitoring appropriate to the clinical condition of the parturient and the fetus should be employed when indicated. When extensive regional blockade is administered for complicated vaginal delivery, the standards for basic intraoperative monitoring[3] should be applied.

GUIDELINE VI

Regional anesthesia for cesarean delivery requires that the standards for basic intraoperative monitoring[3] be applied and that a physician with privileges in obstetrics be immediately available.

GUIDELINE VII

Qualified personnel, other than the anesthesiologist attending the mother, should be immediately available to assume responsibility for resuscitation of the newborn.[2]

The primary responsibility of the anesthesiologist is to provide care to the mother. If the anesthesiologist is also requested to provide brief assistance in the care of the newborn, the benefit to the child must be compared with the risk to the mother.

GUIDELINE VIII

A physician with appropriate privileges should remain readily available during the regional anesthetic to manage anesthetic complications until the patient's postanesthesia condition is satisfactory and stable.

GUIDELINE IX

All patients recovering from regional anesthesia should receive appropriate postanesthesia care. Following cesarean delivery and/or extensive regional blockade, the standards for postanesthesia care[4] should be applied.

1. A postanesthesia care unit (PACU) should be available to receive patients. The design, equipment, and staffing meet requirements of the facility's accrediting and licensing bodies.
2. When a site other than the PACU is used, equivalent postanesthesia care should be provided.

GUIDELINE X

There should be a policy to ensure the availability in the facility of a physician to manage complications and to provide cardiopulmonary resuscitation for patients receiving postanesthesia care.

---

[1]Anesthesia Care Team (Approved by ASA House of Delegates 10/14/87).

[2]Guidelines for Perinatal Care (American Academy of Pediatrics and American College of Obstetricians and Gynecologists, 1988).

[3]Standards for Basic Intraoperative Monitoring (Approved by ASA House of Delegates 10/21/86 and last amended 10/21/92).

[4]Standards for Postanesthesia Care (Approved by ASA House of Delegates 10/12/88 and last amended 10/21/92).

Appendix 3
Standards for Postanesthesia Care

(Approved by House of Delegates on October 12, 1988 and last amended on October 21, 1992)

These standards apply to postanesthesia care in all locations. These standards may be exceeded based on the judgment of the responsible anesthesiologist. They are intended to encourage quality patient care, but cannot guarantee any specific patient outcome. They are subject to revision from time to time as warranted by the evolution of technology and practice. *Under extenuating circumstances, the responsible anesthesiologist may waive the requirements marked with an asterisk (*); it is recommended that when this is done, it should be so stated (including the reasons) in a note in the patient's medical record.*

STANDARD I

All patients who have received general anesthesia, regional anesthesia, or monitored anesthesia care shall receive appropriate postanesthesia management.[1]

1. A postanesthesia care unit (PACU) or an area that provides equivalent postanesthesia care shall be available to receive patients after surgery and anesthesia. All patients who receive anesthesia shall be admitted to the PACU **except** by specific order of the anesthesiologist responsible for the patient's care.
2. The medical aspects of care in the PACU shall be governed by policies and procedures that have been reviewed and approved by the Department of Anesthesiology.
3. The design, equipment, and staffing of the PACU shall meet requirements of the facility's accrediting and licensing bodies.

STANDARD II

A patient transported to the PACU shall be accompanied by a member of the anesthesia care team who is knowledgeable about the patient's condition. The patient shall be continually evaluated and treated during transport with monitoring and support appropriate to the patient's condition.

STANDARD III

Upon arrival in the PACU, the patient shall be re-evaluated and a verbal report provided to the responsible PACU nurse by the member of the anesthesia care team who accompanies the patient.

1. The patient's status on arrival in the PACU shall be documented.
2. Information concerning the preoperative condition and the surgical/anesthetic course shall be transmitted to the PACU nurse.
3. The member of the anesthesia care team shall remain in the PACU until the PACU nurse accepts responsibility for the nursing care of the patient.

STANDARD IV

The patient's condition shall be evaluated continually in the PACU.

1. The patient shall be observed and monitored by methods appropriate to the patient's medical condition. Particular attention should be given to monitoring oxygenation, ventilation, circulation, and temperature. During recovery from all anesthetics, a quantitative method of assessing oxygenation such as pulse oximetry shall be employed in the initial phase of recovery.*† This is not intended for application during the recovery of the obstetric patient in whom regional anesthesia was used for labor and vaginal delivery.

2. General medical supervision and co-ordination of patient care in the PACU should be the responsibility of an anesthesiologist.
3. There shall be a policy to assure the availability in the facility of a physician capable of managing complications and providing cardiopulmonary resuscitation for patients in the PACU.

STANDARD V

A physician is responsible for the discharge of the patient from the PACU.

1. When discharge criteria are used, they must be approved by the Department of Anesthesiology and the medical staff. They may vary depending on whether the patient is discharged to a hospital room, to the ICU, to a short stay unit, or home.
2. In the absence of the physician responsible for the discharge, the PACU nurse shall determine that the patient meets the discharge criteria. The name of the physician accepting responsibility for discharge shall be noted on the record.

---

[1]Refer to *Standards of Post Anesthesia Practice 1992*, published by ASPAN, for issues of nursing care.

[†]To become effective as soon as feasible, but no later than January 1, 1992.

Index

Page numbers followed by *f* indicate figures; those followed by *t* indicate tables.

B

E

F

G

P

Q

R

U